26. 4. 75.

Disease in Infancy and Childhood

ELLIS AND MITCHELL

Disease in Infancy and Childhood

ROSS G. MITCHELL M.D., F.R.C.P.Ed., D.C.H.
Professor of Child Health, University of Dundee

SEVENTH EDITION

CHURCHILL LIVINGSTONE · EDINBURGH AND LONDON · 1973

CHURCHILL LIVINGSTONE
Medical Division of Longman Group Limited

Distributed in the United States of America by Longman
Inc., New York, and by associated companies, branches
and representatives throughout the world

© E. & S. Livingstone Ltd, 1951, 1956, 1960, 1963, 1965, 1968

© Longman Group Ltd, 1973

First Edition	...	...	1951
Reprinted ...	...	...	1952
Second Edition	...	...	1956
Third Edition	...	...	1960
Translated into Spanish	...		1960
Translated into Greek	...		1962
Fourth Edition	...	...	1963
Fifth Edition	...	...	1965
Sixth Edition	...	...	1968
Seventh Edition	...	...	1973
Reprinted ...	...	...	1974

ISBN 0 443 00988 0

PRINTED IN GREAT BRITAIN

Preface

This new edition of the book which Professor R. W. B. Ellis of Edinburgh first wrote in 1951 has been very thoroughly revised but its aim remains unchanged. It is intended as an introduction to the diseases of infancy and childhood for senior medical students who are already familiar with the natural history of disease in adult life and have some knowledge of normal child development. It emphasizes those features of the young and growing individual which determine his response to the impact of disease processes and distinguish this response from the behaviour of the adult whose development is complete.

As far as practicable, the classification of disease by systems has been subjugated to the consideration of disorders occurring in particular age periods, of the reaction of the immature host to different stimuli and of the results of interference with function. Thus emphasis is placed on the perinatal period in describing the fetal and neonatal disorders which constitute such a major field of paediatric endeavour. Congenital malformations of all systems have been discussed in a single chapter and considered in some detail owing to their particular importance in the clinical practice of paediatrics. Disorders causing continuing handicap are grouped because they have so much in common in their effect on the child's life.

Although some of the rarer manifestations of disease have been included when it was felt that these would serve to illustrate the subject, this book is not intended as an inclusive work of reference. It is hoped, however, that it may prove useful also to family doctors and junior hospital staff as a ready source of paediatric information and as a guide to further reading.

Dundee, 1973   R.G.M.

Contents

1 History-taking and Examination

When the patient is an infant or young child, the history of illness will be concerned with observations made by a third party. Subjective symptoms, which figure so largely in the complaints of adults, can often be inferred only from the behaviour of the patient. The history should be taken, whenever possible, from the mother or from whoever is in direct charge of the child. It is most desirable that the mother should be present during school medical examinations, since the teacher can provide only half the picture of the child's life, and may be wholly unaware of such symptoms as bed-wetting or night-terrors which are only manifest at home.

The interpretation of the history will involve assessment of the informant as a witness, remembering that anxiety or the desire to impress or please the doctor may result in exaggeration or suppression of relevant information. A distinction should be made between the mother's own observations (which she is well qualified to make) and the interpretation she offers (which is commonly based on no specialist knowledge). 'A fall' or 'teething' will very commonly be offered as the explanation of a wide variety of unrelated symptoms in young children, since falls are frequent and teeth cut over a long period.

At the beginning of the consultation, the mother should be put at her ease by a few friendly words and then the presenting symptom or complaint should be recorded in her own words. At this stage it is often wise not to pay attention to the child, in order to allow him to get used to the doctor and the unfamiliar surroundings. The mother should be allowed to tell her story with little or no interruption and only after she has disburdened herself should a detailed routine history be taken.

The following scheme for case-taking will provide most of the information generally required, though it will need supplementing in some cases, while in others not all the details can be given by the informant.

GENERAL INFORMATION

Name:
Address:
Date of birth:
Date of first attendance (or admission):
Informant:

HISTORY

Complaint (in informant's own words):
Duration:

PRESENT ILLNESS

Mode of onset and dates of onset of the symptoms. Health immediately before illness. Supposed and possible causes, e.g. injury. Progress of the disease and note of fresh symptoms in their order of onset. State of activity, appetite, bowels, sleep, changes in temperament, before and during illness. Enquiry as to specific physical signs and symptoms if information is not volunteered, e.g. wasting or loss of weight, with reference to weight-card if available, vomiting, pain, cough, convulsions, enuresis.

PREVIOUS HEALTH

Antenatal. Health of mother during pregnancy (medical supervision, diet, etc.). Rubella or other infection, medication, and stage of pregnancy at which it occurred. Vomiting. Toxaemia. Antepartum haemorrhage. (Supplement from antenatal records if indicated, e.g. Wassermann reaction, Rhesus constitution.) Employment during pregnancy.

Natal. Gestational age. Birth weight. Duration of labour and method of delivery. Whether infant born at home or in hospital. (If the latter, supplement from hospital record if indicated, including resuscitation, oxygen administration.)

Neonatal. Whether colour, cry and respiration normal; jaundice; feeding difficulty; rashes; twitching, flaccidity. Any other abnormalities noted. Transfusion or other treatment (confirm from hospital record).

Later life. Exact details of feeding in early months; whether breast-fed, and if so, for how long; type of artificial feeding used; whether vitamin supplements given, and if so, preparation, amount, and duration. Weaning—breast to bottle, or milk to solids: age and ease with which carried out. Appetite in infancy and subsequently.

History of convulsions, skin rashes, diarrhoea, infection, or other illnesses. Enquire specifically re measles, rubella, pertussis, mumps, chicken-pox. Immunization. Operations. Recent contact with infectious disease, especially tuberculosis.

DEVELOPMENT

Ages of head balance, sitting and standing unsupported, walking, talking (words and sentences), reading.

Ages at which gained control of bowel and of urinary bladder (*a*) during day, (*b*) at night. Any special difficulties in toilet-training.

Whether child can feed and dress himself, and if so, how early he began to do so.

School progress, e.g. average age of class and place in class; school report if indicated. Special aptitudes.

Social adjustment with other children at home and at school.

FAMILY HISTORY

Father's age and occupation. Mother's age and occupation. Health of parents and whether any consanguinity. (In familial conditions, include genealogical tree showing affected members, any cousin marriages, etc.) Health of near relatives (especially hereditary and congenital disorders, nervous and mental disease). The children in their order, with details of age and health, and including deaths, stillbirths, and abortions.

SOCIAL HISTORY

Whether mother employed part-time or full-time, and if so, what care provided for children. Size of house, situation, sanitation, ventilation, lighting, access to playground or open air. Details of family income if relevant.

In the event of the child requiring admission to hospital, it is additionally important that the history should be detailed, e.g. including particulars of previous exanthemata and feeding, since it is much more difficult to supplement the history in hospital when the patient is a child than in the case of an adult. Thus if a case of measles appears in the ward, it may be essential to know as promptly as possible which of the children in the ward have already had the disease.

The child himself, however, may prove a valuable additional witness, if certain limitations of his evidence are borne in mind. Firstly, young children are very seldom able to localize pain at all accurately, and their description of symptoms will be limited by their vocabulary and their previous experience. It is exceptional, for instance, for a child under six to complain of sore throat or to localize abdominal pain (as distinct from tenderness) more closely than by placing a hand on the umbilicus. Secondly, most children are even more suggestible than adults, and the answers to leading questions may be correspondingly unreliable. In common with adults, their complaints may be coloured by a desire for sympathy or alternatively by a desire to get out of hospital. But as a general rule children tend to be at least as truthful as adults.

The significance of most of the information included in the scheme of history-taking will be brought out in subsequent chapters: but some aspects of the history will be briefly illustrated here.

Present illness

While most acute infections, e.g. primary pneumonia, will have a clear-cut onset which may even be dated to within a few hours, determination of the duration of more chronic illness is likely to present considerable difficulty. There is often a period during which the child has failed to thrive before the presenting symptoms have appeared, and the assessment of this period will depend on the mother's powers of observation and often on whether she is occupied with the one child or with a large family. Failure to gain weight requires careful assessment, since a child is often thought (wrongly) to have lost weight when he is in fact growing rapidly and losing the rounded contours of later infancy. Retardation of growth is only likely to be noticed when the child has obviously begun to lag behind his contemporaries. This may not be noticed for six months or more after growth has ceased. Against the fact that the mother of an only child will probably observe him closely must be set the fact that the mother of a larger family will know what to expect and will be in a better position to judge what is a deviation from the normal.

The history of the present illness is often inextricably interwoven with the history of the child's previous development. Thus considerable importance may be attached to the fact that a child has passed a normal milestone of development, e.g. being dry at night, and has suddenly regressed to a more infantile phase (nocturnal enuresis). Again, in the case of a child who has learnt to walk at 1 year of age and has subsequently 'gone off his legs' at 18 months, active disease should be suspected.

In older children, a school report is often valuable, though with the large classes commonly found in primary schools, observation of the individual child is often less detailed than might be desired.

Behaviour problems

These represent such an important field of ill health in childhood that their elucidation requires special consideration. It must be realized from the outset that while certain behaviour problems may have a purely emotional basis, the association of physical and emotional ill health is commonly a very close one. While the sick child is likely to behave abnormally as a direct result of physical illness, the child who is emotionally disturbed is equally likely to suffer in physical well-being. The paediatrician, family doctor, or school medical officer will constantly encounter cases where the illness is psychosomatic, and should be able to judge whether the child requires expert psychotherapy or intelligence-testing, whether a physical defect is the basis of the behaviour disorder, and whether the problem is one within his competence to treat.

The psychological history taken in the child guidance clinic or department of child psychiatry is more detailed than the routine history taken by the paediatrician, but much of the relevant information can be obtained by him in cases in which physical and emotional disturbances co-exist. The following scheme is adapted from one designed for the use of psychiatric social workers:

Date of interview:
Name:
Address:
Date of birth:
School. (Including socio-economic status of family in relation to school, e.g. a poor child in a fee-paying school or a child from a wealthy family in a free school.)
Referred by. (Parent, school, youth organization, probation officer, welfare officer, etc.)
Reasons for referral—as given on referral note.
Symptoms—as described by parent, e.g. bed-wetting. Sleep—restless or otherwise, night-terrors, shouting or sleep-walking. Appetite—food fads. Nail-biting and/or finger-sucking. General demeanour, e.g. 'nervous' (ready tears, apprehensiveness, etc.), obstreperous, negativistic, destructive, insolent, solitary or sociable. Tics, temper tantrums, obsessional habits, e.g. hoarding, excessive tidiness or cleanliness. (*Note.* There is frequently a discrepancy between the parent's account and the reason given for the referral by other agencies.)
Informant. Relationship to patient; reliability or otherwise; any other relevant information.

GENERAL IMPRESSION OF PARENTS AND FAMILY

(*Note.* The attitude of the parent to the child will depend on the type of personality.)
Father. Age. Occupation. Type of personality.
Mother. Age. Occupation. Type of personality.
Marriage. Duration; marital relationships. (*Note.* Little information as to marital relationships should be sought at first interview, and most information will be obtained indirectly.)
Family. Including abortions, stillbirths and deaths. Age range between children—was family planned? Any problems in regard to each child, e.g. bed-wetting, attendance at special school. (*Note.* It is rare to find that only the patient is disturbed.) Religion.

SOCIAL CONDITIONS

Financial state, Home conditions, e.g. crowded, furnished rooms, living with relatives. Relationship with neighbours, kind of neighbourhood.

PERSONAL HISTORY

Pregnancy. Conscious attitude of mother; unconscious attitude as gauged by sickness, etc. (Prolonged vomiting throughout pregnancy may indicate rejection.)
Delivery. Details, including gestational age and weight of baby.
Feeding. Breast and/or bottle, with reasons. Weaning (*a*) from breast, (*b*) from bottle, and methods, gradual or

sudden. Reaction of baby to feeds—greedy, unduly slow, etc. Reaction of baby to weaning.

Developmental history.

Habits. Training and reaction of baby to training. Mother's reaction to constipation, soiling, etc., and concern of mother with faeces.

General behaviour of child in first year—e.g. crying, smiling, solemn, etc.

One to 5 years. Timid or reasonably secure and adventurous. Clinging to mother or independent. Admiration by other adults, e.g. grandparents, aunts, neighbours. Reaction to birth of next child, and age of patient when this took place. Relationship with children of own age outside family. Day or residential nursery, and if so, why.

School. Age at beginning. Reaction to first day. Reaction now. Mother's conception of progress (compare with school report at end of history). (*Note.* A school visit may be desirable, to gain impression of teachers and teachers' impressions of child.)

Home. Sleeping arrangements. Participation in household duties and willingness or otherwise to be helpful. Relations between patient and siblings and parents. Separations from parents (e.g. hospital admissions, holidays). Relations with children outside home. Hobbies and leisure occupations. Membership of any youth organization. Pocket money.

Puberty. Age of onset. Sex instruction and if so, by whom.

Illness. With note on age, severity, admission to hospital (and reactions to this).

School report. In addition to the report furnished by the school, a school visit by a psychiatric social worker will provide the following information:

Impression made by headmaster/mistress.

Impression made by child on headmaster/mistress and teachers: (*a*) behaviour and social adjustment, (*b*) intellectual capacity, (*c*) achievements.

Subsequently—correlate intelligence and achievement.

Report from any other Agency concerned—e.g. youth organization, probation officer, welfare officer, etc.

It will be seen that whether the child's disability is primarily physical or primarily emotional (or psychological), emphasis is placed not only on the history of the present illness but also on antenatal and postnatal development, his previous illnesses, family history, and social background. This concept of the child as the product of his heredity and environment is essential for a proper understanding of disease processes when they occur. Unless the history taken is adequate in every particular, essential factors will be overlooked, and therapy undertaken with a misconception of the underlying causes which must be remedied. To take a simple example, prolonged hospital treatment of a child with pulmonary tuberculosis will be largely wasted if he is sent back to the care of an aged grandmother who is expectorating tubercle bacilli about the house and cannot provide him with an adequate diet.

It is time well spent if a history taken at hospital can be followed up by a visit to the home. In this way the child can be seen as a member of a family unit, and the standard of living of the family assessed. Although in practice these home visits are usually undertaken by a social worker or health visitor, the student will find it a very great advantage to make a number of such visits himself to homes of different socio-economic status.

Family history

This may provide the clue to at least three different aspects of disease in childhood, viz. genetic determination of abnormality, source of infection and the emotional impact of other members of the family on the individual child. It is usually best to take the family history after that of the present illness, since the informant may otherwise regard detailed questioning as irrelevant inquisitiveness. Whenever it is desired to indicate the distribution of a disease-process or abnormality within a family group, a pedigree should be constructed, using the standard international symbols. Members of each generation appear on the same horizontal line, and the generations are given roman numerals. Arabic numerals can be used for individual members of each generation. The individual around whom the pedigree is constructed is known as the

□ Unaffected male   ○ Unaffected female   △ Sex unknown

■ Affected male   ● Affected female   ▨ ⊘ Unknown whether individual affected

• Abortion   • or ⚊ Stillbirth   ⋈ or ✝ Death in infancy

□⎯○ Marriage coupling bar   □⚌○ Consanguineous marriage coupling bar

□ ○ ○ Brother and sister relationship (sibship coupling bar)

◈ or ◈ Sibship of which details are unknown or only number is known

□⊓□ or ⌂ Identical twins   □⊓□ or □⊓○ Non-identical twins

× Examined personally   * Examined competently but not personally

propositus, and is indicated by an arrow. The symbols on page 4 are the most commonly required. The standard symbols can be varied in particular instances if a key is given.

The paediatrician is in an exceptionally favourable position for obtaining information of genetic or epidemiological value. Since the informant is normally the mother, she will not only be able to provide equally reliable information with regard to other members of the sibship, but will usually be prepared to bring her other children for examination if the need is explained to her. She will often also be able to give at least some information with regard to the two previous generations (her own and her parents'). Parents will, in addition, usually be prepared to undergo examination themselves if they are convinced that it is relevant to the well-being of the child, or will help to assess the likelihood of healthy children being born subsequently. Human pedigrees concerned with a genetically-determined defect are likely to require expert assessment, and it is important that the information provided should be as full as possible, and that consanguineous (cousin) marriages should be clearly indicated.

In the case of a congenital abnormality, particular attention should be paid to the history of the pregnancy. Maternal medication or the occurrence of infection, e.g. rubella, during the first three months may well be forgotten unless particular enquiry is made.

Source of infection

The importance of determining this is obvious in such a condition as tuberculosis, and the family history will serve as the basis for the examination of immediate contacts. While the family group is the most important source of infection in the case of the infant and young child, enquiry may have to extend beyond it when there are lodgers or in the case of older children attending school. Thus an outbreak of erythema nodosum in a particular class may be found to be due to the teacher suffering from open tuberculosis.

Examples of other conditions in which there is likely to be a high familial incidence of infection within the home are dysentery, threadworm infestation, upper respiratory infection, and scabies. Certain families may suffer from recurrent staphylococcal infections affecting many members of the family over long periods.

Emotional impact of family

Enough has been said of the child's reactions to other members of the family, and to the parents' marital relationship, to indicate the important effect these may have on his mental health. The eliciting of this part of the history often requires considerable tact, since the mother may be unwilling for various reasons to give an objective picture of the child's relationship to the father, grandparents, or to herself. It is often necessary to construct the background piecemeal by indirect questioning. Relationship of the child to siblings is usually more clearly outlined, though the child's reaction to the birth of a subsequent child will be very largely determined by the mother's handling of the situation at the time the event occurred. This latter can often only be inferred from the present mother-child relationship, though certain factual points in the story should be noted, e.g. whether the mother was in hospital for the birth of the infant, and the patient's behaviour to her and the new baby on her return home.

Audience

The examiner must use a certain discretion in taking histories in the presence of the child or of other parties. In the case of many physical disabilities, there may be no objection to doing so, though even here the mother's fears may sometimes be better expressed in private, and she may well be unwilling to give details of the family history in the child's hearing. Where behaviour problems are being discussed, it is often best for the mother to give her story without the child as audience, and the child should also be seen both with and in the absence of the parent. It may also be desirable to interview the father, either to supplement the history or to enlist his co-operation in treatment. Where the mother can be confidently reassured, this is best done in the presence of the child, since the child's anxieties may be quite as important as the mother's, and will often best be allayed if he is convinced that he is not being told one thing and his mother another.

PHYSICAL EXAMINATION

The general scheme of examination of the various systems will be similar to that adopted in the case of adults, and only the difficulties and differences peculiar to infancy and childhood will be discussed. Co-operation on the part of the patient cannot be assumed, but it is a great saving of time if it can be obtained. To do so it is essential that the child should not be frightened and that procedures likely to cause discomfort, e.g. examination of the throat or ears, should be left until last. The organization of the clinic can do much to assist the examiner by eliminating a long wait in cheerless surroundings, and ensuring that preliminary procedures such as undressing, weighing, measuring, and collection of urine are carried out with a minimum of disturbance or embarrassment.

Although every doctor will in time develop his own technique of examining children, and recognize that no single approach is universally applicable, there are certain general procedures which will normally be found satisfactory. It must be remembered that the toddler's reaction to a stranger will almost invariably be hostile if an immediate attempt is made to separate the child from his mother. The time during which the history is being taken provides a valuable opportunity for the child to form an impression of the doctor and to realize that the mother regards him as someone in whom she has confidence. At the same time the child will be assessing his surroundings, and will probably find a toy or book to interest him.

By the time the history has been taken, the child will usually be ready for some attention himself. The older child will naturally expect a more adult approach, while the behaviour of the younger child or infant can usefully be observed for a few minutes after something to examine or play with has been provided. This is the time to make a brief developmental assessment before the physical examination is started. In the case of infants and young children attending as out-patients, as much of the examination as practicable should be carried out with the child sitting or lying on the mother's lap; if examination on a couch is necessary, it should be the mother who lifts the child on to the couch, and she should stand where the child can both see and touch her. The order in which the examination is carried out depends on opportunity, but it is usually wise to examine the abdomen early while the child is co-operative. If the gait of the child is to be observed, the mother should back away from the child who is then encouraged to walk to her; a toddler should not be made to walk away from his mother unless he will do so spontaneously.

General examination

A careful assessment of the general appearance and nutrition of the child should precede systematic examination. This will include particulars of behaviour, posture, cleanliness (including the condition of the skin and hair), muscle tone, subcutaneous fat, and colour of face and mucous membranes. Pulse and respiratory rates and body temperature may be recorded before or after the examination as convenient. At birth the pulse rate is 140 to 120 beats per minute, falling to 115 to 105 between 6 and 12 months, 105 to 90 between 2 and 6 years, and 85 to 75 at 11 to 14 years. It may be temporarily raised by crying or excitement and a transient tachycardia is sometimes observed at puberty. The respiratory rate is extremely erratic during the newborn period, and is influenced by sleep, crying, etc. An average sleeping rate is 30 per minute: by the age of 4 years it has fallen to 25, and from then onward is 25 to 20. Although temperatures taken in the groin or axilla are less reliable than those in the mouth or rectum, the skin temperature is usually preferred in out-patient clinics owing to the risk of cross-infection by other routes. The rectal temperature is approximately 0·5°C higher than the oral temperature. Whichever method is used, it is essential that the thermometer should be kept *in situ* sufficiently long to give a true reading. Urinary examination is considered in Chapter 12.

Blood-pressure readings must be made when the child is quiet and relaxed, using a cuff of appropriate size, i.e. covering two-thirds of the upper arm. The blood pressure is one of the less reliable examinations recorded in infancy and childhood, but if the technique is standardized, serial examinations, e.g. in nephritis, will give a reasonably accurate indication of the changes which may occur in the individual patient. In the newborn infant, estimation of blood-pressure requires special techniques, e.g. the flush method or use of a specially designed sphygmomanometer (Ashworth *et al.*, 1959).

HEAD. The occipito-frontal circumference should be recorded and, if there is any suggestion of an increase above normal, the measurement should be repeated at intervals to detect progressive enlargement. The mean measurements in Table 1.1 are closely similar to those from American sources, the standard deviations for this Edinburgh series being approximately 1·3 cm for both sexes.

The shape of the head should be described, the size of the fontanelles being recorded in infants. Asymmetry of the skull, overriding or separation of the sutures, and presence or absence of a bruit on auscultation should be noted. An unduly small head generally implies microcephaly, though rarely premature fusion of the sutures is a primary condition, in which case there will be signs of increased intracranial pressure. When cerebral agenesis is suspected, it may be revealed by transillumination of the head.

Table 1.1 Mean head circumference of term infants (in cm) (from Edinburgh data of J. Thomson)

	Birth	13 weeks	26 weeks	1 year	2 years	5 years
Male	34·6	40·6	44·0	47·3	49·1	51·2
Female	33·9	39·7	42·9	46·2	47·8	50·2

Height and weight

These should be recorded at each examination. During the first 2 years, crown–heel length is measured by placing the child supine, with legs extended, on a measure fitted with a sliding footpiece. In young infants, crown–rump measurement is more accurate, since it is difficult to keep the legs straight. In older children, it is usual to measure standing height, which is about 1 cm less than supine length. A rigid vertical measuring board with sliding headpiece is used and the child carefully positioned, with weight borne evenly on the two feet, heels and back touching the upright, and the head held so that the eyes look directly forward. For accurate weighing, the child should be naked or in minimal standard clothing, the weight of which can be allowed for.

In assessing the significance of a single measurement, the range of normal must be considered and the child described in terms of his place within that range, which is taken as within 2 standard deviations of the mean or as from the third to the ninety-seventh centile, the middle of the group (median) being the fiftieth centile. There are significant differences between the mean measurements of different populations, e.g. London schoolchildren are taller and heavier than those in Glasgow, and London schoolchildren in 1964 were taller and heavier at all ages than children at school in the same districts in 1938. As far as possible, therefore, comparison should be made with standards obtained from a similar population. Tables 1.2 and 1.3 give cross-sectional type standards for height and weight which are generally suitable for British children, though there are slight regional variations.

Repeated measurements over a period of time are more valuable than a single observation, since they indicate whether a child's growth curve is parallel to the standard or progressively deviating from it. Serial observations can be presented as height or weight attained or, more informatively, as rate of growth (velocity) expressed as cm per year (velocity standards have been published by Tanner, 1970). In the teen ages, individual variation is greater than in early childhood, due to the varying age of puberty (see p. 9).

Growth and development

The changes which take place between birth and adolescence include physical growth, sexual maturation and intellectual and emotional

Table 1.2 Standards for height and weight—London boys, 1965 (from Tanner, Whitehouse and Takaishi, 1966)

Age (years)	Height centiles (cm)							Weight centiles (g)						
	3	10	25	50	75	90	97	3	10	25	50	75	90	97
4·0	93·5	96·1	98·7	101·6	104·5	107·1	109·7	13·0	14·3	15·3	16·6	17·9	19·1	20·4
5·0	99·4	102·2	105·1	108·3	111·5	114·4	117·2	14·4	15·7	16·9	18·5	20·0	21·5	23·2
6·0	104·9	108·0	111·1	114·6	118·1	121·2	124·3	15·9	17·3	18·6	20·5	22·4	24·0	26·5
7·0	110·3	113·5	116·8	120·5	124·2	127·5	130·8	17·4	19·0	20·6	22·6	24·9	26·9	30·3
8·0	115·4	118·8	122·3	126·2	130·0	133·5	137·0	19·1	20·9	22·7	25·0	27·5	30·0	34·4
9·0	120·4	124·0	127·6	131·6	135·7	139·3	142·9	21·0	22·9	25·0	27·5	30·3	33·4	38·8
10·0	125·1	128·8	132·6	136·8	141·0	144·8	148·5	23·0	25·2	27·5	30·3	33·6	37·3	43·3
11·0	129·4	133·3	137·4	141·9	146·4	150·4	154·4	24·9	27·4	30·1	33·6	37·7	42·6	49·5
12·0	133·7	138·0	142·4	147·3	152·2	156·6	160·9	27·1	29·9	33·2	37·7	42·7	49·0	57·2
13·0	138·7	143·4	148·2	153·4	158·7	163·5	168·2	29·6	33·0	37·1	42·6	49·0	56·0	64·4
14·0	145·0	150·0	155·0	160·7	166·3	171·3	176·2	33·3	37·7	42·6	48·8	55·4	62·5	70·9
15·0	152·3	157·1	161·9	167·3	172·7	177·6	182·4	39·0	43·7	48·7	54·7	60·9	68·0	75·9

Table 1.3   Standards for height and weight—London girls, 1965 (from Tanner, Whitehouse and Takaishi, 1966)

Age (years)	Height centiles (cm)							Weight centiles (g)						
	3	10	25	50	75	90	97	3	10	25	50	75	90	97
4·0	92·3	94·9	97·5	100·4	103·3	105·9	108·5	13·1	14·1	15·2	16·3	17·5	18·8	20·3
5·0	98·2	101·1	104·0	107·2	110·3	113·2	116·1	14·6	15·9	17·0	18·3	19·8	21·4	23·3
6·0	103·8	106·8	110·0	113·4	116·9	120·0	123·1	16·2	17·6	18·9	20·4	22·2	24·4	26·8
7·0	109·1	112·4	115·7	119·3	123·0	126·3	129·6	17·8	19·2	20·8	22·6	25·0	27·7	30·6
8·0	114·2	117·6	121·1	125·0	128·9	132·4	135·8	19·4	21·0	22·9	25·1	28·0	31·2	35·0
9·0	119·3	122·9	126·6	130·6	134·6	138·3	141·9	21·0	23·0	25·2	27·7	31·4	35·4	40·6
10·0	124·5	128·3	132·1	136·4	140·6	144·5	148·3	22·7	25·1	27·7	31·1	35·7	41·0	47·7
11·0	129·5	133·7	138·0	142·7	147·4	151·6	155·8	24·7	27·8	31·0	35·2	41·0	47·7	55·7
12·0	135·0	139·6	144·2	149·3	154·4	159·1	163·6	27·8	31·6	35·5	40·5	46·7	54·7	63·3
13·0	142·6	146·7	150·9	155·5	160·2	164·4	168·5	32·0	36·3	40·7	45·8	52·3	60·0	69·3
14·0	147·6	151·4	155·3	159·6	163·9	167·8	171·6	37·0	41·2	45·5	51·0	57·0	63·9	72·3
15·0	150·3	153·9	157·6	161·7	165·8	169·5	173·2	41·7	45·1	49·0	54·4	59·8	66·3	73·7

development. These are all closely interrelated and abnormality of any one is likely to affect the others, though to differing degrees. Each succeeding phase of development is characterized not only by a particular rate of growth, but also by physical proportions which are peculiar to it. Thus the infant has a large head which represents about one-quarter of the total length, a broad trunk, and short legs representing approximately three-eighths of the length. In adolescence, the head represents one-seventh and the legs one-half of the total length, the proportions being slender and longilinear in contrast to the squat brevilinear proportions of the infant. The change from one to the other is not a matter of steady and uniform increase in size, since the growth of individual tissues does not proceed equally. Thus the nervous system develops most rapidly during infancy, while the gonads grow very slowly until the onset of puberty, when sexual development occurs rapidly, accompanied by a characteristic spurt of somatic growth. The amount of subcutaneous fat, determined by measuring skinfold thickness with calipers, increases from birth to about 9 months and then diminishes until about 7 years, when it again increases.

Physical assessment is therefore based not only on height and weight attained but also on rate of growth, bodily proportions, nutritional status and sexual maturity. This last is closely related to skeletal maturity, which can be assessed radiologically by the number and size of ossification centres, a total score being allocated and compared with the Tanner-Whitehouse standards. Dentition will also provide confirmatory evidence, though the correlation with skeletal maturity is not high and individual varia-

tions in the age and order of eruption of the teeth are considerable. An approximate indication of the normal is given in Table 1.4, from which it will be seen that the full set of 20 deciduous teeth is usually present shortly after the age of 2 years. Deciduous teeth erupt earlier in the male than in the female on average, whereas the reverse is true of the permanent dentition.

Table 1.4   Average ages of eruption of teeth

Deciduous teeth	Age in months	Permanent teeth	Age in years
Central incisors		First molars	6
lower	7	Central incisors	6–7
upper	9	Lateral incisors	7–9
Lateral incisors		First premolars	10–11
lower	11	Canines	10–12
upper	10	Second premolars	11–12
First molars	15	Second molars	12
Canines	18	Third molars	17–25
Second molars	26		

Maturation

The considerable physical changes which occur at adolescence may be summarized as a spurt in the rate of growth, changes in endocrine balance, the appearance of secondary sexual characters, and functional maturation of the gonads. These are accompanied by increase in sexual interest and by emotional and personality changes, intensified by the need to adjust to the physical changes and often manifest by self-consciousness, resentment of parental authority and other typical behaviour. In examining older children, evidence of adolescence and the degree of such secondary changes as are present should

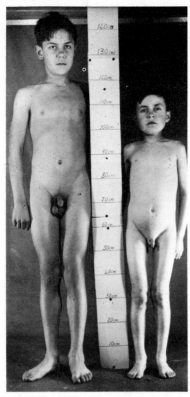

Fig. 1.1   Extreme physiological variations in stature and development. Both boys are aged 10 years 10 months. Boy on left shows unusually early pubescence and is 10 cm above average height for age. Boy on right is 18 cm below average height for age but is normally proportioned; ossification and dentition correspond with the average at 9 years. Both boys are healthy and of similar intellectual development.

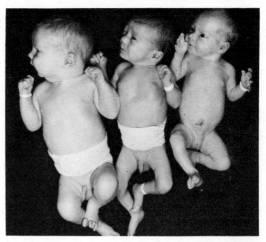

Fig. 1.2   Physiological variation in the newborn period. Three full-term infants aged 1 week weighing respectively 12½lb, 7½lb (average), and 5½lb at birth.

always be recorded: standards for rating genital maturity, pubic hair and breast development are given by Tanner (1970). The age at which these changes occur varies widely, girls being on average about two years ahead of boys. Thus the spurt of growth is at its peak velocity in British girls at an average age of 12 years and in boys at 14 years. Breast development begins in girls on average about 11 years and pubic hair appears shortly after 11, while in boys it appears on average a year later. Axillary hair usually appears after pubic hair. Approximately 95 per cent of British girls begin to menstruate between 11 and 15 years of age, with an average of 13, but the menarche (onset of menstruation) may occur as early as the tenth or as late as the seventeenth year without evidence of disease.

The great variation in the age of adolescent changes means that the whole range of maturation may be seen in a group of girls aged 12 years or boys aged 14, from those who have not yet started to change to fully mature adolescents, with all stages in between and corresponding differences in height, weight and strength. This important fact must be borne in mind in schools and other communities of children, especially where competitive sports are concerned.

Developmental diagnosis

Gesell classified infant behaviour into motor, linguistic, adaptive and social activities and by intensive study of large numbers of normal infants was able to define standard patterns for different ages, which are now used in measuring development. Gesell's four areas of development are now better considered under the headings: locomotion and posture; hearing, language and speech; vision and fine manipulation; and everyday skills and social development. Full details will be found in the many publications of Gesell and of Illingworth; the works of Piaget are also of interest, giving a rather different view of child development.

Within the range of normal there is considerable variation in the age at which different skills are acquired. In clinical work, reliance is usually placed on the mother's memory in establishing past developmental progress, though her recollections may be increasingly inaccurate as time passes. Most mothers remember when their child first walked without holding on and some can recall the ages of sitting unsupported, using three or four single words correctly and stringing three or more words into sentences. Care must be taken to ensure that both mother and doctor mean the same thing by these terms, e.g. sitting unsupported means that the infant can sit on a firm flat surface without using his arms for at least a minute. Table 1.5 gives the normal range of ages at which these developmental milestones' are passed.

Table 1.5   Ages at which Newcastle children passed developmental milestones (modified from Neligan and Prudham, 1969)

Milestone	Age centiles (months)						
	3	10	25	50	75	90	97
Sitting							
unsupported	4·6	5·2	5·8	6·4	7·2	8·1	9·3
Walking							
unsupported	9·7	10·7	11·8	12·8	14·2	15·8	18·4
Single words							
boys	8·7	10·0	11·6	12·4	15·0	18·0	21·9
girls	8·6	9·8	11·5	12·3	14·6	17·3	20·1
Sentences							
boys	17·5	19·1	21·4	23·8	26·8	32·5	36·0+
girls	16·2	18·4	20·4	22·9	25·0	30·8	36·0

To the information elicited from the mother can be added the results of direct observation of the child's abilities, on a single occasion or repeatedly over a period of time. In order to identify potentially handicapping disabilities as early as possible, every infant and young child should undergo periodic developmental screening examinations, the most important ages being 28 and 40 weeks (approximately 6 and 10 months). Simple developmental screening should also form part of the clinical examination of any infant and can be carried out in a few minutes, preferably at the beginning of the consultation when he is not tired. The following are some of the more important items to look for, with the average age of achievement.

4 weeks. Lifts head slightly when held in ventral suspension. Head lag not quite complete when pulled to sitting from supine. Follows object momentarily with eyes. Gives attention to sound.

6 weeks. Smiles responsively. Earliest vocalizing begins.

12 weeks. Holds head erect when upright. Head above plane of body in ventral suspension. Holds object in hand. Eyes follow moving object from side to side.

16 weeks. Little or no head lag when pulled to sitting. Reaches out for objects but fails to grasp.

24 weeks. Grasps cube offered but drops it if offered another.

28 weeks. Transfers cube to other hand if offered a second. Imitates.

32 weeks. Sits without support on a flat surface.

40 weeks. Uses finger and thumb to pick up small bead. Stands holding on.

48 weeks. Walks with support.

13 months. First unaided step. Two or three single words.

18 months. Climbs stairs. Scribbles spontaneously. Five or more words. Builds three blocks. Turns pages of book and looks at pictures.

2 years. Runs. Builds six blocks. Names three to five objects. Short sentences.

In interpreting the results of testing, due regard must be given not only to what the child did but also to how he did it and to his general state of interest in his surroundings; allowance must be made for infants born before term. When initial screening suggests the possibility of developmental retardation, full developmental testing should be undertaken by an expert.

It will be obvious that the pattern of development may be interfered with by a wide variety of causes. If there is fairly uniform retardation in all activities, a general cause such as mental subnormality is likely to be responsible, whereas if one activity is far behind the rest (dissociation), a local cause should be suspected, e.g. deafness when speech only is retarded. In certain cases of developmental delay, the child may have been prevented by emotional or other disturbance from acquiring a skill at the optimum time and becomes more resistant to learning once this 'sensitive period' has passed. Such a mechanism may be operative in some children with enuresis who have difficulty in gaining control of the bladder.

Neurological examination

The techniques of examination of the nervous system which are generally employed in the examination of older children and adults are in many instances inapplicable to the infant and small child. Thus accurate determination of sensory function is based to a large extent on the intelligent co-operation of the patient, while the same applies in some measure to the clinical estimation of motor power. The value of standard testing of reflexes largely depends also on the assumption that these are consistently present in the intact nervous system. In the case of the infant, the central nervous system is not only immature but rapidly changing. Co-operation is absent or minimal, while the presence or character of reflexes (e.g. the plantar response, which is extensor during the first year and flexor later) will be dependent on the stage of maturity reached. The examination is therefore principally based in infancy on the observation of spontaneous activity, muscle tone and posture, and reflexes and responses. In the newborn infant, damage to the central nervous system may be first indicated by colour changes, or disturbances of sleep, respiration, crying, sucking, or swallowing, while throughout infancy the progress of the infant will frequently form a more reliable indication of neurological impairment than will a single examination. Except when there are other confirmatory signs present, such as microcephaly or stigmata of mongolism, it is usually wise to delay a firm diagnosis of mental subnormality until the age of 12 months or even later, although severe subnormality can be suspected much earlier.

REFLEXES. The functional activity of the central nervous system is closely related to its degree of myelinization. Myelinization begins first in the ventral spinal roots at the sixteenth week of fetal life and last in the correlation centres of the cerebral cortex at the twelfth week of postnatal life. The cerebral cortex therefore exerts comparatively little control on the newborn infant's behaviour, which is characterized by lack of true volition or inhibition of the segmental apparatus and by the presence of reflexes not normally present in older infants. Persistence of such reflex activity beyond the usual age of disappearance may indicate delayed cortical development and is commonly found in severe mental subnormality. In the case of preterm infants, reflexes which are present in the baby at term may be absent or atypical and maturity at birth may therefore be estimated by their presence or absence. Testing of reflexes and responses should be carried out under standardized conditions about two or three hours after a feed.

The Moro reflex is consistently present from the twenty-eighth week of gestational age and normally disappears by four or five months after birth. It is elicited either by suddenly striking the couch on either side of the infant or by holding him up with support to his head and suddenly allowing the head to drop a few centimetres. The arms spring outwards in abduction and extension and the legs may show a similar response (Fig. 1.3). Complete absence of the reflex suggests cerebral damage, while a unilateral arm response

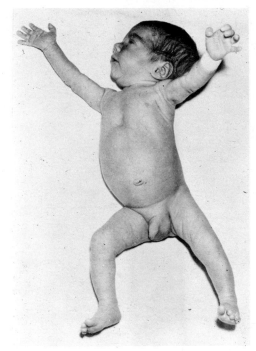

Fig. 1.3   The Moro reflex.

is seen in cases of brachial palsy or fractured clavicle.

The abdominal and tendon reflexes are nearly always present in the newborn infant: a marked difference between the two sides suggests neurological abnormality, as does sustained ankle clonus. Other reflexes constantly present in the newborn are Galant's trunk incurvation response, elicited by paravertebral stimulation, when the trunk curves towards the stimulated side, and the palmar and plantar grasp reflexes, in which flexion of fingers or toes occurs in response to pressing the finger into palm or sole respectively.

The asymmetrical tonic neck reflex, which consists of extension of the limbs on the side to which the face is turned, with flexion of the limbs on the opposite side, is sometimes present at birth but more often at two to three months. Its persistence into later infancy usually indicates extensive cerebral damage.

Reflexes useful in assessing gestational age (Robinson, 1966) are the pupil reaction to light, present from 31 weeks, blinking in response to a tap over the glabella (32 to 34 weeks), arm flexion and head-raising in response to traction on the wrists (33 to 36 weeks) and the neck-righting reflex (36 to 37 weeks). In the last, the head is rotated to one side and the infant rotates the trunk in the same direction.

OPHTHALMOSCOPIC EXAMINATION. Detailed examination of the discs and fundi presents considerable difficulty if an infant is crying or struggling, while even in the case of older children it may require much patience. Where it is essential to obtain evidence of early disc or fundus pathology in an infant, previous sedation and dilatation of the pupils with homatropine may be necessary. There is greater variation in the colour of the normal disc in infancy than in later life, and it is more common to suspect optic atrophy where the disc is a 'pale normal' than to overlook the condition when it is present. Where early papilloedema is suspected, repeated examinations may be required if the first is inconclusive. A common error is to mistake the appearance seen in compound hypermetropic astigmatism for papilloedema, since both cause blurring of the disc margin. Confirmatory evidence of early papilloedema is provided by distension of the retinal veins and filling-in of the physiological cup.

EXAMINATION OF THE THROAT AND EARS. Every effort should be made to obtain the co-operation of the patient when the throat is examined. If this is impossible, the mother should hold the child firmly on her knees, with his back towards her, putting one arm round him and the other on his forehead. A soft wooden tongue-depressor of appropriate size can usually be inserted gradually between the side teeth (not the incisors), when pressure on the back of the tongue will result in opening of the mouth. A rapid examination under these circumstances will usually be sufficient to show whether acute infection of the tonsils or naso-pharynx is present or not, and it will be possible to swab the throat. Decision as to the necessity of tonsillectomy, however, should only be based on a more thorough examination, correlated with the medical history and general physical examination.

When it is necessary to examine the throat and ears of a struggling infant without assistance, the infant can be wrapped tightly in a blanket.

The smallest auriscope should be used for the examination of infants. The external ear is drawn gently upward and backward, and the point of the auriscope inserted, taking particular care not to scratch the wall of the auditory canal. The view of the drum is often obscured by soft wax, and if this is so the wax must be removed by twisted wisps of cotton-wool mounted on a match-stick before the auriscope is reinserted. Hard wax may be better removed by a loop through the auriscope, again taking care not to scratch the wall of the canal, since any bleeding will add to the difficulties of examination.

BIBLIOGRAPHY AND REFERENCES

ACHESON, R. M., KEMP, F. H. & PARFIT, J. (1955). Height, weight, and skeletal maturity in the first five years of life. *Lancet* i, 691.
ASHWORTH, A. M., NELIGAN, G. A. & ROFERS, J. E. (1959). Sphygmomanometer for the newborn. *Lancet* i, 801.
EGAN, D. F., ILLINGWORTH, R. S. & MACKEITH, R. C. (1969). *Developmental Screening: 0–5 Years.* London: Spastics International Medical Publications. Heinemann.
FALKNER, F. (1966). *Human Development.* Philadelphia: Saunders.
FLAVELL, J. H. (1963). *The Developmental Psychology of Jean Piaget.* Princeton: Van Nostrand.
GESELL, A. (1928). *Infancy and Human Growth.* New York: Macmillan.
GESELL, A. & AMATRUDA, C. S. (1947). *Developmental Diagnosis.* New York: Hoeber.
ILLINGWORTH, R. S. (1958). Dissociation as a guide to developmental assessment. *Archives of Disease in Childhood* 33, 118.
ILLINGWORTH, R. S. (1972). *The Development of the Infant and Young Child,* 5th edn. Edinburgh: Churchill Livingstone.
LANGWORTHY, O. (1933). *Development of Behaviour Patterns and Myelination of the Nervous System in the Human Fetus and Infant.* Washington: Carnegie Institute, Pub. no. 443.
LEIGHTON, B. C. (1968). Eruption of deciduous teeth. *Practitioner* 200, 836.
MCGRAW, M. B. (1963). *Neuromuscular Maturation of the Human Infant.* New York: Hafner.
MEREDITH, H. V. (1946). Physical growth from birth to two years: head circumference. Part I. *Child Development* 17, no. 1 & 2.
NELIGAN, G. & PRUDHAM, D. (1969). Norms for four standard developmental milestones by sex, social class and place in family. *Developmental Medicine and Child Neurology* 11, 413.
PAINE, R. S. & OPPÉ, T. E. (1966). *Neurological Examination of Children.* London: Heinemann.

ROBINSON, R. J. (1966). Assessment of gestational age by neurological examination. *Archives of Disease in Childhood* **41**, 437.

SCAMMON, R. E. (1930). The measurement of the body in childhood. *The Measurement of Man*. University of Minnesota Press.

SHERIDAN, M. D. (1968). *The Developmental Progress of Infants and Young Children*, 2nd edn. London: H.M.S.O.

STUART, H. C. & MEREDITH, H. V. (1946). Use of body measurements in the school health programme. *American Journal of Public Health* **36,** 1365.

TANNER, J. M. (1970). In *Child Life and Health*, 5th edn. Edited by R. G. Mitchell. London: Churchill.

TANNER, J. M., WHITEHOUSE, R. H. & TAKAISHI, M. (1966). Standards from birth to maturity for height, weight, height velocity and weight velocity: British children, 1965. *Archives of Disease in Childhood* **41**, 454, 613.

THOMAS, A., CHESNI, Y. & SAINT-ANNE DARGASSIES, S. (1955). *Examen Neurologique du Nourrisson*. Paris.

WATSON, E. H. & LOWREY, G. H. (1967). *Growth and Development of Children*, 5th edn. Chicago: Year Book Medical Publishers.

WOLFF, P. H. & FEINBLOOM, R. I. (1969). Critical periods and cognitive development in the first two years. *Pediatrics* **44**, 999.

2 Social and Environmental Factors in Disease

Since the child has little control of his environment and the infant virtually none, social and environmental influences have an even greater effect on health in the early years than they have in adult life. Usually such factors are inextricably combined and it is impossible to determine the relative importance of any one in the genesis of ill-health. Thus if a particular disease is closely associated with poverty, it may mean that malnutrition, substandard housing, cold, overcrowding, faulty hygiene and lack of parental education all contribute to its causation. Some factors may operate before the birth of the child. The mother's physique and nutritional status, her own upbringing and nutrition as a child, the care and attention she receives during pregnancy and delivery may all affect the infant's chances of survival or subsequent health.

If it is thus difficult to identify the parts played by different environmental and social factors in disease, it is equally hard to devise acceptable measures of these factors and their effects. Mortality rates, social class and family income are all of some value as indices but are of little help in trying to relate the health status of infants to the quality of maternal care, which is probably the most important single determinant of well-being in early life. In most instances, therefore, it is only possible to speak in general terms of particular social and environmental factors as having an adverse influence or otherwise on child life and health: when such factors are considered separately it is with the proviso that it is rare for one to act alone or for its exact importance to be accurately assessable.

National mortality rates

A falling infant mortality rate (deaths during the first year per 1000 live births) is often taken as one index of social and medical progress. In England and Wales, the I.M.R. remained almost unchanged for 50 years during the nineteenth century, being 153 in 1841–50 and the same in 1891–1900. During the next 50 years it declined steadily to 73 in 1921–25 and 36 in 1946–50. Since then the fall has continued, the rate being 18 in 1968. Similar trends have been shown in all the more developed countries, though the rates still vary considerably from country to country. Amongst the lowest rates recorded are those of Finland and the Netherlands, both being 14 in 1968. In the same year the I.M.R. in Scotland was 21, in U.S.A 22, in Italy 32 and in Portugal 61. Some of the underdeveloped countries still have rates of 150 or more.

In the earlier part of the century in Britain the deaths under 4 weeks of age per 1000 live births (neonatal mortality rate) were considerably exceeded by the deaths during the subsequent 11 months of the first year (postneonatal mortality rate). Although both death rates have been substantially reduced, the postneonatal mortality rate has fallen more steeply and since 1945 the ratio has been reversed. Thus in England and Wales in 1968, out of a total infant mortality rate of 18 per 1000 live births, 12 occurred under 4 weeks of age and only six during the subsequent 11 months.

When the I.M.R. falls to a very low level, it loses its sensitivity as a discriminant, and then the perinatal mortality rate (stillbirths plus deaths in the first week per 1000 total births) may be of greater value as a social index, for it too is inversely related to social class.

Socio-economic status

As a crude index of economic status, the Registrar-General's Reports recognize five social classes, based in the case of children on the occupation of the father. Class I includes the financially independent and professional classes, including officers in the armed forces; class III, skilled labourers, including miners; class IV, semi-skilled labourers; and class V, unskilled labourers. Class II comprises those falling between I and III, including those in small businesses, shopkeepers, etc. Classes I and II therefore represent the more affluent and classes IV and V the poorer sections of the community, while the status of class III will vary greatly in different periods depending on the state of industry and mining. Comparison of mortality rates shows striking differences between social classes: for example, in 1968 in Scotland, the perinatal mortality rate in class V was more than double that in class I, being 31·5 and 12·6 respectively. The health of children in later years

is also inversely related to social class. Though much useful information has been gained by using the Registrar-General's social classification, it will be obvious that it is only a very rough guide and there can be great variation in income and mode of life within one class. A better way of measuring 'poverty' is to compare the family income from all sources with a standard recognized as giving a minimal level of subsistence, such as the standard set by the National Assistance Board. Using such a yardstick, it has been shown that poverty is still widespread in Britain today and that many thousands of children live in families with incomes below the subsistence level.

While it is generally true that poverty is likely to be associated with higher perinatal and infant mortality rates, and lower levels of health in childhood, it should be recognized that present income level is not an entirely satisfactory index of social well-being. The manner in which income is used, which depends largely on the cultural and educational backgrounds of the parents, the priorities allocated to food and clothing, material possessions, and entertainment and the domestic capabilities of the mother will all tend to produce wide differences within similar income-groups. Nevertheless, the lower the income level the greater will be the effect of such variations in management, and at subsistence levels mismanagement may be disastrous.

Parental care

The standard of child care in the home, and protection against accident and infection, depend not so much on income level and social status as on the parents' understanding of the child's needs and willingness to meet them. This will clearly be influenced to some extent by a basic economic security, by the size of the family and by the quality of their housing, but it will often be found that an intelligent and understanding mother can rear children successfully on a weekly income and under housing conditions which would reduce another to impotent despair; here the support of a reliable husband with the interest of the family at heart is at least as important as the actual wage he earns.

The establishment of a satisfactory parent–child relationship is essential for the child's emotional well-being and depends primarily on instinctive affection and understanding, the parents' behaviour to their children and their own marital relationship. When deprived of parental care and affection, the young child's emotional development may be adversely affected, leading to disturbed behaviour and, in extreme cases, the later development of a shallow. personality unable to feel deeply or establish satisfactory relationships with others. Deprivation may be the consequence of separation from the parents, as in admission to hospital or removal to residential care, but it must be realized that severe deprivation can occur in the home with the parents present.

Emotional acceptance or rejection of the child by either parent is little influenced by precept but there are few individuals who cannot derive some benefit from instruction before embarking on parenthood. Normally the foundation of this should be laid in their own homes during childhood. The girl who has helped her mother with younger brothers and sisters will obviously start with an advantage over the only child when she comes to have children of her own. For the future mother, training in mothercraft should be part of the school curriculum, and should include infant nutrition and hygiene, home-cooking and various other aspects of child care. Further training should be given at the antenatal and child health clinics and by the health visitor in the home.

The main role of the father is to provide the support and sense of security which is essential to the mother in the rearing of young children and to play an increasing part in the development of their interests and activities and in planning their later careers.

The importance of parental care in the preservation of child health is evident from the condition of children when parents are less than adequate. This may be because they are of poor intellect or simply ill-educated, harassed by the difficulties of dealing with a large family on a low income, and unable to maintain ordinary standards of hygiene and care. Much less commonly, parents are deliberately neglectful or cruel. In such families, the infants fail to thrive and older children are thin and poorly clad. They are prone to infections and may be verminous, often living in filthy home surroundings and perhaps exposed to moral danger. In some cases the parents have refused to have the necessary medical treatment for their children.

A relatively small but socially deplorable group of cases, which may reach hospital or be seen at necropsy, is the result of direct parental violence. This so-called 'battered child syndrome' (Plate 1), in which an infant or young child is found to have multiple bruises and abrasions, fractures, rupture of viscera or other injuries, is being increasingly recognized. A high index of suspicion is necessary if such cases are not to be overlooked or misdiagnosed as accidental injury or failure to thrive. The parents, who are often psychologically disturbed, usually appear to be responsible people and tell a plausible story of accident. In the absence of a true history it is not always possible to prove parental responsibility but, if violence is suspected from the nature of the injuries or the repeated appearance of the child at hospital, immediate admission to hospital should be arranged and the child held there until investigation clarifies the situation.

Broken homes and illegitimacy

Since the family is the biological unit best adapted to the rearing of healthy children, it is to be expected that if this unit is incomplete in any respect the child will suffer. This may happen in some degree if one parent dies or if the child has no siblings, but is intensified if the father has deserted, especially if a period of parental disharmony has preceded the break. The effect will be further increased by the mother's unhappiness subsequently and the associated economic and social disadvantages of a one-parent family. All these factors, and others such as the mother's youth, her rejection by her own parents and the social stigma, combine to render the child of the unmarried mother most vulnerable.

The proportion of births which are illegitimate has been rising steadily during the past decade, and in 1968 they represented 8·5 per cent of all live births in England and Wales. An additionally disquieting feature is that pregnancies in girls under 16 years of age are also increasing rapidly. Even allowing for the fact that a proportion of unmarried mothers will subsequently marry and the child become a member of the family, and that many other illegitimate infants will be adopted, the chances of survival of the illegitimate infant are substantially less than those of the legitimate. This is clearly seen by comparing the infant mortality rates for each year from 1948 to 1968 (Fig. 2.1). In 1968 the I.M.R. for legitimate infants was 18 and for illegitimate infants 23. The ratio of illegitimate to legitimate stillbirth rates is approximately 1:2, indicating

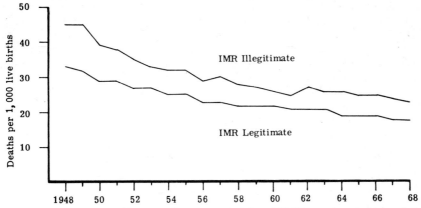

Fig. 2.1 The infant mortality rates for illegitimate infants are still consistently higher than those for legitimate infants (England and Wales, 1948–68).

that even before birth the scales are weighted against the illegitimate infant.

These mortality rates are an indication of society's reaction to the unmarried mother and her child. During pregnancy the mother, and after birth the infant, often receive less care and are exposed to greater risks than those who form part of a normal family unit. The unmarried mother will usually have to work for a greater proportion of her pregnancy and will return to work sooner than the mother who has the support of a wage-earner, while if she tries to keep her baby the economic disadvantage will continue. Social discrimination adds to her difficulties, for though it is diminishing it is by no means a thing of the past.

Although infanticide no longer represents a major cause of death in illegitimate infants, the distinction between this and death by neglect or maltreatment may be an academic one and there are still many infant deaths more or less directly related to illegitimacy. Moreover, a high infant mortality rate is likely to be associated with an excessive morbidity among those surviving, while the psychological effects of illegitimacy on children who are deprived of a normal home background are at least as important as the physical in determining maladjustment and later ill-health.

Nutrition

The clinical manifestations of severe nutritional deficiency are considered in Chapter 6; here we are more concerned with suboptimal nutrition resulting from poverty and faulty feeding habits. Increased prosperity in Britain since 1950 has resulted in better nutritional standards, with greater consumption of meat and dairy products in the poorer socio-economic groups. Milk, a rich source of animal protein and calcium, is cheaply available for infants. Nevertheless increasing unemployment, especially in some areas, and rapidly rising prices suggest that the general improvement may not be maintained. Moreover, data on average consumptions tend to obscure the existence of malnutrition in vulnerable groups, such as very large families, recent immigrants and the socially inadequate. There are probably substantial numbers of children from poor homes whose diets are deficient in first-class protein and fresh green vegetables and who receive the bulk of their calories as carbohydrate. While few of them show overt nutritional disease, their poor nutritional state is likely to interfere with growth, reduce resistance to infection and adversely affect later health, though proof of such effects is difficult to obtain.

The nutrition of the individual child depends not only on the family income but also on how the money is expended, on how the food is prepared and cooked and on the family feeding habits. In addition, variations in appetite and personal preferences are important and may largely offset the value of bulk catering systems such as the school meals service.

Overcrowding

The effects of overcrowding on the child will be both physical and psychological, and will depend on his age, the composition of the group inhabiting the house (e.g. one family, family plus relatives, or lodgers), the time spent in the home, floor space, ventilation and sanitation, as well as on the number of persons per room. Arbitrary standards of what constitutes overcrowding have been laid down for statistical purposes. Thus it must be possible to segregate the sexes at night in the case of children over the age of 10 years and the number of persons sleeping in the house must not exceed that stipulated, which depends on the number of rooms and the floor area.

Close proximity favours cross-infection and the spread of parasitic infestation. The lower standards of cleanliness which are inseparable from overcrowding will frequently result in contamination of food and the spread of infective diarrhoea. Almost equally important is the disturbance of sleep which inevitably results when several children of different ages are sleeping in the same room or in close proximity to a television set or other source of noise. The absence of facilities for play increases the time spent in the street and the consequent exposure to risks of road or other accidents. Lack of privacy in an overcrowded house brings children into contact with their parents' quarrels, anxieties and sex life in a way which may have repercussions on their own emotional development, and where the parents are of low intelligence or inebriate the children are especially liable to suffer. The conflicting authority of parents, grandparents and other relatives in an overcrowded house frequently forms the basis for later emotional difficulties.

Industrialization

The effects of industrialization on child health were seen most dramatically in England during the Industrial Revolution, when a predominantly rural population became converted to a predominantly urban one and increased from 9 million in 1801 to 32·5 million in 1901. Many cities still suffer from the consequences, with their narrow streets and lack of space, inadequately serviced tenement buildings, and smoke pall from domestic and factory chimneys. The drift from the country to the city continues and is clearly seen in Scotland, where the Highlands are becoming depopulated and nearly a quarter of the total population lives in Glasgow. Though town planning and building programmes have improved many British cities, in some parts of the world rapid industrialization and the population explosion are defeating the planners. Cities are

becoming even more crowded in the centre and are surrounded by unsanitary and primitive 'shanty towns' where infant mortality is appallingly high. Moreover, the infant mortality rate is only a crude index of the total effect of urban conditions, for diseases which kill in infancy, e.g. respiratory and intestinal infections, also affect the health of the much greater number of children who survive.

In general, the ill-effects of industrialization on child health can be attributed to unplanned urbanization, overcrowding, poverty due to high rents and periods of unemployment, the abuse of female labour and pollution of the environment. It must be emphasized, however, that these are not inevitable concomitants of industrialization. Well-planned and serviced cities can provide infants and children with all they require for modern healthy living. Child health and social services, the supply of clean water and food, good sanitation and health education are all more readily organized in urban than in rural districts. Within existing industrial towns, rehousing and town planning with provision of open spaces and playgrounds, smoke abatement and improvement of nutritional standards are all practicable. The drift into large cities can be slowed or reversed by establishing new towns and by improving the quality of life in rural areas.

Female employment

Employment in shop or factory is often an economic necessity for the mother from a low-income family, and long hours of work may have repercussions on her health and consequently on that of her children. In addition, however, married women who have adequate means are increasingly seeking outside work for social reasons and to supplement the family income. It is impossible to assess accurately the effects of female employment on child health, since the direct effects may be partly offset when the young child is well cared-for in a day nursery or nursery school, while the economic status of the home will be improved by the increased income. In general, however, the removal of the infant or pre-school child from the home, and the delegation of his care to someone other than the mother for the whole of the working day are likely to have adverse effects on the mother–child relationship and to bring him into contact with infection earlier than if he had been kept within the family unit.

Environmental pollution

Pollution of the environment in industrial areas has become a threat to the health of children. Smoke and fumes from factories and refineries, exhaust gases from countless motor vehicles and radioactivity from nuclear reactors may all contaminate the air they breathe. Effluent from chemical works may enter the rivers and lakes where they swim. Offensive odours may assail their nostrils and soot or dust begrime their skin and clothing.

Air pollution in Britain is mainly due to domestic burning of soft coal, producing black smoke, tar droplets and sulphur dioxide. Chronic respiratory disease is commoner among children living in cities with heavy air pollution than among those from rural areas, the difference being most pronounced in children from poor homes. Very young infants and children who already have respiratory disorders such as asthma or chronic bronchitis are especially vulnerable. Smokeless zones established after the Clean Air Act of 1956 have greatly improved the atmosphere of some cities, but many towns are still without smoke control.

Little is known about the effects of prolonged exposure to background radiation, which may be partly natural and partly due to fallout from military weapons or accidental leakage from industrial installations. Any increase must be considered a health hazard to infants and children, especially as strontium[90] and iodine[131] are concentrated in milk. Children in some areas are known to be accumulating radioactivity from such sources and additional radiation, e.g. from medical diagnostic procedures, must be kept to a minimum. It is doubtful whether there is a critical threshold of radiation below which no adverse effects will occur and above which there will be a rapid rise in the incidence of genetic and somatic damage. Nevertheless, contamination of the environment is likely to continue and there should be international standards for acceptable levels of radiation exposure, beyond which action to protect health would be mandatory.

Season and climate

Many childhood diseases show a seasonal incidence, the pattern often varying from year to year according to the state of the population at risk and the climatic conditions of the particular season. Thus a severe winter favours overcrowding in poorly ventilated rooms and consequent cross-infection, while in hot weather flies increase and the risk of food contamination is greater. Economic factors may be contributory, e.g. the high cost of green vegetables in early spring may result in vitamin or iron deficiency.

Respiratory infections tend to have their highest incidence in winter and spring, when resistance is low and conditions favour cross-infection. Allergic disorders are often most troublesome in the summer months, when the child is sensitive to plant pollens. Some infectious diseases show a seasonal pattern, though this may be obscured by immunization programmes. Thus poliomyelitis used to occur in large epidemics in late summer, especially after a hot dry spell. Improved hygiene and nutrition have also modified the seasonal incidence of disease. Infantile diarrhoea used to assume epidemic form in summer when flies were likely to contaminate unprotected infant feeds. When nutritional rickets was common, its incidence was highest in spring, following the winter deprivation of sunlight. Although many of the disadvantages of season and climate have thus been obviated, careful analysis of seasonal and climatic factors and their relationship to primary cause may be helpful in elucidating the etiology of a disease or in suggesting preventive measures.

War

The effects of war on child health extend far beyond the immediate period of hostilities, while injury and loss of life from enemy action represent only a fraction of the total disability caused. When a country is invaded or suffers civil war, the childhood population is affected first by the immediate preparations for invasion or defence, which commonly involve the food and milk supply of the community; then by the often chaotic movement of refugees; and finally by enemy occupation. In a country attacked by air, many children are likely to be evacuated to foster homes or to suffer the restrictions of a life orientated round air-raid shelters.

The nutrition of children will be severely affected if the measures taken to safeguard their food supplies break down: the distribution of fresh milk is especially liable to sudden disruption. Apart from nutritional deprivation, war conditions of overcrowding in shelters and lack of sanitation and hygiene favour the spread of tuberculosis, scabies and pediculosis, the last facilitating the spread of typhus where this is

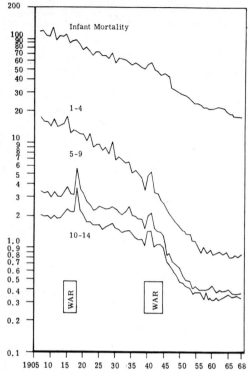

Fig. 2.2   The mortality rates of infancy and childhood from 1905–68 (England and Wales), showing the relative fall in each age group (log scale) and the effects of two wars.
(By permission of the Comptroller, H.M.S.O.)

endemic. The incidence of syphilis almost invariably increases during wars and, although modern treatment has largely offset its effects, some increase in congenital syphilis may follow.

The psychological effects of war on children are as far-reaching as the physical. The most important single factor is probably disruption of the family, leading in some cases to permanent insecurity or delinquency. Separation of parents also results in an increased incidence of illegitimate births and permanently broken homes.

ACCIDENTS AND POISONING

Accidents rank as the commonest cause of child death after the first year of life, being responsible for three times as many deaths in childhood as the next most frequent cause, neoplastic disease, and accounting for one-third of all deaths between the ages of 1 and 15 years (England and Wales). Accident rates and mortality are higher in boys than in girls at all ages but the causes

vary according to sex and age. For every fatality there are many non-fatal accidents, some causing permanent disability. Accident prevention is thus of major importance in the maintenance of child health and is based on knowledge of the epidemiology of accidents, education of parents, children and the general public, and action to remove existing or potential hazards.

Road accidents

About half of all the accidental deaths of children are due to traffic accidents, which thus constitute the most important single cause of death at all ages of childhood and in both sexes. The death rate is highest in children under 4 years of age and thereafter falls in girls but remains high in boys, largely due to increasing deaths among boy pedal-cyclists. Mortality increases after the age of 15 years owing to the high death rate among male motor-cyclists. The loss of child life on the roads is likely to remain heavy until there is greatly improved town-planning, with safe pedestrian crossings, shopping areas and playgrounds, better design of motor vehicles and a greater sense of responsibility among motorists. The training of children in road sense and the provision of road-guides for younger children coming out of school are safety measures which have been widely adopted but their effects have tended to be offset by the greater number and speed of cars.

Other accidents

After traffic accidents, drowning is the most frequent cause of accidental death in boys and burning in girls. Drowning is especially common in sparsely populated areas where there is a long coastline or many lakes and other unprotected water, as in Finland and to a lesser extent in Scotland. Domestic accidents account for a high proportion of fatal accidents to pre-school children and many are burns or scalds, which also cause much disfigurement and disability. The majority of burning accidents could be prevented by such simple measures as providing fireguards, placing hot water and fat out of reach, and turning saucepan handles away from the edge of the stove. The replacement of nightgowns by pyjamas of less flammable material has been a step in the right direction. Manufacturers have a responsibility to produce safe electrical equipment, especially electric fires which frequently cause deep hand burns. Unfortunately, new hazards to children in the home are created by the increasing use of complex household equipment.

In children aged 1 year and under, by far the commonest cause of accidental death is mechanical suffocation, but this term includes not only known inhalation of food or other matter but also a large number of sudden unexpected deaths of infants. These generally conform to a characteristic syndrome, in which a previously healthy infant between the ages of 2 and 5 months is found dead in his cot or pram. Necropsy reveals only petechial haemorrhages in the thorax and slight inflammatory changes in the respiratory tract. Some of these 'cot deaths' may be due to fulminating infection or acute hypersensitivity reactions but in many cases the cause is unknown.

Accidental poisoning

The incidence of accidental poisoning in childhood has increased in recent years, the poisons most frequently fatal in Britain being gases, aspirin, pesticides and ferrous sulphate. Substances commonly ingested by children include medicinal agents, especially aspirin, barbiturates, tranquillizers and antidepressants, household cleaning and disinfecting agents and kerosene (paraffin) but the pattern varies in different localities and is constantly changing. The majority of cases are in the age range 18 to 30 months, when children are normally active and exploratory, and have a strong impulse to put things in their mouths, both for identification and for self-gratification. These characteristics predispose to accidental poisoning, which frequently occurs when parents are inattentive or neglectful, as at times of family crisis. Measures to reduce the incidence of accidental poisoning in childhood include education of parents, wider use of child-proof containers for drugs, and safe storage of poisonous substances in and around the house. When a child is suspected of having swallowed a poisonous substance, immediate emesis should be induced by a finger to the back of the throat or by administering a dessertspoonful of syrup of ipecacuanha, and the child should be taken to hospital as quickly as possible. Emesis should not be induced when paraffin, turpentine or related substances have been ingested, owing to the risk of inhalation.

SALICYLATE POISONING is common in this country, occurring both accidentally and by therapeutic overdosage. Soon after ingestion of a large dose, stimulation of the respiratory centres produces hyperventilation and respiratory alkalosis. Nausea, vomiting, tinnitus and deafness are common complaints. Within a few hours, metabolic acidosis develops, with pyrexia, collapse and sometimes death. Emesis should be induced as soon as possible in salicylate poisoning and may still be effective some hours after ingestion. When symptoms or blood salicylate levels over 50 mg per 100 ml are present, diuresis should be induced by controlled infusion of electrolyte and fluid, with correction of acid-base disturbance. In severe cases, peritoneal dialysis or exchange transfusion may be indicated.

LEAD POISONING is not uncommon in children between 1 and 3 years of age who have chewed lead-containing paint off cots or window ledges or who have swallowed or inhaled lead from other sources, such as old batteries, toys or contaminated domestic water. Clinical manifestations such as pallor, constipation, anorexia and colic are likely if the blood level of lead exceeds 50 μg per 100 ml, while in more severe poisoning there may be convulsions (lead encephalopathy). A history of pica, abdominal pain, behaviour disorder or mental deterioration associated with refractory microcytic, hypochromic or occasionally, haemolytic anaemia should suggest the diagnosis. Deposition of lead in the long bones as a 'lead line', copropor-

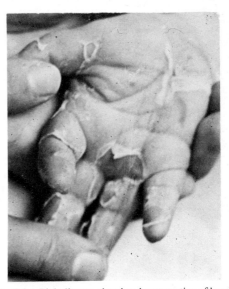

Fig. 2.3   Pink disease, showing desquamation of hand.

phyrinuria and punctate basophilia of the red cells may be present but are not always found in mild cases. Treatment includes eliminating the source of intake. Lead may be removed from the body by a chelating agent such as D-penicillamine (20 mg per kg per day by mouth in two doses) or, in more severe cases, sodium calcium edetate (up to 75 mg per kg daily intramuscularly in 20 per cent solution in divided doses). Repeated blood transfusion may be necessary.

MERCURY POISONING is believed to have been responsible for most cases of pink disease (acrodynia), which is now rare. This condition is characterized by anorexia, loss of weight, sweating, photophobia and extreme irritability. The hands and feet are red and painful with peeling skin and gangrene of the fingers and toes in extreme cases (see Fig. 2.3). An erythematous or macular skin rash commonly occurs. Although mercury in the urine or a history of its ingestion is found in a high proportion of cases, such evidence of mercury poisoning is not invariable. On the other hand, the removal of mercury from teething powders ('grey powders') was followed by the virtual disappearance of the disease. The management of pink disease consists in removing all sources of mercury and treating pain and restlessness with analgesics and sedatives. Tolazoline may help to relieve symptoms but skilled nursing and the maintenance of adequate nutrition are the main needs.

BIBLIOGRAPHY AND REFERENCES

BACKETT, E. M. (1965). Domestic accidents. *Public Health Papers* W.H.O. no. 26.
BACKETT, E. M. & JOHNSTON, A. M. (1959). Social patterns of road accidents to children. *Lancet* i, 409.
BAIRD, D. (1962). Environmental and obstetrical factors in prematurity. *Bulletin of the World Health Organization* 26, 291.
BARLTROP, D. (1969). Lead poisoning. *British Journal of Hospital Medicine* 2, 1567.
BLAKE, P. (1972). The plight of one-parent families. London: Council for Children's Welfare.
BRANSBY, E. R. & ELLIOTT, R. A. (1959). The unmarried mother and her child. *Monthly Bulletin of the Ministry of Health and Public Health Laboratory Service* 18, 17.
DAVIE, R., BUTLER, N. & GOLDSTEIN, H. (1972). *From Birth to Seven*. London: Longman.
ELLIS, R. W. B. (1948). Effects of war on child health. *British Medical Journal* i, 239.
ELLIS, R. W. B. (1955). Social change and child health. *Pediatrics, Springfield* 20, 1041.
FORFAR, J. O. (1965). Prospect and practice in child health. *Lancet* i, 615.
HELFER, R. E. & KEMPE, H. (1968). *The Battered Child*. Chicago: University of Chicago Press.
HOWELLS, J. G. (1969). Separation and deprivation. In *Modern Perspectives in International Child Psychiatry*. Edinburgh: Oliver & Boyd.
MILLER, F. J. W., COURT, S. D. M., WALTON, W. S. & KNOX, E. G. (1960). *Growing up in Newcastle upon Tyne*. Oxford University Press.
MORRIS, J. N. (1955). Social and biological factors in infant mortality. *Lancet* i, 343, 395, 445, 499, 554.
SHERIDAN, M. D. (1959). Neglectful mothers. *Lancet* i, 722.
SPENCE, J. C. (1946). *The Purpose of the Family*. London: National Children's Home.
VALDES-DAPENA, M. A. (1967). Sudden and unexpected death in infancy. *Pediatrics, Springfield* 39, 123.
YUDKIN, S. & YUDKIN, G. (1968). Poverty and child development. *Developmental Medicine and Child Neurology* 10, 569.

3 Constitutional Factors in Disease

Commonly no hard and fast distinction can be drawn between the genetic and environmental influences which have determined the child's individual constitution and susceptibility to disease. Though some conditions, e.g. Down's syndrome or phenylketonuria, are almost entirely genetically determined and others, e.g. accidental injury, are largely of environmental origin, in the great majority of diseases both heredity and environment play a part. Genetic factors are present from conception, though not necessarily active in early life, and may be modified by environmental experiences before as well as after birth. Congenital characters, i.e. those present at birth, cannot therefore be regarded as being necessarily determined by 'nature' as distinct from 'nurture'. If this dual character of 'constitution' is clearly recognized, however, it is useful to consider certain factors influencing the appearance of, or susceptibility to, disease which are primarily the inheritance of the infant, or which characterize him as an individual at any particular period of childhood.

Genetic constitution

This is essentially determined by the contribution made to the individual by the germ plasm of both parents, and is responsible for the inheritance not only of those characters which are common to the species but also certain of those which differentiate one individual from another. These latter may be of little social or clinical importance, e.g. eye colour or the capacity for tasting. They may assume importance under certain circumstances, e.g. the blood group when a transfusion is necessary or the Rhesus constitution in the case of a particular mating; or they may be actively harmful or beneficial. Most recognizable characteristics are determined by multiple gene effects but in some a mutant gene of large effect is responsible. As a general rule, harmful characteristics which are inherited as mendelian dominants tend to die out in a community, either because they are themselves lethal or because they tend to limit the chances of marriage and procreation. (A harmful trait, however, may sometimes be 'corrected' by surgery or other means, so that the individual survives to reproduce.) In the case of recessive characters, there may be no such limitation of procreation by parents in whom the disease is not manifest but who are able to transmit the mutant gene concerned. Consanguineous (cousin) marriages between members of affected families will increase the risk of the condition appearing in the offspring, since there is a greater danger that both parents may be carriers than there would be in a random mating.

With increasing control of disease-producing factors in the environment, the genetic aspects of disease have become relatively more important. There are still many difficulties in applying genetic principles to human material, e.g. definition of the condition studied, random mating, uncontrolled environment, small size or artificial limitation of human families, etc. Thus a clinical condition such as deaf mutism may be due to genetic factors in one patient and environmental factors (e.g. maternal infection) in another, the defect being represented in the genotype and transmissible in the first whereas in the second it is not. Some characters may show low penetrance (the frequency with which the gene effect is shown in a population), while others may arise by a process of mutation in one individual and show a familial incidence in the case of another. A genetically determined predisposition to a disease is more often dependent on the interaction of several genes than on a single gene or chromosomal abnormality, and with such polygenic inheritance the appearance of the disease may depend on a particular environmental experience. It should be remembered that because a disease has appeared in several members of a family it does not follow that it is genetically determined; thus the same environmental or social factors may affect several members of a family and produce the same result, or contact may cause direct infection.

Genetic counselling with regard to the possible genetic hazards of reproduction is becoming increasingly important as more parents and prospective parents practise family planning and understand the principles of genetics and as greater numbers of children with genetically determined abnormalities survive as a result of treatment. Moreover, the availability of early therapy for some disorders makes it imperative to recognize them as early as possible, and parents must be alerted when the birth of an affected infant is anticipated. Genetic counselling can only be reliable if it is based on an accurate family history, precise diagnosis of the condition and knowledge of the way in which it is inherited. There is an increasing number of traits of which the mode of inheritance is sufficiently established to make possible an estimate of the risks of children being affected. This applies to Rhesus immunization, to a number of inborn errors of metabolism, particularly when it is possible to identify 'carriers' by biochemical or other means, and to some congenital malformations (Chapter 5). Thus if parents have had one child with spina bifida, there is about one chance in thirty of a subsequent child suffering from spina bifida, hydrocephalus, or anencephaly. Unfortunately many of the commoner disabilities about which parents are most likely to ask advice, e.g. mental subnormality, are ones where it may be impossible to give a firm prognosis. Probably the most valuable aspect of genetic counselling is still reassurance when parents are concerned about the inheritance of a condition in which the risk of having another affected child is low.

Immunity

The infant or child resists infection partly by non-specific mechanisms, mainly phagocytic activity and local tissue reaction, and partly by specific immunity, which may be established in one of several ways. It may be inborn, i.e. a character of the species or family group; it may be transmitted from the mother; it may be acquired by natural means; or it may be artificially produced by active or passive immunization. The blood plasma in childhood normally contains antibody globulins, comprising three principal immunoglobulins—IgG (immune globulin G), IgM and IgA—and others more recently identified. Most bacterial antigens stimulate the formation of IgG but antibody to colon bacilli is generally IgM.

CONGENITAL IMMUNITY of the newborn infant exists as a passive immunity acquired from the mother by placental transmission of maternal immunoglobulin, mainly IgG. Antibody in the infant's blood at birth therefore reflects the mother's own state of immunity and the newborn infant is thus protected against such diseases as measles, provided that the mother is herself immune. This protection is gradually lost during the first few months of life. Little IgM crosses the placental barrier and so the newborn infant has no specific defences against *Escherichia coli* infection.

ACQUIRED IMMUNITY is normally obtained by exposure to sublethal doses of infection during childhood, and is either built up gradually by repeated minimal exposure, or rapidly during a clinical attack of a particular disease, e.g. measles, pertussis, mumps, chickenpox. Although second attacks of these diseases are rare, they are not unknown, and illustrate the fact that immunity is relative and that it is not necessarily permanent. Other infections, such as streptococcal throat infections and the common cold, may produce only a very partial or temporary immunity. The infant will not only start with little or no immunity to the majority of infections, but during the newborn period is poorly able to produce antibodies. The synthesis of immunoglobulins by the infant increases with age and contact with infection but plasma levels are low during the first year, as maternal IgG disappears and before the infant has had time to form his own. It follows that the young infant is more liable to succumb to infections which would prove of little danger to the older child or adult, e.g. staphylococcal infection of the skin or invasion of the meninges by *E. coli*. That the capacity to produce immune globulins is an inborn character, however, is illustrated by those rare cases of *congenital agammaglobulinaemia* in which a sex-linked recessive deficiency of the normal mechanism results in minimal resistance to bacterial infection.

ARTIFICIAL IMMUNITY may be *passive*, when antiserum or gamma globulin is given to counteract an acute infection such as measles or tetanus, or *active*, when injection of killed or live attenuated vaccine or antigen is carried out in order to stimulate the production of antibodies by the child himself. In the case of passive immunity, the value is only temporary, whereas active immunity will last for a much longer period, though tending to decrease with time unless the production of immune globulin is re-stimulated by a further 'booster dose' or natural exposure. Immunization and BCG vaccination are considered in Chapter 15.

Allergy

This is a condition of changed reactivity or hypersensitivity, which may be associated with a hereditary predisposition (atopy) or arise when no such predisposition can be demonstrated. In 'natural' or atopic allergy, the condition represents an antibody:allergen reaction, and IgE antibodies (or reagins) are present in the blood, being increased by the injection of the appropriate allergen.

Anaphylaxis, which is also a condition of hypersensitivity, is artificially induced by injection of a foreign protein. No hereditary predisposition is present in anaphylaxis, whereas this is present in the atopic types of allergy. The reagins of allergy produce skin sensitivity, whereas the antibodies of anaphylaxis do not. The commoner allergic manifestations in childhood are considered in Chapter 11.

Sex

Since the sex of the individual is itself genetically determined, the male carrying an X and a Y chromosome and the female two X chromosomes, the secondary characters associated with sex may also be regarded as an expression of the genotype of the individual, though liable to variation from endocrine or other influences.

Some disease processes having a genetic basis show strict sex-limitation, though partial sex-limitation, or preference for one particular sex, is a much commoner phenomenon. This may be due to the disease being more readily expressed in one sex, most commonly the male, or may be explicable as the result of the gene itself showing partial or complete sex-linkage. In the case of a sex-linked recessive character such as haemophilia, where the responsible gene is carried on the X chromosome and the chances of an affected male mating with a transmitting female are remote, the disease is only likely to be manifest in males. Where there is unequal penetrance in the two sexes, it is almost always the male who is more commonly affected.

Since we are concerned here only with the clinical effects of sex in the determination of disease, it will suffice that sex provides a constitutional factor which in some instances will explain on a strictly genetic basis the higher incidence, or exclusive appearance, of particular diseases in one sex rather than the other.

We can therefore distinguish three types of sex discrimination: (1) those conditions known to have an hereditary or familial incidence in which the preponderance in one or other sex can be explained on the basis of gene sex-linkage or unequal penetrance; (2) those in which environmental factors will act unequally on the two sexes; and (3) those in which environmental factors might be expected to act equally (e.g. certain infections), but in which the incidence and mortality of the disease are unequal in the two sexes. To these three groups may be added those conditions directly related to the sex organs, though they play a less important part in the etiology of disease in childhood than in later life: thus malignant tumours of the gonads or breasts are extremely rare in childhood, though urethral valves, hypospadias, undescended testicles, balanitis, etc., will be peculiar to the male, and inguinal hernia much commoner in the male than in the female; vulvovaginitis and congenital defects of the vagina and uterus will be peculiar to the female, and urinary infection in childhood, in the absence of demonstrable con-

genital defect, considerably commoner in girls owing to the short urethra.

As an example of genetically determined defects, congenital pyloric stenosis is seen in male infants four to six times as frequently as in females. A condition usually developing rather later and having a heredo-familial incidence is pseudo-hypertrophic muscular dystrophy: when this appears as a sex-linked recessive, the proportion may be as high as 113 males to 3 females (Ford, 1966). Of all deaths from congenital defects occurring during the neonatal period, whether these be genetically determined or not, it will be found that the majority occur in males. Of those resulting in stillbirth, there is also an excess of males, but here there is the interesting exception that anencephaly is three times more common in female than in male fetuses.

When we consider the diseases in which the

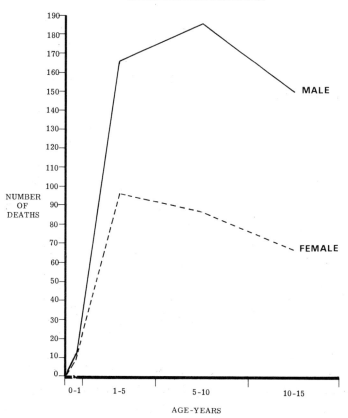

ROAD DEATHS (MOTOR VEHICLE ACCIDENTS) BY AGE AND SEX IN ENGLAND AND WALES, 1966

Fig. 3.1   Road deaths, showing preponderance of male over female deaths at all ages of childhood.

etiological factors affect the sexes unequally, a striking example is furnished by deaths by violence, e.g. road accidents, in which after the age of 1 year the male preponderance is very great (Fig. 3.1). This discrepancy may be attributed, according to inclination, to the timidity or caution of the girl as compared with the recklessness or daring of the male. In the newborn period, it is probably justifiable to attribute at least a small proportion of the excess of male deaths due to birth injury, asphyxia, and atelectasis to the fact that the male infant at birth is on the average slightly larger and has a slightly greater head circumference than the female, though against this purely mechanical theory must be set the fact that the number of deaths attributed to the results of birth before term (with its added risk of injury) is also significantly greater in the male than in the female. The hazards of occupation do not, of course, apply in childhood to nearly the same extent as in later life, though they may become operative during adolescence.

There remains a very great number of diseases showing a preponderance of male over female deaths, for which there is no obvious reason. Indeed, if all the main causes of death during the first year of life are analysed by sex, it will be found that in almost every instance the male deaths substantially exceed the female (except when the infant mortality is very low).

This excessive male mortality, which is not confined to the first year of life, cannot be explained on the basis of the relative number of males and females at risk, although the sex ratio at birth is approximately 105 males to 100 females and the proportion only assumes equality after childhood is passed. It will be found that in most instances the ratio of male to female infant deaths is greater than 1·05 to 1·0. The male appears to be the weaker vessel.

In comparatively few instances is the female mortality greater than the male. Thus in England and Wales, female deaths from pertussis were consistently higher than male deaths from the same cause over a period of many years, while in adolescence and early adult life, tuberculosis accounted for a significantly greater number of female than male deaths. Rheumatic chorea occurs two to three times as frequently in girls as in boys between 5 and 15 years of age. Few diseases of genetic origin appear predominantly in the female, though congenital dislocation of the hip, which is partly genetically determined, is a notable exception.

Race

The attribution of particular characteristics or disease processes to 'race' has given rise to many unjustifiable conclusions. Certainly amongst the inhabitants of Europe the term 'race' can have little significance if an attempt is made to identify it with nationality. When dealing with communities which have remained isolated, and where mixed marriages have been very exceptional, it is possible for gene frequencies in the population to differ from those in communities elsewhere. The likelihood of cousin marriages is also increased where the community is sufficiently small or where cousin marriage is favoured for religious reasons. But the majority of diseases which have been attributed to race as such can usually be explained on the basis of dietetic habits, social and religious customs, hygiene, and climate. Thus a high neonatal mortality may be traced to such various practices as dressing the umbilicus with dung or dirty rags (giving rise to tetanus), to sexual promiscuity and a high incidence of syphilis, to faulty infant feeding, or to the ritual destruction of twins or female (or less commonly of male) infants at birth.

Again, the susceptibility to, and high mortality from, certain infectious and epidemic diseases, such as measles and tuberculosis, in communities where these have been recently introduced, is as likely to indicate a lack of immunity due to the absence of previous exposure, or conditions of living favouring spread, as to represent a true 'racial' susceptibility, though there is some evidence that the latter may exist. Similarly, whole communities may be so heavily infested with malarial or other parasites, owing to climatic and social conditions, that the physical characteristics and resistance of the community to other diseases may be materially affected. Characteristic feeding habits coupled with social practices, e.g. *purdah*, may result in nutritional disorders occurring commonly in one 'race' and not in another when both live side by side, while changing the natural habitat of a dark-skinned race to a northern climate will render infants particularly liable to rickets unless they are adequately protected.

If all such factors which are not truly 'racial' in the genetic sense are eliminated, it will be found that few diseases can confidently be attributed to race as such. Two of the lipidoses (Niemann-Pick disease and Gaucher's disease) occur more frequently, but not exclusively, in Jews, as does amaurotic family idiocy (Tay-Sachs disease) and certain rare inborn errors of metabolism (e.g. pentosuria). Of more practical importance is the distribution of the classical blood groups and Rhesus genes in particular communities, and here there do appear to be true racial differences. Thalassaemia, a genetically determined type of haemolytic anaemia, which was once thought only to affect patients of Mediterranean origin, has now been shown to occur in other stock. Sickle-cell disease, however, is almost exclusively confined to the Negro race.

Age incidence

The field of paediatrics differs from that of adult medicine in that it is largely concerned with diseases of growth and immaturity, whereas the ageing adult is affected primarily with diseases of degeneration. The growing period from conception to puberty can be further subdivided into age periods, each having its particular strains and disabilities, and while many disease processes may act throughout the whole age span under review, the response of the organism is likely to differ somewhat at each stage of development, depending on the immunity it has acquired, the maturity of its organs, and the control of its environment. It will save much mistaken diagnosis if some familiarity is acquired with the manifestations of disease most likely to be associated with each period. For this purpose eight stages of development may be recognized.

THE PRENATAL PERIOD. During this time, from the fertilization of the ovum to the time of delivery, the genotype is established, and the effects of intrauterine environment will operate. The developing embryo and fetus will establish those conditions which are collectively known as 'congenital' and certain infections and toxins are liable to be transmitted from placenta to fetus. Maternal toxaemia, multiple pregnancy and a variety of other causes may result in premature termination of pregnancy, while poorly controlled maternal diabetes is liable to lead to the birth of giant infants, whose prospects of survival are less good than those of normal infants. It is during this period also that the effects of Rhesus incompatibility of mother and fetus will become operative.

The effects of maternal diet during pregnancy

have already been considered. Growth retardation of the fetus may be associated with maternal toxaemia and hypertension, excessive maternal smoking, or poor placental function but in many cases the cause is obscure.

BIRTH. The process of birth is associated with particular hazards, which are principally mechanical. Birth injury is especially liable to occur when there is prolonged or difficult labour, or when breech delivery is effected: but immaturity of the fetus may equally readily result in birth injury when the delivery is easy or rapid. Asphyxia and atelectasis are also to be included in the hazards of birth, while inhalation of infected liquor amnii or meconium during the birth process is liable to cause pneumonia during the neonatal period.

THE NEONATAL PERIOD covers the first month of life. At this time disease established during the prenatal period or during birth will become manifest. The greatest number of deaths during the first week will be due to conditions associated with low birth weight, congenital abnormality, anoxia or birth injury; subsequently infection will play an increasingly important role.

ONE TO SIX MONTHS. During this period, the infant's digestive system is both immature and readily deranged and digestive disorders are particularly common. In addition, the immaturity of the central nervous system renders the infant and young child liable to convulsions, which may be precipitated by a wide variety of provoking causes, including birth injury, infection, and congenital malformation.

Congenital immunity transmitted from the mother will protect the infant, where the mother herself is immune, from some diseases, such as measles, during the earliest months, but this congenital immunity is rapidly lost. Upper respiratory infection, particularly otitis media, begins to assume considerable clinical importance during the first six months of life, and continues to do so throughout childhood.

Intussusception has its maximum incidence in the sixth month, the curve of age incidence (Fig. 6.23) straddling the postnatal period, i.e. 1 to 12 months.

SIX MONTHS TO TWO YEARS. After the first few months, a milk diet becomes inadequate for the infant's needs, and if this is not supplemented nutrition suffers and there is a risk of iron-deficiency anaemia and vitamin deficiencies (rickets and scurvy).

The majority of cases of coeliac disease show the first manifestation of the disease during this period, though earlier introduction of cereals is tending to precipitate symptoms at a younger age.

TWO TO FIVE YEARS (the preschool period). An increasingly high incidence of the common epidemic infectious diseases (measles, chickenpox, mumps) is likely to be seen during the period in which the infant enlarges his social circle. Poliomyelitis, which previously fell particularly heavily on this age group, is seldom seen when immunization is in widespread use. The nephrotic syndrome occurs most frequently between 2 and 5 years, and asthma becomes established. Mismanagement of the child during this age period lays the foundation for future behaviour disturbances.

FIVE TO TEN YEARS. During this period an increasing number of chronic respiratory infections make their appearance. Acute nephritis, though not limited to any one period of childhood, becomes more common during the fifth and subsequent years. Acute rheumatism and chorea occur at this age, the average age of onset of rheumatism being 6 to 9 years.

Tonsillectomy is commonly performed during this age period, though the frequency of the operation cannot be taken as an index of its necessity.

TEN TO FIFTEEN YEARS. The onset of puberty is characterized by the frequency of vasomotor instability, which may be manifested by fainting attacks, and by emotional and behavioural difficulties. The major endocrine readjustment of puberty may give rise to transient imbalance. Cardiac or renal failure is more likely to occur with the added strain of puberty in cases of established disease of the heart or kidneys than it is in earlier childhood.

Maternal age and parity

There is an optimum age for child-bearing, and infants born between the mother's eighteenth and thirtieth years will have a better prospect of survival than those born either later or before the mother's growth is completed. After the thirtieth year, the incidence of certain congenital abnormalities of the fetus, e.g. mongolism, begins to rise. The planning of families so that there is a minimum of two years between successive pregnancies will also reduce the risks run by the fetus and young child. Extreme multiparity, apart from the advancing age of the mother with which it is likely to be associated, will reduce the mother's physical fitness for childbearing, and carries an increased risk to the fetus.

Primogeniture carries certain risks both before and after birth. Not only is the incidence of low birth-weight higher in first-born infants than in second- and third-born, but labour is liable to be more difficult, with greater risk of injury to the child. After delivery, the mother is to some extent serving her apprenticeship with the first infant; although she will be able to give more attention to him than to those born later, she will lack the confidence and understanding which comes from having successfully reared a previous infant. Unless the first child is sympathetically handled when a second child is born, the first is apt to feel displaced and jealous, and his relationship to the mother become seriously upset. This is often reflected in a return to more infantile habits (e.g. enuresis in a child who has previously become dry, or feeding difficulties) or by active hostility to the new baby. It is unfortunate that delivery very often coincides with a period of separation of the first child from the mother. Most of these difficulties can be overcome if the child is prepared beforehand for the birth of the second, allowed to share in the atmosphere of congratulation and possession when it arrives, and given more rather than less affection at the time that the mother's interest becomes shared.

Second-born children are both physically and emotionally the most favoured. The maternal passages will already have become adapted to child-bearing without having lost their full functional capacity. The mother is still able to give a full measure of attention to the child after birth and is not yet overharassed with too large a family. If the relationship to the first child is a satisfactory one, the development of the second child will benefit considerably from the companionship of the first. On the other hand, second- and later-born children are liable to develop communicable diseases earlier than first-born, since these infections are commonly introduced into the home when the first child begins to mix with others at school or elsewhere.

BIBLIOGRAPHY AND REFERENCES

BAIKIE, A. G. (1965). Chromosomal abnormalities. In *Recent Advances in Paediatrics*, 3rd edn. Edited by D. Gairdner. London: Churchill.

CLARKE, C. A. (1964). *Genetics for the Clinician*, 2nd edn. Oxford: Blackwell.

CORNER, G. W. (1944). *Ourselves Unborn*. New Haven: Yale University Press.

CRUICKSHANK, R. (1970). Protection against specific infections. In *Child Life and Health*, 5th edn. Edited by R. G. Mitchell. London: Churchill.

EMERY, A. E. H. (1971). *Elements of Medical Genetics*, 2nd edn. Edinburgh: Churchill Livingstone.

FORD, F. R. (1966). *Diseases of the Nervous System in Infancy, Childhood, and Adolescence*, 5th edn. Springfield: Thomas.

HSIA, D. Y.-Y. (1968). *Human Developmental Genetics*. Chicago: Year Book Medical Publishers.

JANEWAY, C. A. (1966). The immunological system of the child. *Archives of Disease in Childhood* 41, 358, 366.

4 Fetal and Neonatal Disorders

The fetus in the later months of pregnancy and the newly born infant have much in common. Both are in a state of functional immaturity and both depend on the mother for nutrition and protection, though in the case of the newborn substitute care is possible. They are exposed to the common dangers of malnutrition, anoxia, haemolytic disease, infection and haemorrhage, while malformation can cause death either before or after birth. Hitherto the inaccessibility and relative safety of the fetus *in utero* have emphasized the separation of fetal from neonatal life and encouraged the view that the fetus is simply part of the mother. It has become clear, however, that the fetus leads an individual existence in the uterus, that he can be harmed by agents which do not affect the mother and that fetal disease can be diagnosed and treated in an increasing number of ways. The new importance of fetal medicine and the shared interest of obstetricians and paediatricians in disorders arising before, during and immediately after birth, have accelerated the trend towards considering the perinatal period as a whole. By convention, this extends from the 28th week of intrauterine life, after which time the infant is considered viable if birth should take place, until the seventh day of extrauterine life, i.e. including the first few days during which the bulk of neonatal mortality and morbidity occurs. Fetuses who are born dead after the 28th week of gestation (stillbirths) and infants dying in the first week of postnatal life are considered together as representing perinatal loss, and the perinatal mortality rate is thus the number of stillbirths and first-week deaths per 1000 total births (still and live). In 1968 the perinatal mortality rate for England and Wales was 25 and the stillbirth rate 14·3. Although the perinatal mortality rate has fallen from 38·5 in 1948, its reduction has been substantially less than that of deaths during the subsequent 51 weeks of the first year. In 1970, a W.H.O. expert committee recommended the universal adoption of a perinatal mortality ratio, defined as 'Late fetal and early neonatal deaths weighing over 1000 g at birth expressed as a ratio per 1000 live births weighing over 1000 g at birth'.

The causes of perinatal mortality were investigated in a national survey in 1958 carried out under the auspices of the National Birthday Trust (Butler and Bonham, 1963). Figure 4.1 shows the principal necropsy findings in four parity groups, from which it will be seen that antepartum and intrapartum anoxia, cerebral birth injury, and congenital malformation were the most important. (Rhesus immunization, which is not represented in first-born deaths, rises with increasing multiparity.) The mortality rate was lowest in second-born infants and highest in those where the mother had borne four or more previous children.

Detailed analysis of all the perinatal deaths demonstrated the risks of birth before term, nearly half the infants who died being delivered before 37 weeks gestation; of breech delivery; of advanced maternal age; of multiparity; and of adverse social conditions. The lowest mortality rate, which was one-third of the national average, was found in the infants born at term to women aged 20 to 24.

Infection, which previously accounted for some 30 per cent of all neonatal deaths and a higher proportion of those occurring after the first week, has become relatively less important as a cause of death since the introduction of antibiotics. Deaths from intracranial haemorrhage, anoxia, and developmental defects (all of which are liable to kill during the first week of life) have therefore assumed a relatively greater importance, since the reduction of deaths from these causes has been substantially less than from infection.

Prolonged gestation is of greater importance as a cause of stillbirth than of neonatal death, since the senescent placenta allows the fetus a very narrow safety-margin of oxygen-saturation, which may prove insufficient when delivery is

Primary necropsy findings in maternal parity groups

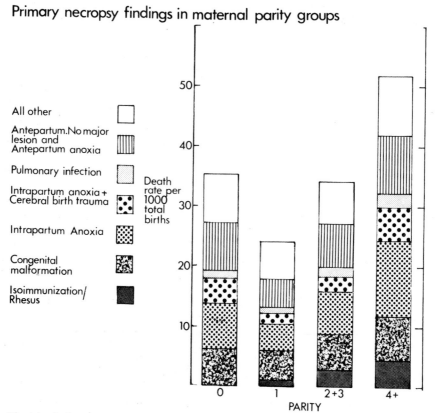

Fig. 4.1   Perinatal mortality with necropsy findings in four maternal parity groups. (From Butler and Bonham, 1963: *Perinatal Mortality*.)

difficult. The liveborn post-term infant is likely to show increased body length, advanced ossification of the skull and rapid drying and desquamation of the skin, all of which are signs of prolonged gestation. He may also show loss of subcutaneous fat and meconium-staining of the vernix, skin, nails and umbilical cord, which may be greenish-yellow or yellow. These signs are attributed to failing placental function and the term *dysmaturity* has been applied to the syndrome. Unfortunately confusion has been caused by the use of this term as synonymous with 'light-for-dates': if used at all, it should be confined to infants who show the stigmata described. These signs of dysmaturity may be found in infants born at or even before term but are most commonly seen in post-term infants and in infants who have grown poorly *in utero*.

PRENATAL INFECTION

The uterine contents are normally sterile until the membranes have ruptured, and it is fortunately exceptional for infection to pass the placental barrier. This is, however, less effective against viruses than bacteria. When infection does penetrate it, the results will depend on the age at which this occurs and the severity of the infection. In early pregnancy, infection is likely to cause the death of the embryo and result in abortion. When the maternal infection, e.g. rubella, is not sufficiently virulent to kill the embryo, it may interfere seriously with organogenesis and result in congenital malformation (see below).

If, however, the fetus is infected later in pregnancy and is not killed, the infection is more likely to reproduce the picture of postnatal infection. Thus, maternal measles, smallpox, chickenpox or herpes simplex infection occurring in later pregnancy may result in the birth of an infant with the characteristic exanthem. Maternal poliomyelitis may also be transmitted to the fetus and result in paralysis or in a state resembling congenital hypotonia (p. 121). Congenital malaria may occur in the infants of infected mothers with little immunity.

Septicaemia

Septicaemia is occasionally demonstrable in stillborn infants of mothers who are themselves suffering from a blood-stream infection or in whom the placenta is heavily infected.

Pneumonia

Pneumonia in stillborn infants will usually be found to be due to premature rupture of the membranes and intrauterine inhalation of infected liquor. Such cases are probably better classified as birth infections rather than prenatal ones.

Congenital tuberculosis

This is rare and is only likely to occur when the maternal infection is of metastasizing type and tuberculous foci are present in the placenta. It is often difficult to establish the prenatal character of the infection with certainty if the infant has subsequently been in contact with the mother.

Toxoplasmosis

Prenatal human infection with a protozoon, *Toxoplasma gondii*, has been recognized with increasing frequency in recent years and may occur as often as once in 1000 births, though in only a small proportion will the fetus be severely affected. The organism is present in various animals and is probably transmitted to human hosts by the ingestion of oocysts from the excreta of domestic animals, especially cats. Infections acquired after infancy are frequent and give rise to little or no disturbance, but the fetus is particularly vulnerable. Signs of congenital toxoplasmosis may be present at birth or appear some time later. These include hydrocephalus or microcephaly, microphthalmos, convulsions, jaundice and hepatosplenomegaly. A maculopapular rash may appear during the neonatal period and chorioretinitis (the most constant clinical manifestation) may be present at birth. Encephalitis occurs in most cases and cerebral calcification, particularly in the region of the basal ganglia, is likely to develop later. The calcified areas consist of multiple rounded deposits (Fig. 4.2) or curved linear markings. The cerebrospinal fluid is either normal or shows an increase of globulin; occasionally it is xanthochromic or turbid. Diagnosis depends ultimately on the recovery of the organism from the tissues or demonstration of toxoplasma antibodies in the infant's serum. Early treatment with large doses of pyrimethamine and sulphadiazine may limit the extent of brain damage. Infants who survive the newborn period are generally mentally subnormal with epilepsy and defective vision.

Cytomegalic inclusion disease

This disease is due to infection with cytomegalovirus, which is thought to be transmitted to the fetus through the placenta. The virus is widely distributed in the general population and congenital infection is not necessarily followed by clinical manifestations of cytomegalic inclusion disease. The infection is associated with the appearance of abnormally large cells with intranuclear inclusions in the salivary glands, kidneys, and other organs. Depending on the tissues principally involved, the clinical picture of cytomegalic inclusion disease may include hepatosplenomegaly, jaundice, purpura and haemolytic anaemia. It may simulate haemolytic disease of the newborn and should be suspected if maternal antibodies to rhesus or other red cell antigens are absent. The disease may also cause microcephaly, hydrocephalus, microphthalmos, chorioretinitis and occasionally intracranial calcification and it must therefore be differentiated from congenital toxoplasmosis. Diagnosis depends on finding the large inclusion-containing cells in the urine of an infant with the typical clinical features, and demonstration of elevated antibody levels in the serum. Cytomegalovirus may be isolated from the urine or saliva. Affected infants may be stillborn, die during the neonatal period or survive, usually though not invariably with signs of permanent brain damage. Corticosteroids have been used in treatment, without notable success: transfusion will be required when there is severe anaemia.

Maternal rubella syndrome

Infection with the rubella virus during the first

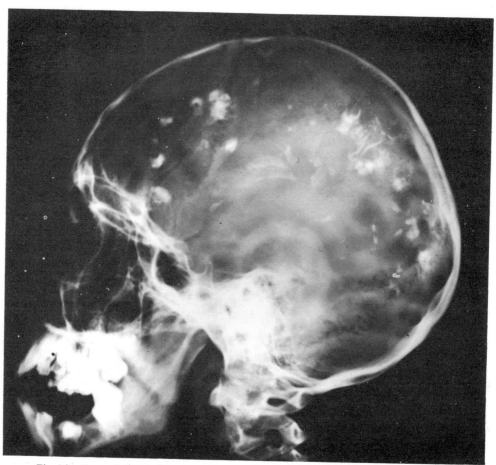

Fig. 4.2   Congenital toxoplasmosis. Multiple rounded areas of cerebral calcification. The condition was associated with mental defect and microcephaly.

16 weeks of pregnancy may cause death or malformation of the fetus. The frequency with which this happens and the type and severity of the malformations vary in different epidemics. Thus in the early Australian epidemics it was believed that as many as 90 per cent of infants at risk had congenital abnormalities, whereas the percentage malformed in subsequent epidemics has generally been in the range 10 to 30 per cent, although higher rates have been reported. It is now known that, in addition to causing malformation, the rubella virus may be responsible for continuing disease of the fetus and the affected newborn infant may be a danger to others because it continues to excrete the virus. Infants with the congenital rubella syndrome are generally small for their gestational age and commonly have multiple congenital abnormalities. These include persistent ductus arteriosus, septal defects and other cardiac malformations; anomalies of the eye, such as cataract and retinopathy; deafness; and microcephaly. Signs of active rubella infection may be present at or shortly after birth. There may be enlargement of liver and spleen, jaundice, thrombocytopenic purpura, myocarditis, rash and lymphadenopathy, while radiological examination of the bones may disclose characteristic changes in the metaphyseal areas. In a small proportion of infected infants there are no clinical manifestations, despite widespread dissemination of virus throughout the body.

Many infants die in the newborn period from the disease and the effect of the major malformations. In the surviving infants, virus can be recovered from the upper respiratory tract and the urine for as long as one year and neutralizing antibodies are present in the plasma of infant and mother. It is evident therefore that pregnant women may contract rubella, not only from overt or subclinical cases during an epidemic, but also from infected infants, with or without malformations, and this should be borne in mind where nurses or other staff are caring for young infants. When there has been known contact with rubella or a rubella-like illness occurs during the first 16 weeks of pregnancy, serum should be taken immediately for antibody tests and a large dose of human immunoglobulin injected, though the protective value of this has not been established. Subsequent occurrence of infection should be looked for by clinical observation, serial antibody tests and attempts to isolate the virus. It is not yet clear whether it is safe to administer rubella virus vaccine to seronegative women in early pregnancy. When there is clear evidence of infection, termination of pregnancy must be considered.

Congenital syphilis

Although congenital syphilis is now rare in Britain, it still remains the most important prenatal infection in many parts of the world. The recent rise in incidence of adult syphilis and the changes in population brought about by immigration, emphasize the continuing necessity for antenatal supervision, and routine serological testing during pregnancy. Since congenital syphilis is preventable if the maternal infection is diagnosed early and adequately treated, every effort should be made to establish treatment before the fetus is damaged.

Infection of the fetus very seldom occurs before the fourth or fifth month of intrauterine life. It may be assumed that infants who show clinical evidence of syphilis at birth have been infected either earlier or more severely than those who appear normal and only show stigmata later. In the case of those infants who are stillborn or show lesions at birth, the placenta will usually be extensively diseased.

CLINICAL MANIFESTATIONS. In those infants who are liveborn it is less common for clinical signs to be present at birth than to appear after two to six weeks. The presence of signs at birth is of bad prognosis, implying very severe infection. Most of these infants are poorly grown, and their prospects of survival are correspondingly reduced. In the majority of cases the newborn

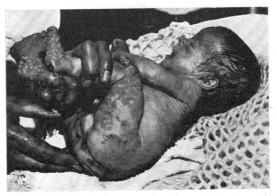

Fig. 4.3   Rash of congenital syphilis on buttocks and thighs, with desquamation of soles.

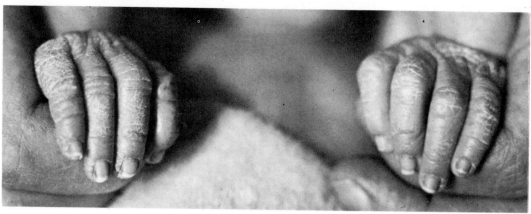

Fig. 4.4   Congenital syphilis. Desquamation of fingers and paronychia. Infant aged 5 weeks.

infant shows no external signs, except possibly low birth weight and diminution of subcutaneous fat, to suggest infection. During the neonatal period, one or more manifestations of the disease appear. The infant fails to thrive, and becomes increasingly wizened. Unless the condition is recognized and treated early, the infant is likely to die or suffer permanent damage.

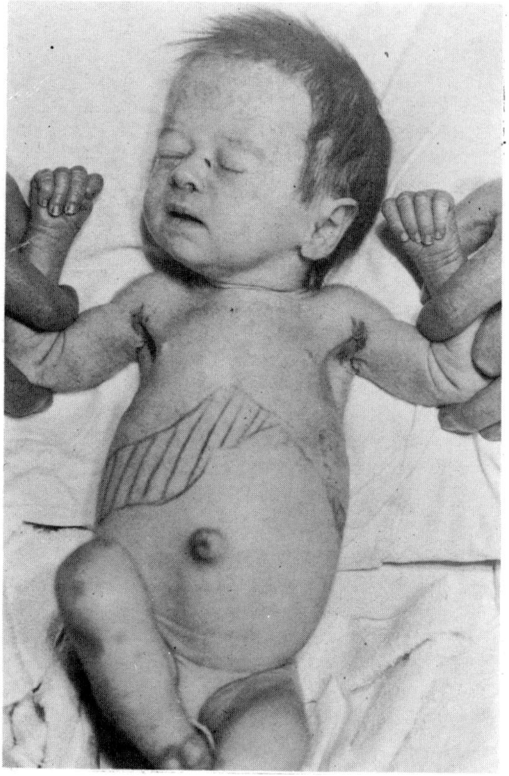

SKIN LESIONS. A great variety of lesions may occur, and only the more typical can be described.

Maculo-papular eruption, either generalized or on the buttocks, back and face, is a characteristic skin manifestation. The lesions vary in colour from pink or copper colour to purple and are frequently associated with annular areas of ulceration, or with bullous lesions. Since the rash often affects the napkin-area, it may be mistaken for a napkin-rash unless the possibility of syphilis is borne in mind.

Syphilitic pemphigus. Bullous lesions which become secondarily infected may occur in any area, but are most characteristic when they affect the palms and soles.

Desquamation. Peeling of the palms and soles should always suggest the possibility of congenital syphilis. Often the desquamation is more widespread, but it is unlikely to occur without other skin manifestations, and can therefore be distinguished from the fine branny desquamation often seen in otherwise normal babies.

Circumoral lesions. Fissuring around the lips and skin infection secondary to snuffles may lead to permanent scarring, the fine scars radiating from the angles of the mouth being known as *rhagades.*

Condylomata. These are flat, sodden-looking lesions, occurring in moist areas at the junction of skin and mucous membrane, particularly around the anus and vulva.

RHINITIS. Syphilitic ulceration and secondary infection of the nasal mucous membrane give rise

Fig. 4.5   Congenital   syphilis,   showing   hepatosplenomegaly.

to one of the most frequent and diagnostic lesions of early syphilis. Nasal discharge, or 'snuffles', appears usually within the neonatal period, and crusting and infection around the nares rapidly follow. Unless the condition is recognized and treated early, the ulceration extends to the cartilage of the nose and subsequently gives rise to a characteristic depression of the nasal bridge.

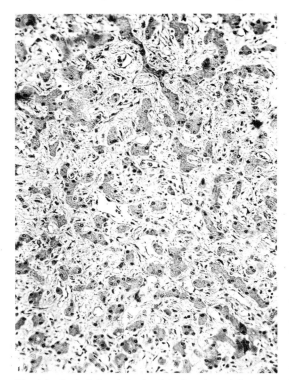

Fig. 4.6   Pericellular cirrhosis of the liver in an infant with congenital syphilis.

VISCERA. Although widespread visceral lesions are likely to be present, only enlargement of liver and spleen is likely to be clinically recognizable. Examination of the liver at necropsy shows fine pericellular cirrhosis, and spirochaetes are present in abundance.

The lungs of infants who are stillborn or die shortly after birth may show a characteristic type of pneumonia, *pneumonia alba*, in which areas of the lung are firm and pale.

BONES AND JOINTS. The radiological appearances due to syphilis are often sufficiently widespread and characteristic to establish the diagnosis with certainty, although periostitis alone will require further differentiation.

Periostitis. An irregular thickening along the shaft gives the long bones the appearance of having a double margin or greatly thickened cortex. The lesions are usually symmetrical, e.g. affecting both radii or both tibiae, and several bones are often involved. The symmetrical and painless character of the periostitis should distinguish the condition from osteomyelitis. The lesions must be distinguished from those of infantile scurvy (p. 157).

A rare condition, *infantile cortical hyperostosis*, in which symmetrical periostitis of unknown etiology affects the long bones, scapulae, clavicles, and mandibles, may be confused with syphilitic periostitis in infancy, and can only be diagnosed with certainty by the distribution of lesions and the absence of other evidence of syphilis or scurvy.

Occasionally, subperiosteal leukaemic deposits may give a radiological appearance bearing some similarity to osseous syphilis, but here the blood picture will distinguish the two conditions.

Bossing of the skull due to syphilis occurs in

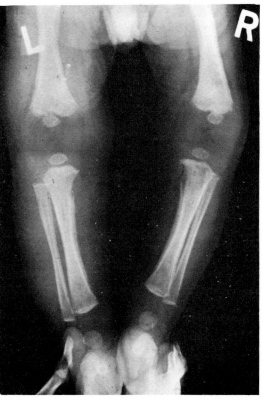

Fig. 4.7   Congenital syphilis. Periostitis of shafts and erosion of ends of tibiae and femora (osteochondritis).

the parietal areas and is caused by localized periostitis.

Osteochondritis. The lesions are diffuse and roughly symmetrical; they occur principally at the ends of the long bones, but both the metaphysis and diaphysis may be involved. The appearance is best described as 'moth-eaten'; the areas of irregular rarefaction may be sufficient to cause fracture through them with displacement of

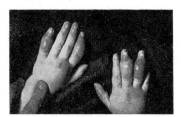

Fig. 4.8   Syphilitic dactylitis.

the epiphyses, giving rise to local swelling and limitation of movement (pseudoparalysis). A very characteristic lesion, which is always symmetrical, is seen at the upper end and inner aspect of the tibia; the bone appears to have an irregular area bitten out of it (Wimberger's sign).

Dactylitis. One or more of the digits may show fusiform swelling (Fig. 4.8), which is usually painless. The radiological appearance is similar to that of the long bones elsewhere. The condition must be distinguished from tuberculous dactylitis, osteomyelitis, and sarcoidosis.

NERVOUS SYSTEM. Although clinical evidence of neurosyphilis is only found in a small percentage of young infants with congenital syphilis, routine examination of the cerebrospinal fluid shows a positive Wassermann reaction in up to 40 or 50 per cent of cases when the mother has been untreated during pregnancy. Blindness, deafness, and hydrocephalus are amongst the manifestations observed.

ANAEMIA. Since the haemopoietic system is likely to be extensively infected, anaemia and a variety of changes in the peripheral blood often occur. The presence of large numbers of nucleated red cells may suggest a diagnosis of haemolytic disease of the newborn, or primitive white cells that of leukaemia.

DIAGNOSIS. Congenital syphilis should be suspected in an infant showing any of the above manifestations, especially when there is a previous history of miscarriages or stillbirths. The association of a rash, snuffles, and splenic enlargement in a young infant is particularly suggestive. If there are open lesions from which serum can be obtained, dark-ground examination should be made for spirochaetes. The mother's Wassermann reaction or Kahn test will be positive unless she has had antisyphilitic treatment or penicillin for other cause. The Wassermann reaction of the infant is unreliable during the first three months of life. A positive reaction at birth may in some cases be due to passive transfer of maternal antibodies, and the reaction subsequently becomes negative. False negative reactions may also be obtained during the first six weeks, and it must be remembered that if penicillin has been given for any reason, e.g. an infected skin rash, it will be likely to modify or negative the reaction. The cerebrospinal fluid should be examined when syphilis is suspected, and if the Wassermann reaction of the fluid is positive it should be repeated after treatment as a test of cure.

TREATMENT AND PROGNOSIS. The infant with early syphilitic lesions must be regarded as infectious and appropriate precautions taken. Treatment should be instituted as soon as possible after birth and early treatment with penicillin gives a good prospect not only of survival but of cure. For infants under three months of age, 250 mg of phenoxymethylpenicillin six hourly by mouth for three weeks or one injection daily of 300,000 units of procaine penicillin in aqueous suspension with aluminium monostearate (PAM) is ample unless relapse occurs. Quantitative serological tests should be carried out monthly for six months after the initial course of treatment, and three-monthly thereafter for at least two years; any evidence of serological relapse should call for further examination of the cerebrospinal fluid and repetition of treatment.

In the case of infants whose mothers have been adequately treated during early pregnancy (e.g. with ten daily injections of 600,000 units of PAM), treatment of the infant is unnecessary. Although the infant's Wassermann reaction is occasionally found to be positive at birth when the mother has been treated later this is almost always due to 'reagin carry-over' rather than transmission of infection, and spontaneous reversal will occur within three months. It is, however, an indication for monthly serological testing and careful observation.

ADAPTATION TO EXTRAUTERINE LIFE

The sudden transition from the intrauterine environment to relatively independent existence involves complex anatomical and physiological changes, including a major readjustment of both respiratory and circulatory systems. During normal parturition, the fetus and placenta are subjected to intense pressure, which interferes with gaseous exchange and causes a moderate fall in pH and Po_2 with a rise in Pco_2 in the fetal blood. These changes can be measured by sampling blood from the scalp and used as a guide to the clinical state of the fetus. Fetal distress is suggested by a large decrease in pH and Po_2, continuing bradycardia and the presence of meconium in the amniotic fluid, obtained if necessary before rupture of the membranes by the technique of amnioscopy.

Once the infant is born, reflex stimulation of the central nervous system by thermal and tactile impulses from the periphery, reinforced by chemical stimuli, initiates rhythmic breathing. Should this fail, asphyxial changes acting on chemoreceptors stimulate lower medullary centres, causing periodic gasps. An infant who does not breathe immediately after birth may be in the stage of primary apnoea before the gasp mechanism comes into operation or in secondary apnoea, when chemoreceptor stimulation can no longer initiate gasping and death will follow unless artificial respiration is instituted. The pressure required to open the lungs is about 30 cm of water; once the lung has opened up, each subsequent breath is easier as the air remaining in the alveoli prevents complete closure between breaths. Formation of the residual capacity is made possible by removal of fluid from the lung, mainly by drainage from nose and mouth aided by compression of the thorax during birth, but also by absorption through the lymphatic system. As soon as breathing starts, the pulmonary arterioles, which were constricted, dilate in response to increased oxygen and decreased carbon dioxide tensions. The resultant lowering of pulmonary vascular resistance allows blood in the pulmonary artery to be diverted from the ductus arteriosus into the lungs and the ductus closes.

Anoxia (hypoxia)

This may be defined as an interference with the oxygen supply of the brain sufficient to cause disturbance of function. *Asphyxia* refers to the condition of anoxia, hypercapnia, and acidaemia present to a varying degree at birth. The relatively slight degree normally occurring is rapidly corrected when breathing starts and produces no after effects, since the newborn infant possesses much greater tolerance of anoxia than is present in later life, due to the ability to metabolize glycogen anaerobically. When anoxia is more prolonged or intense, the function of the respiratory centres is depressed, which in turn tends to prolong and intensify the asphyxia.

Since anoxia is a symptom of a wide variety of pathological conditions rather than a primary disease, it is difficult to estimate accurately its direct responsibility for stillbirth and neonatal death: but it is generally accepted that anoxia is an associated if not the primary cause of death in more than half of all infants dying during birth or within the first 24 hours.

ETIOLOGY. Anoxia has been classified as *anoxic*, when the supply of oxygen reaching the blood is inadequate, and the oxygen-saturation correspondingly low; *anaemic*, when oxygen-saturation is normal but the total quantity of haemoglobin (and hence the oxygen carried) is inadequate; *stagnant*, when the circulation is defective, e.g. from shock, and the transport of oxygen is impaired; and *histotoxic*, when the tissues are so damaged that they cannot utilize the oxygen supplied.

Cerebral haemorrhage or *trauma* during birth is an important cause of anoxia, the function of the respiratory centre being depressed. Anoxia can itself cause intracranial haemorrhage, so that the two conditions are closely interrelated.

Obstruction of the respiratory tract from any cause will result in anoxia. Although inhalation of liquor amnii itself is comparatively harmless and is readily remedied by postural drainage, the substances it may contain (vernix caseosa, meconium or blood) are liable to cause obstruction, while if the liquor is infected its inhalation will result in pneumonia. Obstruction due to mucus should be relieved by aspiration. The mouth should be cleansed gently as soon as possible after delivery, and liquor allowed to drain from the lungs. When aspiration is necessary, it should be undertaken with strict precautions, using a presterilized disposable aspirator. Care must be taken to avoid damage to the mucosa of the infant's mouth or nasopharynx.

Premature separation of the placenta, whether

due to placenta praevia, accidental haemorrhage or the rapid escape of a large quantity of liquor amnii in cases of hydramnios, is an important cause of fetal anoxia, while placental degeneration is liable to interfere with proper oxygenation.

Prolapse of the cord and strangulation by the cord *in utero* are both possible causes of anoxia, but are less important than placental separation.

Maternal conditions associated with anoxaemia, e.g. respiratory disease, convulsions of eclampsia or epilepsy, and inhalation of vomitus during induction of anaesthesia, will tend to produce fetal anoxia.

Analgesic drugs and anaesthesia. The effects on the fetus of the various anaesthetics and analgesics used during labour must be assessed in addition to the maternal hazard. While morphine and its derivatives are the most dangerous to the fetus, and should never be used within four hours of delivery, there are many others which in skilled hands carry little risk. Even prolonged anaesthesia, though affecting the fetus temporarily, may have no permanent ill effects if properly used. The full effects of anaesthesia are often not seen in the infant until some hours after birth.

CLINICAL FEATURES. The newborn infant suffering from the effects of mild anoxia will be cyanosed, with slow full pulses and moderate muscle tone. While he does not breathe immediately, he may respond to stimuli by gasping. In more severe degrees, the infant will be pale and limp, with weak irregular pulses and absence of respiratory effort. He will not respond to any form of stimulation. The clinical distinction between 'blue' and 'white' asphyxia is only one of degree, white asphyxia representing a more severe condition associated with profound shock and frequently with intracranial damage.

The infant's condition at birth can be assessed by means of the Apgar score, in which a value of 0, 1, or 2 is given to each of five signs: colour, heart rate, muscle tone, respiratory effort, and response to stimulation. A total score of 10 indicates that the infant is in very good condition, whereas a severely asphyxiated infant may have a score of 3 or less.

TREATMENT. The first requirement of the anoxic infant is oxygen. Any obstruction of the respiratory passages must be removed by aspiration and the infant should be placed so that fluid can drain from the lungs by gravity. Aspiration of gastric contents is advisable in infants born by Caesarean section. If the first breath is not taken immediately, a stream of oxygen may be played on the infant's face providing both sensory stimulation and a high oxygen concentration when breathing starts. The first few gasps, though relatively inefficient, will usually supply sufficient oxygen to overcome anoxia and respiration will pass into the normal rhythm. In the great majority of cases, no further action will be required.

Superficial stimulation can only be effective when the central nervous system is able to respond to it. It should never be sufficient to cause further risk to an already traumatized infant, and when the central nervous system is severely damaged, vigorous stimulation can only do harm. The use of respiratory stimulants is dangerous and ineffective in severely asphyxiated cases, but in those of milder degree a few drops of vanillic acid diethylamide (Vandid) instilled into the infant's mouth may help to initiate the first gasp. If the mother has been given drugs of the morphine group, 0.02 mg per kg of levallorphan should be injected into the umbilical vein.

Should no spontaneous respiration occur after two or three minutes, it is advisable to take measures to counteract anoxia. The most effective method is to insufflate oxygen through an endotracheal tube passed under direct vision using an infant laryngoscope. Short intermittent puffs of oxygen are given, using a water manometer to ensure that a pressure of 30 cm of water is not exceeded. This method should only be used by skilled staff and in their absence direct mouth-to-face insufflation or delivery of oxygen through a face mask may be attempted, but is only likely to be effective if the infant has already gasped spontaneously. Any method carries the risk of rupturing alveoli if safe pressures are exceeded. The use of hyperbaric oxygen is still in the experimental stage.

Subsequent care must include the avoidance of chilling and rough handling, since the anoxic infant is usually in a state of more or less severe shock. Frequent changes of position are advisable to promote drainage from the lungs, and repeated aspiration may be necessary if there is persistent mucus in the respiratory passages. Oxygen should be used with the necessary precautions when any tendency to colour-change persists. It is also advisable to raise the humidity in the case of infants who have inhaled meconium, and to use antibiotics prophylactically. If sustained spontaneous respiration cannot be achieved, mechanical ventilation may be instituted and continued for several days if necessary.

PROGNOSIS. If the infant survives the first 24 hours, the prognosis as regards life is usually good. Minor degrees of anoxia are unlikely to cause permanent nervous damage, but severe or prolonged anoxia may cause widespread loss of nerve cells from the grey matter and changes in subcortical or periventricular white matter. In such cases there is an abnormally high incidence of mental impairment and of cerebral palsy in later life.

ATELECTASIS

This term is used to describe those conditions of incomplete expansion seen within the newborn period, whereas 'collapse' is preferred for the condition of a lung which has fully expanded and subsequently lost its aeration.

Some degree of atelectasis is normally present in the lungs of newborn infants, since full expansion is not attained with the first breath, or indeed for several days after birth. It is only when the areas of atelectasis are extensive that the condition is pathological. Any condition interfering with the depth of respiration at birth will be responsible for atelectasis. It is doubtful if atelectasis *per se* should ever be regarded as a cause of death; the atelectasis is secondary to some other factor and frequently complicated by secondary infection. Thus any of the conditions causing anoxia are likely to result in atelectasis. These may either be central (dysfunction of the respiratory centre) or peripheral (blockage of the bronchi, hyaline membrane disease).

The pre-term infant is particularly prone to atelectasis owing to deficiency of surfactant, the feebleness of respiratory movement and softness of the thoracic cage (see p. 49).

In addition to the above causes, pressure from an enlarged heart or mediastinal mass, or malformation of a bronchus, may result in atelectasis. When the whole of one lung is atelectatic, the heart is likely to be displaced towards the affected side; blockage of a main bronchus should be suspected, and bronchoscopy will be required in such cases.

The clinical signs will depend on the primary cause. The affected portion of the lung will show diminished or absent air entry or the presence of fine crepitations; it may also be possible to demonstrate impairment of percussion note. One of the more important signs is cyanosis, although gross atelectasis may sometimes occur without cyanosis being obvious. Transient cyanotic attacks may be due to atelectasis, as well as to such causes as intracranial haemorrhage, diaphragmatic hernia or tracheo-oesophageal fistula.

X-ray of the chest may show a localized area of loss of translucency or displacement of the heart, but when atelectasis is diffuse, radiological appearances are often not conclusive.

Treatment is that of the primary cause, particular attention being paid to clearing the respiratory passages. The infant will require oxygen if cyanosis is present.

BIRTH INJURY

Although improved maternal health and better obstetric practice have reduced the dangers to the fetus during delivery, many avoidable birth injuries still occur, and birth injury ranks as an important cause of stillbirth and of neonatal death during the first week. In view of the very great number of possible injuries, only the more common or important types will be considered here. As indicated later, the pre-term infant is not only more liable to birth injury than the term infant owing to the fragility and immaturity of its tissues, but is more liable to succumb to injury when it occurs.

Caput succedaneum

This consists of an oedematous swelling, often associated with ecchymosis, occurring over the presenting portion of the fetus during prolonged labour, when this portion is surrounded by the pressure of the cervix. It is commonly seen over the parietal region in vertex deliveries, but may occur over any presenting portion, e.g. the face, buttocks, or genitalia in other types of delivery. When the face is affected the caput may be very gross and unsightly, and in the case of the genitalia, blistering of the scrotum may occur. In the great majority of cases, the oedema subsides completely within two to three days, and while ecchymosis may result in some staining of the affected area for a longer period, recovery is complete.

Cephalhaematoma

Subperiosteal haemorrhage is a relatively common form of birth injury, but is seldom

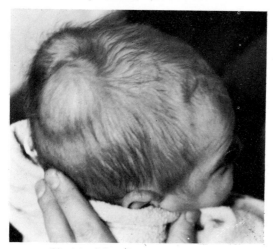

Fig. 4.9   Bilateral cephalhaematoma.

manifest before the second day of life. It causes a large fluctuant swelling, usually over the parietal region, but occasionally in the occipital, frontal, or temporal regions. The haematoma is limited by the attachment of the periosteum at the suture lines to the area of the affected bone, and may be unilateral or bilateral. Unless the scalp is lacerated or the underlying skull fractured, cephalhaematoma is harmless, though unsightly. Aspiration carries a definite risk of infection and is not indicated. Although the swelling may remain obvious for weeks or months, it gradually decreases in size; the remaining swelling undergoes calcification and ultimately resorption.

Palpation of a cephalhaematoma which is undergoing marginal calcification will often give the impression of a surrounding ring of bone with a central soft depression; this may be mistaken for a depressed fracture unless the nature of the lesion is recognized.

Cephalhaematoma differs from caput succedaneum in that the latter is maximum at birth and disappears rapidly; the caput consists of pitting oedema and is not fluctuant; and while cephalhaematoma is limited by suture lines, the caput is not.

Forceps injuries

Forceps injuries of the face or scalp vary from trivial ecchymoses and abrasions to deep lacerations. Local necrosis of tissue is only likely to occur when pressure has been exceptionally prolonged or severe. Localized fat necrosis due to forceps pressure may be noted about three weeks after delivery, commonly over the masseters.

With increasing use of the Malmstrom vacuum extractor in place of low forceps, a variety of scalp lesions may be observed at the site of application. Congenital defects of the scalp or underlying bone are sometimes mistaken in later infancy for the results of birth injury.

Subaponeurotic haemorrhage

Use of the vacuum extractor may cause haemorrhage beneath the epicranial aponeurosis, especially in infants with coagulation deficiencies. When the thrombotest shows less than 10 per cent of the normal adult value, 10 ml per kg of fresh plasma given intravenously may prevent massive bleeding endangering life.

Fractures

Fracture of almost any bone may occur during delivery, when excessive traction or pressure has been applied. The skull is to a large extent protected from fracture by its elasticity and capacity for becoming moulded, and when fractures do occur they are most likely to be small stellate fractures without displacement. Depressed fractures are seldom seen except after forcible delivery in cases of contracted pelvis, although very occasionally fractures occur during an apparently normal delivery without disproportion. Elevation of depressed fractures is not usually necessary.

Fractures of the long bones are likely to be recognized by pseudoparalysis or deformity of the affected limb; greenstick fractures are more common than complete fractures. In the newborn

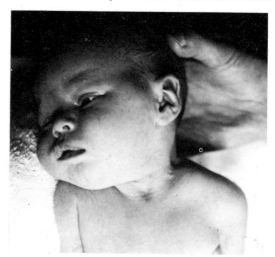

Fig. 4.10   Fractured left clavicle in an 11-day-old infant.

the amount of callus formation is very great, and it is a characteristic of fractures during this period that in the absence of bone disease they heal extremely readily, with little or no permanent deformity. When the clavicle is fractured, disability is often minimal unless there is an associated lesion of the brachial plexus. The fracture easily passes unrecognized at birth and may only attract attention by the subsequent formation of callus. In uncomplicated cases treatment is unnecessary.

Moulding of the head

The application of pressure to the fetal head will normally result in a change in shape, due to the relative elasticity of the skull bones and the fact that these are not rigidly fixed one to the other at their apices. When pressure during delivery is prolonged, the infant is born with an elongated skull which is described as 'moulded'. Though the skull normally allows some degree of adjustment to pressure, excessive moulding is likely to result in damage to the intracranial contents.

INTRACRANIAL INJURIES

These are by far the most important of birth injuries, as a cause of neonatal death and morbidity. While extensive lacerations involving blood vessels and causing gross cerebral haemorrhage are likely to be fatal during or shortly after birth, non-fatal injuries may result in permanent disability, including cerebral palsy, hydrocephalus, and mental subnormality. The obstetric difficulties which produce anoxia will frequently be the same as those that result in intracranial injury; intracranial injury will itself be liable to result in anoxia when the respiratory centre is affected, while severe anoxia from any cause will cause small petechial haemorrhages of the brain. Moreover, the associated engorgement of vessels will increase the liability of these to bleed if they are traumatized, and will predispose to thrombosis and cerebral infarction.

The following classification of intracranial injuries has certain practical applications, although some cases will fall into more than one category, and in others the exact lesion can only be determined at necropsy.

I. INJURIES WITHOUT HAEMORRHAGE
　1. *Insignificant lacerations of tentorium or falx*

　2. *Cerebral contusion, oedema, and intracranial hypertension.*

II. INJURIES ASSOCIATED WITH HAEMORRHAGE
　1. *Subdural haemorrhages*
　2. *Subarachnoid haemorrhages*
　3. *Brain haemorrhages*
　　(*a*) intraventricular
　　(*b*) diffuse or circumscribed.

Injuries without haemorrhage

Injuries without haemorrhage probably account for a large proportion of cases in which there are minor manifestations of cerebral irritation or shock during the first days of life, and subsequent recovery. The infant may be born in a state of white asphyxia and remain flaccid, with a feeble or absent Moro reflex. Alternatively, the infant may be restless and irritable, and show twitchings or more rarely generalized convulsions. Respiration is irregular and colour changes may occur. The temperature is unstable, transient rises in temperature being common, and the infant fails to suck normally. Where cerebral oedema is responsible for the symptoms, the latter are likely to disappear in the first two to three days with the subsidence of the oedema.

It is often impossible to be certain at first whether the infant is suffering from intracranial haemorrhage or contusion. Lumbar puncture is not a certain guide, since blood in the subdural space may not reach the cerebrospinal fluid, while, on the other hand, the likelihood of getting a blood-stained fluid due to the trauma of puncture is considerably higher in the newborn than in older infants. The rapid disappearance of symptoms, however, will favour the diagnosis of injury without major haemorrhage. Twitching and jittery behaviour may also be due to hypoglycaemia or tetany: these can be excluded by biochemical means.

The prognosis in injury without major haemorrhage is generally good. While a small proportion of such injuries may prove fatal, and others result in permanent cerebral damage, the majority are followed by complete recovery. Treatment in the initial stages is designed to combat shock.

Damage to the brain in the first few days after birth may also be caused by hypoglycaemia, hypernatraemia and hyperbilirubinaemia: any of these may give rise to permanent neurological sequelae.

Injuries associated with haemorrhage

While haemorrhage is often the most obvious necropsy finding, it is generally associated with other forms of damage such as cerebral infarction. Since most of our information with regard to the relative incidence of different types of intracranial haemorrhage is derived from necropsies carried out on stillborn infants or on infants dying within the neonatal period, it must be realized that most of the published series represent only the relative incidence of types of fatal haemorrhage. The order of frequency in fatal cases is subdural haemorrhage (with or without tentorial tears), subarachnoid haemorrhage, intraventricular haemorrhage, and haemorrhage into the substance of the brain.

There can be little doubt that in post-mortem series haemorrhage secondary to tentorial tears is seen in a disproportionately high percentage of cases. Subarachnoid haemorrhage, though actually commoner, is much less frequently fatal.

Subdural haemorrhages are most likely to occur in one of three ways. (1) Tearing of the tributaries of the longitudinal sinus at their site of entry, brought about by excessive elevation of the vertex; more rarely, the longitudinal sinus itself may be ruptured. (2) Tearing of the tentorium, with involvement of vessels. This occurs most commonly in breech or instrumental deliveries, and mainly in term infants. (3) Rupture of the straight sinus or great vein of Galen.

The most frequent form of brain damage in the pre-term infant is intraventricular haemorrhage with periventricular cerebral infarction, while the term infant is likely to show infarction and haemorrhage in the cerebral cortex.

CAUSES. Mechanical causes are undoubtedly important, notwithstanding the fact that cerebral haemorrhage is not infrequently observed in infants born by Caesarean section. The dangers of breech delivery are well recognized, since there is not only the likelihood of difficulty in delivery of the after-coming head, but the engorgement of the cephalic end of the fetus with blood during the slow squeezing of the lower portion of the body through the birth canal will increase the likelihood of rupture of intracranial vessels. Manipulations and the use of instruments will increase the dangers to the fetus, while large size of the head or contraction of the maternal pelvis will result in disproportion, making the safe passage of the head difficult or impossible. Pre-

cipitate labour and the abuse of oxytocics carry particular danger to the fetus.

CONTRIBUTORY CAUSES. Venous congestion and thrombosis due to hypoxia predispose to perinatal brain damage, especially in the pre-term infant. In addition to these factors, any condition of the fetus rendering it peculiarly liable to bleed will increase the risk of intracranial haemorrhage from trauma which might prove innocuous to a normal infant. While overt haemorrhagic disease of the newborn is not usually manifest until after birth and probably contributes to only a small proportion of all intracranial haemorrhages, severe prothrombin complex deficiency as indicated by the thrombotest is an important antecedent of intracranial haemorrhage, especially in infants of low birth weight.

Of the infants who do not die at birth but succumb during the neonatal period, it is found that a proportion show pneumonia or atelectatic changes in the lungs. While the pulmonary pathology must be regarded as a complication of the original haemorrhage, it may be sufficient to prove fatal.

SIGNS AND SYMPTOMS. Intracranial haemorrhage should be suspected when the infant appears shocked at birth, is difficult to resuscitate, shows recurrent apnoea and cyanosis, and fails to cry and suck normally. In those infants who cry incessantly, the cry is not the full-throated cry of the healthy newborn, but is more likely to be high-pitched or feebly mewing in character. Twitchings or convulsions may occur, but do not necessarily indicate haemorrhage (see above). The symptoms will be present at birth or arise within a few hours of delivery in the great majority of cases. More rarely they are not manifest until one to two days after birth.

TREATMENT. The immediate treatment of intracranial haemorrhage is similar to that for anoxia, with which it is commonly associated. The infant should be kept warm, handled as little as possible, and if necessary nursed in oxygen. Lumbar puncture may be advisable when there is evidence of raised intracranial tension, and it has some diagnostic value (see above) if its limitations are kept in mind. Sedation with chloral hydrate should be given if the infant is restless, and phenobarbitone or paraldehyde if convulsions occur. Phytomenadione (1 mg) should be injected intramuscularly.

LATE EFFECTS. It is impossible to estimate with any certainty the proportion of infants with minor haemorrhage who survive. Occasionally evidence of old birth injury is found at necropsy in infants dying from other causes, where there has apparently been little or no residual effect. In others, particular neurological disturbances in later childhood can clearly be attributed to birth haemorrhage. Thus a proportion of cases of recurrent convulsions are due to this cause. The following complications of intracranial haemorrhage resulting from birth injury are of particular importance.

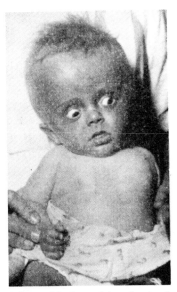

Fig. 4.11   Advanced hydrocephalus showing large globular cranium and downward dislocation of eyes.

Hydrocephalus. Although hydrocephalus may be due to a variety of causes, including congenital abnormality and infection, a certain number of cases are the direct result of birth haemorrhage, in which blood-clot has blocked the ventricular system at some point. The condition is manifested by increased tension of the anterior fontanelle and progressive enlargement of the head, with separation of the sutures. Hydrocephalus from this cause usually progresses rapidly, but occasionally there is a spontaneous arrest of the cranial enlargement (see p. 117).

Chronic subdural haematoma. This may be caused by trauma at any period of infancy or childhood, but the majority of cases seen in infancy are probably due to birth injury. The haematoma is commonly bilateral but may lie over only one hemisphere. Diagnosis is made by inserting a short-bevelled needle through the coronal suture lateral to the angle of the fontanelle, when dark blood spurts out under pressure; in long-standing cases the fluid is serosanguineous and xanthochromic. Clinically, infants with chronic subdural haematoma fail to thrive and are likely to present a picture of extreme wasting. Vomiting, convulsions, inequality of pupils and other focal neurological signs may occur. The fontanelle is enlarged and often bulging, in contrast to the depressed fontanelle commonly seen in other types of infantile marasmus and dehydration, and there is progressive enlargement of the cranial circumference; an appearance of hydrocephalus may develop. When the diagnosis has been confirmed, daily aspiration of up to 30 ml (15 ml from each side) may effect permanent cure in cases of recent onset but a long-standing haematoma must usually be removed surgically.

Cerebral palsy

The important group of cases characterized by cerebral palsy is of mixed etiology, but birth injury is probably the most important single cause. The clinical features, and etiological factors other than birth injury, are considered in Chapter 16.

SPINAL CORD AND NERVE INJURIES

Spinal cord injury

This is considerably less common than intracranial injury, but necropsies on the newborn will sometimes show evidence of haemorrhage into or around the cord. Traction, either on the arms in vertex deliveries, or much more commonly on the legs in breech deliveries, is the cause of cord injury, which is unlikely to occur in unassisted deliveries. When the anterior horn cells alone are damaged, the infant will show flaccid paralysis of the corresponding part. Transection of the cord, if not fatal during the neonatal period, will result in bilateral flaccid paralysis below the injury. In reaching the diagnosis, spina bifida and cord tumour must be excluded and the type of delivery taken into consideration.

Facial paralysis

Although supranuclear paralysis may occur as the result of cerebral trauma, and the facial nerve may also be injured intracranially or as the result of fracture where it emerges through the skull, the great majority of facial birth palsies are due to

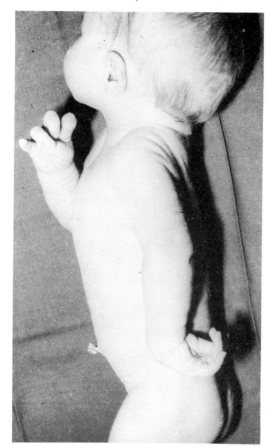

Fig. 4.12   Erb's palsy, showing characteristic position of arm and hand.

The commonest type encountered is the *Erb's* palsy, in which the arm hangs limply to the side, internally rotated, and with the fingers flexed. The Moro reflex and the biceps jerk will be absent on the affected side. The paralysis is accounted for by injury to the fifth and sixth cervical nerves or their roots.

Minor injuries, probably involving only the perineural sheath, are commoner than the more severe, and recovery is usually complete within a matter of weeks. Prolonged immobilization is undesirable, but as a first-aid measure the infant's sleeve may be pinned to the pillow so as to keep the shoulder abducted and the elbow flexed.

A much rarer palsy is *Klumpke's* type, in which the seventh and eighth cervical nerves are involved, and the muscles which they supply in the forearm are paralysed. The clinical manifestations include wrist-drop and flaccid paralysis of the hand. If the first thoracic nerve is also involved, there may be homolateral miosis and ptosis.

Radial nerve palsy, characterized by wrist-drop, is occasionally seen when a contraction ring has involved the shoulder. The hand is

extracranial injuries of the facial nerve caused by the blades of forceps which have been applied obliquely. More rarely, extracranial injury of the facial nerve may occur in the course of a spontaneous delivery.

The condition is easily recognizable, since the mouth is drawn over to the uninjured side when the infant cries, and there is inability to close the eye on the side of the injury. Eye drops should be instilled to avoid corneal damage. It is unusual for sucking to be seriously interfered with, and unless the nerve has actually been severed, function is commonly re-established within two to three weeks of birth.

Brachial palsies

These are usually unilateral; when bilateral, they should suggest the probability of cord injury. In all cases, the possibility of an associated injury to the shoulder should be kept in mind.

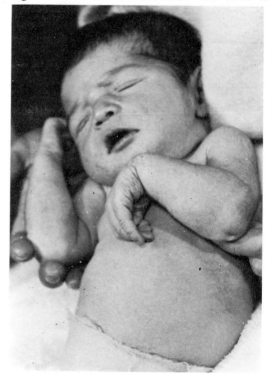

Fig. 4.13   Radial palsy of left arm due to contraction ring (newborn infant).

treated in a cock-up splint. Recovery is usually complete.

INJURIES OF VISCERA AND OTHER ORGANS

Birth injury of the viscera is fortunately rare, and is seldom seen except in difficult breech or assisted deliveries, in which anoxia is likely to represent a contributory factor. The liver or kidneys may show subcapsular haemorrhage, while rupture of the liver, spleen, or bladder occasionally occurs and is likely to prove fatal. The testicles and scrotum may be traumatized in breech deliveries.

Adrenal haemorrhage in the newborn is observed more frequently, particularly in breech deliveries. Massive haemorrhage is likely to prove fatal within a few hours of birth, the infant showing profound shock, cyanosis, and possibly hyperpyrexia; occasionally such haemorrhages may be palpable. Smaller haemorrhages produce a less severe clinical picture, and are not necessarily fatal. Hydrocortisone should be administered if adrenal damage is suspected, and shock should be countered by intravenous fluids and noradrenaline.

The *eyes* and *ears* are occasionally damaged in instrumental deliveries, when the cause and nature of the lesion are usually obvious. Anoxia and any of the conditions leading to intracranial injury will tend to produce retinal haemorrhages, but it is probable that the great majority leave no residual disability.

Sternomastoid muscle. A lesion of this muscle, which presents during the newborn period as a localized swelling, is relatively common. It is often described as a haematoma, but is usually caused by rupture of muscle fibres associated with fibrinous exudate rather than simple haemorrhage. In most cases it resolves without treatment, but the mother may be shown how to put the muscle on the stretch by manipulation and asked to do this gently several times a day, to prevent fibrous contraction which can result in torticollis later.

LOW BIRTH WEIGHT

NOMENCLATURE. In the past, a premature infant has been defined as one weighing 2500 g ($5\frac{1}{2}$ lb) or less at birth, irrespective of the period of gestation. This had statistical convenience for the international comparison of records, but it was not scientifically accurate or clinically reliable, since infants of the same weight may vary greatly in gestational age. Approximately 30 per cent of infants born after 37 completed weeks weigh less than 2500 g, while the infant of a diabetic mother born before 37 weeks may weigh considerably more. The World Health Organization has now recommended the use of the term *low birth weight* to describe any infant weighing 2500 g or less at birth, regardless of the reason for its low weight. Within this general category are included infants who have grown well but are born early and infants born at or before term who are disproportionately small for gestational age, because they are maldeveloped or their growth has been restricted. The recognition of these different groups is important because they differ in morbidity and prognosis and require different management in the newborn period. A satisfactory nomenclature for these varieties of low birth-weight infant has not yet been agreed but here they will be considered in two groups— those born early (before 37 completed weeks) and called 'pre-term' and those of body weight disproportionately low for gestational age (below the tenth percentile) and called 'light-for-dates' or 'small-for-dates'. These groups are not mutually exclusive, since some pre-term infants will also be light-for-dates and consequently liable to the characteristic disorders of both groups. Standards of birth weight for gestational age are given by Thomson and his colleagues (1968): the pitfalls and limitations in using such data have been discussed by Tanner (1970).

Infants of less than 28 weeks gestation are generally considered non-viable but such very immature infants occasionally survive.

INCIDENCE. Recent estimates of the incidence of low birth weight suggest that approximately 7 per cent of all live births would be so classified. Although the majority of babies weighing 2000 to 2500 g can be reared without great difficulty, care of the smaller infants represents one of the major paediatric problems.

CAUSES. In nearly half the cases of low birth weight the cause is unknown. In the remaining 50 per cent, toxaemia and twin pregnancy are the two most important causes, followed by accidental haemorrhage, placenta praevia, fetal deformity, and various maternal conditions (cardiac and respiratory disease, urinary infection, etc.). Toxaemia and hypertension in preg-

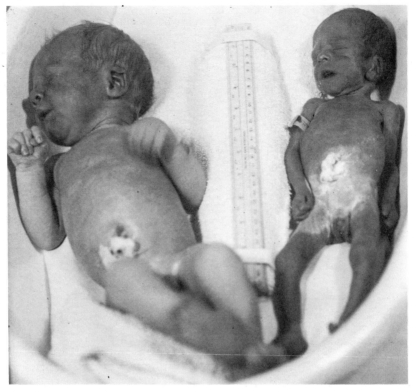

Fig. 4.14   Newborn infant weighing 879 g with newborn control weighing 3175 g. The estimated duration of gestation was less than 28 weeks. At 12 months of age the infant weighed 7·5 kg, and at seven years old was of normal development.

nancy are especially frequent in the histories of light-for-dates infants. The importance of the general physique and nutrition of the mother has been emphasized by many writers, and is related to the higher incidence of stillbirth and neonatal death amongst infants of mothers in the lower income group. There is also a higher incidence of low birth weight in illegitimate pregnancies.

PRE-TERM INFANTS

CLINICAL CHARACTERISTICS. The pre-term infant is not only small but usually shows recognizable stigmata of immaturity. The head and abdomen appear relatively large compared with the limbs. Since the growth of the brain is disproportionately rapid after birth, the shape and size of the head and separation of the sutures may give rise to a mistaken diagnosis of hydrocephalus. Subcutaneous fat is small in amount, and if the infant becomes dehydrated he rapidly assumes a wrinkled and senile appearance. In very immature infants, the skin is thin, red and often appears shiny and translucent: it may be covered with lanugo. These and other physical characteristics can be used to estimate gestational age, which can also be assessed by the presence or absence of certain neurological reflexes (p. 11).

The body temperature of pre-term infants tends to be lower than that of older babies, even when the ambient temperature is high, and a rectal temperature of 36°C (97°F) should probably be considered satisfactory. The infant is particularly liable to become chilled, but since temperature regulation is not well established, there is also a danger of overheating.

Neonatal jaundice is more marked and more prolonged in pre-term than in term infants, due to inefficient hepatic conjugation and excretion of bilirubin (see below). Owing to the possible risk of brain damage from unconjugated serum bilirubin, exchange transfusion will occasionally be necessary. In the absence of Rhesus or ABO incompatibility, hyperbilirubinaemia may result from the injudicious use of vitamin K analogues or sulphonamides in immature infants, the action of sulphonamides being to displace unconjugated bilirubin from its albumin linkage.

The pre-term infant is in general much less active and is more somnolent than the term baby, and reacts badly to excessive handling and the effort of feeding, which may produce transient cyanosis. The sucking reflex is weak or absent and feeding by nasogastric tube may be necessary. Respiration is commonly irregular and interrupted by gasps and short periods of apnoea. Since respiratory movements are shallow and feeble, and crying minimal in the case of small infants, it is understandable that the lungs will only become fully aerated over a period of days or weeks.

COMPLICATIONS

Anoxia and atelectasis

The same causes of anoxia operate in pre-term babies as in all newborn infants, but in addition their general feebleness may make the initial respiratory effort which is necessary to expand the lungs a task beyond their powers. Atelectasis contributes to anoxia because there is increased pulmonary vascular resistance and perfusion of non-ventilated lung. Brief spells of apnoea associated with periodic breathing occur frequently in pre-term infants and are harmless but longer apnoeic episodes lead to anoxia and cyanosis. Such cyanotic attacks occurring after birth may be evidence of cerebral haemorrhage, congenital malformation of heart or diaphragm, severe infection, or obstruction of the respiratory tract, e.g. from hyaline membrane, inhaled vomitus or mucus. Treatment is directed towards the cause but may include the judicious use of oxygen (see below), regular changes of position to facilitate drainage and expansion of the lungs and in some cases assisted respiration. Various alarm devices are in use to alert nurses when an infant stops breathing.

Hyaline membrane disease

This is the most frequent cause of neonatal respiratory distress, which can also be due to pneumonia, pulmonary haemorrhage, pneumothorax and malformations of heart or lungs. Hyaline membrane disease occurs predominantly in pre-term infants weighing less than 2000 g at birth but also in larger pre-term and term infants. Babies of diabetic mothers are predisposed only in so far as they are often born before term.

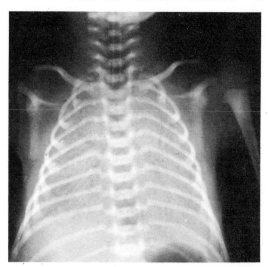

Fig. 4.15 Hyaline membrane disease. Pre-term infant (birth weight 1800 g) two hours after birth. Opacity of both lung fields and air bronchogram effect.

Similarly the higher incidence in infants delivered by Caesarean section is attributable to the reasons for the section rather than to the mode of delivery itself.

The genesis of hyaline membrane disease is complex and not yet satisfactorily explained. The hyaline membrane consists of eosinophilic material lining the smaller bronchioles and alveolar ducts. Its content of cell debris indicates that necrotic respiratory epithelial cells contribute to its formation, while its fibrinous composition suggests that it is partly a transudate from damaged pulmonary capillaries. The lungs of affected infants show diminished activity of surfactant, a surface-tension lowering phospholipid normally produced by alveolar cells from about the twenty-third week of gestation. Its insufficiency in hyaline membrane disease has been attributed to primary inadequacy through immaturity, to damage to alveolar cells by asphyxial changes and to inhibition by the hyaline membrane itslf. Increased pulmonary vascular resistance and consequent hypoperfusion of the lungs occurs in this disease and may be due to vasoconstriction in response to asphyxia. Other possible etiological factors for which there is some evidence are slow clearance of fluid by the pulmonary lymphatics after birth, decreased blood volume and disordered autonomic function. Disseminated intravascular coagulation of blood is commonly found in the lungs at necropsy and may contribute to the pathogenesis but is non-specific, since it is also present in a variety of other diseases, especially those characterized by shock.

CLINICAL FEATURES. The infants usually have difficulty in establishing respiration at birth and within a few hours develop rapid, laboured breathing with rib retraction and expiratory grunting. Cyanosis appears and increases as pulmonary vasoconstriction reduces pulmonary blood flow, and right-to-left shunting of blood occurs. The size of the shunt of unoxygenated blood depends partly on the flow through the ductus arteriosus, which remains patent, and partly on the amount of blood perfusing atelectatic lung. Retention of carbon dioxide and immaturity of renal homeostatic mechanisms combine to produce increasing acidaemia of mixed respiratory and metabolic origin. X-ray shows reticulogranular opacity of the lung fields, the air passages being clearly outlined by air (air bronchogram).

PROGNOSIS. Between one-quarter and one-half of affected infants die in the first week, usually within 36 hours of birth. At necropsy the lungs are dull red and congested, with widespread atelectasis. Intraventricular haemorrhage is a frequent associated finding. Infants who survive the newborn period usually make a complete recovery but in a small number of cases respiratory signs persist and are accompanied by radiological changes consisting of cystic areas progressing to patchy opacities and areas of hyperaeration throughout the lung fields (Wilson-Mikity syndrome). About one-third of such infants die in severe respiratory distress.

TREATMENT. In addition to the ordinary methods of care for pre-term infants, treatment will include the administration of oxygen in sufficient concentration to relieve cyanosis, humidification of the atmosphere to 90 to 100 per cent relative humidity, and antibiotics if infection is suspected. When micro-methods are available for biochemical control of therapy, the acidaemia and associated hyperkalaemia should be corrected as far as possible by intravenous infusion of alkali and glucose or fructose. An attempt should be made to maintain the arterial oxygen tension within normal limits, if necessary by the use of mechanical ventilation.

Anaemia

Anaemia following pre-term birth is thought to be due to a combination of factors, viz. haemolysis, immaturity of the blood-forming organs, rapid post-natal growth, and the relatively small total quantity of available iron. The anaemia can be temporarily corrected by transfusion, but this is only required in cases where the haemoglobin falls below 50 per cent. Iron should be administered to all infants of low birth weight, however, after the fourth week, since it will reduce the degree of early anaemia and expedite recovery. Failure to administer iron is likely to result in a secondary late anaemia, which is hypochromic and occurs during the latter part of the first year. In very small pre-term infants, folic acid deficiency may cause megaloblastic anaemia which can be corrected by giving folic acid.

Inhalation of food or vomitus

Since the cough reflex is poorly developed or absent, the stomach readily overloaded, and the cardiac sphincter a feeble barrier, there is a much greater danger of inhalation of food or vomitus than in the case of the term infant. Particular care is therefore necessary in feeding and handling pre-term infants, and an aspirator should always be available for removal of vomitus regurgitated into the naso-pharynx.

Haemorrhage

Owing to the immaturity of the vascular system and permeability of the capillaries, coupled with the softness of the skull, the pre-term infant is particularly liable to cerebral haemorrhage, even when his small size might be expected to render delivery easy. Hypoxia is an important factor in the genesis of intracranial haemorrhage, especially intraventricular haemorrhage, and it is significant that the lowest mortality occurs in vertex deliveries and rises progressively with breech, mid and high forceps deliveries, and Caesarean section. The abuse of oxytocic preparations also increases the risks to the infant during delivery.

Haemorrhage due to hypoprothrombinaemia is a complication carrying a higher risk than in the term infant. It is the practice in most clinics to administer vitamin K to the mother before delivery and 1 mg to the infant immediately after birth, whenever a pre-term birth occurs. Owing to the risk of some of the vitamin K analogues causing haemolysis and kernicterus (see below), a dosage of 1 mg of vitamin K_1 for the infant should not normally be exceeded.

Oedema

Oedema affecting the extremities or greater part of the body is liable to occur in small pre-term infants, particularly if they have been chilled. A variety of causes may be responsible, viz. deficient renal function, permeability of the capillaries, hypoproteinaemia, and increased body fluid content. While oedema is not necessarily of bad prognosis, it is an indication for special care, and for correction of hypoproteinaemia if this exists.

Hypothermia (*Cold injury*)

The use of a low-reading rectal thermometer registering as low as 29·4°C (85°F) will bring to light cases in which a variety of signs (failure to suck, apathy, reddening, cyanosis and coldness of the skin, oedema or sclerema) are primarily due to hypothermia. Although this may occur in any newborn infant, small feeble babies are particularly vulnerable. The infant's cot should be gradually warmed until the rectal temperature has risen to 36·5°C (97° or 98°F). Administration of glucose by gastric tube and antibiotics to avoid intercurrent infection will be required. Unless the condition is recognized and treated promptly, it may lead to fatal pulmonary haemorrhage or infection.

Dehydration

Dehydration either due to diarrhoea and vomiting (excessive fluid loss) or to deficient fluid intake, may be precipitated with dangerous rapidity. Correction is undertaken in the same manner as for term infants.

Acidaemia

Acidaemia occurs readily in pre-term infants and is predisposed to by immaturity of renal function. It may be associated with gasping respiration, though this is not a constant or reliable sign. Acidaemia may be corrected by the administration of sodium bicarbonate or lactate (see p. 183).

Deficiency diseases

It is probable that the short period of gestation is responsible for a deficient storage of vitamins by the fetus. This, in association with rapid growth after birth, renders the pre-term infant particularly liable to develop early rickets, which is almost invariably seen if active measures are not taken to prevent it. Clinical manifestations of other deficiency diseases are less common, though early administration of vitamin A, vitamin C, and vitamin B complex is advisable (see Feeding).

Retrolental fibroplasia

This retinopathy represented an important cause of blindness before the risks of excessive oxygen administration were fully recognized. It occurs principally, but not exclusively, in infants weighing less than 1500 g at birth, and particularly in those that have been nursed continuously at high concentrations of oxygen for a week or more. The retinal vessels undergo an angioblastic change, which is at first reversible, and subsequently an opaque membrane forms behind the crystalline lens. In cases which do not undergo spontaneous regression, vision is lost. The incidence of the disease has been very greatly reduced by exercise of extreme caution in the use of oxygen.

Congenital malformations

The incidence of congenital malformation is high in pre-term infants, presumably due to the fact that many congenital deformities may be responsible for the fetus failing to go to term. Every infant should therefore be carefully examined to exclude such conditions.

Infection

The pre-term infant has poor resistance to infection due to low levels of immune globulins, reduced phagocytic activity and probably other deficiencies. Severe infection may develop with only slight clinical signs, such as failure to suck and grey pallor. Thrush is liable to prove invasive and must be treated promptly. Respiratory infections, septicaemia, meningitis and diarrhoea are particularly lethal.

LIGHT-FOR-DATES INFANTS

This category includes a number of different kinds of infant. Some appear normal though small while others have long thin bodies and reltively large heads. In yet others, malformations or signs of dysmaturity (p. 33) may be present.

Neurologically, these infants are more advanced than pre-term infants of comparable weight and this probably reflects a generally greater maturity. They are especially liable to develop severe hypoglycaemia in the first days of life, due to low fetal stores of carbohydrate: hypoglycaemia should be corrected by the injection of glucose to prevent damage to the brain. Light-for-dates infants become hypothermic easily and are prone to extensive and sometimes lethal pulmonary haemorrhage. Mental subnormality and epilepsy are common in long-term survivors.

CARE OF INFANTS OF LOW BIRTH WEIGHT

At the time of birth the infant must be received immediately into a warm blanket and transferred to a warmed cot or incubator, preferably in a specially designed and equipped nursery. Whereas formerly such nurseries were used exclusively for infants of low birth weight, and designated 'premature nursery', the present trend is for large obstetric hospitals to have special care infant units for any newborn infant requiring special observation or treatment. Such units are staffed throughout the 24 hours by skilled nurses, a high proportion of whom should be permanently assigned to the unit, and have biochemical, radiological and other services available at all times. The professional skills and technical equipment in special care nurseries contribute in no small measure to the improvement of mortality and morbidity rates in the newborn period and whenever possible infants of low birth weight should be transferred to such a unit immediately after birth. Hypothermia during

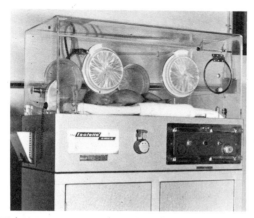

Fig. 4.16   A type of incubator (the 'Isolette') designed to provide microfiltration of air, precise control of temperature, and oxygen concentration, humidification, safety signal and ease of cleaning.

transfer must be avoided by use of a portable incubator or by wrapping the baby in a suit of polyester and aluminium ('the silver swaddler').

Incubators are now generally preferred to thermostatically controlled nurseries, as they provide better isolation and allow a greater degree of humidification (80 to 90 per cent) without discomforting nursing staff. The temperature can be kept constant, e.g. at a selected point between 32° and 35°C (90° to 95°F) for the smaller infants, procedures can be carried out through ports without opening the incubator, and in some models a high degree of air filtration is provided.

Oxygen can be given when required, but its administration should be reduced to a minimum after the immediate hazards of delivery are passed. The concentration should not subsequently exceed 40 per cent except to relieve cyanosis, and should be gradually reduced and discontinued as soon as the infant no longer requires it. Careful records should be made of the oxygen concentration, and the duration of administration.

Infants should be under the constant observation of nurses trained to recognize abnormalities and skilled in the use of the specialized equipment in special care nurseries. Nursing care includes scrupulous cleanliness, a minimum of handling, periodical changes of position, and attention to the skin, which readily becomes excoriated or infected. All unnecessary visitors must be excluded but mothers should be encouraged to visit and handle their babies often during the early days of life and later to participate in feeding and care.

Feeding

The fact that the smallest infants fed on breast milk alone fail to gain weight quite as rapidly as those fed on artificial cow's milk formulae, should not prejudice the use of breast milk when it can be obtained. This may be possible in a large maternity hospital, even if the mother is unable to provide sufficient. In the case of infants weighing less than 1500 g the milk may be fortified by the addition of a protein preparation (e.g. casein hydrolysate if this is well tolerated) to bring the infant's protein intake up to 5 g per kg body weight per day. If the mother wishes to breast-feed, her lactation should be maintained by expression until the infant is able to suck on the breast.

While the pre-term infant will usually require a higher caloric intake to gain weight than will the term baby, it must be realized that there is a risk in giving highly concentrated feeds during the first two to three weeks of life. Good results can be obtained if the infant takes sufficient to maintain weight during this time, after which weight gain is usually rapid and the intake can be correspondingly increased. Feeding is unnecessary during the first few hours but longer periods of starvation are inadvisable as they entail the risk of dehydration and possibly of brain damage. During the first 6 to 12 hours of feeding, 5 per cent glucose or lactose water is given three-hourly in small amounts and there-after milk feeds are given, starting with dilute feeds but quickly increasing the concentration and quantity according to the tolerance of the infant.

It is impossible to work to a rule of thumb in deciding the quantities given in relation to weight, since there is great variation between infants of the same weight in the amounts toler-ated. In general, however, the infant will often take 120 or more calories per kg body weight per day after the third week.

Where breast milk is unobtainable, a half-cream dried milk or evaporated-milk formula should be used in its place. Provided that the infant's capacity is not overtaxed by the volume of the feed, and the technique of feeding is carefully observed, the composition of the for-mula can be similar to that used for term infants though some prefer a more concentrated feed.

TECHNIQUE. The smallest infants, in whom the swallowing reflex is imperfectly developed, must be fed by nasogastric tube, care being taken to avoid distending the stomach with air. Alter-natively, a gastrostomy can be performed and feeds given by this route for two to three weeks. Tube feeding may be alternated with bottle feed-ing in the case of larger infants who become rapidly exhausted. Infants who suck well can feed by bottle with a teat of appropriate size.

It is generally advisable to feed three-hourly, since each feed is a slow process and tends to exhaust the infant. More frequent feeding, e.g. two-hourly, can usually be avoided by the judi-cious use of tube feeding when necessary.

VITAMINS AND SUPPLEMENTS. From the third week, infants should receive an aqueous con-centrate containing 400 units of vitamin D, 20,000 units vitamin A, and 25 to 50 mg ascorbic acid daily. Vitamin B complex is also recommended, though the infant's requirements are less certainly known. Infants of very low birth weight should be given folic acid daily. Supplements of iron are required from the fourth week onward, starting with small doses to avoid digestive upsets. When dried milk fortified with vitamins and iron is used, these additions are unnecessary. Vitamin K_1 in a dose of 1 mg should be given to all infants of low birth weight immediately after birth.

PROGNOSIS OF LOW BIRTH WEIGHT

In the absence of gross congenital malforma-ton or haemorrhage, the immediate prognosis depends to a great extent on the birth weight and maturity of the infant, the mortality rising rapidly as the birth weight falls below 1250 g. Although there are many instances of infants weighing less than 1000 g at birth having been reared, the prognosis of very small infants who survive is generally poor as regards both mental and physical development. Hitherto a high pro-portion of surviving infants weighing less than 1500 g at birth have shown neurological dis-abilities but this proportion may be lower when modern intensive neonatal care has been avail-able.

INFECTION

Before the advent of antibiotics, infection was the most important single cause of neonatal death after the first week. The special susceptibility of immature infants is well illustrated by Edinburgh figures for the years 1939–43, before the use of antibiotics, when the neonatal death-rate due to infection was 5·4 per 1000 full-term live births and 79 per 1000 premature live births. Despite the great decline in its relative importance, infec-tion still causes deaths if unrecognized or in-adequately treated.

It has already been mentioned that while the infant may be born with congenital immunity to certain organisms to which the mother herself is immune, the capacity for independent antibody formation during the neonatal period is poorly developed, particularly in the case of pre-term infants. Most neonatal deaths from infection are attributable to pneumonia, septicaemia or meningitis: gastroenteritis and severe thrush formerly caused many deaths but are now less common causes. Recent reports have drawn attention to fatal Coxsackie group B virus infections with *myocarditis* occurring in this age group. In addition to lethal infections, however, the newborn infant is vulnerable to many minor infections by organisms which are normally saprophytic on the skin or mucous membranes of the adult, e.g. staphylococci. The incidence of all minor infections, however slight, is about 10 per cent in well-run maternity units and considerably higher where staffing is inadequate. The liberal use of skin preparations containing hexachlorophane has resulted in a diminution in the incidence of staphylococcal infections, whereas coliform bacilli, including *E. coli*, *Proteus* and *Pseudomonas*, have increased in importance. On the other hand the majority of hospital staphylococcal infections are now not only penicillin-resistant, but are showing increasing resistance to other commonly used antibiotics.

Apart from the possibility of infection through the maternal blood-stream, the fetus is normally bacteriologically sterile until rupture of the membranes occurs. The fetus may then come in contact with vaginal organisms or inhale infected liquor amnii. At this time, therefore, the infant is liable to be infected with thrush or to contract gonococcal ophthalmia, inhalation pneumonia, or septicaemia. It is now a general practice to cleanse the eyes and drain liquor or mucus from the respiratory passages as soon as the head is delivered. Maternal pyrexia during labour, prolonged rupture of the membranes and offensive liquor amnii are all indications for giving antibiotics to the infant prophylactically.

After delivery, the infant comes in contact with a larger variety of possible sources of infection. While the skin and respiratory tract of the attendants are undoubtedly of first importance, there are additional dangers from feeding and washing utensils, etc. In institutions where there are large numbers of newborn infants, and particularly in special care nurseries, the greatest care must be taken in preventing both cross-infection and multiple infection from a common source (e.g. an attendant with a cold or skin infection, or an infant harbouring pathogens in numerous sites). A strictly observed technique of hand-washing is extremely important, and a liberal supply of dry hand-towels must be provided for attendants, since chapped hands are particularly liable to convey infection. Any infant suspected or known to have an infection should be promptly isolated.

Neonatal septicaemia and pyaemia

Blood-stream infection in the newborn period can be due to a great variety of organisms, the most frequent being *E. coli*, *Pseudomonas*, *Klebsiella*, staphylococci and streptococci. The condition is undoubtedly commoner than generally realized, partly owing to the difficulties of diagnosis and partly to the fact that certification of death will often describe only a local lesion (e.g. pneumonia) when this may be associated with a generalized infection.

SITE OF INFECTION. Occasionally septicaemia in the newborn occurs from an infected placenta after rupture of the membranes, before the cord has been divided. After birth, infection of the stump of the cord and entry of organisms through the umbilical veins is a possible cause. Infections of the skin are easily recognized as possible sites, but it is probable that in the majority of cases the portal of entry is the respiratory or gastro-intestinal tract.

SIGNS AND SYMPTOMS. There is no very clear-cut picture of septicaemia at this age, and some infants simply appear grey and apathetic, and die without developing other signs. Most infants refuse feeds and there may be vomiting with or without diarrhoea. The temperature may be raised but is often subnormal. The spleen is frequently enlarged, unless the infection is very rapidly fatal; hepatomegaly also commonly occurs, and jaundice may develop. Haemorrhage or purpura is a common complication, and haematuria or haemoglobinuria may also occur. Pyaemic abscesses may form in any organ.

DIAGNOSIS. Apart from the clinical picture, secure diagnosis must rest on repeated blood culture; a single negative culture cannot be taken as excluding blood-stream infection.

PROGNOSIS AND TREATMENT. Before the era of antibiotics, the prognosis was extremely poor, and this is still true if septicaemia is associated with deep jaundice and haemorrhage. While it is now possible to save a proportion of cases if the infecting organism is identified and sensitive to therapy and the condition is suspected early, the prognosis is worse in the newborn than in older age groups. The occurrence of cyanosis or respiratory complications is an indication for oxygen administration, while the general measures appropriate for shock and dehydration are likely to be required.

Pneumonia

Four types of pneumonia are encountered in the newborn period:

1. Pneumonia within the first few days, which is usually intrauterine in origin, due to inhalation of contaminated liquor, blood, etc. into lungs affected by atelectasis. This is one cause of respiratory distress occurring within hours of birth.
2. Aspiration pneumonia, due to inhalation of food or vomitus. This is particularly liable to occur in small feeble infants, and its incidence is to some extent an index of the quality of nursing care. The presence of stomach contents in the lung results in destructive inflammatory changes, and leads on to suppuration.
3. Staphylococcal pneumonia, producing rapid suppuration and extensive disorganization of lung tissue, often with pyopneumothorax. This is most commonly seen in the neonatal period, and may occur in association with outbreaks of other staphylococcal infections in a newborn nursery.
4. Bronchopneumonia, due to air-borne infection by the common pathogens of the respiratory tract, including viruses, streptococci, pneumococci, and *Haemophilus influenzae*, or by organisms of the *E. coli* group which do not normally cause pneumonia in older patients.

CLINICAL PICTURE. This is often ill-defined, with the result that neonatal pneumonia may not be diagnosed during life. The temperature may be irregularly raised, but may be normal or subnormal. Dyspnoea is not always obvious, and respiratory embarrassment is more likely to be shown by colour changes than by tachypnoea, although a respiratory rate above 60 per minute is an important sign when present.

Clinical signs in the chest are also often elusive and while fine crepitations are highly suggestive of the diagnosis they are not invariably detected. The general condition of the infant, the colour, and failure to suck or gain weight may be the only indications that the lungs are affected.

Radiological examination will often confirm the diagnosis, but here again it is sometimes impossible to interpret the appearance with certainty or to distinguish between atelectasis and pulmonary consolidation.

TREATMENT. In cases of aspiration pneumonia, an attempt should be made to clear the respiratory passages of aspirated material. Subsequently the position of the infant should be changed at regular intervals to encourage drainage. The infant should be nursed in oxygen. Antibiotic therapy should be instituted promptly, a broad-spectrum antibiotic such as cephaloridine or ampicillin with cloxacillin being given while organism sensitivity is being determined.

Upper respiratory tract infections

The newborn infant is liable to contract upper respiratory infection, most commonly from attendants. Such infection may result in a purulent rhinitis or serve as the prelude to bronchitis or bronchopneumonia. Rhinitis is apt to interfere with sucking. The nose should be cleansed with cotton-wool soaked in saline, and vasoconstrictive drops may be instilled. No oily drops should ever be instilled in the infant's nose, since there is a serious risk of producing aspiration pneumonia by so doing. It is advisable to give antibiotic therapy if there is evidence of bacterial infection.

The middle ears are often involved in upper respiratory tract infection, while there is an added danger of infection if the infant is fed lying flat, since milk or vomitus may pass into the Eustachian tubes.

Thrush

Infection with Monilia (*Candida albicans*) is a more serious condition in the newborn infant than in later infancy, and may occur either during birth or later from attendants' hands or feeding utensils. It is usually limited to the mouth, in which case its principal effect is to interfere with feeding, but it sometimes affects the napkin area and may occasionally extend to the lung, oesophagus, stomach, or intestines. The lesions in the mouth consist of white patches of mycelium and spores situated on the tongue, roof of the mouth, and particularly on the buccal mucosa of the cheek immediately adjacent to the alveolar margin. While the lesions superficially resemble milk-curds, they are found to be adherent to inflamed mucosa, which appears raw if the patches of thrush are scraped away. Microscopic examination will demonstrate the presence of mycelium and spores (Fig. 4.17). Local treatment with nystatin (200,000 units per ml) or with 1 per cent gentian violet is usually effective in oral lesions, but scrupulous cleanliness and isolation are necessary to prevent re-infection or spread in a newborn nursery.

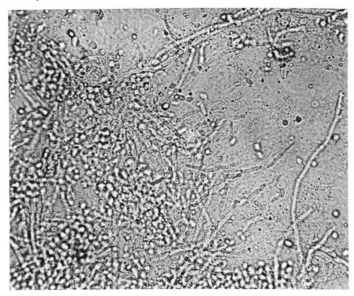

Fig. 4.17   Thrush (*Candida albicans*). ×350. Colony from mouth of newborn infant, showing mycelium and spores.

Diarrhoea and vomiting

Epidemics of neonatal diarrhoea in maternity hospitals are of such serious consequence that immediate isolation of even the mildest case is essential. Various pathogens and atypical strains of *E. coli* have been isolated in different outbreaks. The possibility of a virus being responsible in some epidemics is suggested by the occurrence of an influenza-like infection affecting mothers or attendants.

Whichever the cause, the condition is highly infectious. The mortality differs markedly in different epidemics, but is generally low in comparison with outbreaks of 25 years ago, when it sometimes exceeded 50 per cent of cases. In the newborn, there is not the same difference in case incidence between breast-fed and artificially fed infants as is seen in outbreaks of diarrhoea in older infants.

CLINICAL PICTURE. The disease seldom starts before the fourth or fifth day of life. There may be no premonitory symptoms, or more commonly the infant will refuse his feeds, lose weight abruptly, and appear listless and apathetic before the onset of diarrhoea. This is sudden, with the passage of a watery, explosive stool, followed rapidly by others. In most cases the greenish stools contain very little faecal matter, but the amount of fluid passed is considerable. Mucus may be present, but there is very rarely any blood unless the infecting organism is a dysentery bacillus. Vomiting occurs in the severer cases. The infant rapidly becomes dehydrated and appears collapsed and toxic. The abdomen may become distended, and the temperature is usually irregularly raised.

TREATMENT. The same principles of treatment of shock and dehydration apply as in the case of older infants (Chapter 6). If the infant is able to retain fluids by mouth, saline and glucose should be substituted for milk feeds, and a return to these made gradually when clinical improvement occurs.

Specific treatment must depend on the causative organism when this can be identified. Outbreaks due to atypical strains of *E. coli* may respond to oral neomycin or colistin, or intramuscular gentamicin, and treatment should be extended to carriers and patients at risk. Viral infections must be treated symptomatically.

Conjunctivitis

A purulent discharge from the eyes may be due to a variety of organisms including staphylococci, diphtheroids and streptococci, while in approximately 10 per cent of cases there is strong evidence for regarding a virus as the responsible agent. Gonococci, which account for a high proportion of cases in some countries, are very rare in Britain due to improved antenatal care.

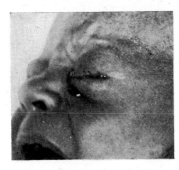

Fig. 4.18 Neonatal conjunctivitis: swollen eyelids and sero-purulent exudate. Infant aged 14 days.

CLINICAL SIGNS. Acute swelling and oedema of the eyelids, which make it impossible for the infant to open the eyes voluntarily, are associated with a thin serous or blood-stained discharge which rapidly becomes purulent. When infection has occurred during birth, the signs usually appear on or about the third day.

Milder degrees of conjunctivitis often show little or no swelling of the eyelids, and the discharge is often very slight, though sufficiently sticky to cause adherence of the lids. Many of these 'sticky eyes' are probably due to chemical irritation rather than to infection.

PROPHYLAXIS. Ideally, prophylaxis should aim at the elimination of vaginal organisms likely to cause infection. Antenatal treatment of gonorrhoea has been highly successful, but with regard to other infections, including viruses, it cannot be said that equal progress has been made. In most institutions, the routine use of silver nitrate has now been abandoned in favour of simple wiping of the eyes after the head is born.

TREATMENT. In all cases the infecting organism and its sensitivities should be determined. The severer forms of conjunctivitis, including the gonococcal cases, respond well to local application of the appropriate antibiotic. If the organism is penicillin-sensitive, an initial irrigation of the conjunctival sac with saline should be followed by instillation of 1 drop of penicillin in a strength of 2500 units per ml at five-minute intervals until discharge has ceased, and then at half-hourly intervals until the swelling has subsided. By this method the great majority of cases are clinically cured within 12 hours. Penicillin is, however, continued at hourly intervals for a further 12 hours and at two-hourly intervals for 24 hours.

The milder cases of conjunctivitis, from which penicillin-insensitive staphylococci are often re-covered, usually respond well to repeated irrigation with saline and instillation of sulphacetamide. Good results have also been obtained with neomycin-bacitracin ointment.

Skin infections

These vary in severity from isolated pustules to generalized exfoliative dermatitis, which is now rarely seen. The great majority of skin infections of the newborn are due to staphylococci.

Pustules may occur in any site, but are most often seen in the folds of the groins; they may be single or multiple, and contain thick pus. *Paronychia*, a low-grade infection around the nails, gives rise to swelling and discoloration of the terminal phalanx of the affected fingers, and a slight local discharge. The infection readily spreads to other parts of the skin and to underlying bone. In *bullous impetigo*, crops of raised vesicles containing a sero-purulent discharge form superficially and tend to increase in size and finally rupture.

Pemphigus is the name given to the most extensive type of vesiculating lesions, which may involve the greater part of the body. The lesions

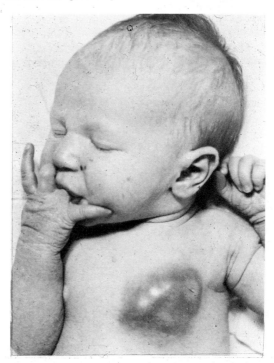

Fig. 4.19 Staphylococcal breast abscess in newborn infant.

spread rapidly, and when they rupture leave a raw reddened surface which exudes thin pus. In staphylococcal *epidermal necrolysis*, there is widespread 'scalding' of the skin due to intra-epidermal cleavage.

Furuncles and *abscesses* occasionally occur and may require incision and drainage.

A true *mastitis* or *breast abscess* may be produced in the physiologically enlarged breast of the newborn if it is squeezed in an attempt to express the contents. This practice is wholly unnecessary, since breast enlargement of the newborn subsides spontaneously; it is not itself inflammatory in origin (though sometimes incorrectly described as 'mastitis neonatorum') and is due to the withdrawal of circulating maternal oestrogens.

Infections of the umbilicus are common, though usually limited to a slight stickiness which clears up with routine treatment. In some cases a granuloma forms, which requires application of silver nitrate. When the infection is more virulent, it may cause septic thrombosis of the umbilical veins, which can be palpated as hard cords. In such cases the vein should be ligated above, and the infected clot evacuated. Infection is a hazard of catheterizing the umbilical vessels, and scrupulous precautions should be taken to avoid introducing organisms.

PROPHYLAXIS. Since the majority of skin infections derive from contact with the attendants, strict attention must be paid to nursing technique, nasal hygiene, and the exclusion of infected adults. Prompt isolation of infected babies is essential. The handling of infants should be reduced to a minimum, and the hands and arms of attendants should be adequately washed and dried before and after touching an infant. It is found that the incidence of infection tends to rise when nurseries are overcrowded, or when nursing standards deteriorate. The risk of infection from washing newborn infants depends to a great extent on the facilities available. It has been greatly reduced by the use of hexachlorophane solution, which should be applied sparingly to the infant's skin and rinsed off afterwards, since absorption is potentially harmful. Daily bathing of newborn infants is not essential and cleansing may be limited to the face and napkin area.

Since a high proportion of newborn infants (without clinical evidence of infection) have been found to harbour staphylococci or haemolytic streptococci in the umbilicus, it is advisable to apply 1 per cent solution of chlorhexidine in spirit (or powder containing hexachlorophane) to the cord stump.

TREATMENT. Infected skin areas should be covered, to prevent as far as possible spread to other parts of the body, after any loose skin has been removed. Since an increasing proportion of staphylococcal infections in maternity hospitals are due to penicillin-resistant strains, it is advisable to treat the more severe infections immediately with cloxacillin or erythromycin, pending the results of sensitivity tests.

Osteomyelitis

This is occasionally seen in the newborn, and when the long bones are affected, the condition must be distinguished from traumatic periostitis. Prompt diagnosis is essential since destruction of bone occurs rapidly. A site which is seldom affected in older infants is the maxilla. Here there is great oedema of the eyelids and face; if the condition is untreated it is likely to cause extrusion of the tooth-buds on the affected side, or result in a sinus opening on the cheek. Good results, avoiding these complications, have been obtained with antibiotic treatment. A more serious complication is *orbital cellulitis*, which may occur in association with osteomyelitis or in

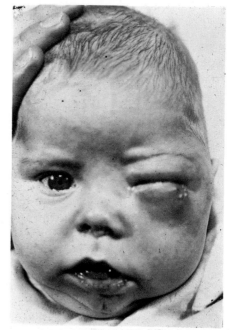

Fig. 4.20   Osteomyelitis of maxilla, giving rise to swelling of left side of face and eyelids. Infant aged 11 weeks.

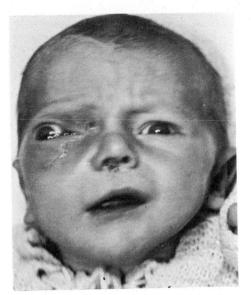

Fig. 4.21   Orbital cellulitis. Infant aged 4 weeks.

the course of a blood-stream infection; unless this condition responds rapidly to antibiotic or chemotherapy, it is likely to result in loss of the eye or death from septic thrombosis.

Meningitis

This may be caused by almost any pyogenic organism but is most frequently due to *E. coli*, which is seldom a cause in older infants. The condition may be predisposed to by complicated delivery or maternal infection, while there is often preceding septicaemia or pneumonia. The infant, frequently of low birth weight, becomes lethargic, refuses feeds and may vomit. Frank signs of raised intracranial pressure, such as bulging fontanelle, head retraction or convulsions, are uncommon although the fontanelle may be full and the infant irritable. Lumbar puncture and blood culture should therefore be carried out readily in any newborn infant with unexplained illness, and particularly in pre-term infants who show unwillingness to feed, diminished activity, grey pallor or colour changes. Antibiotic treatment must be started immediately on diagnosis and, because of the gravity of the prognosis, chloramphenicol and sulphonamide in full doses are often given pending the results of culture and sensitivity tests.

Infection of the urinary tract

This may or may not involve the kidneys and is commonly secondary to a congenital abnor-

mality. Pyelonephritis when present is generally due to haematogenous infection with Gram-negative bacilli. The infant may show little or no evidence of infection but is often pale, anorexic and febrile. Jaundice is not uncommon in severe infection. The diagnosis will be clear if there are many pus cells and organisms in the urine, but in cases of doubt colony counts, if necessary on urine obtained by suprapubic bladder puncture, will be required to establish the diagnosis. Results must be interpreted with care, however, since the incidental finding of bacteriuria in an otherwise healthy newborn infant is a common and transient phenomenon.

When infection is confirmed, the choice of antibiotic will depend on sensitivity tests and treatment should be continued for at least six weeks, followed by repeated examination of the urine to exclude relapse. Pyelography and micturating cystourethrography may demonstrate a congenital abnormality which should be dealt with surgically if necessary.

Tetanus

Tetanus of the newborn is now considered a rare disease in this country, but in the Balkans, China, and elsewhere it has been one of the most important causes of neonatal death; recent north American figures suggest that it is somewhat commoner there than previously supposed. Infection commonly occurs through the umbilicus, due to the use of contaminated dressings. Symptoms usually appear between 3 and 10 days after birth, when spasm of the masticatory muscles and face is followed rapidly by spasms of the limbs, opisthotonos and generalized convulsions. Although some cases respond well to tetanus antitoxin, penicillin, and assisted respiration, the mortality is still generally high.

JAUNDICE

The main precursor of bilirubin is the haemoglobin of erythrocytes which are broken down in the reticulo-endothelial system. Nearly all the bilirubin in plasma is bound to albumin. In the older child, the binding capacity is large and saturation seldom if ever occurs, but in the newborn infant the capacity is far less and saturation may occur with degrees of hyperbilirubinaemia commonly encountered clinically. The binding is reversible, since bilirubin crosses the placenta from fetus to mother, thus preventing the accumulation of unconjugated bilirubin in the fetal circulation. Drugs such as salicylates and sulphonamides may reduce the binding capacity for bilirubin by competing for binding sites on albumin.

Excretion of bilirubin by the liver cell is accomplished by transfer of free bilirubin across the cell membrane, conjugation in the cell and transfer of the conjugated bilirubin into the bile canaliculi. The neonatal liver cells may not be able to conjugate all the bilirubin presented to them because there is insufficient conjugating enzyme. This enzyme, glucuronyl transferase, converts lipid-soluble unconjugated bilirubin to water-soluble bilirubin diglucuronide, by transfer of glucuronide from uridine diphosphoglucuronic acid to bilirubin. A small quantity of bilirubin may also be conjugated by sulphation. Certain steroids may inhibit conjugation and their presence in breast milk may account for higher bilirubin levels in the plasma of breast-fed infants.

The capacity of the liver to transfer bilirubin from blood to bile may also be limited by the rate at which conjugated bilirubin can be transferred across the cell membrane into the bile canaliculi. Some unconjugated bilirubin may find its way directly into the intestinal lumen from the plasma or may pass in the reverse direction (entero-hepatic circulation). The role of this mechanism in the production of jaundice is uncertain.

Kernicterus

This is yellow staining of the basal ganglia and other parts of the brain caused by deposition of unconjugated bilirubin. It is associated with various neurological disturbances, notably lethargy, opisthotonos and convulsions, which are likely to appear within the first week. The mortality rate is high and survivors show athetosis, high-tone deafness and sometimes intellectual subnormality at a later age. The danger of kernicterus increases rapidly as levels of unconjugated bilirubin in the plasma rise above 20 mg per 100 ml, which level is taken as an indication for active measures to lower it. The bilirubin level is only an approximate measure of the risk, however, since the occurrence of kernicterus is determined by other factors in addition, such as the binding capacity of plasma albumin. Hypoxia, acidaemia and infection diminish the binding of bilirubin to albumin and so increase the liability to kernicterus. Levels over 15 mg per 100 ml are

therefore potentially harmful, especially in infants of low birth weight, who must be carefully observed for any manifestations of kernicterus.

DIFFERENTIAL DIAGNOSIS

The differential diagnosis of jaundice in the newborn period often presents some difficulty. The following are some of the important causes in this age group.

Physiological jaundice

Physiological jaundice is observed in more than 50 per cent of normal infants within the first week of life, though it may be of very slight degree and obscured by erythema. Unlike jaundice due to haemolytic disease, physiological jaundice does not appear on the first day of life. It commonly fades within a period of days or, at most, a week or two. If it persists beyond the second week it can hardly be classed as physiological.

Physiological jaundice is due to the limited capacity of the liver for bilirubin excretion during the first few days of life, determined largely by temporary deficiency of glucuronyl transferase. The breakdown of red cells in response to more efficient oxygenation in extrauterine life presents a larger load of bilirubin to the liver, thus adding to the demands made on it.

The infant normally suffers from no symptoms attributable to jaundice, except in cases where it is exceptionally deep. Such infants may be somewhat apathetic and unwilling to feed. It is advisable to postpone operations of choice, such as circumcision, until after the jaundice has cleared. The meconium and stools in infants with physiological jaundice are of normal colour.

Jaundice in the pre-term infant (see p. 48).

Haemolytic jaundice

Haemolytic jaundice associated with Rhesus and other incompatibilities is recognized by the criteria described below and confirmed by serological examination. Prolonged jaundice following haemolytic disease may be due to obstruction caused by liver damage or possibly by inspissation of bile.

Jaundice due to infection

Jaundice due to infection will usually be overshadowed by symptoms of the primary disease. The jaundice in these cases is partly haemolytic and partly toxic in origin. The most marked jaundice is likely to occur following pyogenic umbilical infection when the liver becomes involved, but mild jaundice is quite common in urinary infections in the newborn. In addition to pyogenic infections, toxoplasmosis (p. 33), cytomegalic inclusion disease, and viral hepatitis may be responsible for jaundice at this age. Persistent obstructive jaundice is sometimes caused by neonatal giant-cell hepatitis, which may be of viral origin.

Congenital atresia of the bile-ducts (p. 85)

Here the jaundice is of obstructive type. The meconium or stools are pale or grey in colour, and the urine contains bile. The jaundice tends to deepen progressively, the infant sometimes becoming greenish-bronze in colour. In other cases, however, even when the obstruction is complete, the jaundice is less deep and may vary in intensity over a period of months.

Enzyme deficiencies

Decreased activity of enzymes in the newborn infant's red cells may render them more easily destroyed than in later life. The susceptibility of neonatal red cells is greatly increased when the enzyme glucose-6-phosphate dehydrogenase (G-6-PD) is deficient, for the cells are then easily lysed when challenged by agents such as primaquine or sulphonamides (p. 245). This is an important cause of jaundice in Mediterranean and eastern countries and exchange transfusion may be required to prevent kernicterus.

Very rarely, jaundice in the infant may be due to a genetically determined defect of glucuronidation (Crigler-Najjar syndrome).

Hereditary spherocytosis

This condition occasionally causes jaundice or anaemia during the newborn period, but is more often recognized when the condition is suspected on account of the family history (p. 243).

Congenital syphilis

This is a rare cause of unexplained jaundice in the newborn, associated with splenomegaly.

TREATMENT

The treatment of jaundice due to haemolytic disease is considered below. In most other types of neonatal jaundice, treatment will be that of the underlying condition. Except in small pre-term infants, jaundice due to hepatic enzyme immaturity seldom reaches dangerous levels but may occasionally do so, necessitating exchange transfusion. Exposure of jaundiced infants to artificial light (phototherapy) is effective in preventing hyperbilirubinaemia in a proportion of cases and may thus obviate the need for exchange transfusion. Administration of phenobarbitone to the mother in late pregnancy or to the infant has also been advocated to prevent jaundice in high risk cases.

HAEMOLYTIC DISEASE OF THE NEWBORN (*Erythroblastosis fetalis*)

Haemolytic disease of the newborn is the result of incompatibility between maternal and fetal blood, the great majority of severe cases being due to differences in Rhesus constitution and many milder ones to ABO incompatibility.

Rhesus constitution

The term 'Rhesus factor' (or Rh) was coined following the discovery that the injection of the red blood cells of Macacus Rhesus monkeys into laboratory animals would produce agglutinins which would also agglutinate the red cells of approximately 85 per cent of humans (Landsteiner and Wiener, 1940). The agglutinogen present in human cells, and so responsible for this reaction, was described as the Rhesus factor. Those whose cells were agglutinated were classified as Rhesus-positive, and those where no agglutination took place as Rhesus-negative.

The original conception of the Rhesus factor as a single specific antigen capable of producing immunization and antibodies in a Rhesus-negative individual into whom it was injected, was soon modified. It was first recognized that alleles at three loci were involved in determining the Rhesus constitution of an individual. The principal gene pairs (and their corresponding antigens) at the three loci were described by the letters Cc, Dd, Ee. Eight combinations are possible, each of which has been given a 'short title'. In most Caucasian populations the frequencies are:

Fisher notation	Short notation	Frequency %
CDe	R_1	42
cde	r	39
cDE	R_2	14
Cde	r'	1
cdE	r''	1
cDe	R_0	3
CDE	Rz	Rare
CdE	Ry	Very rare

Eight chromosomes can be paired in 8/2(8+1) or 36 different ways, but other less common alleles have been described, e.g. C^w at the C locus and D^u at the D locus, etc., which greatly increases the number of possible Rh genotypes.

Thus while it is theoretically possible for each antigen to stimulate the production of antibodies which have been named respectively anti-C, anti-D, and anti-E; anti-c, anti-d, and anti-e, one of these (anti-d) has not been conclusively demonstrated. The antigen which is most potent and causes over 95 per cent of cases of immunization is D. Anti-D serum is therefore used for routine typing of patients as Rhesus-positive or Rhesus-negative. Where D is concerned, it is a convenient shorthand to use the symbols dd for Rhesus negativity, and DD (homozygous) and Dd (heterozygous) for Rhesus positivity, if it is

remembered that D is only one part of the complete Rhesus system.

Maternal Rhesus constitution. Since the great majority of cases of severe haemolytic disease of the newborn occur in infants of Rhesus-negative mothers who have become sensitized to the red cells of a Rhesus-positive fetus, it is with Rhesus-negative women that we are principally concerned. It is the practice in antenatal clinics to carry out routine Rhesus-typing early in pregnancy, and to follow up women found to be Rhesus-negative. The follow-up will include testing for the presence of antibodies, and if these are found to be present, repeating the test to determine whether the titre is rising. It should be emphasized that only a comparatively small proportion of Rhesus-negative women become immunized even when the fetus is Rhesus-positive,

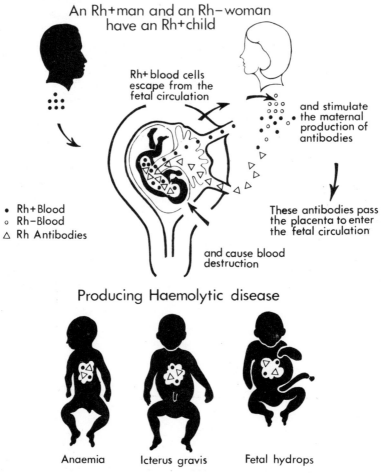

Fig. 4.22   The etiology of haemolytic disease. (Adapted from *Rh* by E. L. Potter, 1947. Chicago: Year Book Medical Publishers.)

and repeated pregnancies are often necessary for immunization to occur. A previous transfusion with Rhesus-positive blood, however, will greatly increase the likelihood of immunization and the further production of antibodies when the fetus is Rhesus-positive, and may result in haemolytic disease occurring in a first-born child.

Incompatibility of blood groups of the ABO series between mother and fetus, on the other hand, appears to have some inhibitory effect on the occurrence of Rhesus immunization, though the mother may become immunized to an incompatible fetal blood group (particularly if the mother is group O and the baby A_1) and this immunization may then be responsible for haemolytic disease of the fetus. Immunization may also occur from a number of other blood-group antigens, e.g. Kell, Duffy, Kidd, etc., which are not of the Rhesus system, or from previous transfusions of Rhesus-positive women.

Paternal Rhesus constitution. In the case of a Rhesus-positive man married to a Rhesus-negative woman, great importance attaches to the question as to whether the man is homozygous (DD) or heterozygous (Dd), i.e. whether both members of the D gene-pair or only one are liable to stimulate antibody formation in his wife. Since the fetus receives half a gene-pair from each parent, it is inevitable that if the father is DD the fetus will inherit D and so be Rhesus-positive. If, on the other hand, the father is Dd, the chances are equal that the fetus will inherit D and be Rhesus-positive, or d and be Rhesus-negative, the mother who is dd contributing d in all cases. The practical application of this lies in the fact that if the mother has already been sensitized and borne a child affected with haemolytic disease, it is certain that if the father is homozygous later children will be affected, whereas if he is heterozygous normal children may be born subsequently.

Rhesus sensitization

Since the fetal blood contains a factor which the mother's blood does not possess, an escape of fetal cells into the mother's circulation is capable of stimulating the production of antibodies by the mother. Such transplacental haemorrhages may occur at any time during pregnancy but most large ones take place at delivery. Exactly how transplacental haemorrhage occurs is not clear, and it is certain that in many such matings maternal antibodies are either not produced at all or not produced until several pregnancies have occurred. With the exception of sensitization to the A and B antigens, when the disease is usually mild, and the comparatively rare sensitization to antigens of the Kell, Duffy, or Kidd series, the conditions most likely to produce severe haemolytic disease in a family are sensitization of a Rhesus-negative mother by repeated Rhesus-positive pregnancies or by previous transfusion with Rhesus-positive blood. (Unless an incompatible blood transfusion has been given, less than 10 per cent of Rhesus-negative women become sensitized when the husband is Rhesus-positive.)

Once the mother has become sensitized to Rhesus-positive cells, however, subsequent Rhesus-positive infants are likely to increase the production of maternal antibodies; these are at first agglutinins and may later be incomplete antibodies. (Incomplete antibodies differ from agglutinating antibodies in that they can cross the placental barrier, do not cause agglutination of Rhesus-positive cells suspended in saline, are more thermostable, and persist longer. They combine directly with the Rhesus-positive cells, and are a greater danger to the fetus than are agglutinating antibodies.)

With the mother sensitized, the antibodies she has produced will pass into the fetal circulation, and an antibody–antigen reaction will occur between the maternal antibodies and the fetal Rhesus-positive cells, causing haemolysis of the latter.

It will be seen that since sensitization of the mother is likely to be cumulative, the first children are often unaffected or only slightly affected even if they are Rhesus-positive, and that the disease tends to become more severe with successive pregnancies, though exceptions to this occur.

CLINICAL TYPES. The three major clinical manifestations of the disease are haemolytic anaemia, jaundice, and oedema. These features commonly co-exist in the same infant, but any one of the three may dominate the picture. Erythroblastosis is a frequent but not an invariable finding, and since erythroblastosis may occur in a variety of other diseases during the newborn period, the name 'erythroblastosis fetalis' is not an altogether satisfactory one for the condition.

On the basis of these three manifestations, three clinical types of the disease are recognized, though it must be emphasized that they are not different disease entities.

1. *Congenital haemolytic anaemia.* Here the anaemia is more in evidence than either jaundice or oedema. It may be relatively mild if it occurs in the first child to be affected; before Rhesus-typing of the mother during pregnancy became a routine practice, many of the mild cases were liable to pass unrecognized. In its severer forms, however, haemolysis may occur with remarkable rapidity, leading to profound anaemia which may cause death if untreated.

2. *Icterus gravis neonatorum.* Intense jaundice occurring within one to three days of birth (occasionally manifest actually at the time of birth) is characteristic, and may mask the anaemia with which it is associated. A temporary obstructive phase is common in severe cases. As the jaundice deepens, there is an increasing risk of kernicterus (see p. 60).

3. *Hydrops fetalis.* General oedema of the fetus, which may be sufficient to make normal delivery impossible, is usually only seen when previous children have been affected, or occasionally when the mother has already been sensitized by a transfusion of Rhesus-positive blood. Such infants are commonly stillborn or live only a short time after birth. The placenta is also found to be greatly enlarged and hydropic.

GENERAL FEATURES. In all three types the spleen and liver are likely to be enlarged, and at necropsy these organs and also the kidneys show localized areas of haematopoiesis.

In liveborn infants, whether deeply jaundiced or not, a striking feature is the rapidity with which the haemoglobin level and red-cell count can fall within 24 hours. It is important, therefore, that these infants should be under close observation, with facilities for bilirubin and haemoglobin estimation, until their blood count has stabilized and active haemolysis is no longer likely to occur. The length of time during which maternal antibodies are detectable in the circulation is usually a matter of weeks unless they are removed by exchange transfusion.

Deeply jaundiced infants are likely to show the effects of cholaemia, viz. lethargy, disinclination to suck, and a tendency to haemorrhage. These infants are the ones in whom kernicterus is most liable to occur. A serum bilirubin of approximately 20 mg per 100 ml is regarded as the danger level in term infants but the occurrence of kernicterus will be determined by other factors as well as the bilirubin level, such as the binding capacity of plasma albumin.

DIAGNOSIS. Routine Rhesus-typing during pregnancy will determine which mothers are Rhesus-negative, and though only a small proportion of these are likely to give birth to infants suffering from haemolytic disease, they will form a group requiring special observation. The Rhesus-negative mother's serum should be examined for antibodies at least twice during pregnancy, including examination at first attendance and at the thirty-sixth week in her first pregnancy; in subsequent pregnancies the test should be performed at the thirtieth week in addition. (Repeated examination may serve to demonstrate a rising titre, though in general the titre of maternal antibodies is not a very reliable indication of severity of the disease.) Amniocentesis at the thirty-second week can be used to assess the severity of the condition when a previous child has been affected. In this technique the yellow pigment in the liquor is measured spectroscopically. The results of consecutive estimations are of value as a guide to the need for intrauterine transfusion and to the optimum time for delivery.

At the time of birth, the direct Coombs' test (designed to demonstrate the presence of maternal antibodies in the infant's circulation) should be carried out on the umbilical cord blood. If the test gives a positive reaction, the infant will be affected, although clinical evidence of haemolysis may not appear until some hours or days after birth. The Coombs' test is of great value in diagnosing haemolytic disease, and if this test is negative, and the fetal ABO blood groups compatible with those of the mother, some other cause for neonatal jaundice should be sought (p. 60).

PREVENTION. Selected unsensitized Rhesus-negative women can be protected against sensitization in subsequent pregnancies by the intramuscular injection of 1 ml of anti-D gamma globulin immediately after the birth of a first Rhesus-positive child. The antibody will coat the antigenic sites on any Rhesus-positive cells which have entered her circulation from the fetus and so prevent their stimulating antibody production. The exact indications for this technique are not yet clear but it holds out great hope of diminishing the number of infants affected by haemolytic disease.

When a fetus is severely affected, the likelihood of death *in utero* is high. In carefully selected cases, repeated transfusion of compatible red cells into the fetal peritoneal cavity may allow survival of the fetus until a stage when there is a reasonable prospect of successful treatment after birth.

TREATMENT. Although the mildest cases may recover spontaneously, all infants severely affected at birth are likely to require exchange transfusion though the need may be avoided in a few cases by phototherapy. Neither the mother nor the father is a suitable donor (the father's blood being liable to haemolysis, the mother's containing antibodies). Rhesus-negative blood from a donor who has not been sensitized is therefore required, and must be compatible with the maternal serum, and less than five days old.

Exchange transfusion, by means of which up to 90 per cent of the infants' red cells can be replaced by non-sensitized adult cells thus correcting anaemia and removing some bilirubin and maternal antibody at the same time, has proved a life-saving procedure in severely affected infants, and has greatly reduced the incidence of kernicterus in survivors. There is still considerable difference of opinion as to the indications, optimum time of transfusion and amount of blood to be exchanged. Immediate exchange transfusion via the umbilical vein is employed in some clinics if the Coombs' test is positive and the cord haemoglobin is less than 14·8 g per cent or the unconjugated serum bilirubin is high, e.g. over 7 mg per 100 ml. Others claim equally good results if exchange transfusion is reserved for those cases where the Coombs' test is positive, the cord haemoglobin is less than 10 g per cent and the unconjugated serum bilirubin is more than 4 mg per 100 ml at birth. Subsequently a rising unconjugated serum bilirubin approaching 20 mg per 100 ml will be a further indication for exchange transfusion in term infants and 18 or even 15 mg per 100 ml in pre-term infants. Criteria based on measuring residual binding capacity of plasma albumin may prove more reliable but have not yet come into general use. Exchange transfusion, which is not without risk, requires considerable technical skill. The danger of cardiac failure is greatest in those infants who are severely anaemic, and is increased if the procedure is carried out too rapidly.

At birth it is advisable to clamp the cord at once after the delivery to avoid the further transfusion of approximately 100 ml of placental blood which occurs when the cord is clamped late. Delivery before 37 weeks is generally contraindicated except in selected cases, owing to the increased risk of kernicterus and poorer prognosis in pre-term infants. Infants who are severely anaemic should be digitalized early if there is evidence of incipient cardiac failure.

Since persisting maternal antibodies are likely to cause haemolysis for two to three weeks after birth, and in some cases up to six weeks, it may be necessary to repeat exchange transfusion during the first seven days if the unconjugated serum bilirubin approaches 20 mg per 100 ml, or to give a simple transfusion of packed cells later if the haemoglobin falls below 7·5 g per cent.

PROGNOSIS. There is still an appreciable mortality from haemolytic disease of the newborn, which accounts for about 4 per cent of all perinatal deaths. When modern methods of prevention and treatment are practised, however, the mortality rate is lower and very few infants born alive at term should die. When there is no evidence of central nervous system involvement, the prognosis in those that survive the newborn period is good.

HAEMORRHAGE

Loss of blood is badly supported by the young infant, and may easily prove fatal if it is not promptly recognized and treated. Apart from haemorrhage before delivery or resulting from birth trauma, bleeding may occur from improper clipping or tying of the cord, from a circumcision wound, or as a result of infection, jaundice, or haemorrhagic disease of the newborn, while the vomiting of swallowed maternal blood may cause confusion shortly after birth. Neonatal haemorrhage may be due to thrombocytopenia. This can result from decreased production of platelets, as in congenital leukaemia and primary hypoplastic disorders, or from increased destruction of platelets by maternal antibody, as in idiopathic thrombocytopenic purpura of the mother or platelet incompatibility with isoimmunization. Sequestration of platelets in a large haemangioma is a very occasional cause of thrombocytopenia in the newborn period. Haemophilia is rarely responsible for haemorrhage at this age.

Bleeding from the umbilical cord

Bleeding due to a loosely tied or slipped ligature, or to tearing of the cord by a clip, is a danger immediately after birth, and the stump should be inspected frequently. Bleeding may occur later from the same site as a result of local sepsis. If any considerable loss of blood has occurred, transfusion will be necessary.

Infection

Any severe neonatal infection may cause haemorrhage, and treatment is that of the infection with replacement of blood if necessary. Cytomegalic inclusion disease is a rare cause of purpura with jaundice.

Jaundice

Deep jaundice from any cause is likely to result in an increased tendency to bleed, particularly in the case of pre-term infants. Even physiological jaundice when more than slight is a contraindication to operations such as circumcision which can be delayed until after the jaundice has faded.

Vaginal haemorrhage

Although bleeding from the vagina may be due to any of the causes mentioned, a blood-stained vaginal discharge occurring shortly after birth is usually an effect of maternal hormones in the circulation, and is not regarded as pathological.

Haemorrhagic disease of the newborn

Haemorrhage, which is commonly external but which may also involve closed cavities, occurs on the third or fourth day of life (more rarely the second or fifth). It is typically associated with a prolonged coagulation time and a fall in the prothrombin level of the blood.

The condition is by no means clearly defined, but probably comprises a number of different coagulation defects caused by accentuation of the various clotting factor deficiencies normally present in the newborn infant.

Bleeding may occur from any site, the most common manifestations being melaena, haematemesis, bleeding from the umbilical cord or vagina, and haematuria. The onset is sudden, and when bleeding occurs from the gastro-intestinal tract, the infant either vomits bright blood or passes a bloody stool which is readily distinguished from meconium by the blood-staining of the napkin around it. When the amount of blood lost is considerable the infant will show evidence of shock and pallor.

Bleeding into closed cavities is fortunately rarer; there may be delay in its recognition, and the prognosis is considerably worse than in the case of external haemorrhage.

TREATMENT. The injection of phytomenadione (vitamin K_1) will raise the prothrombin level of the blood, and will usually control haemorrhage within 6 to 12 hours. The dosage is 1 mg intramuscularly, repeated if necessary.

When the infant has lost any considerable amount of blood, however, as may occur in bleeding from the gastro-intestinal tract when there is a time-lag before the blood is vomited or passed by rectum, or in the occasional case of haemorrhagic disease which is not responsive to phytomenadione, blood transfusion is required. The urgent indications for this will be collapse, pallor, and rapid pulse, but it is much safer to transfuse early than to risk delay and possible collapse later. The blood should be fresh, since the prothrombin content falls when blood is kept for any length of time.

The prognosis in cases with external bleeding is good, if the condition is recognized and treated promptly; even without treatment a proportion of the milder cases would recover spontaneously. When haemorrhage occurs into a closed cavity, the mortality is high.

NEONATAL TETANY

Convulsions, twitching or laryngeal and carpopedal spasm associated with low serum calcium and raised phosphorus occasionally occur in artificially-fed infants during the first two weeks of life. The etiology is still obscure, but is thought to be related to excessive phosphorus intake during cow's-milk feeding and to relative parathyroid insufficiency. Symptoms are relieved by the administration of calcium, and the prognosis is good.

Rarely, similar signs may be due to hypomagnesaemia and corrected by the injection of magnesium sulphate intramuscularly.

SKIN AND SUBCUTANEOUS TISSUE

In addition to infection (p. 57) and congenital defect (p. 124), there are several conditions of the skin or subcutaneous tissue which are particularly liable to occur in the newborn period, though not in all instances limited to this age.

Localized fat necrosis

Areas of fat necrosis may become obvious at about the third week of life, and appear as localized depressed areas, situated over the masseters, shoulders, or buttocks. The infants are usually well nourished and otherwise healthy. In most, if not all instances, the fat necrosis occurs as the result of localized pressure during delivery. Spontaneous recovery is the rule within two to four months.

Sclerema

This condition represents a more or less extensive change in the subcutaneous fat, which becomes hardened and has a lard-like consistency. The overlying skin is not involved in the process, but often appears waxy or livid. The areas most commonly involved are the extremities, cheeks, buttocks, and back. The onset is usually within the first two weeks of life, and small feeble infants are those most likely to be affected. In some cases the condition follows prolonged hypothermia.

On palpation, the lesions are strikingly hard and are obviously subcutaneous although the skin may be firmly adherent to them. They are discrete, non-tender, and non-fluctuant. The absence of pitting is characteristic. Affected infants show apathy, subnormal temperature, and anorexia.

TREATMENT. The infant should be nursed in an incubator, and antibiotics used if there is any evidence of infection. Cortisone is thought to be of value in treatment. Although many affected infants succumb, it is possible for the condition to regress under treatment.

Oedema neonatorum

Much confusion exists in the literature between this condition and sclerema. It is unfortunate that the term scleroedema has been introduced, since it is used by different authors to describe sclerema, sclerema plus oedema, or oedema.

Oedema in the newborn period is liable to occur in small feeble infants, and in those who have undergone severe chilling. Often the oedema affects the extremities, particularly the feet and calves. It is often harder than the oedema commonly seen in later age periods, but unlike sclerema, pits on firm pressure. The skin can be raised from the subcutaneous tissue.

The prognosis is not necessarily serious, though some of the more feeble infants in whom it occurs are likely to succumb from other causes. The possible relationship to hypoproteinaemia has been mentioned (p. 51). Generalized oedema is occasionally due to cardiac failure or, in females, to Turner's syndrome.

Napkin rash (*Ammoniacal dermatitis*)

A rash occurring in the napkin-area, affecting the inner surface of the thighs, the buttocks, and genitalia, is common during early infancy; it is erythematous at first but may become ulcerated and secondarily infected. Napkin rash is due in most instances to irritation from contact with napkins soaked with ammoniacal urine, or in some cases napkins that have been washed in soda. Occasionally a rash in this area may be due to thrush.

Local treatment consists of the application of benzalkonium cream. The napkins must be frequently changed and the infant carefully dried after bathing.

Intertrigo

Intertrigo is closely similar to the above, but occurs in the flexures, particularly of the groins and neck, of fat and dirty babies. It varies in severity from an erythema to exuding and crusted lesions, which may become secondarily infected. Treatment consists of general hygiene, frequent bathing, and the application of calamine lotion or dusting powder.

Milia

Minute yellowish-white vesicles situated on the nose or cheeks are extremely common in the newborn infant. They represent small cysts, but require no treatment and disappear spontaneously.

Miliaria

A rash consisting of innumerable red papules or vesicles, of pin-head size, may occur as the result of excessive perspiration; it is commonly followed by desquamation.

If the cause is recognized, the rash responds rapidly to bathing and the application of a bland lotion or dusting powder.

Erythema toxicum

Erythema toxicum may appear during the first week and consists of minute raised white spots on an erythematous base. Histologically the lesions contain large numbers of eosinophil leucocytes. The eruption quickly disappears without treatment.

Drug rashes

Although relatively uncommon in the newborn period, drug rashes are occasionally seen as the result of medication given to the infant (penicillin, phenobarbitone) or more rarely due to the secretion of drugs in the milk of a nursing mother.

INFANTS OF DIABETIC MOTHERS

In pre-insulin days the fertility rate of diabetic women was extremely low (1 to 6 per cent); if pregnancy did occur, both perinatal and maternal mortality rates were high, the latter having been estimated as approximately 30 per cent. With the introduction of insulin, the fertility rate increased greatly and the maternal mortality fell to less than 1 per cent. Unfortunately the perinatal mortality has not shown a corresponding general improvement, being still about 20 per cent overall, with stillbirths outnumbering first-week deaths. A lower rate may be expected when diabetic control is good, but when there is poor antenatal supervision the mortality will be substantially higher. The obstetric histories of diabetic mothers also show a high perinatal mortality in the pre-diabetic period and a high incidence of overweight infants. In fact, a history of one or more infants weighing over 5 kg at birth will sometimes reveal an early diabetic state in the mother which has been unsuspected clinically.

It is probable that the abnormal weight attained by these infants is due largely to subcutaneous fat resulting from increased fetal insulin-secretion in response to maternal hyperglycaemia. Necropsy often reveals beta-cell hyperplasia in the islets of Langerhans and their increased production of insulin can be demonstrated at birth. Infants born to diabetic mothers remove glucose from their plasma more rapidly than do infants of normal mothers and so become hypoglycaemic more quickly. The high neonatal mortality cannot be explained on the basis of hypoglycaemia, however, since correction of hypoglycaemia does not necessarily ensure survival.

The infants are often delivered before term, with the result that an infant may weigh more than 3 kg at birth and yet be very immature. When control of maternal diabetes is excellent, the infant at birth often appears little different from normal though he may be fat and rather plethoric. With less good control, these features are more pronounced and the baby may be cyanotic and shocked. In some cases respiration is established with difficulty and hyaline membrane disease may follow. Even those infants who first appear well may subsequently develop sudden apnoeic attacks, with or without convulsions, so that careful observation is essential in all cases. Surviving children grow satisfactorily but show an increased incidence of diabetes and of major congenital malformations.

TREATMENT. The maternal diabetic condition should be strictly controlled throughout pregnancy, and the mother should be in hospital for several weeks before the expected date of delivery. The frequency with which intrauterine death occurs in late pregnancy, the large size of the fetus and the poor fetal tolerance of prolonged or complicated labour led to Caesarean section commonly being practised at about the thirty-seventh week of gestation, and this is still advocated for primiparous women. The smaller size of the infant and the improved survival rate which have followed very strict carbohydrate control in pregnancy, however, now make induced vaginal delivery practicable in an increasing percentage of cases. Immediately after delivery, the infant's stomach should be aspirated to remove swallowed liquor, any necessary resuscitation given, and vitamin K_1 administered. For the first few days the infant should be nursed in an incubator and must be under continuous supervision. If respiratory distress appears, the treatment outlined on page 50 is indicated. Early hypoglycaemia may be countered by intravenous glucose or fructose. Glucose-water feeds are started at 6 hours if the infant's condition is satisfactory. Inhalation of fluid may occur if the infant is fed too early, but dehydration and jaundice become more marked if feeding is commenced late. Milk feeds may follow the conclusion of 12 hours successful feeding with glucose-water. Infants who survive this period usually progress normally in the absence of severe congenital malformation.

CONGENITAL ABNORMALITIES

These are considered in more detail in Chapter 5. Since many congenital abnormalities prove fatal in the newborn period unless promptly recognized, and others are incompatible with a prolonged extrauterine life, they assume a particular importance at this time. The possibility of a malformation should always be borne in mind when there is hydramnios, a single umbilical artery or a family history of congenital abnormalities. Every newborn infant should be carefully examined as soon as possible after birth to determine the presence of any correctable abnormality, and particular attention paid to the following signs during the first two days of life.

Failure to pass meconium

Atresia of the gastro-intestinal tract at any site (duodenum, ileum, rectum, or anus) is usually associated with failure to pass meconium, although excretion of a little pale material does not rule the diagnosis out. In low obstruction, there is progressive abdominal distension and vomiting occurs late. Straight X-ray shows dilated loops of bowel and areas without gas shadows, giving some indication of the probable level of obstruction. Prompt surgical intervention will be required if the infant is to survive. Constipation with abdominal distension may also be due to meconium ileus, Hirschsprung's disease or, in ill pre-term infants, functional ileus or necrotizing entero-colitis. In this last, there may be small blood-stained stools and the bowel may perforate, leading to peritonitis and death.

Vomiting

Although normal infants may vomit liquor or blood swallowed during delivery, persistent vomiting during the first two days of life, unless due to intracranial injury or infection, should suggest the possibility of obstruction. If the vomitus is forceful and bile-stained, stenosis or atresia of the duodenum below the ampulla of Vater, and volvulus, are the most likely causes. The vomiting of pyloric stenosis very seldom occurs before the second or third week of life and the vomitus is not bile-stained. Obstruction may also occur from strangulated hernia, meconium ileus, intussusception, Hirschsprung's disease, and atresia of the lower bowel. Occasionally the neonatal intestine is obstructed by the curds of dried milk. A straight X-ray will often indicate the site of the obstruction, since if it is complete the gut below it will contain little or no air. If a contrast medium is used, gastrografin is now generally preferred.

Failure to pass urine

During the first 24 hours this may be normal if the bladder has been emptied during delivery, but should suggest the possibility of obstruction of the urinary tract. If obstruction is the cause, it is likely to have given rise to hydronephrosis during intrauterine life.

Cyanosis

Deep cyanosis persisting after delivery, in the absence of evidence of intracranial injury or respiratory difficulty, is most likely to be due to congenital malformation of the heart.

When deep cyanosis occurs immediately after a feed, it may be due to the presence of a tracheo-oesophageal fistula or to a diaphragmatic hernia, though the former should be suspected before a feed is given by a history of hydramnios and the bubbling of mucus from the

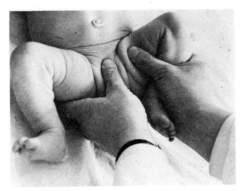
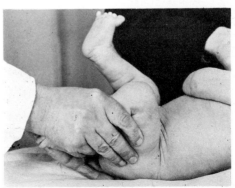

Fig. 4.23 & Fig. 4.24   The test for congenital dislocation of hip.

mouth and nose. In the case of diaphragmatic hernia the cyanosis is sometimes dramatically relieved by a change of position, e.g. holding the infant face downward.

Failure to suck

While this may be due to general causes such as immaturity or shock, failure to suck should call for special examination of the mouth to exclude thrush, cleft-palate, hypomandibulosis, or other deformities of the mouth or jaws. Nasal obstruction is also a possible cause, while mental subnormality is often first suspected by the infant's reaction to feeding.

Instability of hips

Routine examination of the hips should be carried out on all newborn infants, particular attention being paid to females and infants born by the breech and to any family history of hip dislocation. With the baby supine the hip is flexed to a right angle with the examiner's middle finger over the greater trochanter and thumb on the medial aspect of the thigh. The hip is then slowly abducted and if it is dislocated, the head of the femur can be lifted into the acetabulum by presure with the middle finger, sometimes producing a noticeable and palpable 'clunk' as the head snaps over the socket wall (*Ortolani's sign*) (see also p. 129).

BIBLIOGRAPHY AND REFERENCES

AHUJA, G. L., WILLOUGHBY, M. L. N., KERR, M. M. & HUTCHISON, J. H. (1969). Massive subaponeurotic haemorrhage in infants born by vacuum extraction. *British Medical Journal* iii, 743.

AMERICAN ACADEMY OF PEDIATRICS (1964). *Standards and Recommendations for Hospital Care of Newborn Infants.*

AMERICAN ACADEMY OF PEDIATRICS (1967). Nomenclature for duration of gestation, birth weight and intrauterine growth. *Pediatrics, Springfield* 39, 935.

AVERY, M. E. (1968). *The Lung and Its Disorders in the Newborn Infant*, 2nd edn. Philadelphia: Saunders.

BANKER, B. Q. (1967). Neuropathological effects of anoxia and hypoglycaemia in the newborn. *Developmental Medicine and Child Neurology* 9, 544.

BARRIE, H. (1963). Resuscitation of the newborn. *Lancet* i, 650.

BIRNBAUM, G., LYNCH, J. I., MARGILETH, A. M., LONERGAN. W. M. & SEVER, J. L. (1969). Cytomegalovirus infections in newborn infants. *Journal of Pediatrics* 75, 789.

BLATTNER, R. J. (1961). Syphilis is still a problem. *Journal of Pediatrics* 59, 625.

BRITISH MEDICAL JOURNAL (1970). Transmission of toxoplasmosis. i, 126.

BRYANT, G. M., GRAY, O. P., FRASER, A. J. & ACKERMAN, A. (1970). Fate of surviving low birth-weight infants with coagulation deficiencies on the first day of life. *British Medical Journal* iv, 707.

BUTLER, N. R. & BONHAM, D. G. (1963). *Perinatal Mortality*. Edinburgh: Livingstone.

COLTART, T. M., TRICKEY, N. R. A. & BEARD, R. W. (1969). Foetal blood sampling. *British Medical Journal* i, 342.

CORNER, B. (1960). *Prematurity: The Diagnosis, Care and Disorders of the Premature Infant*. London: Cassell.

CRACCO, J. B., DOWER, J. C. & HARRIS, L. E. (1965). Bilirubin metabolism in the newborn. *Proceedings of Staff Meetings of the Mayo Clinic* 40, 868.

CROSS, K. W. & DAWES, G. S. (1966). The fetus and the newborn: recent research. *British Medical Bulletin* 22, 1.

DAWKINS, M. & MACGREGOR, W. G. (1965). *Gestational Age, Size and Maturity*. London: Heinemann.

DRILLIEN, C. M. (1964). *The Growth and Development of the Prematurely Born Infant*. Edinburgh: Livingstone.

DUDGEON, J. A. (1967). Maternal rubella and its effect on the fetus. *Archives of Disease in Childhood* 42, 110.

FARQUHAR, J. W. (1965). The influence of maternal diabetes on fetus and child. In *Recent Advances in Paediatrics*, 3rd edn. Edited by D. Gairdner. London: Churchill.

FARQUHAR, J. W. (1969). Prognosis for babies born to diabetic mothers in Edinburgh. *Archives of Disease in Childhood* 44, 36.

FINLAY, H. V. L., MAUDSLEY, R. H. & BUSFIELD, P. I. (1967). Dislocatable hip and dislocated hip in the newborn infant. *British Medical Journal* iv, 377.

FINN, R., WALKER, W. & ELLIS, M. I. (1970). *Rh* haemolytic disease. *British Medical Journal* ii, 219.

FORFAR, J. O., GOULD, J. C. & MacCABE, A. F. (1968). Effect of hexachlorophane on incidence of staphylococcal and Gram-negative infection in the newborn. *Lancet* ii, 177.

GRIN, E. I. (1953). Epidemiology and control of endemic syphilis. *World Health Organization Monograph Series*, no. 11.

HODGMAN, H. E., MIKITY, V. G., TATTER, D. & CLELAND, R. S. (1969). Wilson-Mikity syndrome. *Pediatrics, Springfield* 44, 179.

HORGER, E. O. & HUTCHINSON, D. L. (1969). Diagnostic use of amniotic fluid. *Journal of Pediatrics* 75, 503.

HUGHESDON, M. R. (1946). Congenital tuberculosis. *Archives of Diseases in Childhood* 21, 121.

HULL, D. (1971). Asphyxia neonatorum. In *Recent Advances in Paediatrics*, 4th edn. Edited by D. Gairdner and D. Hull. London: Churchill.

JAMES, L. S. (1966). Symposium on the newborn. *Pediatric Clinics of North America* 13, 573, 943.

JAMES, L. S. (1967). Scientific basis for current perinatal care. *Archives of Disease in Childhood* 42, 457.

KEEN, J. H. (1969). Hypoglycaemia in neonatal convulsions. *Archives of Disease in Childhood* 44, 356.

LANCET (1970). Phototherapy for neonatal jaundice. i, 825.

LANCET (1971). Jaundice of the newborn and phenobarbitone. i, 119.

LANDSTEINER, K. & WIENER, A. S. (1940). *Proceedings of the Society for Experimental Biology and Medicine* 43, 223.

MCDONALD, A. (1967). *Children of Very Low Birth Weight*. London: Heinemann.

MACGREGOR, A. R. (1960). *Pathology of Infancy and Childhood*. Edinburgh: Livingstone.

MORISON, J. E. (1970). *Foetal and Neonatal Pathology*, 3rd edn. London: Butterworths.

NELIGAN, G. A. (1965). Idiopathic hypoglycaemia in the newborn. In *Recent Advances in Paediatrics*, 3rd edn. Edited by D. Gairdner. London: Churchill.

NELSON, N. M. (1970). On the etiology of hyaline membrane disease. *Pediatric Clinics of North America* 17, 943.

OSKI, F. A. & NAIMAN, J. L. (1966). *Hematologic Problems in the Newborn*. Philadelphia: Saunders.

POCHEDLY, C. (1971). Thrombocytopenic purpura of the newborn. *Obstetrical and Gynecological Survey* 26, 61.

REYNOLDS, E. O. R., ROBERTON, N. R. C. & WIGGLESWORTH, J. S. (1968). Hyaline membrane disease, respiratory distress and surfactant deficiency. *Pediatrics, Springfield* 42, 758.

REYNOLDS, E. O. R. (1970). Hyaline membrane disease. *American Journal of Obstetrics and Gynecology* 106, 780.

ROBINSON, R. J. (1966). Assessment of gestational age by neurological examination. *Archives of Disease in Childhood* 41, 437.

SEVER, J. L. (1969). Cytomegalovirus infections in newborn infants. *Journal of Pediatrics* 75, 789.

SEVER, J. L. (1969). Immunological responses to perinatal infections. *Journal of Pediatrics* 75, 1111.

SMITH, C. A. (1959). *The Physiology of the Newborn Infant*, 3rd edn. Oxford: Blackwell.

TANNER, J. M. (1970). Standards for birth weight or intrauterine growth. *Pediatrics, Springfield* 46, 1.

THOMSON, A. M., BILLEWICZ, W. Z. & HYTTEN, F. E. (1968). The assessment of fetal growth. *Journal of Obstetrics and Gynecology of the British Commonwealth* 75, 903.

TIZARD, J. P. M. (1964). Neuromuscular disorders in infancy. In *Disorders of Voluntary Muscle*. Edited by J. N. Walton. London: Churchill.

TOWBIN, A. (1970). Central nervous system damage in the human fetus and newborn infant. *American Journal of Diseases of Children* 119, 529.

WALKER, W. (1961). Early exchange transfusion. *British Medical Journal* ii, 1513.

WORLD HEALTH ORGANIZATION (1964). Endemic treponematoses of childhood. *WHO Chronicle* 18, 403.

WORLD HEALTH ORGANIZATION (1970). The prevention of perinatal mortality and morbidity. *WHO Technical Report Series*, no. 457.

5 Congenital Malformations

This title includes all the disorders of structural development which arise during fetal life but not abnormalities which are the direct result of the birth process. In discussing incidence, the type and degree of malformation must be stated, since the inclusion of minor defects or of disorders demonstrable only in later life which are considered to have a congenital basis will greatly increase the rate. The incidence of major congenital malformations in Britain is approximately 15 per 1000 total births, though later recognition of some not apparent in the newborn period will increase this rate to over 20 per 1000.

Congenital malformations represent an important cause of abortion, stillbirth, and neonatal death. At least 20 per cent of human zygotes are lost in early pregnancy and as many as one-third of these have chromosomal or structural abnormalities. Infants who survive the neonatal period may succumb later as the direct or indirect result of their deformity, or may carry a more or less severe disability throughout life. The stillbirths and first-week deaths from this cause therefore only represent a fraction of the total interference with health for which congenital malformations are responsible, but even so form a hard core of perinatal mortality (approximately 6 per 1000 births) which has not reflected the general reduction in infant deaths from other causes. Of low birth-weight infants dying in the first week, approximately 20 per cent are likely to show congenital malformation.

It has already been emphasized that because a condition is 'congenital', i.e. present during fetal life, it is not necessarily due to any single etiological factor. This is true of congenital malformations, and many of the observations which have been made with reference to 'constitution' apply to them. Thus there are congenital malformations which are clearly genetically determined; others which are due to maternal medication, radiation, or intrauterine infection; and others again which are almost certainly due to mechanical causes. It is also clear that different causes may produce similar malformations, environmentally-induced imitations of genetic defects being called *phenocopies*. The great majority of malformations, however, are of multifactorial etiology, caused by the interaction of several genetic and environmental factors, which can seldom be identified. Congenital deformities can be produced not only by abnormalities of development but also by degeneration of pre-formed structures in later pregnancy under the influence of factors such as infection or irradiation.

In the present state of knowledge, no classification of congenital malformations on a strictly etiological basis can be complete, while a purely morphological classification is equally inadequate. The more important etiological factors will therefore be considered individually and, where possible, illustrated by malformations occurring in different systems. From the morphological viewpoint, the following classification provides a means of grouping malformations which may have some practical value.

1. FAILURES OF DEVELOPMENT
   (*a*) Complete absence of an organ or part of an organ—e.g. anencephaly, absence of digits, single kidney.
   (*b*) Small size of an organ or part of an organ—e.g. microcephaly, hypomandibulosis, microphthalmos, micromelia.
2. FAILURES OF FUSION—e.g. cleft lip, cleft palate, spina bifida.
3. FAILURES OF DIFFERENTIATION—e.g. syndactyly, fusion of ribs, horseshoe kidney.
4. FAILURES OF ATROPHY—e.g. imperforate anus due to persistent anal plate, urethral valves, persistent inguinal hernial sac, Meckel's diverticulum, thyroglossal cysts, branchial cysts.
5. FAILURES OF INVAGINATION—e.g. absence of anus or vulva.
6. FAILURES OF MIGRATION—e.g. pilonidal sinus, undescended testicle, ectopic thyroid, malrotation of the intestine.
7. FAILURES OF CANALIZATION—e.g. hypospadias, congenital atresia of bile-ducts.
8. REDUPLICATION—e.g. polydactyly, cervical rib, double ureter.
9. HYPERTROPHY—e.g. local gigantism of digits, hemihypertrophy, adrenal hypertrophy with pseudohermaphroditism, congenital pyloric stenosis.
10. UNCONTROLLED GROWTH—e.g. angioma, hamartomas. (Malignant tumours present at birth are considered in Chapter 9.)
11. ABERRANT DEVELOPMENT AND DISPLACEMENT
Under this heading may be included a variety of malformations in which an organ has developed in a manner which is atypical, but which does not fall into one of the above categories, e.g. cystic fibrosis of pancreas, or where otherwise normal tissue is found in an abnormal position, e.g.

gastric mucosa in a Meckel's diverticulum, or where a whole organ or part of an organ is displaced. Congenital dextrocardia is perhaps better described as a displacement than a failure of migration, while other congenital cardiac abnormalities may combine displacement, e.g. transposition of the great vessels, with one or more of the morphological types described above.

It is comparatively common to find an association of several congenital malformations in the same subject; these may have a common etiology but do not necessarily fall into the same morphological categories.

Detection of congenital abnormalities before birth may be possible by radiology or by examination of cells from amniotic fluid. A family history of malformation or the presence of hydramnios raises the possibility of the infant's being malformed. In the neonate, a single transverse palmar crease and a single umbilical artery are both associated with increased frequency of congenital malformations and a high perinatal mortality.

Early diagnosis may be important in instituting prompt therapy or in genetic counselling. Parents who have had one affected child should receive informed advice to help them decide about future pregnancies. Although the risk of a second malformed infant is high in only a few conditions, genetic counselling should always be based on sound appraisal of all the available information, and in difficult cases the advice of an expert geneticist should be sought.

ETIOLOGICAL FACTORS
Genotype

From what has been said of the genetic constitution of the individual it will be clear that certain congenital malformations are likely to be genetically determined. Amongst those that have been most systematically studied from this angle are the inherited abnormalities of the skin, which have the advantage of being readily visible and recognizable in forebears and collaterals; cleft lip and cleft palate; mongolism (Down's syndrome); and anencephaly, meningomyelocele, etc. In such studies the inherent difficulties of human genetics at once become obvious. For example, the chances of survival from particular abnormalities may be radically altered within a generation. Thus the introduction of Caesarean section has made it possible for female achondroplastics to bear living children, while the treatment of congenital pyloric stenosis has so improved during the past 50 years that a much higher proportion of affected infants is likely to survive and procreate than previously.

Since it is easy to overlook minor manifestations of many malformations (e.g. oxycephaly, arachnodactyly, osteopetrosis), it is understandable that many of the earlier pedigrees published are inaccurate where the incidence of the disease in collaterals is based on hearsay or has not been confirmed by radiological or other special examinations. The number of congenital malformations of which we can state with certainty (a) that they are genetically determined and (b) the manner in which they are transmitted, is therefore much less than might be expected. But the number is nevertheless considerable, and it is probably true that genetic constitution accounts for more congenital malformation than does any other single factor.

Chromosome defects

The establishment of techniques for the direct examination of human chromosome structure has already demonstrated the relationship of certain abnormalities of chromosome number or structure with specific malformations or syndromes. Thus Turner's syndrome and Klinefelter's syndrome (p. 212) are likely to show an abnormal number of sex chromosomes, which can generally be demonstrated by counting the nuclear chromatin bodies in cells from a buccal smear, the number being one less than the number of X chromosomes. Of the autosomal chromosome defects, trisomy of chromosome 21 (giving a total of 47 chromosomes, or more rarely 46 if the additional 21 becomes translocated and joined to one of another chromosome pair) is most important, since it is associated with mongolism (Down's syndrome, p. 114), and is relatively common. Trisomy 18 is characterized by poor fetal growth, malformation of the heart and ears, flexion and overlapping of the fingers, a small jaw and a short sternum. Trisomy 13–15 may be suspected when an infant has abnormalities of the eyes, especially anophthalmia, with capillary haemangioma of the forehead, cleft lip and palate, and other malformations. Infants with autosomal trisomies are generally mentally subnormal and seldom survive long. Deletion of fragments of chromosomes has been found in some malformed children. In the 'cri-du-chat' syndrome, characterized by low birth weight, a weak 'mewing' cry, microcephaly and hypertelorism, there is partial deletion of the short arm of a chromosome 5. An increasing number of syndromes associated with chromosome defects is being recognized.

Mechanical factors

Pressure on the fetus (associated with oligohydramnios) results in a variety of deformities which can best be understood if the newborn infant is refolded into the position he has occupied *in utero*. Of the commoner deformities,

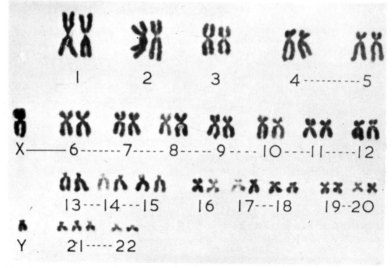

Fig. 5.1   Karyotype of a male mongol (Down's syndrome) showing trisomy 21 and XY chromosomes. (Courtesy of Professor P. Polani.)

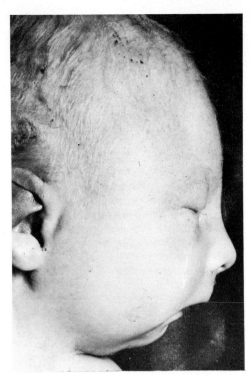

Fig. 5.2   Micrognathia in trisomy 18.

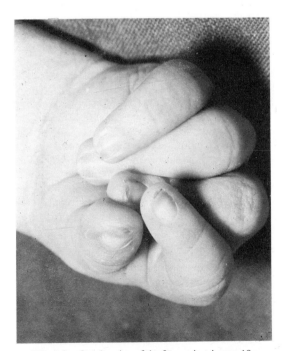

Fig. 5.3   Overlapping of the fingers in trisomy 18.

talipes equino-varus is most logically explained by pressure on the crossed legs, the foot that has been on the outer side being invariably more affected than the inner one. The occurrence of increased intrauterine pressure is often suggested by the presence of dimples over bony points or thinning of the skin at the site of local pressure.

Infection

Rubella occurring during the first three months of pregnancy may cause a variety of congenital deformities, of which malformations of the eye, ear, and heart are the most common (p. 35). The infection must occur during the period of organogenesis if it is to have an effect on the development of the organ, and hence infections occurring later in pregnancy will not affect the fetus in the same way. Other maternal viral infections occurring during the early months of pregnancy can have similar effects. Fetal infection with toxoplasmosis or cyto-megalic inclusion disease occurring after the early period of organogenesis can also produce malformations such as hydrocephalus and micro-cephaly, but these are due to changes in organs already formed, though still undergoing some differentiation.

Maternal medication

It is well recognized that maternal poisoning, e.g. with carbon monoxide or barbiturates in cases of attempted suicide in early pregnancy, might be followed by fetal malformation, probably as the result of severe hypoxia. More recently it has been shown that certain drugs administered in therapeutic dosage to the mother during the first three months of pregnancy may also be responsible for fetal malformation. The widespread use of thalidomide in Germany and Britain was followed by the birth of a large number of infants showing severe deformities of the limbs (micromelia, phocomelia, etc.), associated with naevi of the upper lip. The proprietary preparation of thalidomide has been withdrawn from the British market in consequence. There is suggestive evidence that other drugs, e.g. mer-captopurine, cyclophosphamide and aminopterin, are also teratogenic. Malformations attributed to salicylates may have been caused by the illness for which the drug was given. Androgens and the androgenic progestagens given to the mother may cause masculinization of the female fetus, while thiouracil may produce goitre.

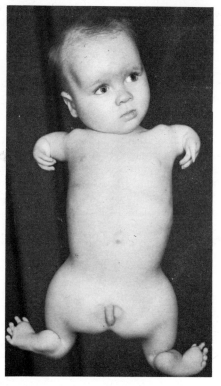

Fig. 5.4 Infant of mother who had received thalidomide during early pregnancy, showing characteristic deformities of limbs.

Maternal age and parity

It is well known that mongolism is more frequently observed amongst infants born towards the end of the reproductive period than amongst children of young mothers. The incidence per 1000 births increases in the offspring of mothers aged 30 and over, and rises steeply in those where the maternal age is over 40. Twin studies, now confirmed by chromosome examination (see above), have indicated that the ovum is at fault, and it is reasonable to suppose that there is a greater likelihood of abnormal ova being produced by elderly than by young women unless the latter themselves show translocation of chromosome 21.

Primogeniture appears to be related to the incidence of certain congenital abnormalities such as pyloric stenosis, and possibly also to that of anencephaly and spina bifida, but multiparity is generally regarded as a more important etiological factor in the majority of congenital malformations.

Hydramnios

Maternal hydramnios is frequently associated with abnormality of the fetus, particularly anencephaly and tracheo-oesophageal fistula, but it cannot be assumed from this that hydramnios is itself responsible for congenital malformation. It is more probable that fetal abnormality is responsible for hydramnios, or that both are due to the same etiological factors.

Hormonal factors

The infants of diabetic, or pre-diabetic, mothers are often abnormally large and the neonatal mortality of such infants is high (p. 68). In addition to this congenital inferiority, the incidence of congenital malformations amongst them has been found to be higher than amongst the offspring of non-diabetic mothers. Congenital abnormality of the genital organs can be produced by abnormal hormones from hyperplastic fetal adrenal glands. Rare cases have been described where a similar endocrine disorder has appeared in both parent and child (e.g. exophthalmic goitre, precocious puberty).

Irradiation

Exposure of the embryo to ionizing radiation during the early phases of development may produce malformation of the tissues which would normally be most active immediately following exposure. While most of our knowledge of the effects of such exposure comes from animal experiment, malformations have inadvertently been produced in the human embryo by excessive irradiation of the pelvis during pregnancy. Now that the dangers are recognized, congenital malformations from this cause should be almost entirely avoidable.

A more serious risk to the community is the danger that irradiation of the gonads of either parent may result in mutation of genes. Since such mutations are more likely to result in recessive than in dominant characters, it may take several generations for congenital abnormalities to appear.

Nutritional factors

Animal experiment again has shown that nutritional deprivation in early pregnancy can produce congenital malformations of the eyes, ears, and palate (Kalter and Warkany, 1959). In human subjects, however, the degree of deprivation in early pregnancy will seldom if ever be comparable to the experimental diets employed in animals. There is little direct evidence that nutritional factors are a significant cause of human congenital malformations but several studies have shown higher malformation rates among infants of poorly nourished mothers than among those of mothers on good diets.

Other factors

There remain many cases of congenital malformation where the causation is at present unknown. There is little evidence that social factors materially influence the incidence of most malformations, since there is no constant variation in the death-rate from this cause between social classes. Defects of the central nervous system may show a marked social class distribution, however, having a higher incidence in the lower income groups in Scotland, though not in Birmingham or South Wales.

In spite of the inherent difficulties of prospective studies of the first trimester of human pregnancy, the advances which have already been made in knowledge of embryology and fetal growth during the present century provide considerable cause for optimism. With a clearer understanding of the etiology of congenital malformations, there is at least a hope that the mortality and disability from this cause may ultimately be reduced.

UNDIFFERENTIATED TWINS

Although considerable confusion has existed in the older literature between teratomata, which should be regarded as neoplasms (Chapter 10), and undifferentiated twins, there should be no real difficulty in distinguishing the two conditions. True fusion of twins is rare. When it occurs, the organs of a second individual are clearly recognizable. In the most striking examples, two infants, both more or less completely formed, are joined anteriorly or laterally. In a few instances (e.g. the famous Siamese twins) both have been liveborn and survived for many years. More commonly, both are stillborn or die shortly after birth, although separation in selected cases is now a surgical possibility.

In other instances, one twin, or part of a twin, is much smaller than the other and is carried as an appendage having no separate viability on the chest or side of the other. Again, there may be incomplete differentiation of the heads of the two infants, or one may be incompletely represented.

MULTIPLE MALFORMATIONS

In some cases, congenital malformations are multiple and so gross as to be incompatible with life. When several organs are actively differentiating and therefore equally sensitive to teratogenic action, multiple primary malformations are likely to occur. These are commonly associated with hypoplasia of the whole body and may be due to chromosomal abnormalities, occasionally constituting recognizable syndromes (see p. 74). In other cases, a primary defect leads to secondary maldevelopment of other organs. Such single primary defects are usually of polygenic origin, e.g. anencephaly, in which defective formation of the neural tube gives rise to multiple secondary abnormalities such as malformation of brain and skull, cleft palate and hypoplasia of adrenal and pituitary glands.

CONGENITAL MALFORMATIONS OF THE MOUTH AND GASTRO-INTESTINAL TRACT

Cleft lip (Hare-lip)

This is one of the commoner malformations, occurring either alone or in association with cleft palate, and not infrequently with other malformations. There is frequently a familial incidence.

The deformity varies in degree from a slight notching of the red margin of the lip to left or right of the mid-line, to a complete cleft running up to the nostril. When the cleft is bilateral and combined with complete cleft palate (see below), the premaxilla is displaced forward (Fig. 5.5). Since the cleft or clefts follow the normal lines of fusion, it is extremely rare for a cleft lip to be central.

Repair of cleft lip is usually undertaken early,

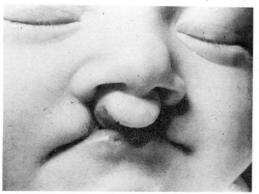

Fig. 5.5   Bilateral cleft lip and palate.

and may be carried out after the first two months of life if the infant is thriving. With skilled surgery, the cosmetic results are often remarkably good even in cases with bilateral clefts and displacement of the premaxilla.

Cleft palate

Failure of fusion in the midline of the roof of the mouth may occur independently of cleft lip, and is then much less likely to be a heredo-familial disorder. The cleft may be of any magnitude, from a bifurcation of the uvula extending only a short distance into the soft palate, and causing little disability, to one involving the hard palate and so allowing communication between the mouth and nose. Where the cleft is complete, and involves the alveolar ridge, it will pass anteriorly to the left or right of the midline. When it is associated with bilateral cleft lip, the anterior portion of the cleft is divided by the vomerine process which lies in the midline.

Since surgical repair of the palate is usually postponed until the age of 18 months, and can only be undertaken in the absence of infection, the nursing and feeding of infants with this deformity require particular care. With the more extensive lesions the infant is unable to suck, and must be fed by spoon or tube, care being taken to avoid regurgitation or choking. There is a particular danger of the nasopharynx and middle ear becoming infected. Some surgeons use an oral prosthesis in complete cleft palate from birth until operation is undertaken. Speech training and orthodontic treatment are required after operation.

Arched palate

A high arched palate is frequently associated with other congenital abnormalities, particularly mental defect. It may result in nasal obstruction and nasal discharge, and if the palatal deformity is not recognized as the primary cause of this, adenoidectomy is sometimes uselessly performed. It is not amenable to surgical treatment.

Hypomandibulosis (*Micrognathia*)

Minor degrees of failure of development of the mandible are not uncommon. When the mandible is excessively small, there is a danger of suffocation from falling back of the tongue, and considerable ingenuity is required in nursing the infant so that this does not occur. Usually if the neonatal period is survived, the deformity does

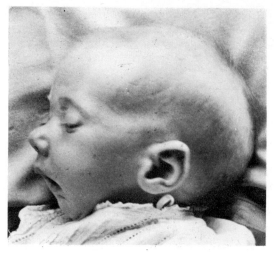

Fig. 5.6   Hypomandibulosis.

not constitute a danger to life, though it is a greater risk when associated with cleft palate (*Pierre Robin anomaly*).

Ranula

A cystic swelling below the tongue, due to obstruction of the sublingual duct, may occur as a congenital abnormality. As it is liable to increase in size and interfere with sucking, or to become infected, the cyst should be resected.

Tongue-tie

A degree of tongue-tie sufficiently severe to interfere with sucking or later with speech is extremely rare. In the great majority of cases in which the fraenum is cut, the interference is both unnecessary and dangerous.

Oesophagus

Congenital deformities of the oesophagus include atresia, stenosis, tracheo-oesophageal fistula without atresia, and congenital pouches. (The condition sometimes described as 'congenital short oesophagus' is considered under hiatus hernia.) The most frequent type of atresia encountered is one in which the upper end of the oesophagus ends blindly, and the cardiac end of the stomach has a fistulous connection to the trachea (Fig. 5.7). Much rarer types of atresia are: upper oesophagus ending blindly below and lower segment blindly above; upper segment having a fistulous connection to the trachea, and lower segment ending blindly above; and both upper and lower segments connecting with

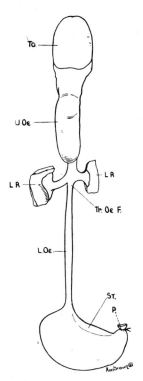

Fig. 5.7   Atresia of oesophagus, showing upper third ending in a blind pouch and lower oesophagus connecting with bifurcation of trachea.

the trachea. It is most important to establish the diagnosis before food has been taken, since regurgitation and inhalation of milk into the lungs will prejudice operative treatment. Oesophageal atresia is commonly associated with hydramnios, and may be suspected when excessive mucus bubbles from the mouth, the infant becomes cyanotic, or moist sounds are heard in the lungs. If fluid has been given, it will cause choking and regurgitation with increased cyanosis. The diagnosis can be confirmed by the passage of a large rubber catheter into the upper pouch. Straight X-rays will show the presence of air in the intestinal tract when a fistula connects the lower segment of the oesophagus with the trachea. The use of contrast media should be avoided, since the inhalation of even gastrografin is dangerous. Closure of the fistula with reconstruction of the oesophagus may be possible but in infants of low birth-weight or when difficulty is anticipated, it is preferable simply to close the fistula and feed the infant through a gastrostomy. End-to-end anastomosis of the oesophagus or

colonic transplantation can be carried out later as a planned procedure. The prognosis in uncomplicated cases is good but many babies die from associated anomalies.

Congenital pyloric stenosis

This is one of the commonest malformations of the digestive tract, the incidence having been estimated as 1 in 357 live births (Newcastle) and 1 in 250 (Sweden). Approximately 85 per cent of affected infants are male, and 40 to 60 per cent are first-born. A number of cases in monozygous twins have been reported. Consanguinity of parents of infants with pyloric stenosis has been found to be significantly more frequent than amongst the general population, and the condition is thought to be due to multifactorial genetic inheritance, though environmental factors probably also play a part in its genesis.

The abnormality consists of hypertrophy of the circular muscle of the pylorus, which forms a hard tumour the size of an almond, and causes a variable degree of obstruction to the passage of food from the stomach. If the condition is not recognized early and treated, the stomach becomes dilated and hypertrophied, and a secondary mucous gastritis occurs. The presenting symptom is vomiting, which starts with the regurgitation of small amounts of feed but rapidly (within 48 hours) becomes projectile. The vomited milk does not contain bile but may be blood-stained. Vomiting is seldom observed before the tenth day; in many instances it is not established until the third or fourth week, and sometimes much later. The type of vomiting is characteristic. The infant feeds hungrily until the stomach has become distended and the milk is then violently shot from the mouth in a copious volley which may travel one or two feet. Unless a secondary gastritis has already occurred, the infant will feed again immediately after vomiting, indicating the absence of nausea and the mechanical nature of the vomiting. The infant ceases to gain weight or, if little food is passing the pylorus, rapidly loses weight. He appears restless and anxious, and becomes constipated, the stools being small, infrequent, and dark in colour. If the condition is unrecognized and severe, the infant becomes dehydrated and occasionally jaundiced. The loss of chloride from the stomach may be sufficient to produce alkalaemia.

The signs which confirm the presence of hypertrophic pyloric stenosis are *visible gastric*

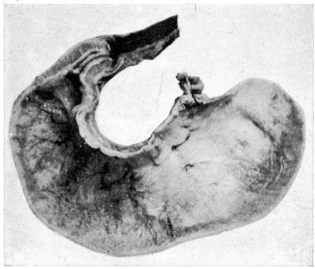

Fig. 5.8   Congenital pyloric stenosis, showing hypertrophy of circular muscle fibres of pylorus. The duodenum is unaffected, but the stomach shows secondary gastritis.

peristalsis and the presence of a *palpable tumour*.

Gastric peristalsis occurs as the stomach begins to fill, and the infant's abdomen should therefore be carefully observed while a feed is given. At a certain stage in the feed, a rounded elevation, which has been compared to a golf ball rolling below the abdominal wall, travels across from the left hypochondrium to a point approximately one inch above and to the right of the umbilicus, where it subsides. These alternating waves of contraction and distension of the stomach wall may follow each other in rapid succession, until the stomach contents are suddenly ejected and the peristalsis subsides.

The abdomen should be carefully palpated during the feed to determine the presence of a tumour, which is usually felt to the right of the umbilicus. It may be necessary to exert continuous gentle pressure before the tumour is felt as a small firm knob which appears and disappears. With time and patience it is possible to feel a tumour in 80 per cent or more of cases, but there are some in which the position of the pylorus makes its palpation impossible. It may then be necessary to confirm the diagnosis radiologically, using a small quantity of contrast medium to visualize the pylorus and demonstrate the characteristic narrowing of the aperture. Washing out the stomach will often demonstrate a considerable gastric residue. Alkaline fluids should never be employed for the purpose, owing to the danger of precipitating tetany.

Treatment may be either medical or surgical, the choice being influenced by the availability of a skilled surgeon, the duration of symptoms, and the condition of the patient. While there are some who advocate a trial of medical treatment

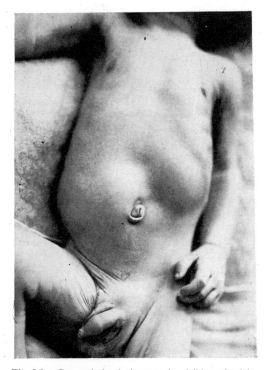

Fig. 5.9   Congenital pyloric stenosis: visible peristalsis.

in the first instance, this policy carries the risk that if medical treatment fails to relieve the vomiting, the prospects of successful surgical treatment subsequently are reduced by the delay. It is now the general practice to recommend surgery in every case diagnosed early, after any existing dehydration has been corrected by intravenous administration of fluid and electrolyte, and the stomach has been washed out with physiological saline.

Pyloromyotomy (the Fredet-Ramstedt operation), in which splitting of the circular muscle fibres is carried out along the length of the pylorus, not only relieves the obstruction completely but causes a minimum of shock and disturbance of feeding. Under good conditions the mortality should be less than 1 per cent, as compared with a mortality of over 50 per cent before this operation was introduced. The infant should be nursed in isolation to avoid risk of cross-infection. Post-operative feeding with equal parts of glucose and physiological saline can be started 3 to 4 hours after operation, 5 ml being given half-hourly for 2 hours. Then dilute milk feeds are given hourly in gradually increasing amounts, reaching 30 to 50 ml per feed at about 12 hours, and are continued two-hourly for a further 36 hours. Thereafter normal feeding can usually be resumed and no further disability need be expected. The infant may go home about the fifth day, returning to have stitches removed on the tenth day, though some surgeons prefer to keep the infant in hospital until that time. In a small proportion of cases, persistent post-operative vomiting and failure to pass stools suggest obstruction, which may be due to incomplete myotomy, though a second operation is seldom necessary.

Where the infant is seen for the first time at the age of 10 to 12 weeks, medical treatment may be advisable since the duration of the disease is self-limited, and spontaneous remission of symptoms is likely to occur at about 12 weeks. Medical treatment includes frequent small feeds thickened with cereal (which is less readily expelled from the stomach than a fluid feed) and the administration of eumydrin (atropine methyl nitrate), one to three drops of 0·6 per cent alcoholic solution being placed on the infant's tongue 20 minutes before a feed, or skopyl (methyl scopolamine nitrate) 0·1 mg in alcoholic solution being given 15 minutes before each feed. Correction of dehydration by parenteral fluids

is essential, and a slow-drip blood transfusion should be given to anaemic infants.

The prognosis depends largely on early diagnosis, skilled surgery, and prevention of infection. Although a much greater proportion of cases is now recognized early, it is still too common to find that feeds have been frequently changed before the true cause of the vomiting is suspected.

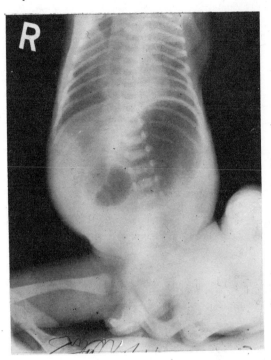

Fig. 5.10   Duodenal atresia in a newborn infant. Plain film showing air in stomach and dilated first part of duodenum, with none below the obstruction.

Atresia and stenosis of the duodenum and small intestine

Congenital obstruction of the duodenum or small intestine is less common than pyloric stenosis. The duodenum is most often the site, followed by the ileum and the jejunum. In the small intestine, multiple occlusions are not infrequent. Atresia signifies complete occlusion of the intestinal lumen, whereas in stenosis the lumen is narrowed and obstruction only partial. The nature of the occlusion ranges from complete loss of continuity between segments of bowel, which may be joined by a fibrous cord, to a simple septum with or without an opening in it. The most common cause is considered to be a vascular lesion of the fetal intestine with subsequent resorption of the necrosed area, though duodenal atresia may sometimes be due to failure of canalization in early intrauterine life. There is frequently a history of hydramnios during pregnancy and other malformations may be present, the association of duodenal atresia or stenosis with Down's syndrome being particularly common.

Congenital intestinal atresia or stenosis presents with vomiting in the first 24 hours after birth, the more proximal and complete the obstruction, the earlier the onset. The vomitus is usually bile-stained: in small intestinal atresia, the abdomen becomes distended, whereas in duodenal atresia there is only minimal distension in the upper abdomen. When obstruction is complete, little or nothing is likely to be passed by the bowel but the appearance of a small amount of pale or even normal-looking meconium does not exclude atresia. Prompt diagnosis is essential, since the results of early surgical treatment are good in uncomplicated cases and untreated atresia is invariably fatal, usually within the first week. Stenosis may be compatible with longer life but here too the earlier the diagnosis, the better the outlook.

Congenital atresia of the small intestine must be distinguished from other forms of intestinal obstruction, notably Hirschsprung's disease and meconium ileus (see p. 310). Since duodenal obstruction due to either atresia or stenosis is sometimes misdiagnosed as pyloric stenosis, the similarities and differences should be emphasized (Table 5.1).

Malrotation of the intestine

Failure of the intestine to rotate in the normal manner during intrauterine development is a rare disorder but one which may affect more than one member of a sibship. Malrotation may occur as a single abnormality or be associated with atresia. In either case it is likely to give rise to obstruction, particularly of the third part of the duodenum, and is an important cause of volvulus occurring during the neonatal period. When malrotation is part of a complete transposition of the viscera (see p. 85), the position of the appendix in the left iliac fossa may cause confusion if this organ becomes inflamed.

Volvulus

Volvulus, or the twisting of one portion of intestine on itself, is occasionally present at birth but more frequently occurs later as the result either of an abnormality of the intestine or of an abnormally long mesentery. The symptoms are those of obstruction, viz. vomiting, distension, and constipation. Ladder-patterning or peristalsis above the obstruction may be seen. Older children will complain of abdominal pain, and

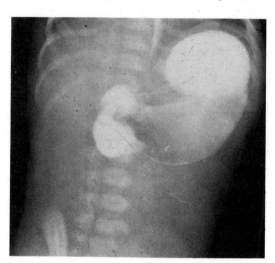

Fig. 5.11   Volvulus in newborn infant. The contrast medium has not passed beyond the duodenum and the intestine below the obstruction is airless.

Table 5.1

	Pyloric stenosis	Duodenal stenosis	Duodenal atresia
Onset of vomiting	2nd to 4th week	Usually within 24 hours of birth	Within 24 hours of birth
Type	Projectile	Projectile	Projectile
Bile in vomitus	Absent	May be present	May be present
Gastric peristalsis	Visible	Visible	Visible
Tumour	Usually palpable	Absent	Absent
Straight X-ray	Air in intestine	Air below obstruction minimal	Air below obstruction absent
Meconium	Normal	Minimal or absent	Minimal or absent
Stools	Small, infrequent	Minimal or absent	None

often localize it to the umbilicus. Occasionally blood-stained mucus or faecal matter is passed by the rectum.

Since a volvulus may reduce itself spontaneously, but is then likely to recur, the diagnosis should be considered in any child showing evidence of recurrent obstruction and abdominal pain. Between attacks, a barium meal or enema may reveal a redundant or displaced intestinal loop, but opaque media should not be given during an acute attack when operation is likely to be necessary. Usually straight X-rays of the abdomen will serve to confirm the presence of obstruction. The volvulus may involve the small or large bowel, though the former is more commonly affected.

If the condition is not recognized and the volvulus does not become reduced spontaneously, the intestine will become gangrenous with the likelihood of rupture and peritonitis.

Diverticula

The commonest diverticulum of the intestine is that described by Meckel. It is seen more frequently in males than females. This abnormality represents a persistent portion of the omphalomesenteric duct, which in embryonic life runs from the mid-gut to the yolk-sac. It is commonly found projecting from the lower portion of the ileum, and when it is a small blind pouch it may produce no symptoms. Since even a small diverticulum, however, may contain aberrant gastric mucosa, it is a possible site of ulceration and a cause of umbilical pain and rectal bleeding in childhood. When the diverticulum is more extensive, it may connect with the umbilicus and form an umbilical fistula, or cause intestinal obstruction, or be the site of diverticulitis. Operation will be necessary in any of these complications.

Hirschsprung's disease

This abnormality consists essentially of hypertrophy and dilatation of part or the whole of the large bowel proximal to a narrowed segment which shows little or no peristaltic activity. The condition gives rise to vomiting, abdominal distension, delay in the passage of meconium, constipation, reluctance to feed and failure to thrive. In the great majority of cases, these clinical features are evident in the first weeks of life, when the diagnosis should be made. In the narrowed segment, which extends for a variable

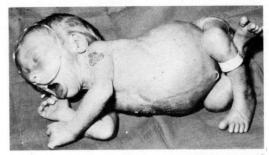

Fig. 5.12   Hirschsprung's disease in a newborn infant.

distance upwards from the anus and rectum, the parasympathetic ganglion cells are deficient and spasticity results from unopposed sympathetic action. The diagnosis is confirmed by low barium enema, which usually shows a normal or small rectum, above which a narrowing of the bowel leads to a funnel-shaped expansion leading in turn to the greatly dilated colon. In a few cases the narrowed, aganglionic segment is situated above the sigmoid while in others it is limited to the recto-anal junction. Injection of a barium enema must be undertaken with great caution, since attempts to fill the dilated intestine may result in death from shock or perforation. In the newborn infant, the typical radiological appearance is often not demonstrable and biopsy to show the absence of ganglia and the presence of nerve trunks is necessary.

Treatment consists of decompression by colostomy in the newborn period, followed by resection of the narrowed area together with the lowest portion of the dilatation at the age of about 1 year. The results of this operation have been good.

Idiopathic megacolon

In contradistinction to true Hirschsprung's disease, a second group of cases has been distinguished as *idiopathic megacolon*, occurring mainly in older children. This shows either a simple dilatation of the lower bowel, forming a pear-shaped terminal reservoir above the anus, or a tubular dilatation in which the rectum is dilated and the pelvic colon both longer and larger than normal. This group is of mixed etiology, some cases being psychogenic in origin and others due to anomalies of the internal sphincter.

SYMPTOMS AND SIGNS. The presenting symptom is constipation, which may be of extreme degree, patients sometimes going for weeks without a natural bowel action. The constipation, however, is less likely to date from early infancy than it is in Hirschsprung's disease. In cases where there is a terminal reservoir, large masses of faeces tend to accumulate in the rectum, and liquefy, the constipation then being masked by faecal incontinence (see p. 393).

Palpation of the abdomen will usually demonstrate the presence of scybalous masses, which can be indented through the abdominal wall and must be distinguished from neoplastic masses. Rectal examination will also commonly show the presence of scybala in a dilated rectum, in contrast to the narrow, empty rectum in Hirschsprung's disease.

TREATMENT. This must depend on the underlying cause. Impaction of faeces may necessitate the use of oil-retention enemata, or even removal under an anaesthetic, but these procedures should not be used unnecessarily. Where megacolon is found to be secondary to a local lesion, surgical treatment or dilatation of the anus may give good results.

The treatment of functional constipation and faecal incontinence is considered in Chapter 17.

Imperforate anus and rectal atresia

The anus may be completely absent, due to failure of invagination of the proctodeum; it may not communicate with the rectum either on account of failure of absorption of the anal plate or owing to a failure of development of the rectum; and it may be displaced. Anorectal anomalies are classified as low, intermediate or high, according to the relationship of the bowel to the puborectalis sling of the levator ani muscle. In anorectal agenesis, there is often a fistulous connection between the rectum and the bladder or vagina.

Failure of the newborn infant to pass meconium will usually draw attention to an

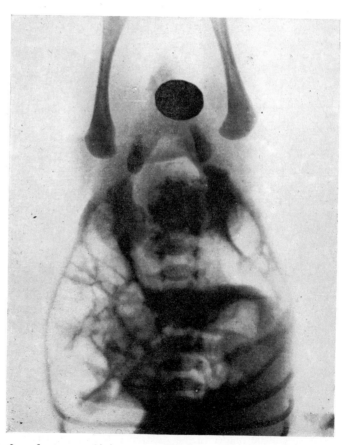

Fig. 5.13   Imperforate anus. Air in rectum, which forms a blind pouch. Site of anus marked by coin.

imperforate anus within the first 24 hours. If the anal orifice is sufficiently patent to admit the finger-tip, the site of the obstruction can be determined. The infant should be X-rayed with the head downward, a metal marker being placed over the anus. The air which is present in the large intestine within 24 hours of birth will rise to the obstruction, and the distance separating the portion of the rectum that is patent from the anus can be determined. The urine should be examined for the presence of meconium, indicating a recto-vesical fistula. Where only a persistent anal plate is present, its perforation presents little difficulty, but when there is atresia of any considerable portion of the rectum, major surgery in a neo-natal surgical centre will be necessary.

Congenital stenosis of the anus

This is commonly due to incomplete absorp-tion of the anal plate. It is evidenced by abdomi-nal distension, and by the dribbling of meconium; confirmation is obtained by digital examination. Treatment consists in repeated dilatation of the anal canal.

Ectopic anus

Displacement of the anus may be perineal, marginal to the vulva, or within the vagina in the female, or in connection with the urethra in the male. It is likely to be associated with kinking of the lower bowel, chronic distension of the abdomen, and constipation. The posterior margin of the anus should be incised and the orifice dilated.

Prolapse of the rectum

This is commonly due to a congenital mal-development of the perirectal tissues associated with redundant rectal mucosa. Malnutrition, cystic fibrosis, constipation, and rectal polypi are predisposing causes. During defaecation the rectal mucosa becomes everted and projects as a pink or purple mass from the anus. It can be seen to be continuous with the anal mucosa, and so is distinguishable from an intussusception present-ing at the anus. The prolapse is readily replaced but tends to recur. The buttocks should be strapped together between defaecations, and if possible the infant should defaecate when lying on the back or side. The general nutrition should be improved if the child is wasted, and constipa-tion corrected. In the majority of cases surgical treatment is unnecessary, and the prolapse ceases to occur as the child grows older.

Rectal polypi

These consist of rounded masses up to the size of a cherry, red in colour, and covered with mucosa. They are usually single and attached by a pedicle to the rectal mucosa. They give rise to rectal bleeding if they become ulcerated, and when mobile may present at the anus. More rarely, there is a generalized *congenital polyposis* involving the rectum and colon.

DIAGNOSIS is made readily by proctoscopic examination.

TREATMENT. Single polypi should be snared under direct vision and removed. Since general-ized polyposis is a more serious condition, resec-tion of the affected area will usually be necessary.

Cysts and reduplication

A cyst may arise from a persistent portion of Meckel's diverticulum, when the duct has be-come occluded at either end; the cyst is then usually attached by a fibrous cord both to the umbilicus and the ileum. Cysts are also occasion-ally found in the omentum or mesentery. They are unlikely to cause symptoms unless they are of large size or become infected.

Reduplication of any portion of the intestine is a rare cause of haemorrhage or peritonitis (due to the rupture of a blind pouch).

CONGENITAL MALFORMATIONS OF THE LIVER, GALL-BLADDER, BILE DUCTS, AND PANCREAS

Although minor abnormalities of lobulation of the liver are comparatively common, they seldom cause symptoms. Occasionally the liver will be found transposed, the situs inversus occurring either alone or as part of a general transposition of the viscera (including the heart, stomach, and intestine). Transposition of the viscera is due to a single autosomal recessive gene. The incidence of congenital cardiac malformation is considerably higher in partial than in complete transposition, and males are affected more commonly than females.

Congenital atresia of the bile ducts

This is the commonest abnormality of the hepatic system, and while the mortality is very high, occasional cases are found which are amen-able to surgery.

The extent of the atresia varies considerably in different cases, but commonly the whole bile duct system is involved, the bile ducts being reduced to fibrous cords. Some degree of hepatic cirrhosis is invariably present, associated in long-standing cases with generalized enlargement of both liver and spleen. The presenting sign is jaundice, which may at first be mistaken for physiological icterus but which instead of fading during the first three weeks of life becomes gradually deeper. Although the increase in jaundice is not always steadily progressive, the skin eventually assumes a greenish-bronze tint which persists. A characteristic feature of the disease is the pallor and putty-like consistency of the stools. It might be expected that these would be completely white, but while they are always paler than normal they may acquire a secondary yellow tinting from the passage of the bile-free faecal matter down the deeply bile-stained intestine.

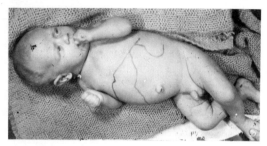

Fig. 5.14   Congenital atresia of bile ducts, showing hepatosplenomegaly. Infant aged 10 weeks.

Since it may be impossible to distinguish clinically between biliary atresia and hepatitis and a few cases of atresia occur where it is possible to perform an anastomosis of the existing gall-bladder or bile ducts to the intestine, laparotomy and biopsy of the liver should be carried out as soon as possible, since delay will increase the degree of cirrhosis. Haemorrhage, which is liable to occur due to the extensive liver damage, should be guarded against by administration of vitamin K and transfusion. The differential diagnosis is described under jaundice in the neonatal period (p. 60).

The majority of affected infants die within the first year but a few survive in reasonably good health into the second year, though rarely longer.

Malformations of the gall-bladder

Malformations of the gall-bladder vary from complete absence to reduplication, are rare and are of little clinical importance.

Cystic dilatation of the common bile duct

This is a rare cause of upper abdominal pain, nausea, and recurrent jaundice. Treatment consists in drainage and anastomosis to the duodenum.

Malformations of the pancreas

Malformations of the pancreas are rare, though annular pancreas may occasionally be associated with duodenal stenosis or atresia. There are two important disturbances of development which occur during intrauterine life and which can be considered as malformations in the wider sense. One of these, *hypertrophy of the islets of Langerhans*, is often seen in the infants of diabetic mothers, and is commonly associated with excessive prenatal growth. The other, *cystic fibrosis (fibrocystic disease of the pancreas)*, is considered on p. 310.

HERNIA AND EVENTRATION

An abdominal hernia is a projection of some portion of the viscera through an abnormal opening in the wall of the abdominal cavity, or through an opening within the abdominal cavity itself, e.g. the foramen of Winslow. The term 'eventration' is sometimes used to describe a massive escape of bowel to the exterior, or an extensive ballooning of the diaphragm, which in effect corresponds to a hernial sac. The principal danger of hernia is obstruction of the portion of bowel involved, though in the case of diaphragmatic hernia there is also risk of respiratory embarrassment.

Strangulation of hernial contents will give rise to acute abdominal pain, usually followed rapidly by vomiting and other signs of obstruction. In the case of inguinal hernia, the external swelling is tense and painful. Surgical relief of strangulation is a matter of urgency, though where the hernia is incarcerated but not strangulated conservative treatment may be given a trial at least for a matter of hours. Here an attempt is made to obtain complete relaxation and reduction of the hernia by raising the foot of the bed or suspending the infant by the feet before proceeding to operation.

Umbilical hernia

This is extremely common in infancy, the projecting umbilicus being covered with skin and lined with peritoneum. It may reasonably be objected that the term 'hernia' is really a misnomer, since in most cases the sac contains neither intestine nor omentum, but the term is commonly used to describe the sac itself. The smaller sacs will frequently disappear without treatment but when the sac is more than 1·5 cm in diameter operative repair will be required. The age of choice for operation is 18 months to 2 years. If there is any primary cause of abdominal distension, however, this should be corrected before operation is attempted. It is common to see umbilical hernia in cretinism and other conditions associated with chronic constipation.

Divarication of the recti

Separation of the recti may give rise to herniation of omentum above the umbilicus. The condition seldom requires treatment, and is usually corrected spontaneously with growth and improvement in muscle tone and nutrition.

Omphalocele (*Exomphalos*)

Occasionally infants are born with a very large sac present at the site of the umbilicus, which is covered only with peritoneum and which contains a large part of the intestine or other viscera. Surgical treatment should be undertaken immediately after birth. Primary

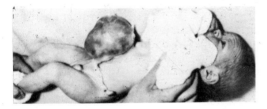

Fig. 5.15   Exomphalos in a newborn infant. Operation was successfully effected six hours after birth.

repair of the abdominal wall may be possible if the defect is small, but with larger ones the skin is merely closed over the sac and the ventral hernia is repaired later. If skin cover cannot be achieved, plastic sheeting may be used or the sac can be painted daily with 2 per cent mercurochrome, which causes it to shrink gradually.

Inguinal hernia

The descent of the testis from the abdominal cavity to the scrotum is effected by way of the internal and external abdominal rings, through which passes an extension of the abdominal peritoneum. This peritoneal tube is normally

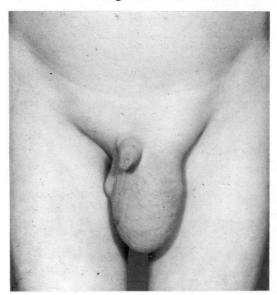

Fig. 5.16   Left inguinal hernia.

obliterated before birth, with the exception of the portion forming the tunica vaginalis of the testis, and the inguinal canal becomes functionally closed. When the testis fails to descend (cryptorchidism) or when the peritoneal tube remains patent after descent of the testis, this sac provides a route through which abdominal contents may herniate into the inguinal canal or scrotum. The depth to which the hernia can descend will depend on the extent to which the process of peritoneum remains patent. Inguinal hernia may therefore be regarded as due to a congenital malformation (or failure of atrophy), although the actual herniation of abdominal contents may not occur until long after birth.

Inguinal hernia in infancy and childhood is almost invariably of the indirect type described, and is nine times as frequent in boys as it is in girls. It is also more frequently seen on the right than left side.

SYMPTOMS. In the uncomplicated case symptoms are often minimal, the recurrent swelling in the inguinal canal or scrotum being the reason for the child coming under observation. In other cases there is complaint of abdominal discomfort and disturbance of appetite.

DIAGNOSIS. Careful examination, with the child in the erect position, will often reveal the hernia before palpation is attempted, or a swelling may appear when the child coughs or cries. Palpation over the swelling will show whether it is reducible, and so help to distinguish it from hydrocele.

TREATMENT. Obliteration of the sac occasionally occurs spontaneously during the first three or even six months of life, but the majority of cases will require operation, and this is best undertaken at a few months of age when the infant is thriving, or on diagnosis in older infants and children.

Femoral hernia

This is very much rarer than inguinal hernia, but should be remembered in the differential diagnosis of swellings appearing in the region of the femoral triangle. Since there is considerable risk of strangulation occurring, operation should not be unduly delayed.

Diaphragmatic hernia and eventration

Herniation of abdominal contents through the diaphragm occurs most frequently on the left side, the viscera either passing directly into the thorax through a defect in the postero-lateral part of the diaphragm or being covered by a hernial sac. Eventration of the diaphragm will produce the same signs, but there is less likelihood of the abdominal contents being strangulated by the ballooned diaphragm than by the margins of a hernial opening.

SYMPTOMS. There may be respiratory difficulty necessitating resuscitation at birth but frequently the infant breathes spontaneously and appears normal for some hours. Air and later the first feed entering the stomach increase the volume of the displaced viscera, compressing the lungs and causing acute respiratory embarrassment, which may be rapidly fatal. Cyanosis is frequently noted and is characteristically relieved by altering the infant's position. In cases in which dyspnoea and cyanosis are less severe, there is commonly failure to thrive and intermittent vomiting.

SIGNS. On auscultation of the chest, bowel sounds are seldom heard in the newborn infant though this is a useful sign at a later age. Breath sounds will be weak or absent and the heart will be displaced. The movement of the side of the thorax into which the hernia has occurred is likely to be reduced, and in cases of left-sided hernia the left lung is frequently hypoplastic.

DIAGNOSIS. A straight X-ray will usually confirm the diagnosis without the necessity of using contrast media, and a combination of views indicates the site and extent of the hernial orifice.

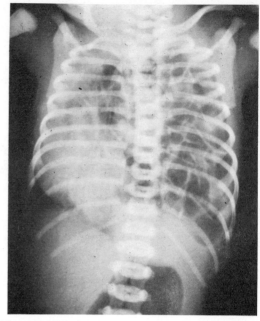

Fig. 5.17 Diaphragmatic hernia in a newborn infant. Bowel shadows in left side of chest and mediastinum displaced to right.

TREATMENT. A nasogastric tube should be passed at once and the stomach contents aspirated. Administration of oxygen should be delayed until the larynx has been intubated, so that the expansion of the lung is under control. There is otherwise a real risk of inflation of the left lung and fatal displacement of the mediastinum before operation.

Surgical repair should be carried out as soon as possible. The mortality in diaphragmatic hernia is high because affected infants are often born before term and associated malformations are frequently present.

Hiatus hernia

In this condition part of the stomach is displaced into the chest through an abnormally wide oesophageal hiatus in the diaphragm. This is facilitated by deficiency of the crural muscle surrounding the hiatus. The disorder occurs about once per 1000 live births and should be suspected when there is persistent vomiting from early infancy, especially when it starts in the first week of life. The vomits are large and occur during or just after feeds. The vomited material contains slimy mucus and may be stained brown with altered blood, due to associated reflux oesophagitis. Weight gain is often poor and in severe cases there will be failure to thrive, dehydration and constipation.

Hiatus hernia is diagnosed by barium swallow with fluoroscopy, which may have to be repeated before the thoracic part of the stomach can be demonstrated. Oesophagoscopy, which is seldom necessary, shows gastric mucosa above the level of the diaphragm and ulceration may be visible. Treatment consists in nursing the infant in the sitting position throughout the 24 hours, with thickening of the feeds if necessary. On this regimen vomiting usually ceases within a few days or weeks; when the baby is thriving and has not vomited for many weeks, postural treatment may be stopped and in the majority of cases there will be no further symptoms. If vomiting persists or recurs, the possibility of pyloric stenosis must be considered, since the incidence of this is increased in infants with hiatus hernia. However, in some uncomplicated cases vomiting may take months to settle despite treatment.

When there is persistent vomiting or recurrent bleeding, oesophageal stricture may develop, causing increasing dysphagia, nocturnal vomiting and failure to gain weight. If it seems likely that such a stricture will develop, surgical correction of the hiatus hernia is advisable. Occasionally symptoms of stricture arise in an older child previously considered healthy but nearly always a history of vomiting in infancy can be elicited, indicating that a hiatus hernia has been overlooked.

MALFORMATIONS OF THE CARDIOVASCULAR SYSTEM

As in the case of other congenital malformations, cardiac anomalies may arise from genetic or environmental causes, or more usually from complex interaction between the two (Campbell, 1965). Association with other malformations or syndromes (e.g. arachnodactyly, mongolism and other chromosomal anomalies) is well known, but more commonly cardiac defect occurs as an isolated malformation. Maternal rubella in the first three months of pregnancy has been clearly shown to be a cause of cardiac malformation, but other infections appear relatively unimportant. In the great majority of cases the cause is unknown.

A congenital cardiac malformation usually represents an arrest of development of some portion of the heart, aortic arches, or adnexa at a particular point in time, and a subsequent attempt by the remainder of the heart to develop along normal lines. In many instances the primary abnormality will result in an uneasy compromise, in which the functional disturbance caused will be met by further malformation or failure of development. In the great majority of instances, however, the heart will at least swing to the left and be found in approximately the normal position, a point of considerable practical importance when fluoroscopy is employed as an aid to diagnosis and assessment of size of the respective chambers. Since the formation of the heart occurs between the third and eighth weeks of intrauterine life, major malformations are likely to be established during this time, and environmental factors which may play a part in etiology must be looked for in the early months of pregnancy.

DIAGNOSTIC METHODS

Although accurate diagnosis in infancy presents formidable difficulties and is frequently only made at necropsy, improved techniques are rapidly increasing the number of lesions which can be diagnosed with confidence during the early months of life. Unaided physical examination of the heart in this age period is particularly unreliable. Thus significant degrees of cardiac enlargement are often not appreciated, and the accurate determination of site, distribution, and character of precordial murmurs may prove extremely difficult. Transient systolic murmurs which are not indicative of malformation may be heard during the newborn period, while loud murmurs due to malformation may only appear after the neonatal period is passed. Usually, however, malformation is suspected at birth if a loud systolic murmur is present, particularly if the murmur is accompanied by a precordial thrill; in some cases these signs will be associated with dyspnoea and cyanosis, which must be distinguished from cyanosis of peripheral or pulmonary origin. Occasionally an infant with a major malformation presents in cardiac failure, although there will usually have been premonitory signs such as increase in respiratory rate and enlargement of the liver.

During early infancy, failure to thrive is a common manifestation of cardiac malformation and deformity of the left chest is often observed when cardiac enlargement and embarrassment are present while the thorax is still soft. The presence or absence of cyanosis will depend on the nature of the abnormality, but even when intense cyanosis is present it is rare for clubbing of the fingers to occur during the first six months of life.

Examination of the character of the pulse should be made as a routine in both femoral and radial arteries. Acceleration of the pulse rate during inspiration and slowing during expiration constitute sinus arrhythmia, which is physiological in childhood and disappears on exercise. The nervous tachycardia associated with crying and the tachycardia of fever must be distinguished from that due to cardiac abnormality and from paroxysmal tachycardia (see p. 99). A pulse rate of less than 50 per minute occurs in congenital heart block, due to an abnormality involving the conducting mechanism. Incomplete heart block with prolongation of the P–R interval occurs in rheumatic or infective carditis. Very occasionally, heart block gives rise to syncopal or convulsive attacks (Stokes-Adams syndrome). Bradycardia may also occur as the result of jaundice or raised intracranial pressure, or during convalescence from prolonged illness. In all these variations of pulse rate, electrocardiography will help to establish the diagnosis. Blood-pressure readings on infants necessitate the use of a narrow cuff (the width not less than two-thirds the length of the upper arm), and repeated examination may be necessary with the infant at rest before consistent readings are obtained; even so, accurate estimation of the diastolic pressure is seldom possible in infancy, and in the newborn special techniques are necessary for determining systolic pressure.

Heart sounds and murmurs are usually well heard through the relatively thin tissues of the child's chest wall. Splitting of the first or second heart sound and a low-pitched third heart sound can often be heard in healthy children and are generally to be considered normal unless very pronounced. A venous hum is sometimes audible below the clavicle, usually the right, in young children. It varies with the position of the head and neck, sometimes almost disappearing if the head is turned in one direction. It is of no clinical importance and must not be mistaken for the murmur of a persistent ductus arteriosus.

A short localized systolic murmur is heard over the precordium in many normal children and can generally be identified as of no clinical

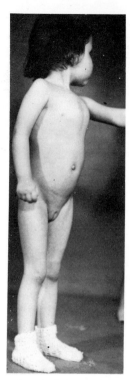

Fig. 5.18 Congenital malformation of the heart (large ventricular septal defect with dextroposition of aorta) showing deformity of thorax.

importance by its character and from the past history, though in some cases the patient must be followed up for some time before a confident opinion can be given.

In interpreting the radiological findings, the differences between the child and adult hearts must be borne in mind. Thus in infancy the thorax is wider than it is high and the heart lies more horizontally; in the adult the thorax is higher than it is wide and the heart lies more vertically. In childhood the thorax is approximately as wide as it is high, and the heart lies between the infantile and adult positions. Fluoroscopic examination should include anterior-posterior and left and right anterior oblique views, supplemented by barium swallow, to determine the relative size of the chambers and great vessels.

Electrocardiographic findings should be compared with standard normals of approximately the same age, the unipolar chest leads giving the most useful information. The E.C.G. patterns characteristic of particular malformations will be helpful in diagnosis when correlated with the clinical and radiological findings.

Special investigative procedures such as cardiac catheterization and selective angiocardiography may be essential for precise diagnosis, especially when complex malformations are present. Details of these and other techniques are given in standard textbooks of paediatric cardiology (e.g. Keith, Rowe and Vlad, 1967; Watson, 1968). While such diagnostic methods are finding increasing application, especially in infancy, it must be emphasized that they carry an appreciable mortality rate and should only be

undertaken by fully trained teams working in hospitals which are properly equipped for cardiological investigation.

INCIDENCE

Figures for the incidence of congenital cardiac abnormality are likely to be unreliable, since necropsy findings are apt to be overweighted with infants and routine clinical examinations of school children may fail to distinguish minor abnormalities. Recent surveys indicate that

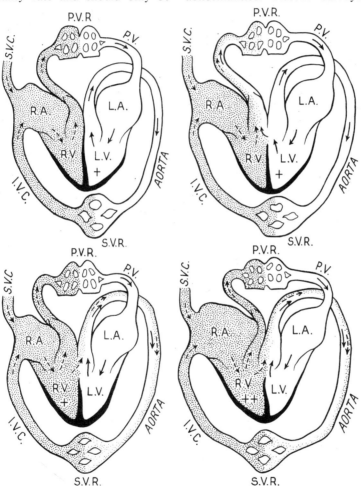

Fig. 5.19   Course of the circulation: I. Under normal conditions, and in cases without abnormal communication, but in which the anomaly may become the seat of strain. II. In cases of arterio-venous shunt (compensated septal defects). III. In cases of arterio-venous shunt with terminal reversal of flow (decompensated septal defects). IV. In cases of the cyanotic group with permanent venous-arterial shunt with raised pressure at periphery (pulmonary stenosis with defect of ventricular septum and dextroposition of aorta). Abbreviations: P.V.R.=pulmonary venous reservoir; I.V.C=inferior vena cava; S.V.R.=systemic venous reservoir; S.V.C.=superior vena cava. (After M. E. Abbott.)

about 6 per 1000 newborn infants have cardiac malformations, the most common being septal defects, transposition of the great arteries and coarctation of the aorta. The death rate in infancy is high and the incidence in children of school age is about 2 per 1000. Among these older children, ventricular septal defect is the most frequently encountered anomaly, while atrial septal defect, pulmonary stenosis, persistent ductus arteriosus and Fallot's tetralogy are also common. Cyanotic heart disease in the newborn infant is thus most likely to be due to transposition of the great arteries, whereas in older children the most probable cause is Fallot's tetralogy. The risk of a later sibling of a child with cardiac malformation being similarly affected is nearly 2 per cent.

CLASSIFICATION

In view of the very great number of malformations or combinations of malformations which may occur, no classification is likely to be wholly satisfactory to both embryologist and clinician. Only those malformations which are relatively common and of clinical importance will be considered here. The work of Gross, Taussig, Blalock, Brock, and others, however, has shown that certain types of abnormality which were previously considered beyond the reach of medical aid can be relieved by surgery, and this result was only achieved by an intensive study of all types of congenital cardiac defect on a functional basis. The development of hypothermic anaesthesia and cardio-respiratory by-pass techniques has made it possible to arrest the circulation and operate on the open heart. This has been a major advance, and as surgical skills develop with this help the field of corrective cardiac surgery can be expected to expand.

Broadly, cardiac abnormalities may be grouped into those which are incompatible with survival of the fetus; those which are compatible with survival of the fetus but not with independent existence; those in which the infant survives a matter of months and succumbs before the age of 2; and those where childhood or adult life may be reached. This last group may be further subdivided into cases where the cardiac function is seriously impaired, those in which there is little or no functional incapacity for a long period but where the risk of intercurrent infection (bacterial endocarditis or

pulmonary infections) or excessive strain lessens the expectation of life, and those in which there is no functional disability.

Abbott's (1936) classification of cases into three main groups, viz. (1) cases without abnormal communication but the seat of strain, (2) cases of arterio-venous shunt with possible terminal or transient reversal of flow and (3) cases of venous-arterial shunt, has been widely used (Fig. 5.19). However, the emphasis placed on the presence or absence of cyanosis (which is variable in the second group, and which may not be clinically detectable in some patients with a significant right to left shunt) has disadvantages, and the following anatomical classification of Marquis provides an alternative:

I. SIMPLE OBSTRUCTIVE MALFORMATIONS

   A. *Right-sided*
   Pulmonary valve stenosis
   Subvalvular (infundibular) stenosis
   Pulmonary atresia
   Tricuspid stenosis
   Tricuspid atresia.

   B. *Left-sided*
   Aortic valve stenosis
   Subaortic stenosis
   Aortic atresia
   Coarctation of aorta
   Mitral stenosis
   Mitral atresia.

II. SIMPLE LEFT TO RIGHT SHUNTS

   Atrial septal defect
   Ventricular septal defect
   Aorto-pulmonary artery septal defect
   Persistent ductus arteriosus.

III. SIMPLE DISPLACEMENTS

   Dextrocardia (isolated or with situs inversus)
   Dextroposition of the aorta
   Transposition of the great arteries
   Anomalous pulmonary venous drainage into right
     atrium (partial or complete)
   Anomalous drainage of vena cava
   Displacement of tricuspid valve into right ventricle
     (Ebstein's anomaly).

IV. COMPLEX MALFORMATIONS

   (a) Any combination of two or more of the above three
       groups, e.g. pulmonary stenosis, ventricular septal
       defect, dextroposition of aorta with associated
       right ventricular hypertrophy (tetralogy of Fallot).
   (b) Developmental arrests, e.g. persistent truncus
       arteriosus, single ventricle, atrio-ventricular
       cushion defects.
   (c) Acquired haemodynamic changes, e.g. the Eisen-
       menger syndrome.

To this classification must be added the rare examples of congenital enlargement of the heart such as *cardiac glycogenosis* (p. 200) and *fibro-elastosis* (p. 98).

SIMPLE OBSTRUCTIVE MALFORMATIONS

Pulmonary stenosis

Stenosis of the pulmonary valve without other abnormality is one of the commoner isolated obstructive lesions. The clinical picture varies greatly in different patients, depending on the degree of obstruction to the outflow of blood from the right ventricle. When the stenosis is slight or moderate, the condition may be virtually asymptomatic and associated with normal growth during infancy and childhood, being discovered only on routine examination. More severe stenosis will lead to right ventricular and atrial hypertrophy and cardiac embarrassment, with impaired exercise tolerance.

SIGNS. The condition is typically acyanotic in early life, but when the pulmonary circulation is very seriously impaired, some degree of peripheral cyanosis (due to the low cardiac output and consequently increased extraction of oxygen by the tissues) may be detected.

A harsh systolic murmur, ejection in type and often accompanied by a thrill, is heard over the second left intercostal space adjacent to the sternum, and is conducted over the precordium.

RADIOLOGICAL EXAMINATION may show the heart to be of normal size or demonstrate right ventricular hypertrophy, with prominence of the pulmonary artery. The lung fields are likely to appear ischaemic when the stenosis is severe.

OTHER INVESTIGATIONS. Cardiac catheterization will demonstrate a raised pressure in the right ventricle associated with a low or normal pressure in the pulmonary artery. The electrocardiogram is the best guide to the severity of the stenosis. When there is evidence of right ventricular hypertrophy the stenosis is severe and cardiac catheterization is advisable. It is of great value in confirming the diagnosis and in measuring the degree of the stenosis.

TREATMENT. Patients with apparently mild stenosis do not require treatment but should be kept under review. Development of right ventricular hypertrophy may necessitate revision of the original assessment. Patients with severe stenosis require surgical treatment. The results of pulmon-ary valvotomy are good, and operation should not be delayed until symptoms develop.

Coarctation of the aorta

Two types of coarctation of the aorta have been described, known as the preductal and postductal types respectively, although there is considerable variation in the type of aortic narrowing and its relationship to the ductus. Coarctation of the aorta occurs twice as frequently in males as in females.

The *preductal type* is characterized by narrowing of the aorta between the root of the left subclavian artery and the entry of the ductus. The diameter of this aortic isthmus is normally less than that of the rest of the aorta at birth but may be further reduced by a narrow segment or by diffuse hypoplasia. This type of coarctation represents a complex malformation, since the ductus generally remains patent, and there are frequently other malformations. These usually obscure the diagnosis during life, and cause cardiac failure and death in early infancy. Coarctation with persistent ductus occasionally causes cyanosis of the lower but not of the upper extremities, due to the shunt of blood which passes from the pulmonary artery to the aorta through the ductus instead of in the reverse direction. The flow into the aorta may be sufficient to prevent reduction of blood pressure in the femoral vessels.

The *postductal type* of coarctation shows a localized constriction of the aorta below the site of entry of the ductus and most commonly immediately distal to it. The ductus is usually found closed, and a collateral circulation to the lower limbs is established from the subclavian arteries by way of the arteries of the shoulder girdle, the intercostal arteries, and the internal mammary arteries. Blood is delivered by the two former routes to the descending aorta below the constriction, while the internal mammary joins the deep epigastric artery and so delivers blood to the internal iliac arteries.

DIAGNOSIS. Palpation of the femoral pulses should form part of the routine examination of all infants and children, for the diagnosis of coarctation of the aorta depends on finding weak or absent femoral pulses and a difference in blood pressure between the upper and lower limbs. The blood pressure in the upper limbs may be normal in infancy (becoming raised later), whereas the pressure in the femoral vessels is reduced. Evidence of collateral circulation is most likely to be found in the posterior axilla, above the clavicles, and in the interscapular region, where enlarged pulsatile arteries may occasionally be seen and felt. A systolic murmur may be heard and strong suprasternal pulsation is a confirmatory sign. Erosion of the ribs by enlarged intercostal arteries (an important radiological finding in older patients) is unlikely to be seen in early childhood. Radiologically there is generally cardiac enlargement with left ventricular hypertrophy and the normal aortic knot may be small or absent. The coarctation may be visualized by angiography if necessary. When coarctation occurs proximally to the left subclavian, the pulse will be forcible in the right and feeble in the left wrist.

COMPLICATIONS. Although coarctation of the aorta is compatible with good health and long life, signs of cardiac failure appear in early infancy in most cases. In patients who do not manifest symptoms, there is a considerably increased risk of cerebral haemorrhage and of bacterial endocarditis, usually when the age of childhood is passed.

TREATMENT. Surgical removal of the local aortic constriction with reconstruction of the aorta is the treatment of choice in all young patients presenting with symptoms. Simultaneous correction of associated anomalies such as persistent ductus may be necessary. A short period of pre-operative medical treatment is advisable for infants presenting in failure. In the asymptomatic case without significant hypertension or cardiac enlargement, operation is best postponed until 7 to 10 years of age when the aorta is well developed.

Aortic stenosis and other types of obstructive malformation

Aortic stenosis may occur with other cardiac anomalies or as an isolated malformation. It is generally detected by hearing a rough systolic murmur in the aortic area on routine examination of an apparently normal child. The murmur is transmitted into the neck and accompanied by a systolic thrill. A small number of children present with fainting attacks liable to be misdiagnosed as epileptic. Surgical treatment should be considered in children who have symptoms or show left ventricular hypertrophy.

Stenosis or atresia of the mitral or tricuspid valves are relatively rare congenital lesions, which generally cause death in the first year.

SIMPLE LEFT TO RIGHT SHUNTS
Atrial septal defects

While the foramen ovale is patent during intrauterine life, it normally becomes functionally closed when respiration is established, and subsequently is anatomically closed also. Persistent patency is regarded as an abnormality, though frequently it occurs as a necessary adaptation to some other defect. As an isolated lesion it is clinically unimportant.

The simplest and most common form of atrial septal defect lies in the fossa ovalis. It is known as an ostium secundum, and usually occurs as an isolated cardiac lesion. It is commonly a large defect allowing a considerable shunt from left to right atrium. There is thus no cyanosis but there is secondary enlargement of the right side of the heart and pulmonary vessels. Symptoms are seldom severe in childhood and under the age of 20 years cardiac enlargement is usually moderate in degree.

A less common form of atrial septal defect occurs adjacent to the atrio-ventricular valves. This defect, known as an ostium primum, is commonly associated with deformity of the mitral valve with resultant incompetence. Symptoms are often severe and cardiac enlargement marked in childhood.

SYMPTOMS, if they occur, will be dyspnoea and tachycardia, leading ultimately to cardiac failure. In some instances, however, the patient reaches adult life without the condition being suspected.

SIGNS are inconstant, but the heart tends to be enlarged, and there is increased systolic pulsation up the left sternal border; a systolic murmur maximal in the second left intercostal space and a split second sound are commonly heard. Radiologically there is enlargement of the right ventricle, right atrium, main pulmonary artery and hilar vessels. The latter show marked expansile pulsation on screening. The electrocardiogram will show right ventricular hypertrophy and partial bundle branch block.

TREATMENT. Ostium secundum defects can be closed surgically with brief circulatory arrest permitted by hypothermic anaesthesia. This operation has now been proved safe and satisfactory. The operation is best performed in childhood and should not be delayed until the development of symptoms.

Ostium primum defects are less often amenable to surgical correction; their repair necessitates prolonged circulatory arrest and the use of a cardio-respiratory by-pass.

Ventricular septal defects

These may occur in a variety of positions but most commonly are situated in the outflow area of the right ventricle close to or in the membranous part of the septum. The characteristic sign is a loud harsh systolic murmur heard to the left of the sternum in the third and fourth intercostal spaces, and usually accompanied by a palpable thrill. When the defect is small there are no symptoms and the heart is small in spite of an impressive murmur. Larger defects lead to severe disability and considerable cardiac enlargement, sometimes causing death in early childhood. The presence of a left to right shunt through a ventricular septal defect can be established by demonstrating an increase in oxygen saturation on passing a catheter from the right atrium to the right ventricle.

COMPLICATIONS. When there is a high pulmonary vascular resistance, the shunt may become reversed, so that blood passes from right to left and cyanosis appears (Eisenmenger syndrome). Rarely the margin of the defect or the right ventricular wall is affected by bacterial endocarditis.

TREATMENT. The small defects do not require treatment and indeed many close spontaneously. The larger defects can be repaired surgically but the operation necessitates the use of a cardio-respiratory by-pass and the risk is still considerable, though it may be reduced by careful selection of cases. Diminution of pulmonary blood flow by banding the pulmonary artery is a useful palliative procedure in infancy.

Complete congenital heart-block

Unlike bundle branch block, complete congenital heart-block is rare as a complication of either ventricular or atrial septal defects. It occurs more frequently in the high type of ventricular defect than with a simple septal perforation, and sometimes complicates an ostium primum type of atrial septal defect. The condition should be suspected in a young infant when the pulse rate is 80 or below. The diagnosis is confirmed by electrocardiogram, which is similar to that in acquired heart-block.

Persistent ductus arteriosus

The ductus arteriosus, which transmits blood from the pulmonary artery to the aorta in fetal life, becomes functionally closed within a week after birth, and more gradually anatomical closure and occlusion take place. A distinction must be made between infants in whom the ductus is found to admit a probe at necropsy (anatomical patency) and those in whom there is evidence of functional patency, i.e. a shunt of blood between the aorta and pulmonary artery.

This functional patency may persist in a considerable proportion of infants without giving rise to symptoms, and natural closure may probably occur at least as late as the second year. When the ductus remains persistently patent, symptoms seldom occur during infancy and early childhood, except occasionally when the ductus is unusually large. There may then be recurrent respiratory infections and bouts of congestive heart failure before school age, and the characteristic murmur (see below) may be present before the end of the first year. In most cases, however, the diagnosis is made on routine examination, often at school entry.

CLINICAL SIGNS. At a variable time after birth (usually in the first year and nearly always before the fifth year) a characteristic continuous murmur develops which is almost pathognomonic. The murmur, which is best heard in the second left interspace with the child lying supine, characteristically starts with the first heart sound, rises in a crescendo up to the second sound, and thereafter decreases rapidly but is usually audible throughout diastole. The pulmonary second sound is loud but is often lost in the maximum intensity of the murmur. This *humming-top* or *machinery murmur* is usually accompanied by a thrill which may be confined to the second half of systole but sometimes continues into early diastole.

In the uncomplicated case the child is not cyanosed and the heart is usually of normal size. The pulse pressure will depend upon the quantity of blood leaving the systemic circulation through the ductus into the low-pressure pulmonary circuit. When the ductus is large, pulsation may be demonstrable in the nail-beds, or a characteristic pistol-shot sound heard over the femoral arteries. The general development of the child will be normal when little blood is passing through the ductus, but when the amount is large there may be interference with growth and exercise tolerance, and in cases of great severity signs of right-sided heart failure.

RADIOLOGICAL SIGNS. The heart shadow may appear normal, or the left atrium and left ventricle slightly enlarged. The most characteristic appearance (which is not invariably present) is enlargement of the pulmonary arc, while the lungs often show increased vascularity. On fluoroscope examination there is increased pulsation of the heart and a characteristic see-saw movement between the left ventricle on the one hand and the aorta and main pulmonary artery on the other. Expansile pulsation in hilar vessels ('hilar dance') is only present when the ductus is unusually large.

ELECTROCARDIOGRAM. This may show no abnormality, but there is often evidence of left ventricular hypertrophy in the chest leads. The finding of isolated right ventricular hypertrophy casts doubt on the diagnosis of persistent ductus.

DIAGNOSIS. When the characteristic murmur is present the diagnosis of persistent ductus arteriosus is readily made. The diagnosis should also be suspected in infants and young children with pulmonary systolic murmurs when the peripheral pulses are full.

PROGNOSIS AND TREATMENT. Although the prognosis as regards survival is good, life expectancy is reduced in untreated persistent ductus. Hazards include bacterial endocarditis, cardiac failure, pulmonary vascular disease and retarded physical development.

Surgical occlusion of the uncomplicated persistent ductus should be recommended in all cases. In expert hands the operative mortality is less than 1 per cent and the risk is less than the risks of bacterial endocarditis and other complications in the untreated case. The optimum time for operation is before school entry, but it is sometimes therapeutically necessary in infancy.

SIMPLE DISPLACEMENTS
Transposition of the great arteries
This is one of the commoner causes of cyanosis in the neonatal period, occurring twice as commonly in males as in females. When the transposition is complete, the pulmonary artery arises from the left ventricle and the aorta from the right. Unless there is communication between the two circuits (e.g. persistent patency of the foramen ovale or ductus arteriosus), the condition is incompatible with life. There are, however, a number of intermediary types with which the infant may survive for a variable time after birth. Deep cyanosis, occurring at or shortly after birth and increased by crying, is the charac-

teristic feature and is commonly associated with dyspnoea and failure to suck or thrive. Radiologically the heart may appear normal at birth but soon enlarges and assumes an egg shape, with a vascular pedicle which appears narrow anteroposteriorly but wide in oblique views. Murmurs and other clinical findings are inconstant. The prognosis is poor in untreated cases, the great majority of patients dying in early infancy, usually in congestive failure. The creation of an artificial atrial septal defect by the Rashkind technique may be life-saving in selected newborn infants and may permit survival until definitive surgery can be undertaken. The Mustard operation is a promising procedure but experience with it is still limited and the prognosis for these children must remain very guarded.

Dextrocardia
In dextrocardia, the heart is wholly or mainly in the right side of the chest. The term should be reserved for cases of congenital origin and should not be applied to those in which displacement has been caused by postnatal disease. In isolated dextrocardia, the heart is generally maldeveloped, but when there is associated situs inversus of the abdominal viscera, there is no gross malformation of the heart in most instances, although the relative position of atria and ventricles is reversed. The clinical features and prognosis depend on the state of the heart but often there are no symptoms and the anomaly is only recognized on routine examination.

COMPLEX MALFORMATIONS
Fallot's tetralogy
Fallot's tetralogy consists of: (1) pulmonary stenosis, (2) patent interventricular septum, (3) dextroposition of the aorta, and (4) hypertrophy of the right ventricle. The functional disability consists essentially of a defective blood supply to the lungs, and the passage of a large volume of unoxygenated blood into the systemic circulation. The arterial oxygen saturation is commonly in the region of 70 per cent at complete rest, but may fall much lower on exertion, the lack of aeration resulting in polycythaemia, with a red-cell count of 7 millions per mm^3 or more. The haemoglobin may be within the normal range due to hypochromic anaemia, which may be obscured by the high red-cell count.

CLINICAL SIGNS. Cyanosis may not be present in the neonatal period but generally appears during early infancy. It may be episodic at first but later is intense and persistent. Clubbing of the fingers and toes is marked. A loud systolic murmur is heard in the third and fourth left interspaces, is conducted over the precordium and may be heard posteriorly. The exercise tolerance is so low that dyspnoea occurs on slight exertion and cyanosis is increased. The adoption of a squatting position after any activity is so characteristic as to be an aid in diagnosis.

Cerebral thrombosis or abscess is a relatively common cause of death in the tetralogy of Fallot and in malformations in which the aorta arises from both ventricles. Cerebral anoxia may also cause brain damage or death. Bacterial endocarditis is a danger in older children.

Radiologically the heart is usually of normal size and enlargement casts doubt on the diagnosis. In the anterior view, elevation of the apex and concavity in the region of the pulmonary artery give the heart a characteristic boot shape, but in older children this is less common because of the lower position of the diaphragm. The lung fields are ischaemic. The aortic arch is right-sided in 20 to 25 per cent of cases, and this finding is of value in suggesting the diagnosis. Cardiac catheterization and selective angiocardiography make more accurate diagnosis possible.

Electrocardiography shows right ventricular hypertrophy.

TREATMENT. In 1945 Blalock and Taussig designed an operation for increasing the pulmonary circulation by the construction of what was virtually an artificial ductus arteriosus. A branch of the aorta (e.g. the subclavian) is selected for anastomosis to the pulmonary artery, and the stenosed area is thus by-passed. In the Potts operation, which may sometimes be preferred, a similar communication is established by direct anastomosis of the aorta to the pulmonary artery. The development of open-heart surgery has made it possible to attempt complete correction of the deformity. This has proved most successful in the less severely cyanosed cases, but the operative risk remains considerable and the indirect Blalock-Taussig type of operation is still the procedure preferred in some cases.

GENERAL CONSIDERATIONS

It will be seen that congenital malformations of the heart may vary from those in which the disability is minimal to those in which the lesion is incompatible with life, or where activity is so limited that life is one of chronic invalidism. Advances in cardiac surgery have radically altered the prognosis for a proportion of affected patients, but for surgery to be successful it must be highly selective and based on accurate and early diagnosis. Since operative treatment may be essential to survival beyond childhood in some cases, and since surgery is increasingly being undertaken successfully in infancy, responsibility rests with the paediatrician for seeing that cases amenable to treatment are not overlooked. In infancy and early childhood the problem is made more complex by the greater frequency of very complicated malformations and the limitations of the ordinary diagnostic methods. Amongst the acyanotic malformations the finding of a full collapsing pulse should raise the question of a persistent ductus even in absence of the typical continuous murmur. When cyanosis is obvious in the neonatal period, transposition of the great arteries is the commonest lesion but when the heart is small and the lung field is ischaemic the tetralogy of Fallot must be considered. In the early school years the diagnostic problem is less difficult. A parasternal systolic murmur and thrill in an acyanotic child is usually due to pulmonary stenosis, a ventricular septal defect, or aortic stenosis. The distribution of the murmur, the quality of the cardiac impulse and the second heart sound at the base, the radiological features, and the electrocardiographic pattern will help to distinguish between the three. A less impressive murmur especially when combined with cardiac enlargement and plethoric lung fields will suggest an atrial septal defect. Routine palpation of the femoral pulses will lead to the recognition of significant degrees of coarctation of the aorta. The tetralogy of Fallot is the most frequent cause of cyanosis in this age period but cardiac enlargement, prominence of the main pulmonary artery and plethoric lung fields cast doubt on this diagnosis. When the clinical diagnosis suggests the possibility of surgical treatment, further investigation by cardiac catheterization and angiocardiography is often necessary to define the abnormality and determine the nature of the surgical procedure. There should be no undue hesitation in advising these investigations in infants with symptoms, for the risks of investigation and surgery may be less than the risks of conservative management and some infants may be saved who would otherwise die. When the clinical condition permits selection, the optimum age for occlusion of a persistent ductus is about 3 years. In the tetralogy of Fallot, operation should be postponed to over 3 years of age whenever possible. The timing of operation in coarctation of the aorta, pulmonary stenosis and aortic stenosis depends on detailed investigation of the individual patient. The electrocardiographic finding of ventricular hypertrophy and strain is an indication for this investigation even when symptoms are not striking.

MANAGEMENT

The management of cases of congenital cardiac malformation which are either unsuitable for surgery or in which surgical intervention has been refused, will depend principally on the child's exercise-tolerance. When this is seriously impaired, the child himself will limit his own activity, and medical treatment can do little to relieve the disability. In acyanotic cases where a lesion is discovered on routine examination (e.g. a ventricular septal defect) and where there is no functional disability, no useful purpose will be served by turning the child into an invalid. Normal activity should be allowed so long as it can be readily undertaken; even in cases of coarctation of the aorta, it is doubtful if any limitation of activity in childhood will materially affect the prognosis. But since the child runs a greater risk than does a normal individual of developing bacterial endocarditis, it is advisable to maintain careful supervision to detect the earliest signs of such infection during childhood. The possibility of bacterial endocarditis should be considered whenever such a child presents with infection, and the possibility of pulmonary infarcts from this cause simulating pneumonia should be borne in mind. Such procedures as dental extractions should be carried out under routine antibiotic cover, given for 24 hours before and 48 hours after the extraction. Apart from bacterial endocarditis, any condition such as pneumonia or pertussis throwing an exceptional strain on the right heart may produce cyanosis in cases where there is normally a left-to-right shunt and the appearance of cyanosis should be regarded as a danger signal.

CARDIAC ENLARGEMENT

Enlargement of the heart in infancy and early childhood is most commonly due to congenital malformation and cardiac murmurs are usually, though not invariably, audible. In a small proportion of cases, however, cardiomegaly is due to disease of the heart without anatomical malformation. Among the disorders associated with such cardiac enlargement are myocarditis, usually caused by Coxsackie group B or other virus infection but occasionally of unknown etiology; endocardial fibroelastosis; and cardiac glycogenosis. Cardiomyopathies encountered in other parts of the world include parasitic myocarditis in the Americas and endomyocardial fibrosis in Africa, though the latter seldom affects young children. In some cases the nature of the cardiomyopathy is not clear and in many the cause is unknown.

Endocardial fibroelastosis may be present to a variable degree in malformed hearts while extensive fibroelastosis unassociated with malformation is a frequent cause of cardiomegaly without murmurs in infancy. The etiology is unknown and the condition is no longer considered to be the result of fetal endocarditis. It has been attributed by some to a disorder of development and by others to congenital myocardial weakness.

Progressive cardiac enlargement occurs during the first few months of life and signs of congestive failure appear early, sometimes preceded by respiratory tract infection. Radiological examination shows only general increase in heart size. The electrocardiogram shows evidence of left ventricular loading but the changes are not diagnostic. Cardiac enlargement due to an anomalous left coronary artery or to other forms of cardiomyopathy must be considered in the differential diagnosis.

If death does not follow within a few weeks, the infant fails to thrive. Prolonged treatment with digoxin and a low salt diet may allow survival into childhood or even early adult life in a very small number of cases.

CARDIAC FAILURE

Infants with serious cardiac malformations may pass rapidly and almost imperceptibly into congestive failure and a careful watch must be kept for the earliest manifestations. Difficulty with feeds, caused by slight breathlessness on sucking, is one of the first indications. Careful examination at this stage reveals that the liver is firm and slightly enlarged: this is the most useful clinical sign of heart failure in infancy. As the condition deteriorates, dyspnoea and tachycardia increase, cyanosis may appear and eventually oedema becomes evident.

Infants in incipient failure should be digitalized promptly, digoxin (Lanoxin) being given by mouth, or parenterally if necessary. The total digitalizing dose in infancy averages about 0·08 mg per kg and in emergency half this dose (0·04 mg per kg) may be given intravenously or intramuscularly, followed by 0·02 mg per kg every 6 hours until full digitalization has been achieved. A good response will be indicated by slowing of the pulse rate and disappearance of the signs of failure. In less urgent cases, a slower dosage schedule may be adopted. The maintenance dose will usually be about 0·02 mg per kg per day, although requirements vary widely: in general, infants require relatively more digoxin than older children, in whom the dose may be proportionately lower.

Infants in cardiac failure should be nursed in a semi-upright position in 40 to 50 per cent oxygen. Restriction of sodium intake can be achieved by the use of low-sodium milk. Diuretics, e.g. frusemide, 0·5 mg per kg, chlorothiazide 20 mg per kg or hydrochlorothiazide in one-tenth of this dosage, are indicated in the presence of oedema not responding to digoxin. While these drugs are being used, potassium depletion may require correction. In some cases, failure may have been precipitated by an acute infection, which will require antibiotic therapy.

When congestive heart failure in the first few months of life does not respond readily to medical treatment, full and detailed cardiac investigation should generally be undertaken as a matter of urgency.

DISORDERS OF CARDIAC RHYTHM

Congenital malformations of the heart are often accompanied by disorders of rhythm, which may also occur without malformation. In general, the prognosis is worse if the dysrhythmia occurs in early infancy and if there is associated anatomical abnormality.

Paroxysmal atrial tachycardia is characterized by an abrupt onset of tachycardia, the pulse-rate changing suddenly from the normal to over 200 beats per minute, usually about 240, with regular rhythm. The infant becomes pale and quiet and will not feed. Distress increases and cardiac dilatation and failure supervene if the attack continues. The duration of the attacks varies from a few minutes to many hours or days. In some cases the electrocardiogram shows an associated Wolff-Parkinson-White pattern, with a very short P–R interval and a wide QRS.

Attacks usually cease as abruptly as they have begun. In some cases it is possible to terminate them by vagal compression, by forced expiration against a closed glottis or by other means. In the absence of cardiac disease the prognosis in older children is usually good, and when the attacks are infrequent and of short duration they cause little interference with normal activity. In infants in whom there is a much greater danger of cardiac failure, digoxin therapy should be used.

Extrasystoles, which may occur at regular or (more commonly) at irregular intervals, are only of significance when associated with organic heart lesions. Diagnosis is usually clear on clinical examination, but when extrasystoles occur frequently and when the cause is obscure an electrocardiogram is indicated. This will distinguish clearly between frequent extrasystoles and atrial fibrillation. In uncomplicated cases no treatment is indicated.

Atrial flutter, in which a circular contraction wave occurs in the atria causing an atrial rate of 300 or more, is rare in childhood, but should be considered in the differential diagnosis of paroxysmal tachycardia, and excluded by electrocardiogram. Treatment is by digitalization.

Atrial fibrillation also is very much less common in childhood than in adolescence and adult life. Since contraction of the atrial muscle fibres is completely irregular, the ventricular response and pulse are correspondingly erratic. The prognosis in childhood is bad, and though the condition may be temporarily relieved by digitalization, it usually represents a state of terminal cardiac failure.

BACTERIAL ENDOCARDITIS

This represents such an important complication of congenital malformation of the heart that it will be considered here, although it will be realized that it may also occur as a complication of acquired valvular disease, and often arises after childhood is passed. It is very rare before the age of 5 years.

The commonest infecting organisms are the *Streptococcus viridans* and the staphylococci, though other organisms may rarely be responsible. The lesions are likely to occur at a site of lowered resistance, such as the wall of the pulmonary artery opposite a persistent ductus

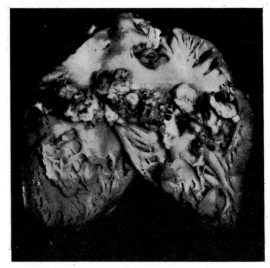

Fig. 5.20   Bacterial endocarditis. Heart opened to show vegetations and ulceration.

arteriosus or the right ventricular wall opposite a septal defect.

A positive blood culture will establish the diagnosis, though blood culture may be repeatedly negative, particularly in the more chronic cases.

CLINICAL SIGNS. In the acute fulminating cases the clinical picture is one of septicaemia. In the more chronic cases the diagnosis may remain unsuspected or uncertain for many weeks. The temperature may be only slightly raised or remain normal for considerable periods. Enlargement of the spleen occurs sooner or later, but is often slight unless splenic infarcts occur, when the spleen becomes large, painful and tender. The urine must be examined for the presence of red cells, pus cells and organisms.

The child's general condition is sometimes surprisingly good for long periods, though loss of weight, anorexia, lassitude, tachycardia, dyspnoea, and pallor are more characteristic of the disease. The cardiac signs will depend on the site and nature of the lesion. A valuable though uncommon diagnostic sign is the appearance of red painful nodes in the pulp of the fingers and toes (Osler's nodes). Small 'splinter haemorrhages' are sometimes seen beneath the nails, and petechiae may appear at any site. In long-standing cases a *café-au-lait* coloration of the skin is occasionally seen.

TREATMENT AND PROGNOSIS. Until the advent of chemotherapy, bacterial endocarditis was fatal in well over 90 per cent of cases. There is now at least reasonable chance of recovery if intensive antibiotic therapy is given early. Good results have been obtained in cases where a persistent ductus was affected, by the combination of ligation and antibiotic therapy. If the immediate response to antibiotic therapy is good, however, it may be found best to postpone ligation of the ductus in such cases until the disease has been arrested.

ANEURYSMS

Congenital aneurysms are rare, but may affect the arteries of the circle of Willis and cause intracranial haemorrhage, usually in later life. Arterio-venous malformations are also occasionally encountered in various sites, particularly in the distribution of the middle cerebral artery. They may give rise to a cranial murmur or thrill and papilloedema and cardiac failure may also occur.

General or focal convulsions, often followed by transient local paralysis or hemiplegia, are the commonest presenting symptoms. These tend to become progressively more severe, though in some cases the course is very protracted, or the lesion may remain latent for a number of years. Subarachnoid haemorrhage is a frequent complication, and is manifested by sudden onset of severe headache associated with the appearance of blood in the cerebrospinal fluid. Such haemorrhages may occur a number of times during childhood before a massive haemorrhage proves fatal. The immediate treatment is complete rest and sedation.

The prospects of successful surgical treatment of arterio-venous aneurysms depend on the site and nature of the lesion. Symptoms will often be relieved by decompression, when there is evidence of raised intracranial pressure, even when more radical treatment is impracticable.

ANGIOMATA

Angiomata should be regarded as congenital malformations rather than 'tumours' in the pathological sense, though in some instances they may enlarge or occasionally become the site of malignant change. Spider naevi may also appear after birth in association with cirrhosis of the liver. Cutaneous angiomata (or naevi) are amongst the commonest congenital abnormalities.

Four pathological types are recognized, depending on the degree of differentiation which has occurred.

Solid haemangiomata

Solid haemangiomata consist of endothelial cords containing no lumen and consequently having no blood-flow through them. These usually require no treatment.

Capillary ('port-wine') naevi

In these, endothelial channels have been formed, but the channels do not connect with the main vascular system and they contain few blood cells. The lesions do not blanch readily on pressure. Port-wine naevi are relatively common and may be extremely unsightly when they occur on the face or other exposed area. Their colour is dark red or purple. They are usually unilateral, and vary greatly in size.

TREATMENT. The success of treatment will depend on the extent and depth of the lesion. Small lesions can often be satisfactorily removed surgically, or by treatment with electrolysis, or solid carbon dioxide. Treatment of the larger facial lesions may be attempted with radiotherapy, but carries a considerable risk of scarring or infection. The less unsightly lesions are probably best left alone. This applies particularly to the small naevi often seen on the forehead or occipital region in newborn infants, where the growth of hair will subsequently render them inconspicuous.

Cavernous haemangiomata ('*Strawberry marks*')

Here there is a direct connection with the vascular system, and blood flows through the fully formed capillaries. This may result in the formation of sinusoids and rapid increase in size of the lesion following birth.

These naevi have a characteristic appearance, since they are elevated, sharply demarcated, and bright red in colour. When multiple, they may appear lobulated. After remaining stationary in size for some months or years, many 'strawberry marks' regress spontaneously and disappear by 4 or 5 years of age. Surgical removal may be feasible in some of those persisting after this age.

Cirsoid aneurysms

A direct connection between the arterial and venous systems renders these lesions of serious prognosis. When they occur in the limbs, they are likely to result in gross hypertrophy of the affected extremity. While surgical correction may be possible in some cases, the more extensive lesions may necessitate amputation.

Sturge-Weber syndrome

The association of a facial capillary (port-wine) naevus and epileptiform seizures is of considerable interest. Here the facial naevus involves the cutaneous distribution of the ophthalmic division of the fifth nerve (Fig. 5.21), and

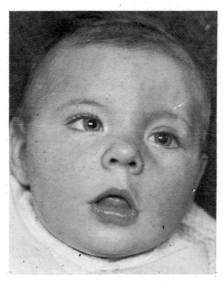

Fig. 5.21 Sturge-Weber syndrome. Trigeminal naevus (left) associated with right-sided Jacksonian epilepsy.

may extend over a greater part of the trigeminal area. On the same side is situated a more or less extensive area of telangiectasis of the pia-arachnoid, while the underlying area of cerebrum or cerebellum is sclerosed. The epileptiform attacks may be Jacksonian in type, involving the opposite side of the body, or become generalized. The intracranial telangiectases ultimately result in deposition of calcium in the immediately adjacent cerebral tissue. This calcium deposition gives rise to a characteristic radiological picture (Fig. 5.22) in which festoons of parallel lines of calcification are seen. There may also be asymmetry of the face.

The intracranial lesions are usually too diffuse to be amenable to surgery. The diagnosis should be suggested by the occurrence of epileptiform attacks in a child with a trigeminal naevus.

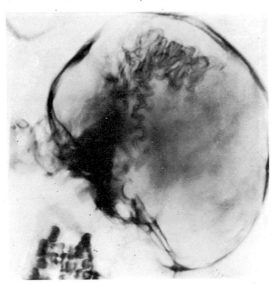

Fig. 5.22 Sturge-Weber syndrome. Cerebral calcification giving a festooned appearance, and the characteristic double-linear configuration.

Hereditary telangiectasis

The occurrence of multiple spider naevi in many members of a family should be borne in mind in the differential diagnosis of epistaxis or other spontaneous bleeding which is familial. The condition can legitimately be regarded as a congenital malformation, although the naevi are not always clinically obvious at birth, and may be confined to the mucous membranes, e.g. of the nose. They should be distinguished from spider naevi occurring as the result of hepatic disease.

LYMPHANGIOMA AND CONGENITAL LYMPHOEDEMA

Cystic masses of lymph vessels may occur alone or in association with haemangiomata. In lesions affecting the whole or part of a limb, causing hypertrophy, there may be overlying areas of vascular naevus, associated with an underlying haemo-lymphangioma.

Cystic hygroma

This consists of a localized cystic dilatation and overgrowth of lymph vessels, and is most frequently seen at birth as a large swelling in the neck, which is soft and fluctuant. It is not malignant, but frequently invades neighbouring tissues and may recur if surgical removal is not complete.

More diffuse types may involve the limbs, producing oedema which subsides when the limb is raised but which recurs when activity is resumed. Surgical treatment of these cases is seldom wholly successful.

Milroy's disease (*Congenital elephantiasis*)

This is a form of congenital and familial oedema of the lower limbs of which the etiology is obscure. The oedema is harder than that due to other causes, and there is little pitting on pressure. Although unsightly, the condition does not affect normal activity.

CONGENITAL MALFORMATIONS OF THE RESPIRATORY SYSTEM

Minor anomalies of the respiratory system are common but major malformations are infrequent and are responsible for fewer cases of clinical importance than those of any other system.

Obstruction of the posterior nares (*Choanal atresia*)

An obstruction which is occasionally observed at birth giving rise to difficulty in sucking and breathing. Lipiodol injected into the nose will demonstrate the obstruction, which can be relieved surgically.

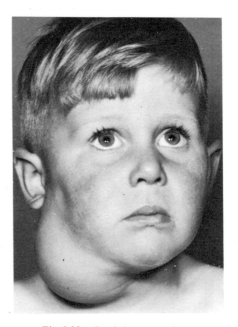

Fig. 5.23 Cystic hygroma of neck.

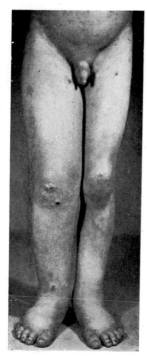

Fig. 5.24   Congenital lymphoedema, with hypertrophy of right leg.

Congenital laryngeal stridor

This condition is due to a variety of causes, the most frequent of which is an exaggeration of the infantile folding-round of the epiglottis ('omega epiglottis'), with partial laryngeal collapse. Occasionally cysts, papillomata or partial webbing of the larynx may be responsible.

The infant is noticed to have stridor from birth; this becomes more evident on crying. It is unlikely to be associated with cyanosis, and often gives rise to no symptoms; it is rare for the obstruction to be so severe as to prove fatal unless secondary infection occurs.

The larynx should be examined and the chest X-rayed. If the condition is due to an exaggeration of the infantile omega form of the epiglottis, it requires no treatment. Webbing will require immediate surgical relief if obstruction is severe. When the child is first seen some time after birth, it is important to determine whether the stridor really is congenital, and to exclude inhaled foreign body, infection, and tetany. Although laryngeal diphtheria is most unlikely to occur within the first weeks of life, the possibility should be remembered in any case where the cause of the stridor is obscure.

Trachea

Stenosis and atresia of the trachea are very rare. Tracheo-oesophageal fistula has already been described (p. 78).

Lungs

Although abnormalities of the lobes and fissures of the lungs are comparatively common, they are unlikely to cause symptoms except in cases where a portion of a lower lobe receives an abnormal blood supply from the aorta and also shows cystic malformation. An azygos lobe at the apex of the right lung, due to an abnormal situation of the azygos vein, is sometimes seen radiologically, but is rarely of clinical importance. Agenesis (complete absence of lung and bronchus), aplasia (absence of pulmonary tissue and rudimentary bronchus), and hypoplasia of a lung or part of a lung, are all rare abnormalities. Compensatory emphysema or hyperplasia of the remaining lobes is likely to occur.

Congenital cysts

Congenital cysts of the lung, which may be large single cysts containing air or fluid, or more commonly multiple small cysts giving a honeycomb appearance in the X-ray, seldom give rise to symptoms unless they become infected. Occasionally, however, an air-containing cyst may cause pressure symptoms requiring relief by deflation with or without lobectomy, while rupture of a cyst into the pleural cavity will give rise to pneumothorax. Infection of multiple cysts will result in a clinical picture which is likely to be confused with true bronchiectasis, since in some cases these cysts connect with a bronchus. Frequently, however, the cystic condition of the lung is only observed on routine radiological examination.

Bronchiectasis

It is probable that at least some of the cases diagnosed as 'saccular bronchiectasis' are in fact congenital cysts of the lungs which connect with the bronchial system and in which infection has occurred. Cystic fibrosis is also associated with pulmonary changes which become bronchiectatic (see p. 310).

Mediastinal cysts

These include cysts of widely different origin, and have been classified as epidermoid, dermoid, pericardial, bronchial, gastric and enteric cysts, teratomata, and cystic lymphangiomata.

Gastric, enteric, and bronchial cysts lie immediately adjacent to the oesophagus, trachea, or main bronchi, and are seen radiologically to occupy the posterior mediastinum. The other types of cysts are more likely to be found in the anterior mediastinum. All types are liable to cause pressure symptoms; in most instances they can be removed surgically.

CONGENITAL MALFORMATIONS OF THE GENITO-URINARY SYSTEM

These are of very great importance, and account for a high proportion of the cases of urinary infection seen in infancy, particularly in male babies. Of the cases of chronic pyuria seen in later childhood, many are due to congenital abnormalities which have passed unrecognized until secondary infection has caused irreversible damage to the kidneys.

In addition to those malformations which are clinically important, minor abnormalities of the kidneys or ureters which have caused no disability are frequently observed at necropsy. Approximately one-third of all cases of congenital malformation of the external genitalia show associated malformations of the upper urinary tract.

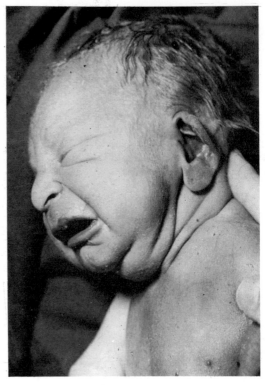

Fig. 5.25   Facies of bilateral renal agenesis (Potter facies).

KIDNEYS

Agenesis and dysplasia (*Hypoplasia*)

Complete absence of both kidneys is incompatible with life, and may be indicated at birth by the characteristic facial appearance (Fig. 5.25). Agenesis of one kidney occurs sufficiently often to make it advisable to determine that one functional kidney is present before any operative procedure is attempted on the other. In most cases of unilateral agenesis, the ureter will be absent on the same side, but occasionally a rudimentary ureter is present.

Dysplasia of one or both kidneys may be symptomless if sufficient renal tissue is present to give adequate renal function but is frequently complicated by pyelonephritis. Renal failure is likely when both kidneys are affected. It is probable that many cases of renal rickets and dwarfism, in which the symptoms date from infancy, are due to congenitally dysplastic kidneys, with or without other malformation of the genito-urinary tract. It may, however, be difficult to distinguish between congenital under-

development and contracture due to pyelonephritic scarring.

Hypertrophy

Hypertrophy of one kidney is usually secondary to agenesis or dysplasia of the other, and is to be regarded as a compensatory malformation.

Fusion of kidneys

This may be seen in a variety of forms, the commonest being fusion of the lower or upper poles in the mid-line to form a horseshoe kidney. Fused kidneys are frequently displaced, and may also show abnormalities of blood supply. While they may be symptomless, they are likely to become infected and hydronephrotic.

Displacement

Anomalous location of one or both kidneys is liable to give rise to distortion of the renal vessels or ureters and hydronephrosis. Very occasionally, a kidney is found to be freely mobile. Malrotation of the kidney during embryonic life may also result in hydronephrosis.

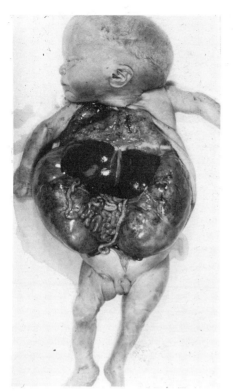

Fig. 5.26 Bilateral polycystic kidneys causing great abdominal enlargement.

Cystic kidneys

In polycystic disease, both kidneys are affected in the great majority of cases, and occasionally the liver and spleen also. The kidneys are greatly increased in size, and made up of innumerable small cysts containing yellow-brown fluid and separated by renal parenchyma. In infantile polycystic disease, which is inherited as a mendelian recessive, the kidneys may be so large as to cause difficulty in delivery of the fetus. In other cases, the presence of large bilateral intra-abdominal masses should suggest the diagnosis, especially if previous siblings have been affected. Intravenous pyelography may help to confirm the diagnosis. Those patients who survive infancy are liable to renal failure at any time, depending on the degree of destruction of the parenchyma or on the occurrence of secondary infection. It is doubtful if any form of therapy is effective. Adult polycystic disease differs from the infantile type, being inherited as a mendelian dominant.

Multicystic kidney disease is caused by embryonic dysplasia and is generally unilateral.

The cysts are of varying size and are united by fibrous tissue. Solitary renal cysts are simple serous cysts, and are rare in childhood. Multicystic kidney or solitary cyst seldom gives rise to symptoms but it is desirable to remove the kidney surgically to confirm the diagnosis.

Aberrant renal vessels

These occur very commonly, in most instances causing no ill effects, but in others resulting in obstruction of the ureter and hydronephrosis.

PELVIS AND URETER

Abnormalities of the pelves and ureters occur frequently, the commonest formations (on one or both sides) being (1) double pelvis uniting to form a single ureter, (2) double pelvis and double ureter, the upper ureter entering the bladder below the lower one, or opening ectopically in the urethra or vagina, (3) double pelvis with one complete ureter and one ureter ending blindly above the bladder. The first two of these may function normally, but there is an increased likelihood of obstruction and infection, especially in the lower, larger segment of the kidney; in the third type, the blind ureter commonly becomes dilated and secondarily infected.

Congenital stenosis

Congenital stenosis of the ureter, ectopic opening into the bladder, or complete atresia of the orifice, are important causes of obstruction. When the ureter is obstructed at its lower end, hydronephrosis will be associated with hydro-ureter.

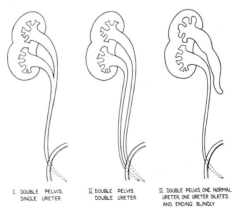

I. DOUBLE PELVIS, SINGLE URETER   II. DOUBLE PELVIS, DOUBLE URETER   III. DOUBLE PELVIS, ONE NORMAL URETER, ONE URETER DILATED AND ENDING BLINDLY

Fig. 5.27 Types of reduplication of pelvis and ureter.

Congenital megaureter

This occurs without organic obstruction but there may be functional obstruction comparable with that in Hirschsprung's disease, with which it is occasionally associated. In such cases, contrast medium injected into the bladder will sometimes reflux readily into one ureter when the condition is unilateral, the normal ureter showing no reflux Damage to the kidney from back pressure and infection will usually indicate nephrectomy but in less severe cases reconstructive surgery with reimplantation of the ureters is successful.

Ureteral valves, kinking, ureterocele

Ureteral valves, kinking, and ureterocele (a cystic dilatation of the lower end of the ureter, which will occasionally prolapse through the ureteric orifice into the bladder) are also possible causes of obstruction.

BLADDER

The bladder capacity in childhood averages 250 ml but there is wide variation. Enlargement of the bladder may be due to polyuria or to obstruction and back pressure, when there will usually be residual urine after micturition. In *megacystis*, which may be associated with megaureters, the bladder is very large but empties completely and seldom requires treatment.

Exstrophy

In the severest degrees of this malformation, the lower abdominal wall and the anterior wall of the bladder are absent, and the posterior wall of the bladder presents in the suprapubic region. The penis is spatulate, and may show complete *epispadias*, i.e. the urethra lying open anteriorly. In the female a similar deformity of the clitoris occurs. Herniae are common and there may be other associated malformations. Since there can be no control of micturition, urine dribbles to the exterior through the ureteric orifices.

Operative treatment is usually advisable. The ureteric orifices can be transplanted into the sigmoid, and an attempt made to close the anterior abdominal wall, but infection of the ureters and kidneys commonly occurs. An ileal bladder with ileostomy is more satisfactory and is usually combined with orthopaedic surgical treatment of the pelvic bones.

Persistent urachus

Failure of the lumen of the allantois to close will result in a fistula connecting the fundus of the bladder to the umbilicus. The condition is easily recognized in its complete form by the fact that the newborn infant passes urine through the umbilicus.

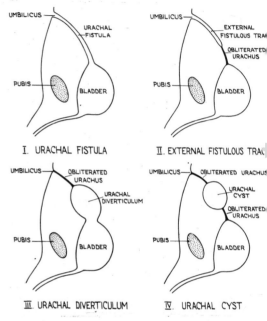

Fig. 5.28   Types of persistent urachus.

When closure is incomplete, the remains of the urachus may form a large diverticulum from the bladder, closed at its umbilical end, or if closure occurs both at the umbilical and vesical ends of the urachus but not centrally, a cyst lying between the fundus of the bladder and the umbilicus will be formed. A blind fistulous track opening externally at the umbilicus will occur when the urachus is closed at the vesical end only (Fig. 5.28). Surgical closure or removal is usually effected readily.

Diverticula

These may be congenital or arise as the result of back pressure. In either case they are liable to result in stagnation of urine, secondary infection, and calculus formation. They may also cause pressure symptoms and obstruction of the adjacent ureter. The diagnosis can usually be made readily by cystogram or cystoscopy. Surgical removal of the diverticulum is indicated.

Trigonal bar

Occasionally obstruction of the outlet of the bladder is caused by a fold of redundant trigonal mucosa, which should be excised.

URETHRA

Owing partly to its greater length, the male urethra is much more commonly the site of malformation and obstruction than the female. While stenosis or congenital narrowing of the central portion of the urethra is rare, obstruction of the posterior urethra by valves or of the meatal orifice by stenosis are both common, and give rise to back pressure affecting the bladder and ultimately the ureters and kidneys.

Urethral valves

These are situated in the posterior urethra, and have been classified into three types. In type I, the common type, folds of mucosa run from the verumontanum above to the urethral walls below; in type II, the obstruction lies above the verumontanum, the folds running from the urethral walls above to the verumontanum below. The folds may be unilateral or bilateral. In both of these types, attempts to pass urine from the bladder will cause ballooning of the mucosal

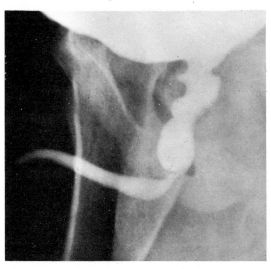

Fig. 5.30   Micturating cystogram showing a posterior urethral valve.

folds or 'curtains', and result in partial obstruction. In type III, the valve represents a partial diaphragm across the lumen of the urethra (Fig. 5.29).

SYMPTOMS. Although the patient may only come under observation when back pressure has already caused extensive damage to the bladder and upper renal tract, the history will usually reveal previous difficulties in micturition. Of these the most common are: difficulties in starting micturition; a feeble stream; and dribbling incontinence following micturition, which may masquerade as diurnal enuresis. Since the bladder is seldom completely emptied, nocturnal enuresis frequently occurs also.

DIAGNOSIS. Urethral valves are frequently overlooked both during life and at necropsy unless their presence is previously suspected. Thus it will often be found that a catheter or probe passed from the meatus into the urethra will not be obstructed by the valve, which only causes obstruction to urine passing in the reverse direction. The site of the obstruction can sometimes be demonstrated if contrast medium is injected into the bladder and an X-ray taken while the patient is attempting to micturate. Satisfactory diagnosis can only be made, however, by direct urethroscopy. This should always be undertaken when the history suggests the presence of valves or when there is evidence of bilateral dilatation of the ureters or residual urine. Bladder neck obstruction may also be

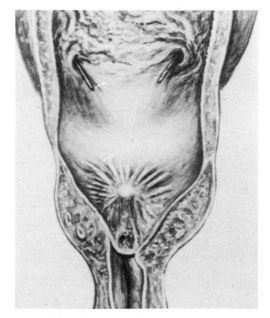

Fig. 5.29   Posterior urethral valve. Specimen from boy aged 9 years showing renal rickets, bilateral dilatation of ureters, and renal dysplasia.

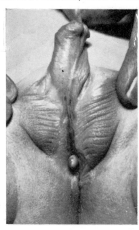

Fig. 5.31 Hypospadias (bulbous type) showing bifid scrotum and failure of canalization of urethra.

caused by fibrous changes in the posterior urethral wall.

TREATMENT. Excision of the valve will usually be necessary, though the partial diaphragm type of valve can sometimes be broken down by dilatation.

Meatal stenosis

Stenosis of the urethral meatus occurs in both sexes, but its frequency has probably been over-estimated by misinterpretation of the radiological appearance of the normal urethra. The symptoms are similar to those of urethral valves. Once the condition is recognized, the stenosis is readily overcome by enlargement of the meatal orifice.

Diverticula of the urethra

These are rare, but may occasionally cause obstruction. The diverticulum is likely to fill during micturition, and may be recognized as a fluctuant swelling adjacent to the urethra.

Hypospadias

This is a common malformation, though the majority of cases are of minor degree and require no treatment. The opening of the urethra, instead of lying in its normal position in the glans, lies at some point along the normal course of the urethra. The most common site is at the base of the glans (glandular type), but the opening may occur at some point down the shaft of the penis (penile type), at the base of the penis or between the two halves of a bifid scrotum (penoscrotal type), or in the perineum (bulbous type). In the glandular type the prepuce and glans are deformed, but apart from dilatation of the meatus if this is constricted, no treatment is required. In the other types the malformation of the penis and scrotum is likely to be more severe, and there may be associated cryptorchidism. The operation performed will have to depend on the type of the deformity, and should be undertaken between 4 and 5 years of age. The principal object is to reconstruct a functional urethral opening situated as nearly as possible on the glans but correction of the penile curvature (chordee) may be required first.

PREPUCE
Phimosis

Extreme phimosis is a very rare cause of obstruction and back pressure. Ballooning of the prepuce on micturition or narrowing of the urinary stream due to a small preputial orifice are definite indications for circumcision, while if the prepuce remains non-retractile in later childhood and the stenosis cannot be overcome by dilatation, circumcision may be advisable.

The majority of circumcisions are quite unnecessary, however, and are performed simply from ignorance of the anatomy of the newborn infant. The prepuce is not normally fully retractile at birth, and is frequently adherent to the glans. In the great majority of children it subsequently becomes retractile, and the adhesions separate spontaneously; when the prepuce remains adherent after the age of 2 or 3 years, separation of adhesions with a blunt probe will often correct the condition without the necessity of operation. Circumcision is not without risk and should be reserved for those cases where it is necessary in order to prevent accumulation of smegma, interference with micturition, or paraphimosis. The operation should never be recommended in a patient with hypospadias in whom the deformed prepuce may be required for reconstruction of the urethra, and should not be undertaken in the presence of ammoniacal dermatitis.

The operation may be followed by the formation of a *meatal ulcer*, micturition then causing pain or slight bleeding due to separation of the scab. Although the condition is troublesome, it will ultimately yield to local treatment. Particular care should be taken after circumcision to keep the infant as dry as possible, since continual contact with cold wet napkins will delay the healing of an ulcer if this should form.

Paraphimosis

An abnormally tight prepuce when retracted may cause constriction and oedema of the penis, with the result that the retraction cannot readily be reduced. If pressure after the local injection of hyaluronidase is unsuccessful, the dorsum of the prepuce should be incised longitudinally (i.e. across the contraction ring) and the distal and peripheral ends of the incision brought together, or circumcision performed.

URINARY OBSTRUCTION

It will be realized from the above that a wide variety of congenital malformations may cause urinary obstruction. These are shown diagrammatically in Figure 5.32. Stenosis of the opening of a single renal calyx will cause a localized cyst, which may remain silent, or be the site of calculus formation. The various types of obstruction occurring between the renal pelvis and the bladder will all tend to produce unilateral *hydronephrosis* (dilatation of the pelvis with destruc-

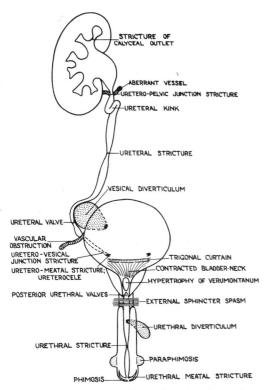

Fig. 5.32 Congenital malformations causing urinary obstruction. (After Campbell, M. F. (1937). *Pediatric Urology*. By courtesy of the author.)

tion of renal parenchyma) and some degree of *hydroureter* (dilatation of the ureter above the obstruction).

Obstruction occurring below the ureteric orifices will result in back pressure which will affect both sides, and one may expect to find bilateral dilatation of ureters and pelves, with involvement of the bladder also. Infravesical obstruction is therefore even more important from the point of view of early diagnosis than supravesical, since bilateral renal damage, if it occurs, will greatly reduce the prospects of survival. Since the obstruction is present before birth, however, secondary hydronephrosis and hydroureter may themselves appear as congenital abnormalities.

Urinary obstruction at any site carries the risk of secondary infection, and the majority of cases do not come under observation until after this has occurred. With the methods of therapy now available, it is often possible to disinfect the urinary tract before operative correction of the obstruction is undertaken.

In all cases of chronic urinary infection or recurrent pyelonephritis in childhood, the likely possibility of congenital malformation being the responsible factor should be remembered, and the patient investigated with this in mind.

OTHER GENITAL MALFORMATIONS

Adhesion of the labia

This condition is recognizable at birth, and should be corrected as soon as possible. When the labia are simply adherent and not fused, they can usually be separated without difficulty, using a blunt probe.

Occlusion of the vaginal orifice

The vaginal orifice may be entirely absent, in which case there is likely to be partial or complete failure of development of the vagina itself, or the vagina may be occluded by an imperforate hymen or by a membrane above it. The latter condition frequently escapes recognition until the onset of menstruation, when haematocolpos results from the retention of menstrual fluid. Occasionally, however, hydrocolpos or pyocolpos secondary to occlusion of the vagina has been observed even in the newborn and has resulted in urinary obstruction. While hymenectomy is a minor surgical procedure, attempts to reconstruct an imperfectly developed vagina should not be made before puberty.

Bicornuate uterus, double vagina

Bicornuate uterus and more rarely double vagina both occur as congenital malformations but are unlikely to cause symptoms during childhood.

Congenital hydrocele

In the female, hydrocele of the canal of Nuck occasionally occurs but seldom requires treatment. In the male, hydrocele is comparatively common, and several varieties occur. In communicating hydrocele, fluid surrounds both the testicle and spermatic cord, and the sac in which the fluid is contained communicates directly with the peritoneal cavity above. The swelling can be

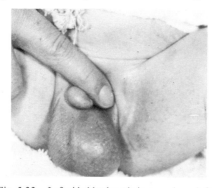

Fig. 5.33   Left-sided hydrocele in a newborn infant.

reduced by pressure unless the communicating tract is obstructed. In some instances this type of hydrocele is associated with hernia. The so-called infantile type of hydrocele consists of a fluid-containing sac which surrounds only the testicle and is closed above. Where the hydrocele surrounds the cord but not the testicle, the sac may be closed above and below (encysted hydrocele of the cord) or, more rarely, communicate with the peritoneal cavity above. The majority of cases of congenital hydrocele recover spontaneously, but when there is a large communication with the peritoneal cavity or an associated hernia exists, operation is likely to be required.

Cryptorchidism and maldescent of the testicle

A clear distinction must be made between the testicle which is *retractile* in childhood, i.e. which is drawn up above the scrotum but can be brought down by manipulation, the testicle which is retained within the abdominal cavity or inguinal canal, and the testicle which has descended to occupy an abnormal position. The term *cryptorchidism* should, strictly speaking, be applied to the testicle lying within the abdominal cavity, but it is not always easy in young children to distinguish clinically between this condition and retention of the testicle within the inguinal canal. The testicle which occupies an abnormal position after having passed through the inguinal canal is an *ectopic* testicle; it may lie superficially in the inguinal region above the canal or in the perineum.

The condition of *retractile testicle* can hardly be regarded as pathological in childhood. If by firm pressure downward from the internal ring towards the neck of the scrotum, and by gentle manipulation through the invaginated scrotum, the testicle can be brought from the superficial inguinal pouch into the scrotal sac, treatment is not only unnecessary but may be harmful.

In the case of an ectopic testicle which cannot be brought down by manipulation into the scrotum, it is probable that an anatomical malformation is preventing the normal course of descent, and operation will be required.

When the testicle lies within the abdominal cavity or the inguinal canal at birth, it may descend into the scrotum within the next two to three months, but spontaneous descent rarely if ever occurs thereafter. The undescended testis remains small and maldeveloped, so that in bilateral cryptorchidism sterility is almost certain. Even in unilateral maldescent, the incidence of infertility is high. There is therefore every reason for bringing the testes down by orchidopexy at an early age, usually about 5 or 6 years, in both bilateral and unilateral cases.

In a considerable proportion of cases, maldescent of the testicle is associated with inguinal hernia and the surgical correction of both may be undertaken in infancy.

Pseudohermaphroditism

While true hermaphroditism (the existence of an ovary and testis in the same individual) occurs extremely rarely, there is sometimes difficulty in determining the sex of an infant at birth owing to malformation of the external genitalia of a male or masculinization of a female during intra-uterine life. In the case of a male, the association of bilateral cryptorchidism, a bifid scrotum, and a perineal hypospadias may simulate a female. A similar difficulty arises in the case of female infants who have fusion of the labia and hypertrophy of the clitoris.

When it is impossible to decide the sex of an infant from examination of the external genitalia aided by rectal examination, nuclear sexing should be carried out in order to determine whether the infant is genetically male or female. If a laparotomy is subsequently considered necessary, the gonads and adrenals should be examined, and the presence or absence of a uterus determined.

Nuclear sexing and chromosome studies have served to define a number of types of human intersex, including at least two varieties of male and female pseudohermaphrodite and cases of gonadal dysgenesis in which the chromatin structure is either abnormal or indicates an opposite sex to the phenotype.

Hyperplasia of the adrenal cortex during intrauterine life produces masculinization of the female to such an extent that the sex may appear ambiguous. Estimation of 17-ketosteroids and pregnanetriol in a 24 hour sample of urine will show elevated levels in this condition.

The etiology and treatment of congenital adrenal hyperplasia are considered in Chapter 8.

CONGENITAL MALFORMATIONS OF THE CENTRAL NERVOUS SYSTEM

Defective development of the central nervous system has probably greater social importance than any other single manifestation of disease in childhood. The majority of cases of the severest grades of mental subnormality are due to this cause, and also a proportion of cases of cerebral palsy and epilepsy. Anencephaly, hydrocephalus and spina bifida occur six or seven times in every thousand births, the incidence varying in different parts of the country. They thus rank amongst the commoner congenital malformations, and are important causes of stillbirth and neonatal death. After the birth of a first affected child, the risk of a second similarly malformed is increased, being about 1 in 30.

Since any part of the nervous system may show defects of development, a very wide range of clinical manifestations may be met with, and only some of the more classical types can be discussed. These will usually be classifiable as failures of development (agenesis); failures of fusion (e.g. failure of closure of the neural tube); failures of differentiation; and local overgrowth. The first two of these are the most important clinically. Using 'congenital malformation' in the widest sense, some degenerative and heredofamilial nervous disorders might also be included, since nerve cells showing a constitutional inferiority and degenerating prematurely could be considered as malformed at birth.

MENTAL SUBNORMALITY (MENTAL RETARDATION, MENTAL DEFICIENCY)

The term 'mental deficiency' has been replaced in the Mental Health Act (England & Wales, 1959) by (1) severe subnormality, defined as 'a state of arrested or incomplete development of mind which includes subnormality of intelligence and is of such a nature or degree that the patient is incapable of living an independent life or of guarding himself against serious exploitation, or will be so incapable when of an age to do so'; and (2) subnormality, representing a state of arrested or incomplete development of mind (not amounting to severe subnormality) 'of a nature or degree which requires or is susceptible to medical treatment or other special care or training of the patient'. While these two broad categories have a certain value for administrative purposes in emphasizing degrees of social inadequacy and need for special care or training, the following subgroupings are still commonly employed as being more precise.

Idiots

Idiots are those in whom the degree of subnormality is so great that they are 'unable to guard themselves against common physical dangers'. These represent the severest grade of subnormality, having an intelligence quotient of less than 25, and including complete aments, where even the most primitive manifestations of intelligence are absent, and less complete types.

Imbeciles

Imbeciles are those who are less defective than idiots but are 'incapable of managing themselves or their affairs, or, in the case of children, of being taught to do so'. According to American definition, the intelligence quotient is from 25 to 49. The educability of imbeciles is low though they may be trainable in the activities of daily life; they are incapable of earning a living as adults, and as children are likely to require constant supervision.

Feeble-minded

Feeble-minded (or morons) are those where the degree of mental subnormality falls short of imbecility, but is such that they require care, supervision, and control for their own protection or for the protection of others, or, in the case of children, that they appear permanently incapable of receiving benefit from the instruction in ordinary schools. The range of intelligence quotient is 50 to 74.

It will be obvious that this classification simply describes *degrees* of mental subnormality, in the same way that the higher ranges of intelligence might be divided in terms of social adequacy and intellectual capabilities, e.g. I.Q. 70 to 85—capable of unskilled labour; I.Q. 85 to 115—skilled labour; and I.Q. above 115—professional occupations. The evaluation of a particular child is better expressed in terms of his capacity for self-help and social adjustment as well as his intelligence than by arbitrary categorization. While the defined degrees of mental subnormality are useful for certification, selection for occupational or training centres, or education in special schools, they bear no relation to causation or clinical types. The distribution curve of intelligence in the community does not show an abrupt transition from 'low normal' to feeble-mindedness on the one hand, or from 'high normal' to genius on the other. The percentage of the most severely subnormal, however, is higher than would be expected from a normal distribution curve. This has been compared to the distribution curve of height, where the number of individuals in the community of very small stature is greater than might be expected from a normal distribution, by the addition of dwarfs whose condition is due to various causes, such as achondroplasia and rickets. It is found that a greater proportion of the most severely subnormal show gross structural cerebral abnormalities, and associated congenital malformations, than is the case in the feeble-minded group. Neurological and psychiatric abnormalities are also found more frequently in children of very low intelligence. While there is no social class gradient for the prevalence of these severely subnormal children, mild degrees of subnormality are markedly over-represented in social classes IV and V.

PREVALENCE OF MENTAL SUBNORMALITY

It has been estimated that mental subnormality as administratively defined affects about 1 per cent of the population, though psychometric testing of all children aged 8 to 10 years suggests that the true prevalence at this age is between 2 and 3 per cent. Since the definitions of the various grades imply that the mentally subnormal are those requiring special care and protection, it will be seen that they represent a very serious burden to the community. While many can be trained for simple duties under supervision, and adapt readily to conditions in which the demands made on them do not exceed their capabilities, the severely subnormal are likely to require institutional care or a quite disproportionate amount of maternal attention in the home.

ETIOLOGY

Even if one excludes those cases due to birth injury (which probably represents the etiological factor in only about 5 per cent of the total), and the relatively small group in which mental subnormality has developed after birth as the result of infection (e.g. meningitis, encephalitis), trauma, metabolic error, intoxication, degeneration, or other causes, the determination of etiology in the truly 'congenital' cases is an extremely complex problem. Mental subnormality cannot be considered as a single disease entity and hereditary and environmental factors are inextricably mingled in the etiology of most cases. We know that before birth the nervous system of the fetus may be subjected to a wide variety of noxious stimuli, including drugs and toxins, radiation, malnutrition, anoxia, and infection, which may interfere with its normal development, while the genetic constitution of the ovum and spermatozoon is no longer considered to be beyond the reach of environmental influences. Even those cases which can confidently be attributed to heredity will represent a mixed group in which the mode of inheritance will require separate analysis in different cases or types of case. A small proportion of the mentally subnormal population conforms to clinical syndromes in which there is more or less constant association with certain physical features and/or metabolic errors, e.g. mongolism, homocystinuria, etc. Mental abnormalities occurring in association with haemolytic disease of the newborn, low birth-weight, lipidosis, cretinism, dyspituitarism, and epilepsy are referred to elsewhere.

The problem of inheritance is one of great importance which is still a long way from complete solution. The parents of a mentally subnormal child will usually wish to know whether they should limit their family for fear of a subsequent child being similarly affected. It will be possible, when the condition is clearly due to birth injury or infection, to say that subsequent children are unlikely to be affected unless exposed to the same risk, e.g. delivery through a contracted pelvis or infection with toxoplasmosis. Similarly, when the case falls into a well-defined clinical type having a familial incidence, and particularly when there is consanguinity, it may be possible to give some indication of the likelihood of the condition recurring. In the majority of cases, however, it is impossible to advise with any degree of confidence.

MANAGEMENT

With the exception of a small proportion of cases due to infection, cretinism and possibly some metabolic disorders, e.g. phenylketonuria (p. 188), mental subnormality is not amenable to treatment aimed at raising a low intelligence quotient to normal. A great deal can be done, however, for children with lesser degrees of subnormality by appropriate management. Training including handicraft should be at a level commensurate with the child's intelligence. This is usually best undertaken in a special school or day centre. Where there is an associated physical disability, careful consideration should be given to the best means of overcoming it. There is, for instance, little purpose in embarking on elaborate operations on the spastic child if he is not capable of benefiting by subsequent training. The question will frequently arise as to whether a mentally subnormal child should remain in his home or be admitted to a hospital or residential home. Here consideration must be given to the economic status of the family, the character of the parents themselves, and the effect on other children. If a child with severe subnormality is one of a family in which the other children are normal, they may suffer from deprivation of the maternal attention given to the subnormal one and in such a situation it is usually advisable for the subnormal child to be removed to a foster home or family group home. In general, however, the mentally subnormal child needs the same affection and security as other children and develops best in a stable family environment, with such professional advice and practical help as are necessary. With the passage of time his needs are likely to change and the provision made must be kept under constant review.

ASSOCIATED CEREBRAL MALFORMATIONS

A very great variety of cerebral abnormalities is found in association with severe mental subnormality, many of them clearly developmental, others probably degenerative. In addition to the types described below, there may be more or less extensive areas of agenesis of the cortex or cerebellum, excessively large or small or undifferentiated gyri, failure of differentiation of the cerebral hemispheres, and absence or maldevelopment of the corpus callosum.

Microcephaly

Microcephaly implies a head circumference more than 2 s.d. below the mean for age and sex. The brain in this condition is often similar to that of a fetus of three or four months' gestation, and development appears to be arrested. At birth, the cranium is usually abnormally small, e.g. 30 cm circumference, and the fontanelle may be closed; the condition must be differentiated from craniosynostosis (p. 131). Growth of the brain and skull is extremely slow, and the discrepancy from the normal becomes more obvious with increasing age. The appearance is very characteristic, since the face is of approximately normal size and is in marked contrast to the small cranium with its flattened occiput.

The condition may be familial and genetically determined, or due to prenatal irradiation or infection, e.g. toxoplasmosis or cytomegalic inclusion disease. The degree of mental defect varies considerably in different cases, some children never learning to walk, talk, or become continent, others being able to carry out simple duties and a small proportion being mentally normal. Convulsions occur in rather less than half the cases. Many patients die during infancy or childhood from intercurrent infection, but others may reach adult life.

Megalencephaly

Though hypertrophy of the brain giving rise to *macrocephaly* is a much rarer condition than microcephaly, the incidence is probably underestimated owing to cases being misdiagnosed as hydrocephalus. The patients are mentally subnormal and the brain shows either a generalized

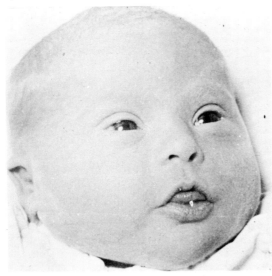 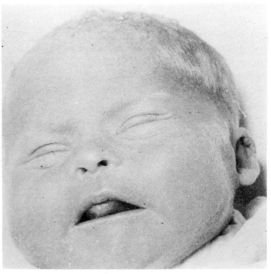

Fig. 5.34   Facies in mongolism (Down's syndrome).

enlargement or an enlargement of one portion at the expense of another, the increase in size being due to a diffuse proliferative gliosis.

Porencephaly

In the type of porencephaly occurring as a unilateral or bilateral congenital malformation, a wide depression of the cerebral cortex communicates with the lateral ventricle. The same term is applied to cystic areas of cerebral degeneration resulting from birth injury. The condition is commonly associated with severe mental subnormality and cerebral palsy.

Hydranencephaly

In this anomaly, virtually the whole of the cerebral hemispheres is absent and the head glows on transillumination in a dark room.

Mongolism (*Down's syndrome*)

This clinical type of mental subnormality is both relatively common, with an estimated incidence of approximately 1 in 600 births, and readily recognized. The established name is misleading since the condition is quite unrelated to racial stock. Substitution of the term Down's syndrome has been advocated.

ETIOLOGY. The characteristic physical defects are established early in pregnancy, and the finding of a supernumerary autosomal chromosome in mongols (who typically have 47 instead of the normal 46 chromosomes) is due to nondisjunction when the germ cell is formed, result-ing in an ovum with two chromosomes 21 which therefore has three after fertilization (trisomy 21). In exceptional cases in which the chromosome number is apparently 46, it has been found that trisomy has occurred but that the additional chromosome 21 has become translocated and joined to one of the other chromosomes, e.g. the D group (13–15) or the G group (21–22). In such cases, one parent may also show translocation and appear to have 45 chromosomes. Translocation occurring in a parent may account for more than one mongol child in a family. In about 2 per cent of all mongols, the body contains two types of cell, one with an extra chromosome and the other chromosomally normal (mosaicism).

Maternal age. Mongolism occurs with increasing frequency amongst the infants born to mothers over the age of 30 years. It is by no means limited to such infants, however, and may occur in infants of mothers in their teens or early twenties, particularly if there is chromosomal translocation in a parent. Paternal age is typically unrelated to incidence.

Place in family. A considerable proportion of mongols are last-born infants. This is related to increasing maternal age, and also possibly to the tendency to limit families after the birth of a mongol child.

Abnormalities of pregnancy. It is found that a history of previous abortions and of uterine bleeding during pregnancy is higher in the mothers of mongols than in normal controls. Numerous other abnormalities of early pregnancy, including attempted abortion, have been recorded.

Maternal endocrine imbalance. Benda (1947) has stressed the high incidence of relative infertility, and thyroid or ovarian abnormalities, which led him to conclude that the mongol might be regarded as the 'survivor of a threatened abortion'.

Familial incidence. Although it is exceptional for more than one case of mongolism to occur in a sibship, a considerable number of examples have been recorded where this has occurred. The likelihood of this being due to chromosomal defect in a parent is referred to above. Monozygotic twins are likely both to be affected. When twins arise from two ova, it is much less likely that both will be affected, but mongolism in fraternal twins has been observed.

CLINICAL FEATURES. Mongols resemble one another quite as closely as do normal brothers and sisters, the resemblance being due to the association of a number of physical stigmata which occur with surprising regularity, though some are more constant than others.

The skull is small and brachycephalic with a flattened occipital region. The face and nose are flattened and the nostrils in consequence are abnormally obvious.

The slanting palpebral fissures, which originally suggested the name of the condition, are characteristic, and usually smaller than normal. There is a prominent epicanthic fold on either side. The iris may show a spotted appearance (Brushfield's spots). With increasing age, there is a tendency for the thin eye-lid to become infected and for the eyelashes to be shed; cataract may develop early. Strabismus very frequently occurs, and nystagmus is often present.

The mouth is small and the mucosa of the alveolar margins thickened. The tongue usually protrudes, and after early infancy becomes fissured (the so-called 'scrotal tongue') in the great majority of cases. Dentition is commonly delayed.

The hands are usually short, and the terminal phalanx of the little finger is incurved. A deep transverse crease is seen across the palms (Fig. 5.35) and study of the epidermal ridge patterns (dermatoglyphics) shows that the palmar triradii are abnormal. The feet are broad and short, with wide deviation of the great toe, and a plantar crease running between the first and second toes.

The general physical development of mongols

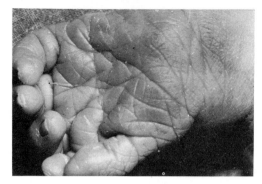

Fig. 5.35   Transverse palmar crease.

is retarded, and the generalized hypotonia gives them an abnormal flexibility. The hypotonia, as well as the mental defect, is partly responsible for the delay in sitting up and walking. Although secondary sexual characters appear, the genitalia and breasts are commonly underdeveloped. After puberty, many mongols become excessively fat. The voice is husky, and often of low pitch even in childhood. Speech is always delayed, and commonly very defective.

Between 40 and 50 per cent of mongol infants are born with congenital malformations of the heart. Since many of these infants die early, the proportion of older mongols showing evidence of congenital heart lesions is lower than that of infants.

While the association of the above features is quite diagnostic, it must be emphasized that not all the stigmata are present in every case, and in rare cases the diagnosis can only be made confidently by examination of the chromosomes.

INTELLIGENCE. Typical mongols do not reach a mental age of more than 7 years. While they may learn to speak in simple sentences, become habit-trained, and show an obvious enjoyment of music, they are unable to learn a trade and will ultimately require institutional care. They are usually happy and biddable children, and if they remain in the home the parents often become very attached to them, making subsequent separation more difficult.

PATHOLOGY. The brain of the mongol is smaller than normal. With increasing age, the brain appears increasingly immature in comparison with the normal; the cerebellum is often more affected than the cerebral hemispheres, but abnormalities of the cerebral convolutional pattern occur. Degeneration in the cortex and white matter is described.

DIAGNOSIS. Although mongolism is sometimes confused with cretinism, the two conditions are widely different. The stigmata of mongolism are present at birth, whereas the cretin is likely to appear normal at birth and only show evidence of thyroid deficiency after a period of weeks. The skull of the cretin is normal in shape, and the facies, though heavy and dull-looking, does not show the oblique palpebral fissures or epicanthic folds characteristic of the mongol. The cretin is sallow, whereas the mongol is of normal or high colouring. The mongol, though mentally defective, appears mobile, observant, and happy, whereas the cretin is peculiarly dull and uninterested. Other features characteristic of the cretin are considered subsequently.

Achondroplasia should not be confused with mongolism if the characteristic shortness of the limbs and relatively large skull are observed. Rickets bears only the most superficial resemblance to mongolism, though both conditions are characterized by hypotonia and developmental delay. The other signs of rickets should establish the distinction. Turner's syndrome and hypertelorism may both be confused with mongolism when they are associated with mental defect, but the facial appearances are not closely similar and the other stigmata of mongolism are absent.

PROGNOSIS. The expectation of life in mongolism is greatly reduced. Many of these infants are born prematurely and have a correspondingly reduced survival rate. In others, congenital heart lesions are responsible for early death. There is an increased incidence of leukaemia, and also of duodenal atresia. In all cases there appears to be an increased susceptibility to infections of all kinds, and the mortality from infection is high in infancy and childhood. Those who survive puberty may live to middle age.

TREATMENT. Much disappointment is caused to parents if they are led to believe that any significant improvement can be obtained by thyroid or other endocrine therapy. Since mongolism is determined early in intrauterine life, it is unlikely that any form of therapy given after birth will do more than modify symptoms and it is unwise to hold out any prospects of improvement other than that which can be expected with age and training.

De Lange syndrome (*Amsterdam dwarfism*)

Certain mentally and physically retarded children show features which warrant the diagnosis of de Lange syndrome. Birth weight is low and the infant has a characteristic facies, with confluent eyebrows, anteverted nostrils and long upper lip. The head is small and brachycephalic and there is general hirsuties. Single palmar creases, syndactyly and other anomalies may be present. The cause of the syndrome is unknown.

Tuberous sclerosis (*Epiloia*)

This uncommon condition is characterized by local areas of cerebral sclerosis giving the affected portion of the brain an appearance similar to that of a peeled walnut. These areas are firm and may be associated with mesodermal tumours elsewhere. A condition of adenoma sebaceum occurs on the face, the lesions being pink or red in colour and distributed over the cheeks, nose, and chin. There is also commonly a pigmented 'shagreen' area on the skin of the trunk. Examination of the fundi may show the presence of whitish retinal plaques (phakomata). Epileptic attacks are a frequent and early symptom. While mental defect is the rule, some patients show little or no mental retardation during early childhood, though tending to regress subsequently. The condition is thought to have some affinity with neurofibromatosis (von Recklinghausen's disease), in which multiple neurofibromata occur in relation to the peripheral

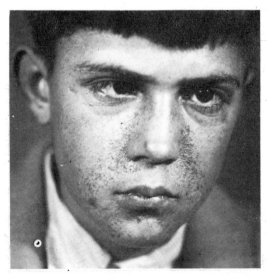

Fig. 5.36 Tuberous sclerosis and adenoma sebaceum, showing distribution of lesions on cheeks and chin. The patient, a boy aged 12 years, had suffered from epileptiform attacks since early childhood.

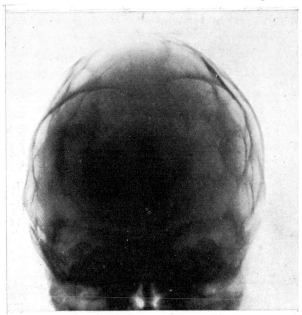

Fig. 5.37   Lacunar skull. Newborn infant with spina bifida, large myelocele and talipes.

nerves, and the skin shows scattered pigmented areas known as 'café-au-lait spots'. Both conditions are inherited as mendelian dominants and may occur in different members of one family. They are sometimes grouped with Sturge-Weber syndrome (p. 101) and other rare angiomatous conditions as the phakomatoses.

Cerebral palsy

The group of cerebral palsies is considered in Chapter 16, but it must be emphasized that some of these cases must be regarded as congenital failures of development. As already indicated, mental subnormality is frequently associated with cerebral palsy, but the degree of paresis is no measure of the intelligence, which may be normal even with severe physical disability.

HYDROCEPHALUS AND SPINA BIFIDA

The various combinations of abnormalities of the nervous system which may be grouped under this heading constitute a major cause of chronic handicap in childhood. Many affected infants die in early life but some survive with or without treatment and the proportion of survivors is increasing with better therapeutic methods and a more optimistic outlook as regards their future. This raises difficult ethical problems but, since an infant who survives untreated is likely to have a

far greater disability than if he had been treated vigorously from the beginning, such infants should be given the benefits of early and comprehensive treatment, although discretion must be exercised if there are multiple gross malformations.

Hydrocephalus

Excess of fluid within the ventricular system or over the surface of the brain may represent simply the replacement of atrophic cerebral tissue by fluid, but the term hydrocephalus should be restricted to those cases in which the fluid is under increased pressure. Congenital hydrocephalus with excess of fluid within the ventricles may arise from defects of the aqueduct, of the foramina of the fourth ventricle, or of the subarachnoid spaces and cisternae. In the last of these types the fluid in the ventricles is in communication with the lumbar fluid, while in the first two (non-communicating types) it is not. It is possible that excessive production of fluid may also occasionally occur from abnormalities of the choroid plexuses, but the great majority of cases are due to interference with circulation and absorption.

Hydrocephalus not infrequently occurs in association with spina bifida. In such cases there is likely to be malformation of the cerebellum and medulla (the Arnold-Chiari malformation), in

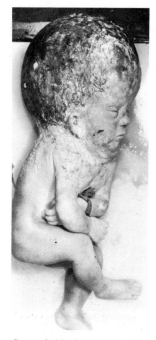

Fig. 5.38   Congenital hydrocephalus (stillborn infant).

which a tongue composed of these elements protrudes through the foramen magnum and by so doing obstructs the canal or subarachnoid space. There is frequently an associated malformation of the skull (*lacunar skull*), which shows multiple fenestrations either widely distributed (Fig. 5.37) or limited to the temporal areas.

In addition to malformation, possible etiological factors in the production of congenital hydrocephalus are prenatal intracranial haemorrhage and prenatal infection, especially toxoplasmosis or cytomegalic inclusion disease. Hydrocephalus becoming manifest in the neonatal period may be due to any of these causes, or may be a sequel of haemorrhage at birth or postnatal meningitis.

CLINICAL FEATURES. In some cases, hydrocephalus has already advanced during intrauterine life to an extent which makes normal delivery impossible or results in stillbirth. In others, cranial enlargement is relatively slight or absent at birth and subsequently progresses until the condition is unmistakable. Measurement of the head circumference should be recorded for all infants at birth and repeated at frequent intervals if there is reason to anticipate hydrocephalus, e.g. if the circumference is unduly large, if the

fontanelle is full or the sutures widely separated, or if there is spina bifida. Serial measurements should be charted against normal standards, so that an excessively rapid increase will be detected before hydrocephalus is clearly evident clinically.

Established hydrocephalus is easily recognized by the large globular cranium protruding above the orbits, the wide anterior fontanelle and separation of the cranial sutures. Although intracranial pressure is not greatly increased at first, owing to the readiness with which the sutures open up in infancy, papilloedema leading ultimately to optic atrophy may appear in the later stages of progressive hydrocephalus.

DIFFERENTIAL DIAGNOSIS. Enlargement of the head in early infancy is commonly due to hydrocephalus or to subdural haematoma and the latter should be excluded by subdural taps. Rare causes include intracranial neoplasm and brain abscess. Rapid growth of the brain, especially in the pre-term infant, may cause temporary separation of the sutures, which must not be attributed to hydrocephalus, since the sutures soon narrow again as ossification of the cranial bones proceeds. Other congenital malformations such as macrocephaly and hydranencephaly are usually easily distinguished.

TREATMENT AND PROGNOSIS. Hydrocephalus without spina bifida generally progresses inexorably and spontaneous arrest is rare. Prompt surgical treatment is therefore indicated, a valve being inserted to drain the cerebrospinal fluid from the ventricles into the blood-stream. The Holter and similar types of one-way valve prevent blood from flowing up the tube and permit the removal of slight obstructions by pumping the valve through the intact skin. When functioning satisfactorily, the valve prevents further enlargement of the head and the child can lead a comparatively normal life with little or no handicap. Sometimes, however, low-grade infection with *Staphylococcus albus* becomes established in the valve and cannot be eradicated by antibiotic therapy. In such cases the valve may have to be changed; in others, a variety of technical difficulties leads to disappointing results.

In untreated primary hydrocephalus, the head generally enlarges to a great size and death usually occurs early. Surviving children are likely to develop neurological disorders such as spasticity, ataxia, tremor, paralysis and blindness, and to suffer intellectual deterioration. Nevertheless, in a few patients arrested hydrocephalus is compatible with normal intelligence, even when ventricular enlargement is great.

Failure of fusion of the neural tube

Anencephaly (p. 77), encephalocele and spina bifida with or without hydrocephalus are related malformations having a common origin in failure of fusion of the neural tube. These disorders are strongly familial: predisposition appears to be polygenically determined, the malformation being precipitated in the susceptible embryo by an unfortunate combination of geographical location, social class, maternal age and parity, and other factors. Thus incidence is higher in the north and west of Britain, in social classes IV and V, when conception has occurred during the winter months, in urban areas and with high parity and advanced maternal age, although the effects of these factors seem to undergo secular variation. In south Wales, the incidence of neural tube malformations is about 8 per 1000 births, comprising anencephaly 3·5, spina bifida and encephalocele 4·1 and hydrocephalus 0·5 (Laurence, 1969); it is higher than this in parts of Ireland and lower in south-east England. These malformations are much less common in some ethnic groups, especially the African races.

Cranium bifidum. When here is a midline gap in the cranium, the meninges may protrude in the form of a sac (meningocele) filled with cerebrospinal fluid and covered with normal or atrophic skin. If neural tissue is not included in the sac, there is a prospect of successful excision but when the meningocele contains brain tissue (encephalocele) there are often associated malformations and the prognosis, even with surgical treatment, is poor.

Spina bifida. Failure of closure at the lower end of the neural tube can result in a variety of malformations ranging from spina bifida occulta to complete rachischisis, in which the neural tube is laid open on the surface of the back. The general term spina bifida includes these extremes and various degrees of meningocele and myelomeningocele. In some cases there is great dilatation of the central canal of the cord (syringomyelocele). Spina bifida may occur at any level but is most common in the lumbosacral region. It is frequently associated with hydrocephalus and with characteristic deformities of the lower limbs, including hyperextension

of the knees and calcaneous talipes. Genitourinary malformations are also common. When the spinal cord is involved in the defect, the nerve supply to the lower limbs and the sphincters is affected and varying degrees of paralysis and loss of sensation result.

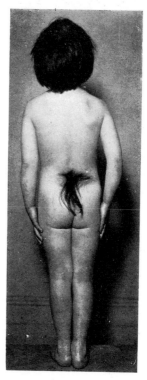

Fig. 5.39   Spina bifida occulta, showing profuse growth of dark hair over site of deformity.

Spina bifida occulta is a defect of the posterior wall of the spinal canal which is of common occurrence but little importance unless the nervous system is involved. It may not be visible externally but its site is often marked by a pad of fat, pigmentation of the skin or a tuft of dark hair. In a small proportion of cases there is weakness or atrophy of one or both lower limbs. There may be urinary incontinence if the bladder is involved but this is rare and spina bifida occulta demonstrated by radiological examination cannot be advanced as an explanation for enuresis in the absence of evident neurological involvement.

In many infants a small depression or sinus is seen in the lower sacral or coccygeal region, representing a remnant of the caudal end of the neural tube. Such a *pilonidal sinus* may com-

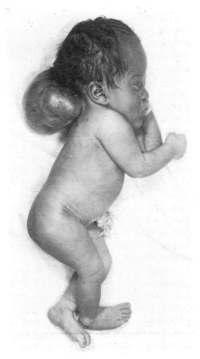

Fig. 5.40 A newborn infant with a large occipital encephalocele.

municate with the spinal canal, with consequent risk of meningitis, but usually the vestigial tube ends blindly or in a small cyst. While slight depressions are of no consequence, extensive ones are liable to infection and require surgical treatment.

Myelomeningocele. When an infant is born with meningocele or myelomeningocele, an appraisal should first be made of the extent of the defect, the nature and quality of any covering tissue, and the probability that neural tissue is included in the meningocele. Then attention should be turned to the presence or absence of hydrocephalus, the power and sensation in the lower limbs, the competence of the urinary and anal sphincters and any associated malformations (Plate 10).

Surgical treatment of the defect in the back should be undertaken as early as possible, preferably within 24 hours, the aim being to provide the area with a good covering of skin. Careful watch is then kept on the head circumference and, if there is rapid increase, it will generally be necessary to establish a ventriculo-atrial shunt. The urgency is not so great as in primary hydrocephalus, however, since spontaneous arrest

occurs more frequently in hydrocephalus associated with spina bifida. Assessment of the degree of ventricular dilatation by radiological measurement of the thickness of the cerebral mantle and estimation of the cerebrospinal fluid pressure may help to determine the need for a shunt. Intravenous pyelography should be carried out in the neonatal period to exclude renal malformation; the development of urinary infection is an indication for cystourethrography, the relief of any obstruction to free drainage and continuous administration of prophylactic antibiotic, since the infant's survival ultimately depends on avoiding pyelonephritis and consequent renal damage.

If there are deformities of the lower limbs, orthopaedic treatment will be required early and anomalies of the hip joint should be excluded, for they occur in about one-third of children with spina bifida.

In continuing care, attention must be paid to the functioning of the valve, watching for signs of bacterial colonization and of increased intracranial pressure, such as papilloedema; the urine must be examined regularly for evidence of infection; the achievement of locomotion may require intensive physiotherapy and the aid of calipers; incontinence of urine may necessitate a urinal or the formation of an ileal bladder; faecal incontinence is not usually troublesome when the internal sphincter is intact but occasionally it creates a major social problem and colostomy may be required. As with any chronically handicapped child, sympathetic support for the parents and co-ordination of arrangements for education and medical care are essential (see Chapter 16). With modern methods of management, about half of all liveborn children with spina bifida survive to adult life and of these about one-third are educable.

Spinal dysraphism

In addition to spina bifida, many other malformations affect the mid-line tissues of the lower back and the collective term spinal dysraphism is applied to them. One of the common forms consists of a cleft of the spinal cord (diastematomyelia), the caudal ends of which are tethered, preventing ascent of the cord as growth proceeds. If there is increasing pressure from a midline bony spur or trauma to the immobilized cord from spinal movements, progressive neurological signs ensue, e.g. weakness, sensory loss and inequality of the lower limbs. Myelography followed by surgical treatment will usually be necessary to prevent further damage. Other forms of spinal dysraphism include dermal sinuses, lipomata, and dermoid cysts, which tend to occur in combination and may enlarge to produce increasing disability at any age. There is often an overlying dimple or patch of hair.

OTHER CONGENITAL NEUROLOGICAL DISORDERS

Failures of development

Congenital absence of individual cranial nerve nuclei, central pathways, or cortical centres is not very uncommon; the defects may be unilateral or bilateral.

Congenital ptosis, congenital strabismus

Both are liable to occur as familial defects, and both may appear in more than one generation.

Congenital nystagmus

Though seldom noticed at birth, this is a heredo-familial disorder which in some families has been found to be limited to males and transmitted by females, and in others to affect both sexes equally. The nystagmus is rapid, horizontal, and affects both eyes synchronously. It should be distinguished from the nystagmus seen in *spasmus nutans*, which is asymmetrical and associated with rhythmic rolling and tilting of the head. Spasmus nutans is a transient disorder in the maturation of ocular fixation and co-ordination of voluntary movements of head and eyes. It may be associated with poor lighting in the home and with rickets in a minority of cases.

Congenital inequality, congenital immobility of the pupils

Confusion may be caused in neurological examinations made in later life, but these conditions are not otherwise of clinical importance.

Congenital facial paralysis

This may be unilateral or bilateral, but more commonly the latter. It must be distinguished from facial paralysis due to birth injury (which is rare except in forceps deliveries), since the prognosis in the latter is usually good. In congenital facial paralysis the upper facial muscles and forehead are principally affected.

Congenital deafness

There are several clinical types of congenital deafness due to malformations, the type depending on whether the middle ears, labyrinths, eighth nerves, or brain are affected. In some instances, malformations of the ears have been caused by maternal infection with rubella. Cretinism may be associated with congenital deafness, and is an important cause in those areas where cretinism is endemic. Deafness may be familial or occur with a familial incidence of mental subnormality. The clinical type most commonly seen is cochlear deafness, in which the cochlear branch of the eighth nerve and the ganglion are also atrophic.

Congenital deafness is of considerable importance, since normal development and particularly acquisition of speech are dependent on auditory perception. The condition therefore becomes one of deafmutism.

While an observant mother may notice even during early infancy that the baby fails to respond normally to noise, deafness is often not suspected until there is an obvious delay in acquiring speech or attention to the spoken word. Diagnosis is difficult in infancy, since simple deafness has to be distinguished from mental defect and from mental defect plus deafness. In later infancy it should be possible to determine whether the infant is behaving normally in other ways, i.e. has acquired skills not dependent on auditory perception, and whether he fails to react to noises produced outside his visual field. It is also sometimes found that deafness is limited to the upper ranges of sound, so that speech is only partially defective. All young children should be routinely screened for deafness: audiometry is required for accurate diagnosis.

When the diagnosis has been made, intensive speech-training should be begun as soon as practicable. Good results have been obtained by special methods when training is started early and when intelligence is normal (see also p. 298).

Congenital hypotonia (*The floppy infant syndrome*)

Severe hypotonia dating from birth or appearing during the first months of life represents a syndrome rather than a disease entity. It includes cases of Werdnig-Hoffmann disease (see below), myasthenia gravis and non-progressive congenital myopathies such as central core disease, in all of which there is pronounced muscular weakness. Hypotonia in infancy is also characteristic of cerebral abnormality such as severe mental subnormality, cerebral palsy, mongolism, cerebral

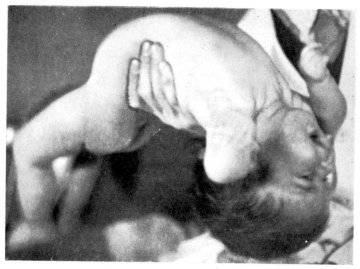

Fig. 5.41   Congenital hypotonia. Infant aged 5 months, showing general flaccidity and inability to support head.

lipidoses and other disorders in which there is little or no reduction in muscle power. Newborn infants may be limp following birth injury, while severe illness or malnutrition will cause temporary hypotonia. When the floppy infant is held in ventral suspension or raised from the supine position, the head and limbs hang down (Fig. 5.41), and when he is lifted by the axillae he seems to slip through the hands. The tendon reflexes may be present or absent, depending on the primary disease. Hypotonia in infancy without muscular weakness or apparent associated disease may be described as essential hypotonia (benign hypotonia). Recovery is complete in some cases, though all motor skills are acquired late, but others later show Prader-Willi syndrome (p. 193).

Werdnig-Hoffmann disease (*Infantile spinal muscular atrophy*)

This is due to a congenital paucity and degeneration of the anterior horn cells of the spinal cord. It is often familial, and is progressive and fatal, usually before the age of five years. The hypotonia may be evidenced before birth by the absence or paucity of fetal movements, or the infant may appear normal at birth, the hypotonia appearing gradually during the first months of life. The tendon reflexes are absent and contractures may develop early. Muscle biopsy shows denervation atrophy. Many of these infants succumb to intercurrent infection, and no treatment has been found to arrest the progress of the disease.

MALFORMATIONS OF THE EYE

Owing to the very great number of possible abnormalities, and their specialized interest, only a few examples will be quoted to illustrate their conformity with congenital malformation elsewhere. Abnormalities of the optic nerve and retina may co-exist with cerebral malformations or mental defect (e.g. retinitis pigmentosa in the Laurence-Moon-Biedl syndrome), while characteristic ocular malformations appear more or less constantly with particular errors of bony development, e.g. dislocation of the lens with arachnodactyly, congenital cataract with punctate epiphyseal dysplasia, corneal opacities with mucopolysaccharidoses, and blue sclerotics with fragilitas ossium. The eyes are displaced in cranial malformations such as oxycephaly and hypertelorism, while the retinae may be involved in malformations affecting other organs, e.g. Sturge-Weber syndrome and neurofibromatosis. Some types of ocular malformation have been shown to be genetically determined, while in others maternal rubella during the period of organogenesis has been found to be responsible.

Failures of development

The whole globe may be absent (anophthalmia), excessively small (microphthalmia), or represented by one or more cysts. More limited failures of development are exemplified by absence of the anterior chamber, absence of the iris, absence of the lens, microcornea, and coloboma, i.e. local defect of the iris, lens, macula, optic nerve, or eyelids. Red-green colour blindness, which is related to defective development of the cones of the retina, is inherited as a sex-linked recessive character.

Failures of canalization

The commonest of these is defective canalization of the naso-lachrymal·duct, which results in failure of drainage of tears from the conjunctival sac with consequent overflow. In most instances only the foramina are blocked, and the ducts become patent either spontaneously or after repeated pressure over the inner angle of the orbit.

Congenital glaucoma

Congenital glaucoma, or increased intraocular tension, may arise from malformation of the angle of the anterior chamber and canal of Schlemm, interfering with the flow of aqueous. In contrast to the findings in acquired glaucoma, pain is not usually an outstanding symptom in congenital glaucoma. The condition is usually progressive.

Overdevelopment

Generalized enlargement of the globe (buphthalmia) is usually bilateral and secondary to glaucoma; the globe may reach two or three times the normal size. Unilateral buphthalmia should raise the suspicion of an intraocular tumour.

Failures of involution

Of these, one of the commonest is *persistent hyaloid artery*, the vessel running as an opaque cord from the posterior surface of the lens into the vitreous. It varies from a small remnant which is of little clinical importance, to a complete artery reaching the optic disc.

Persistent pupillary membrane, persistent tunica vasculosa lentis

Both may occur together, though the former is considerably more common and more innocuous than the latter. When a persistent vascular membrane is present on the posterior surface of the lens, it interferes seriously with vision and cannot easily be removed. Persistent pupillary membranes are often present only as very fine strands and can be surgically removed if necessary.

OTHER MALFORMATIONS

Errors of refraction

There are three types: hypermetropia, in which the image is focused behind the retina; myopia, in which it is focused in front of the retina; and astigmatism, in which the curvature of the cornea or lens is unequal in the horizontal and perpendicular planes. Hypermetropia can hardly be regarded as a congenital malformation, since the small eye of the young infant is always to some extent hypermetropic, and 'normal' vision is only attained gradually. Mild degrees of hypermetropia in childhood are unlikely to require correction unless associated with convergent strabismus. Myopia, on the other hand, shows a much more striking familial incidence, and when it occurs as a congenital abnormality will always require early and complete correction. There is a considerable danger of congenital myopia leading to juvenile glaucoma. Astigmatism is of minor importance if it occurs alone, and though it will result in some blurring of vision there is not the same necessity for correction.

Since there is a tendency for many physicians to attribute a great variety of symptoms to minor errors of refraction discovered on routine examination, it must be emphasized that correction of such errors is not likely to disperse symptoms due to other causes, nor do errors of refraction other than myopia which are not causing symptoms necessarily call for correction at all. It is important that a presenting symptom such as headache should not be attributed to a minor error of refraction unless other possible causes have been excluded. At the same time, it is quite understandable that an error of refraction which has previously caused no symptoms may begin to do so following an acute illness or period of anxiety or fatigue. Careful judgement should therefore be exercised in the recommendation of glasses, and the handicaps which they impose in childhood weighed against their necessity.

Congenital cataract

Opacities of the lens are of common occurrence but are usually small and do not then interfere with vision. When the whole lens is opaque, other malformations are usually found in association. Congenital cataract 'is a feature of rubella embryopathy.

Opaque optic nerve fibres

Myelinization of optic nerve fibres gives rise to a characteristic picture which if not recognized may lead to confusion on retinoscopy. Dense white strands are seen running out from the margin of the disc, but are unlikely to cause an appreciable interference with the field of vision.

MALFORMATIONS OF THE SKIN AND ITS APPENDAGES

Minor abnormalities of the skin, hair, teeth, nails, and ears are so common that most individuals have distinguishing 'birth marks' which may at least be of cosmetic or medicolegal importance. The majority of these are naevi, of which the vascular types have already been considered. A great number of other congenital abnormalities of the skin occur, which are of interest to the geneticist but are so rare as to be of little general clinical importance.

FAILURES OF DEVELOPMENT

Ectodermal dysplasia

In the fully developed syndrome, patients show partial or complete absence of hair, defective development of the nails and teeth, chronic rhinitis, and absence of sweat-glands. These children are often small and poorly developed. Absence of sweat-glands renders them peculiarly susceptible to the effects of high temperature,

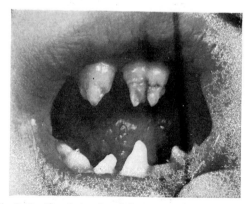

Fig. 5.42   Dysplasia of teeth in a boy aged 5 with chondroectodermal dysplasia (*Journal of Bone and Joint Surgery*, 1962, vol. 44b, p. 626.)

while the chronic rhinitis may lead to depression of the nasal bridge. There are at least two types of the complete syndrome, one a sex-linked recessive and the other a dominant. The linkage of ectodermal dysplasia with other defects in *chondroectodermal dysplasia* is described on page 135.

Isolated ectodermal defects may occur alone, e.g. congenital alopecia, in which the lack of hair may be partial or complete, failures of dentition (in which there may be a familial incidence of absence or defect of particular teeth of the first or second dentition), anidrotic defects, and absence or incomplete development of the nails.

Cutis laxa (*Ehlers-Danlos syndrome*)

The skin in this condition is extremely elastic and fragile, so that it tears readily, and the patients often show multiple scars over the knees, forehead, etc. There is an abnormal tendency to bruising and haemorrhage. The primary defect is probably one of connective tissue development.

Epidermolysis bullosa

In this hereditary disorder, widespread bullae appear from birth, which rupture leaving denuded areas and often heal with scarring. While varying in severity, the condition may cause death in infancy. Only supportive treatment is possible.

FAILURES OF INVOLUTION OR FUSION

Pre-auricular sinus

This is situated on the cheek, anteriorly to the external auditory meatus, at the site of fusion of the maxillary and mandibular processes. Malformation of the external ear may occur in association with it.

Branchial cysts, sinuses

Branchial cysts and sinuses represent persistence of some part of a branchial cleft, most commonly the second. They are situated immediately anterior to the sternomastoid muscle. Owing to the risk of infection, surgical removal will usually be required. Occasionally a cervical fistula will be found to communicate between the skin of the neck and the pharynx.

Thyroglossal cyst

This represents a persistent portion of the thyroglossal duct which runs from the thyroid gland to the base of the tongue. The cyst usually lies superficially in the midline, in close association with the thyroid gland.

Dermoid cyst

While these cysts may occur at any point of fusion, e.g. in the midline of the back, the commonest site for one to be found is at the upper and outer margin of the orbit. A cyst in this site must be distinguished from a meningocele, which is in communication with the cranial cavity and becomes tense on crying. It is usually advisable for a dermoid cyst to be removed surgically.

HYPERTROPHY

Hypertrophy of the nails

This may occur as a congenital malformation, though it is also produced by postnatal trauma or infection of the nail-bed. When the deformity is gross it may be necessary to remove the nails in order to allow normal use of the fingers.

Hypertrichosis

The normal growth of body hair varies considerably in different individuals and in different races, and is subject to a variety of postnatal influences. Congenital hypertrichosis is rare: in the generalized type it may affect almost the whole of the body.

Hyperkeratosis

Excessive development of the horny layer of the skin appears in a number of clinical forms, the most striking being keratosis palmaris et plantaris in which the palms and soles are affected. This type is inherited as a mendelian dominant.

Keratosis follicularis (Darier's disease) affects the pilosebaceous orifices, where hard papules form which subsequently become crusted. The condition is usually localized and symmetrical; the nails are almost always hypertrophied at birth, though the skin lesions may appear later. The condition is thought to be a dominant depending on the presence of two genes.

REDUPLICATION

Supernumerary nipples

These are of common occurrence, though usually vestigial. They are likely to escape recognition until the areola becomes pigmented at puberty. Most commonly they are symmetri-cal and situated below the normal nipple. They require no treatment.

Supernumerary auricles

These also are of relatively common occurrence, and may be multiple. They lie immediately anterior to the external auditory meatus. If sufficiently unsightly, they may be removed surgically.

ABNORMALITIES OF PIGMENTATION

Pigmented, hairy and warty naevi

These are among the commoner congenital malformations, and vary from small pigmented 'moles' or spots to enormous hairy pigmented areas involving the whole of the bathing-drawers area or trunk. They are usually multiple.

Considerable difference of opinion exists as to the advisability of removal of pigmented naevi, but if surgical removal is undertaken a wide excision should be made. When the naevus is not situated on an exposed area or subjected to constant trauma it may be left alone. It is important to distinguish between naevi which have been present from infancy and pigmented naevi which appear suddenly in later life. The incidence of malignant change in true congenital naevi has probably been overestimated, though any change in colour or size is an indication for removal and examination.

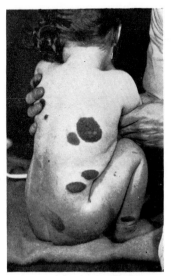

Fig. 5.43   Large pigmented naevi. The patient was microcephalic and mentally defective.

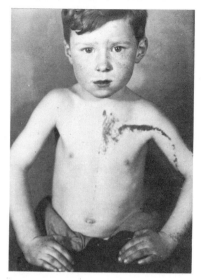

Fig. 5.44   Pigmented naevus, showing linear distribution and limitation to left side of midline.

Mongolian blue spots

These are not, strictly speaking, 'congenital malformations' since they are seen in a high percentage of newborn infants of Chinese, Japanese, and African parentage. In Europeans they are uncommon, and their presence raises the suspicion of other racial inheritance. The mongolian spot has much the same appearance as an ecchymosis, for which it may be mistaken; the commonest site is over the sacral region or buttocks, the size varying from one to several centimetres in diameter. The spots are best seen in the newborn period, and subsequently fade.

Albinism

Deficiency of pigmentation may be partial or almost complete, affecting the hair, skin, and eyes. It is not confined to the white races, though albinism in coloured races is often incomplete. Recessive, dominant, and sex-linked recessive forms have been described. The typical albino has white hair, pink eyes, white skin, and nystagmus. The skin is readily affected by exposure to the sun, and visual defect is very common. The choroid shares in the general deficiency of pigmentation.

Vitiligo (*Leucoderma*)

This condition is not observed at birth but there appear to be a hereditary predisposition and a possible association with autoimmune disease. Areas of skin, which may increase in size, are characterized by disappearance of melanocytes and consequent loss of pigmentation which becomes very obvious when surrounding areas pigment from exposure to sun. Treatment is unsatisfactory, and some patients resort to camouflaging the exposed areas with cosmetic colouring creams.

OTHER MALFORMATIONS

Malformations of the auricle

Malformation or malposition of the external ear is relatively common, and may affect any part of the organ; minor variations in structure are normal. Low-set malformed auricles are sometimes associated with renal malformation. Plastic surgery is indicated when the deformity is very unsightly.

Ichthyosis

A number of distinct conditions are included under this description, all of them characterized by dryness and scaling of the skin. While ichthyosis vulgaris (simplex) is not usually manifest until later infancy, there are congenital and fetal types in which the infant is born with a hard covering which splits and desquamates shortly after birth. In true ichthyosis congenita, which is very rare, the eyelids are everted and sucking may be interfered with; these cases are usually stillborn (*harlequin fetus*) or die within a few hours of birth.

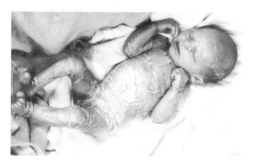

Fig. 5.45   Ichthyosis in a newborn infant (benign type).

Benign forms seen in the newborn are thought to be due either to an accumulation of vernix (ichthyosis sebacea) or to persistence of a fetal membrane, which subsequently splits and desquamates.

CONGENITAL ABNORMALITIES OF THE MUSCLES

Failure of development

Partial or complete absence of individual muscles is not very uncommon, and usually gives rise to little disability. The pectoralis major is the muscle most commonly affected. Absence of the abdominal muscles in males may be associated

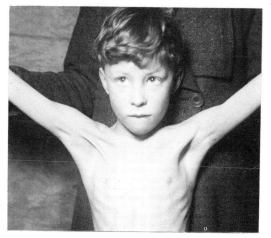

Fig. 5.46 Congenital absence of right pectoralis major.

with other more serious malformations, e.g. ectopia vesicae, megaureter, renal dysplasia, and has been called 'prune belly syndrome' from the wrinkled appearance of the abdominal skin. Defects of the diaphragm are likely to result in eventration or diaphragmatic hernia.

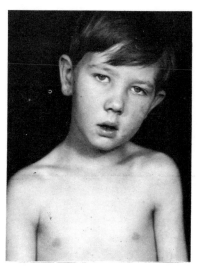

Fig. 5.47 Congenital torticollis.

Contractures

Secondary contractures of muscles occur with a number of the bony abnormalities considered below, and are an important factor in the maintenance of talipes deformities.

Congenital torticollis

While it is often difficult in later childhood to be certain whether a torticollis deformity, in which the cervical spine is flexed to one or other side, has been brought about by birth injury or is truly congenital, there is little doubt that prenatal factors are responsible in some instances. When there is an associated deformity of the cervical spine this becomes obvious on radiological examination. In other cases the only abnormality found may be a contracture of the sterno-mastoid muscle. Correction can usually be obtained by exercises or stretching of the muscle, but occasionally operative correction is necessary.

Arthrogryposis multiplex congenita

In this condition the infant is born with extensive fixed deformities of the joints associated with extreme maldevelopment of the limb muscles. The latter may be largely or entirely replaced by fibrous tissue. Individual joints, e.g.

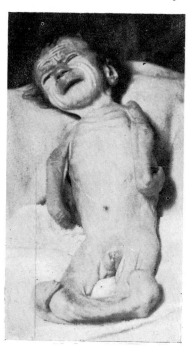

Fig. 5.48 Arthrogryposis multiplex, showing flexion deformities.

the knees, may be fixed in extension, but generalized flexion deformities are more common. The condition is not a disease entity but some cases are probably due to a primary defect of the nervous system. The muscular changes are far advanced at the time of birth and the condition has actually been diagnosed *in utero*. The most severely affected patients die early or suffer permanent crippling; orthopaedic correction of deformities may be possible in milder cases. Survivors are usually mentally normal.

Trigger thumb and finger

Flexion deformity of the thumb or finger, which yields suddenly to pressure, is occasionally seen as a congenital deformity due to localized stenosis of the tendon sheath. It is readily corrected by section of the stenosis.

MALFORMATIONS OF THE BONES AND JOINTS

Almost any part of the osseous system may show partial or complete failure of development, hypertrophy, reduplication, or failure of differentiation. In addition, a number of well-defined malformations and syndromes are observed which cannot readily be classified on this basis. Some of the generalized osseous dystrophies show a heredofamilial or familial incidence, and can be classified as dominants or simple reces-

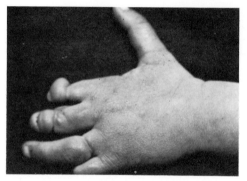

Fig. 5.49   Deep transverse grooves on fingers, occurring as congenital abnormalities.

sives; but the mode of inheritance is often less simply defined, and it is becoming increasingly obvious that intermediary types and familial variants occur, and that even the classical clinical types may behave differently in different families.

The etiology of the deep transverse furrows which are occasionally seen on the fingers (Fig. 5.49) or limbs is uncertain. They may be associated with intrauterine amputation and were previously attributed to mechanical causes, e.g. bands.

FAILURE OF DEVELOPMENT

The most striking examples of failure of development of the limbs are those in which the

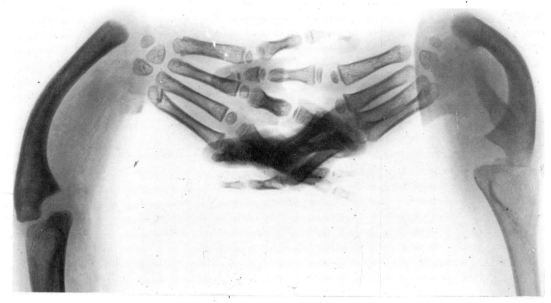

Fig. 5.50   Absent left radius and vestigial right radius, with curvature of ulnae.

infant is born with absence of one or more limbs (*amelia*) or partial absence (*ectromelia*). A congenitally defective limb may show a rudimentary hand or foot at the extremity, or a well-developed hand may spring from the shoulder with failure of development of the intermediary portion of the limb (*phocomelia*). The great increase in incidence of these deformities in 1960–62 in West Germany and Britain was associated with the widespread use of thalidomide in early pregnancy (see Fig. 5.4).

When one of a pair of bones, e.g. radius and ulna, is absent or underdeveloped, the other is likely to show a secondary deformity, e.g. ulnar deviation of the wrist (Madelung's deformity). Figure 5.50 illustrates bilateral underdevelopment of the radius. When one of the lower extremities is underdeveloped, it is often possible for the child to compensate for a slight degree of shortening by tilting the pelvis, but major degrees make walking impossible without artificial support.

Skull

Defective development of the skull occurs in craniocleidodystosis and osteogenesis imperfecta (see below), and secondarily to defective development of the brain (anencephaly, microcephaly).

Congenital parietal foramina (Fig. 5.51) represent a localized defect of development, in which symmetrical foramina occur in the parietal bones, separated by a ridge of bone in the midline. The condition is a mendelian dominant, though since it usually gives rise to no symptoms, familial cases may pass unrecognized.

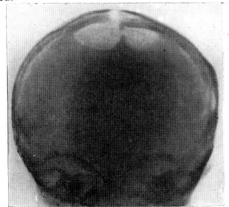

Fig. 5.51   Congenital parietal foramina in an infant. The mother was also affected.

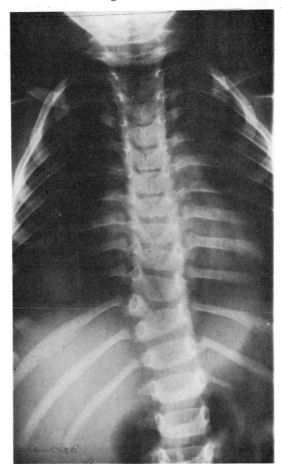

Fig. 5.52   Failure of development of tenth thoracic vertebral body, causing hemivertebra with scoliosis.

Partial absence of vertebra

Failure of development of one-half of the body of a vertebra will give rise to a severe degree of scoliosis, which will require orthopaedic treatment, e.g. with a Milwaukee brace.

When the body of a vertebra is defective or absent, both sides of the vertebral body being affected equally, the defect will cause kyphosis, i.e. an acute angulation of the back. This deformity is seen characteristically in the mucopolysaccharidoses, in which one or more of the lower lumbar vertebrae are hook-shaped, due to failure of development of the upper and anterior portion of the body.

Congenital dislocation of hip

This important abnormality may be unilateral or bilateral. It is commoner in girls than in boys, and a family history of dislocation may be

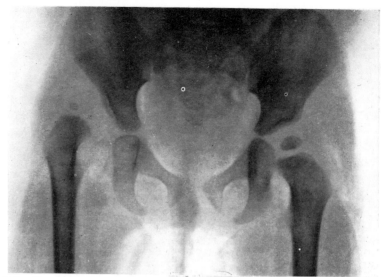

Fig. 5.53   Congenital dislocation of right hip, showing defective acetabulum and head of femur.

obtained. The incidence has been estimated as 2 to 2·5 per 1000 births though the incidence of instability of the hip joints at birth may be 5 per 1000 or more. Defective development of the acetabulum and surrounding structures results in mechanical dislocation of the head of the femur backward and upward. Laxity of ligaments and capsule surrounding the joint is probably a contributing factor. Early diagnosis is the most important single factor in determining the end result of congenital dislocation of the hip. Diagnosis of hip instability in the newborn enables treatment to commence before the development of secondary changes which frequently complicate reduction in the older child. Unless newborn infants are examined routinely (p. 70) to detect instability of the hip, it is often not until the child attempts to walk that the diagnosis is made. A limp or characteristic waddling gait then draws attention to the defect. Radiological examination in the newborn is made with each femur abducted to at least 45 degrees and with appreciable inward rotation. In the normal hip the line of the femoral shaft will be directed towards the edge of the acetabular roof but in the dislocated hip it will point to the anterior superior iliac spine.

Congenital dislocation of the hip when diagnosed within the first few days of life can be successfully treated without admission to hospital by a simple splint maintaining the hips in abduction and flexion for a few months.

Treatment in early childhood consists essentially in bringing the head of the femur within the acetabulum by manipulation, and maintaining it in position. When adequate treatment is carried out early, the functional results are usually excellent, becoming less good the longer it is delayed.

HYPERTROPHY

Hemihypertrophy

Hemihypertrophy affecting the whole of one side of the body seldom gives rise to functional disability unless the asymmetry is great. The pelvis is tilted to compensate for the increased length of one leg, and there may be an associated

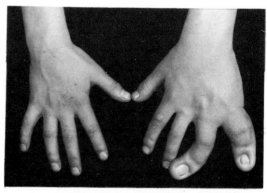

Fig. 5.54   Local gigantism, affecting principally the area of distribution of the left ulnar nerve and resulting in curvature of the left ring finger. Right hand unaffected.

scoliosis. Hemihypertrophy may be associated with Wilm's tumour or neuroblastoma and is also a feature of a rare type of low birth-weight dwarfism with asymmetry (Silver's syndrome).

Local gigantism

This is most commonly found affecting one or more digits (*macrodactyly*), which may be of almost adult size at birth. When the area supplied by the ulnar nerve is involved, the little finger and lateral half of the ring finger are curved towards the midline of the hand (Fig. 5.54). Surgical removal of the affected digit may be necessary in order to give adequate use of the hand or foot.

Hypertelorism

In this condition, the eyes are widely separated, due to overgrowth of the lesser wing of the sphenoid. The condition is frequently but not invariably associated with mental defect, and

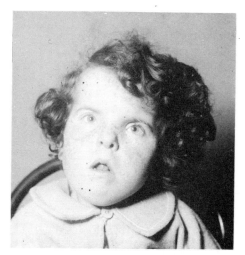

Fig. 5.55 Hypertelorism, showing wide separation of eyes. Patient was mentally retarded.

appears as a dominant. A similar separation of the eyes may occur in other conditions including hydrocephalus, and associated with other facial defects in the median cleft face syndrome.

REDUPLICATION
Cervical rib

The presence of an extra rib attached to the seventh cervical vertebra is one of the commoner congenital abnormalities. In most instances the rib is rudimentary and causes no symptoms.

Pressure symptoms when they occur are likely to affect the brachial plexus and result in wasting of the intrinsic muscles of the hand. In such cases the rib should be removed surgically.

Polydactyly

The presence of one or more extra digits is not very uncommon, though as these are usually rudimentary they are generally removed shortly after birth. These digits may be attached to either side of the hand or foot, and may be present on

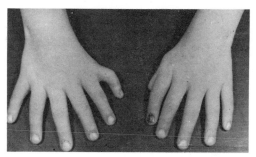

Fig. 5.56 Polydactyly in a child of 7 years.

all four extremities. They vary in size and structure from rudiments attached by a small pedicle, to fully formed digits with separate metacarpal or metatarsal. Examples of both dominant and recessive inheritance have been recorded, and polydactyly also occurs in association with other deformities (e.g. Laurence-Moon-Biedl syndrome and chondroectodermal dysplasia).

FAILURES OF DIFFERENTIATION

Partial or complete fusion of ribs is of common occurrence, and is usually of no clinical importance. When partial fusion of paired bones such as the radius and ulna occurs, it is likely to cause some limitation of movement.

Craniosynostosis (stenocephaly)

Absence of one or more of the cranial sutures will cause deformity of the skull which will be forced to expand unequally. Several clinical types are described, depending on the sutures involved. Premature fusion of the sagittal suture (scaphocephaly) results in a boat-shaped skull, while total or unilateral closure of the coronal suture produces antero-posterior shortening (brachycephaly) or asymmetry (plagiocephaly) respec-

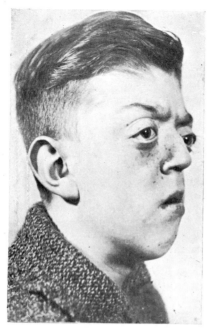

Fig. 5.57   Cranio-facial dysostosis: acrocephaly with exophthalmos, hypoplasia of maxilla, and protruding lower lip. (*Proceedings of the Royal Society of Medicine*, 1937.)

tively. Fusion of the coronal and another suture causes *acrocephaly* (oxycephaly), which may be associated in some cases with syndactyly (acro-cephalo-syndactyly), or with hypoplasia of the maxilla and a peculiarly beaked nose and projecting lower jaw (*cranio-facial dysostosis* or *Crouzon's syndrome*). In acrocephaly the skull is abnormally high anteriorly, and may be raised to a peak. Radiologically, it usually shows extreme digital markings. In the more severe cases, exophthalmos is very obvious and is associated with optic atrophy. Raised intracranial pressure gives rise to headache and occasionally convulsions: the patient may be mentally subnormal.

Multiple synostoses preventing normal enlargement of the head are associated with signs of greatly increased intracranial pressure and surgery is required urgently to allow brain growth to continue. In other cases, surgery may be indicated for cosmetic reasons or to correct persistently elevated intracranial pressure which might cause optic atrophy.

Fusion of vertebrae

Fusion of one or more vertebrae frequently occurs in the lumbar or lumbo-sacral regions, and usually causes no disability. A deformity known as the *Klippel-Feil syndrome* is characterized by fusion and partial absence of the upper cervical vertebrae, giving rise to an abnormally short neck. Other malformations, including webbing of the neck and congenital elevation of

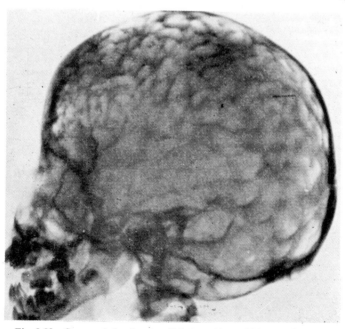

Fig. 5.58   Stenocephaly, showing digital markings. Girl aged 5½ years.

the scapula (*Sprengel's deformity*), are often associated and the patient may be mentally subnormal.

Syndactyly

Failure of differentiation of the digits varies in degree from the complete form in which the hand or foot is represented by a flat plate on which the digits are barely indicated, to partial fusion of two or more metacarpals or metatarsals, associated with webbing of the fingers or toes. (A slight degree of syndactyly of the second and third toes is very commonly seen in otherwise normal individuals.) The occasional association of syndactyly with acrocephaly has been mentioned. A peculiar variety of the malformation is *cleft hand* (*lobster hand*), in which syndactyly is associated with a deep central cleft dividing the hand into two parts; this is usually inherited as a dominant trait.

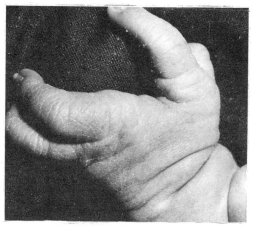

Fig. 5.59 Cleft hand.

While separation of digits in which only the soft tissues are involved can be undertaken, surgery offers little prospect of improvement when there is extensive bony fusion. Some children, however, attain considerable manual dexterity even when there is gross deformity.

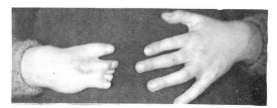

Fig. 5.60 Syndactyly of right hand.

MALFORMATIONS OF MECHANICAL ORIGIN

It has already been mentioned that a variety of congenital malformations can best be explained by mechanical factors depending on the position of the infant *in utero*, and that 'refolding' the newborn infant into the intrauterine position may make their etiology obvious. Thus dislocation of the hip, while depending on maldevelopment of the acetabulum, will occur when the appropriate force is applied either before or after birth. Congenital dislocation of the jaw may also be produced when the feet lie on either side of the mandible *in utero*. Secondary contractures or defective development of muscles will tend to maintain such deformities.

Talipes equino-varus (*Club-foot*)

This represents a dislocation at the talonavicular joint. The forefeet are inverted (varus deformity), and there is equinus (downward displacement of the forefoot) at the ankle, the latter increasing in degree if the tendo Achillis becomes contracted. It is most important to recognize and treat the deformity early, before secondary muscular contractures and bony changes have advanced.

Diagnosis should present no difficulty if the patient is seen at birth or during infancy, though cerebral palsy must be excluded. In patients seen for the first time in childhood it is necessary to distinguish congenital talipes from deformities secondary to poliomyelitis.

In infancy, treatment consists of manual overcorrection, with the knee flexed, into the calcaneo-valgus position, and application of a Denis-Browne splint to both feet.

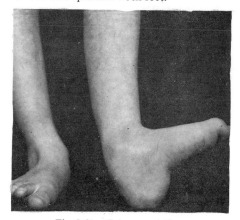

Fig. 5.61 Calcaneous talipes.

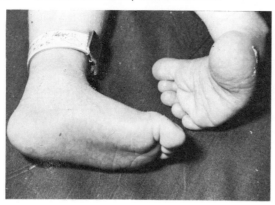 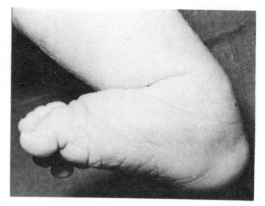

Fig. 5.62   Variations of neonatal talipes.

The functional result in cases treated early is excellent if maximal use of the splinted feet is allowed, and splintage and repeated manipulation are adequately carried out.

Talipes equino-valgus, in which the foot is deflected outward, is less common than the varus form.

Calcaneous talipes

Here the forefoot is deflected sharply upward. The severest type of deformity occurs in association with hyperextension of the knees and gross spina bifida. When calcaneous talipes occurs as an isolated deformity, it is usually not severe, and yields satisfactorily to repeated manipulation.

Overriding of toes

It is sometimes found at birth that one toe is depressed and overridden by the adjacent one (most commonly the fourth toe by the fifth). The deformity can be corrected by lifting the depressed toe in an adhesive plaster sling.

OTHER MALFORMATIONS

Funnel sternum

This consists of a deep depression at the lower end of the sternum, often occurring as a heredofamilial malformation. Minor degrees cause no disability and require no treatment. More severe degrees should be corrected surgically because the unsightly appearance can cause emotional problems in later childhood and adolescence. Occasionally the deformity is so great that the heart and mediastinum are displaced, and there may be cardiac embarrassment and ventilatory disturbance.

GENERALIZED OSSEOUS DYSTROPHIES

Achondroplasia (*Chondrodystrophia fetalis*)

This condition is inherited as an incomplete mendelian dominant, although isolated cases often arise by new mutation. It affects both sexes, and is due to a disturbance of endochondral bone growth. The long bones of the limbs are much shorter and broader than normal, and show mushrooming of the ends. The cartilage bones of the cranial axis and nasal septum are also affected, resulting in depression of the nose; since growth of the cranial vault proceeds from an abnormally small base, the appearance of the skull bears a superficial resemblance to hydrocephalus. While the vertebrae are little affected, and the trunk is of almost normal proportions, some degree of lordosis is always present.

Clinically, the striking feature of achondroplasia is the dwarfing and shortness of the extremities in relation to the size of the trunk and

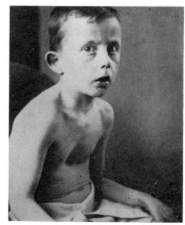

Fig. 5.63   Funnel sternum.

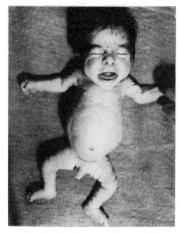

Fig. 5.64 Achondroplasia. Newborn infant, showing facies and short limbs with multiple creases due to 'telescoping' of the normal musculature of the extremities.

head. Since muscular development is normal, the thighs are thrown into folds by the amount of muscular tissue confined within their reduced length. The proximal segments of the limbs are affected to a greater degree than the distal. Achondroplastics can usually jump from the sitting to the standing position without using their hands, and have been popular as performing dwarfs throughout the ages. The gait is usually somewhat waddling. The short 'trident' hand with wide separation of the fingers is characteristic.

While many achondroplastics are stillborn or die shortly after birth, the condition is compatible with normal life-span, good health, and fecundity; females, however, can only bear children by Caesarean section, and when both parents are achondroplastic the gene is likely to prove lethal. Mental development is usually normal, though mental defect is probably commoner in those patients who die early than in those who survive.

Diastrophic dwarfism

This is inherited as an autosomal recessive and is characterized by short limbs, scoliosis, deformities of hands and feet, joint contractures and a normal head and face. There may be cleft palate and cystic swellings of the external ear. Radiologically the long bones are shortened and there are characteristic spinal changes. Handicap is likely to be severe and survivors into adult life are severely dwarfed. The condition must be distinguished from achondroplasia and other forms of dwarfism such as Morquio's osteochondrodystrophy.

Chondroectodermal dysplasia (*Ellis-van Creveld syndrome*)

The syndrome of chondrodysplasia, polydactyly of the hands, congenital malformation of the heart and ectodermal dysplasia affecting principally the nails and teeth occurs as an autosomal mendelian recessive. The skeletal changes differ from those of achondroplasia in that the shortening of the limbs is most marked in their distal segment and includes the fibula.

Arachnodactyly (*Marfan's syndrome*)

The essential features of this condition, which may appear as a dominant, are the extreme length and slenderness of the digits and, to a less extent, of the limbs and trunk, laxity of the ligaments, and dislocation of the lens. The antero-posterior diameter of the skull is abnormally long (dolichocephaly), and the jaw prominent. Abnormalities of the cardiovascular system include medionecrosis in the aorta, septal defects and valvular anomalies. Other deformities such as funnel sternum and pes planus may co-exist. Many patients die early from respiratory infections or as the result of dissecting aneurysm.

Cleidocranial dysplasia (Fig. 5.66)

In this rare heredofamilial disorder there is defective development or absence of the clavicles, resulting in abnormal mobility of the shoulders, which may sometimes be made to meet anteriorly; defective development of the vault and base of the skull, giving rise to a characteristic facies and radiological picture; and frequently absence of the pubic ramus also. There is hypoplasia of the maxilla, and dentition is often incomplete. The fontanelles remain patent, and there is a wide gutter separating the frontal bones. The defect of the clavicles seldom gives rise to serious disability, but these patients are often poorly developed and generally somewhat feeble.

Multiple exostoses (*Diaphyseal aclasis*)

This condition is heredofamilial, affecting both sexes, and has been described in four successive generations. Multiple exostoses appear first as buds projecting from the diaphyses, and later form large bony tumours. The long bones, ribs, clavicles, and scapulae are particularly affected. Although in mild cases the lesions may

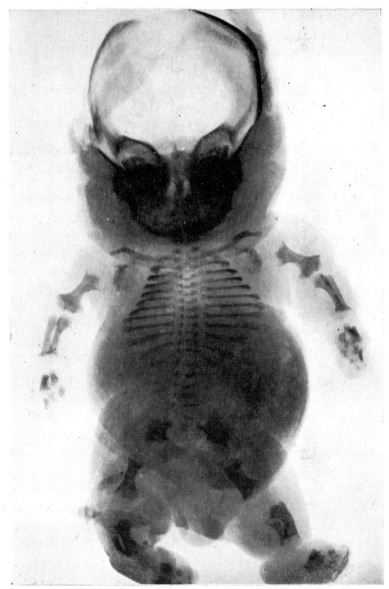

Fig. 5.65   Achondroplasia. Newborn infant, showing the short, thick femora and humeri with 'mushrooming' of extremities.

be limited to a few small exostoses, in cases showing widespread involvement the condition is likely to become extremely crippling. Unfortunately, surgical removal of individual exostoses is of little value.

Enchondromatosis (*Ollier's disease*)

This is a disease of the growing ends of the bone in which normal ossification of cartilage fails to take place. There is no hereditary or familial tendency. The lesions are usually first recognized in childhood, though the condition is probably congenital. The uncalcified areas of cartilage are clearly recognizable on X-ray examination, both within the bone and extending as large excrescences, which only gradually become calcified. They are likely to cause great deformity, particularly when the phalanges are affected, and may become sarcomatous in later life or result in spontaneous fractures.

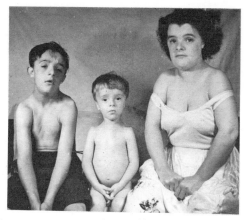

Fig. 5.66 Cleidocranial dysplasia occurring in two generations (a mother, son, and mother's brother). All showed the characteristic cranial defect and facies, with maldevelopment of the clavicles. The older boy illustrates the abnormal mobility of the shoulders.

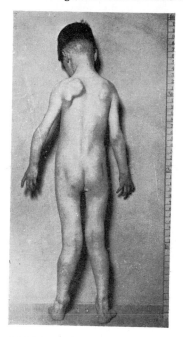

Fig. 5.67 Multiple exostoses around scapulae, wrists, knees, and ankles, with resultant deformity. The patient's mother was less severely affected.

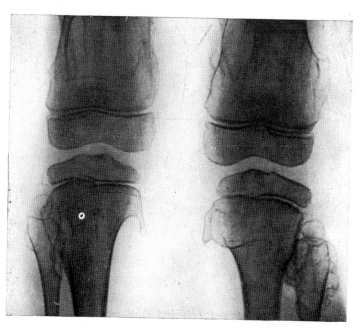

Fig. 5.68 Multiple exostoses of knees. Boy aged 7 years, shown in Fig. 5.67.

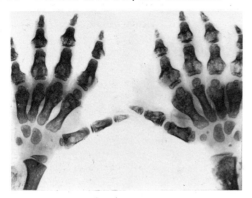

Fig. 5.69   Enchondromatosis. Translucent areas of carti-lage lying within, and extending beyond, the bony contour.

Fragilitas ossium (*Osteogenesis imperfecta: Osteopsathyrosis*)

Extreme fragility of the skeleton, resulting in spontaneous fractures and deformities, is some-times divided into two types, depending on the age at which the fractures occur. In the fetal type, generally described as *osteogenesis imperfecta congenita*, the infant may be born with multiple fractures of every bone in the body. The skull is made up of wormian bones, and ossification of the long bones has not extended beyond the cortex. These patients seldom survive more than a few weeks.

In the cases in which fractures occur for the first time in infancy or childhood, the severity varies considerably. Although callus formation and healing occur, there is likely to be increasing deformity and dwarfing. The skull may show a lateral bulging, as though it were collapsing under pressure. The scerotics are thin and slate-blue in colour, due to pigment showing through them.

Radiological examination will confirm the presence of previous fractures, and demonstrate the slenderness of the long bones and reduction of cancellous tissue in the shafts.

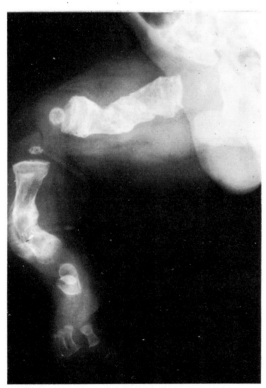

Fig. 5.70   Osteogenesis imperfecta, showing deformities of bones due to multiple fractures.

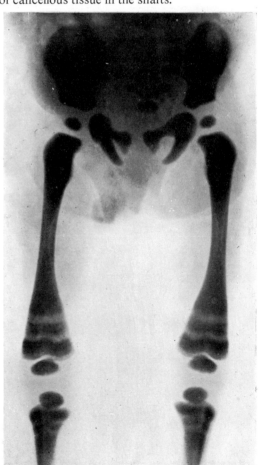

Fig. 5.71   Osteopetrosis in a young infant, showing dense calcification; transverse areas of more normal bone in long bones. (Courtesy of Dr John Thomson.)

A heredofamilial incidence is common in the childhood type, which is inherited as a mendelian dominant with a wide range of expressivity. The congenital type is thought to be a recessive disorder, at least in some cases. Otosclerosis often occurs in the family histories of the childhood group. Many of the patients who are only mildly affected reach adult life, but they are usually of poor physical development, apart from the likelihood of deformities. Since the etiology is unknown, treatment can only aim at the prevention or treatment of fractures.

Osteopetrosis (*Albers-Schönberg's disease*)

This rare disorder is characterized by excessive calcification and defective ossification of the skeleton, which render it abnormally fragile and liable to spontaneous fracture. The condition is hereditary and both sexes are affected. Gradual obliteration of the marrow cavity may ultimately result in progressive anaemia and enlargement of the liver, spleen, and lymph nodes. Encroachment on the optic foramina causes optic atrophy.

Radiologically, the affected portions of the skeleton show extreme opacity. The long bones frequently show clubbing of the extremities, i.e. abnormality of tubulation, and in some cases horizontal bands of opacity alternate with bands of more normal density (Fig. 5.71).

Apart from its genetic character, the etiology of the condition is unknown, though there appears to be a gross increase in calcium absorption. The blood calcium, phosphorus, and phosphatase values are typically normal.

The most severely affected patients usually die in early life, but milder forms of the disease may only be recognized later when spontaneous fractures occur. No form of treatment has been found consistently effective in arresting the progress of the disease, but promising results have been obtained with a calcium-depleting regimen (Dent *et al.*, 1965).

BIBLIOGRAPHY AND REFERENCES

GENERAL

AINSWORTH, P. & DAVIES, P. A. (1969). Single umbilical artery. *Developmental Medicine and Child Neurology*, 11, 297.
BAIKIE, A. G. (1965). Chromosomal abnormalities. In *Recent Advances in Pediatrics*, 3rd edn. Edited by D. Gairdner. London: Churchill.
CLARKE, C. A. (1964). *Genetics for the Clinician*, 2nd edn. Oxford: Blackwell.
CREW, F. A. E. (1970). Genetical aspects of child health and development. In *Child Life and Health*, 5th edn. Edited by R. G. Mitchell. London: Churchill.
GATES, R. R. (1946). *Human Genetics*. New York: Macmillan. (With extensive bibliography to that date.)
KALTER, H. & WARKANY, J. (1959). Experimental production of congenital malformations. *Physiological Reviews*, 39, 69.
NORMAN, A. P. (1971). *Congenital Abnormalities in Infancy*, 2nd edn. Oxford: Blackwell.
RICHARDS, I. D. G. (1969). Congenital malformations and environmental influences in pregnancy. *British Journal of Preventive and Social Medicine*, 23, 218.
SMITH, D. W. (1970). *Recognizable Patterns of Human Malformation*. Philadelphia: Saunders.
SMITHELLS, R. W. (1966). Drugs and human malformations. *Advances in Teratology*, 1, 251.
SWAN, C. (1948). Rubella in pregnancy as an etiological factor in stillbirth. *Lancet*, i, 744.
WOLSTENHOLME, G. E. W. & O'CONNOR, C. M. (1960). Congenital malformations. *Ciba Foundation Symposium*. London: Churchill.

MOUTH AND GASTRO-INTESTINAL TRACT

CARRÉ, I. J. (1969). Hiatal hernia in infants and children. *Clinical Proceedings of the Children's Hospital, Washington*, 25, 123.
DOUGALL, A. J. (1969). Infantile pyloric stenosis. *Scottish Medical Journal*, 14, 156.
FRASER, G. C. & WILKINSON, A. W. (1967). Neonatal Hirschsprung's disease. *British Medical Journal* iii, 7.
RICKHAM, P. P. & JOHNSTON, J. H. (1969). Neonatal Surgery. London: Butterworths.
SANTULLI, T. V., KIESEWETTER, W. B. & BILL, A. H. (1970). Anorectal anomalies. *Journal of Pediatric Surgery*, 5, 281.

GALL-BLADDER AND BILE-DUCTS

CAMERON, R. & BUNTON, G. L. (1960). Congenital biliary atresia. *British Medical Journal*, ii, 1253.
THOMSON, J. (1892). On congenital obliteration of the bile-ducts. *Edinburgh Medical Journal*, 37, 523.

CARDIOVASCULAR SYSTEM

ABBOTT, M. E. (1936). *Atlas of Congenital Cardiac Disease*. New York: American Heart Association.
BROCK, R. (1961). The surgical treatment of pulmonary stenosis. *British Heart Journal*, 23, 337.

CAMPBELL, M. (1965). Causes of malformations of the heart. *British Medical Journal*, ii, 895.

COLEMAN, E. N. (1965). Serious congenital heart disease in infancy. *British Heart Journal*, 27, 42.

KEITH, J. D., ROWE, R. D. & VLAD, P. (1967). *Heart Disease in Infancy and Childhood*, 2nd edn. New York: Macmillan.

MUSTARD, W. T. (1964). Successful two-stage correction of transposition of the great vessels. *Surgery*, 55, 469.

NADAS, A. S. & FYLER, D. C. (1968). Ventricular septal defect. *Archives of Disease in Childhood*, 43, 268.

ROSE, V., BOYD, A. R. J. & ASHTON, T. E. (1964). Incidence of heart disease in children in the city of Toronto. *Canadian Medical Association Journal*, 91, 95.

ROWE, R. D. & MEHRIZI, A. (1968). *The Neonate with Congenital Heart Disease*. Philadelphia: Saunders.

SELLERS, F. J., KEITH, J. D. & MANNING, J. A. (1964). The diagnosis of primary endocardial fibroelastosis. *Circulation*, 29, 49.

SIMCHA, A. & BONHAM-CARTER, R. E. (1971). Paroxysmal atrial tachycardia. *Lancet*, i, 832.

WATSON, H. (Ed.) (1968). *Paediatric Cardiology*. London: Lloyd-Luke.

WATSON, H. & RASHKIND, W. J. (1967). Creation of atrial septal defects by balloon catheter in babies with transposition of the great arteries. *Lancet*, i, 403.

RESPIRATORY SYSTEM

AVERY, M. E. (1968). *The Lung and its Disorders in the Newborn Infant*. 2nd edn. Philadelphia: Saunders.

FERENCZ, C. (1961). Congenital abnormalities of pulmonary vessels and their relation to malformation of the lung. *Pediatrics, Springfield*, 28, 993.

FIELD, C. E. (1946). Pulmonary agenesis and hypoplasia. *Archives of Disease in Childhood*, 21, 61.

GENITO-URINARY TRACT

BONGIOVANNI, A. M. & ROOT, A. W. (1963). The adreno-genital syndrome. *New England Journal of Medicine*, 268, 1283.

INNES WILLIAMS, D. (1968). *Paediatric Urology*. London: Butterworths.

SCORER, C. G. (1955). Descent of the testicle in the first year of life. *British Journal of Urology*, 27, 347.

SMITH, D. R. & DAVIDSON, W. A. (1958). *Symposium on Nuclear Sex*. London: Heinemann.

WAHLQUIST, L. (1967). Cystic disorders of the kidney. *Journal of Urology*, 97, 1.

NERVOUS SYSTEM

BIRCH, H. G., RICHARDSON, S. A., BAIRD, D., HOROBIN, G. & ILLSLEY, R. (1970). *Mental Subnormality in the Community*. Baltimore: Williams & Wilkins.

FORD, F. R. (1966). Prenatal diseases of the nervous system. *Diseases of the Nervous System in Infancy, Childhood and Adolescence*, 5th edn. Springfield: Thomas.

GUTHKELCH, A. N. (1967). The treatment of infantile hydrocephalus by the Holter valve. *British Journal of Surgery*, 54, 665.

HILLIARD, L. T. & KIRMAN, B. H. (1965). *Mental Deficiency*, 2nd edn. London: Churchill.

LAURENCE, K. M. (1969). Recurrence risk in spina bifida cystica and anencephaly. *Developmental Medicine and Child Neurology*, Supplement 20, 23.

LORBER, J. (1971). Medical and surgical aspects in the treatment of congenital hydrocephalus. *Neuropädiatrie*, 2, 239.

MARTIN, H. P. (1970). Microcephaly and mental retardation. *American Journal of Diseases of Children*, 119, 128.

NASH, D. F. E. (1968). Spina bifida and allied disorders. *Hospital Medicine*, 2, 439.

PENROSE, L. S. (1938). A clinical and genetic study of 1280 cases of mental defect. *Special Report Series, Medical Research Council*, no. 229.

PENROSE, L. S. (1963). *The Biology of Mental Defect*. 3rd edn. London: Sidgwick & Jackson.

RECORD, R. G. & McKEOWN, T. (1950). Congenital malformations of the central nervous system: maternal reproductive history and family incidence. *British Journal of Preventive and Social Medicine*, 4, 26, 217.

SMITH, E. D. (1965). *Spina Bifida and the total Care of Spinal Myelomeningocele*. Springfield: Thomas.

STARK, G. D. (1971) Neonatal assessment of the child with myelomeningocele. *Archives of Disease in Childhood*, 46, 539.

TILL, K. (1968). Spinal dysraphism. *Developmental Medicine and Child Neurology*, 10, 470.

TREDGOLD, R. F. & SODDY, K. (1970). *Mental Retardation*, 11th edn. London: Baillière.

EYE

DOGGART, J. H. (1951). Eye, hereditary diseases. In *British Encyclopaedia of Medical Practice*, vol. 5, p. 381. Edited by Lord Horder. London: Butterworths.

HOEFNAGEL, D. & BIERY, B. (1968). Spasmus nutans. *Developmental Medicine and Child Neurology*, 10, 32.

JAYALAKSMI, P., SCOTT, T., TUCKER, S. H. & SCHAFFER, D. B. (1970). Infantile nystagmus. *Journal of Pediatrics*, 77, 177.

MANN, I. (1937). *Developmental Abnormalities of the Eye*. London: Cambridge University Press.

SKIN AND MUSCLES

BLATTNER, R. J. (1968). Hereditary ectodermal dysplasia. *Journal of Pediatrics*, 73, 444.

BOWERS, R. E., GRAHAM, E. A. & TOMLINSON, K. M. (1960). The natural history of the strawberry naevus. *Archives of Dermatology*, 82, 662.

COCKAYNE, E. A. (1937). *Congenital abnormalities of the skin and its appendages.* London: Oxford University Press. (With comprehensive bibliography to that date.)

DUBOWITZ, V. (1969). The Floppy Infant. *Clinics in Developmental Medicine.* No. **31.** London: Heinemann.

FISHER, R. L., JOHNSTONE, W. T., FISHER, W. H. & GOLDKAMP, O. G. (1970). Arthrogryposis multiplex congenita. *Journal of Pediatrics*, **76,** 255.

BONES AND JOINTS

BRAILSFORD, J. F. (1953). *Radiology of the Bones and Joints*, 5th edn. London: Churchill. (With extensive bibliography.)

DEMYER, W. (1967). The median cleft face syndrome. *Neurology, Minneapolis*, **17,** 961.

DENT, C. E., SMELLIE, J. M. & WATSON, L. (1965). Studies in osteopetrosis. *Archives of Disease in Childhood*, **40,** 7.

ELLIS, R. W. B. & ANDREW, J. D. (1962). Chondroectodermal dysplasia. *Journal of Bone and Joint Surgery*, **44B,** 626.

FAIRBANK, Sir T. (1951). *An Atlas of General Affections of the Skeleton.* Edinburgh: Livingstone.

GREIG, D. M. (1924). Hypertelorism. *Edinburgh Medical Journal*, **21,** 560.

MACKENZIE, I. G. (1972). Congenital dislocation of the hip. *Journal of Bone and Joint Surgery*, **54B,** 18.

Nomenclature for constitutional (intrinsic) diseases of bones (1971). *Journal of Pediatrics*, **78,** 177.

WILSON, D. W., CHRISPIN, A. R. & CARTER, C. O. (1969). Diastrophic dwarfism. *Archives of Disease in Childhood*, **44,** 48.

6 Disorders of Nutrition and Digestion

(See also diabetes mellitus, p. 184; cystic fibrosis, p. 310; deficiency anaemias, p. 246.)

During the first few months of life, when the infant is taking a largely fluid diet, and during the subsequent year, when he is gradually becoming accustomed to a variety of solid food, nutritional and digestive disorders are of major importance as causes of infant death and morbidity. The immaturity of the gastro-intestinal tract and digestive organs renders the infant particularly liable to diarrhoea and vomiting, which may be initiated by comparatively minor stimuli, either enteral or parenteral. The age period 6 to 18 months is that in which the majority of cases of vitamin deficiency occur, while anaemia of nutritional origin is still relatively common in infants aged 3 months to 2 years living under poor conditions in urban districts. Severe undernutrition in the first year of life retards physical growth and may also adversely affect the rapidly developing brain, possibly permanently reducing intellectual capacity. The importance of faulty nutrition in relation to ill-health of the community is difficult to assess accurately in later childhood under the conditions at present prevailing in Britain, but in periods of emergency or economic depression the childhood population is likely to be the first to suffer unless special measures are taken for its protection. Even in normal times, digestive disorders of organic or psychological origin provide a substantial proportion of the cases of ill-health in childhood seen in practice.

Nutrition may be adversely affected in one of several ways. The diet itself may be *deficient* in total quantity or in one or more of its essential constituents; or it may be *ill-balanced*, with an excess of a particular ingredient. Alternatively, the diet provided may be adequate, but *absorption* or *digestion* may be interfered with, or food intake may be inadequate owing to disturbances of appetite or feeding habits. Thus failure of fat absorption occurs in coeliac disease and cystic fibrosis, while diarrhoea or infection of the gastro-intestinal tract will also interfere with absorption and cause secondary malnutrition. Deficiency of essential enzymes will result in failure of digestion or metabolism, while diabetes mellitus will interfere with the normal utilization of particular food factors. Severe or generalized infections are likely to have secondary effects on nutrition, due partly to interference with digestion and absorption, partly to disturbance of metabolism, and partly to loss of appetite.

The investigation of any individual case of nutritional disorder should therefore be based on the assumption that the cause may prove to be multifactorial, and that the clinical picture of a deficiency disease may be produced if the normal processes of food intake, digestion, absorption, and metabolism are interfered with at any point.

FEEDING DIFFICULTIES IN INFANCY

While it is not intended to discuss in detail the physiology and technique of infant feeding,* faulty feeding is responsible for so much ill-health in infancy and so much maternal anxiety that the main principles of infant feeding must be briefly reviewed.

FLUID AND CALORIE REQUIREMENTS

The volume of fluid needed to make good the loss in the urine and faeces and from the respiratory tract and skin, and to provide for growth, averages 150 ml per kg (approximately $2\frac{1}{2}$ fl oz per lb) body-weight per day. Any abnormal loss of fluid rapidly leads to dehydration unless the fluid intake is increased.

The calorie requirements of the young infant are normally supplied as milk, both human and cow's milk giving approximately 70 calories per 100 ml (20 cal per fl oz). Since the diet must provide for both metabolism and growth, the daily requirement of the young infant per unit of body-weight is more than double that of the adult in whom growth has ceased. About 110 calories per kg (50 cal per lb) per day will usually be required by younger infants and only slightly less during the second six months of life. There is, however, considerable individual variation in the requirement of different infants. Estimation of the caloric value of the diet is only a rough indica-

* See 'Nutrition and feeding' by R. G. Mitchell in *Child Life and Health*, 5th edition (1970), London, J. & A. Churchill; *Infant Feeding and Feeding Difficulties* by R. C. MacKeith and C. Wood, 4th edition (1970), London, J. & A. Churchill; *Infant Feeding* by M. Gunther (1970), London, Methuen.

tion as to whether the amount is likely to be adequate and a better guide is progress as assessed by weight gain and general well-being.

FAT, CARBOHYDRATE AND PROTEIN

A comparison of human and cow's milk gives the following average values shown in Table 6.1, although there will be considerable variation especially in fat content between individual samples:

Table 6.1   Comparison of human and cow's milk (average values)

	Human milk %	Cow's milk %
Fat	3·5 to 4·0	3·5 to 4·0
Carbohydrate (lactose)	7	4·75
Total protein	1·25	3·4
lactalbumin	0·75	0·4
caseinogen	0·5	3·0

The proportions present in human milk may reasonably be taken as those best suited to the human infant. It will be seen that the percentages both of total protein and of caseinogen differ considerably in cow's milk. The curd of unmodified cow's milk is thus tougher than that of human milk and in addition the buffering action is greater. It is also found that the proteins, and to some extent the fat, of human milk are better utilized than those of cow's milk.

Fat and carbohydrate are the principal sources of energy and have a protein-sparing effect. Protein contains essential amino acids which cannot be synthesized from fat or carbohydrate. It follows that minimal protein requirements must be covered and that these will be greater when the intake of fat and carbohydrate is restricted. The young infant on a diet of breast milk thrives on about 2 g of protein per kg per day, while the infant on cow's milk normally takes 3 g per kg or more, though such a high intake may not be necessary.

INORGANIC ELEMENTS

The two principal inorganic elements required by the growing infant are iron, for haemoglobin formation, and calcium, which is required both for the growth of the skeleton and for the maintenance of the blood calcium level. In addition, small amounts of iodine, magnesium, phosphorus, sodium, potassium, sulphur, chlorine and copper, and minute amounts of other elements, are essential. All of these are provided in both human and cow's milk, the total mineral contents being 0·2 per cent and 0·73 per cent respectively. Many dried and evaporated milks used for feeding infants now contain additional iron. A diet of unfortified milk alone, whether human or cow's, will not provide adequate iron during the latter part of the first year and it is therefore essential to add to such a diet iron-containing foods, e.g. meat and green vegetables, from the age of 4 or 5 months onward.

VITAMINS

Vitamins are required for normal growth and development and their lack is manifested by the appearance of the deficiency diseases described below. It is rare for human milk to be grossly deficient in vitamins A and C unless the mother's diet is extremely abnormal, but under urban conditions it may be deficient in vitamin D. Fresh cow's milk is also likely to be deficient in vitamin D, but modern dried and evaporated milks often have vitamins added during processing. Unless it is quite certain that the infant is receiving adequate vitamins from this source, however, it is a wise precaution to give vitamin supplements from the age of 1 month to all infants.

KINDS OF MILK

Many infants can tolerate fresh whole cow's milk from an early age but it is advisable to modify cow's milk for infant feeding by dilution or by the processes of drying or evaporation. Dried and evaporated milks have become increasingly popular in Britain and their use has helped to lower the incidence of underfeeding, which was commonly due to too-dilute cow's milk formulae. In addition, their fortification with iron and vitamins is important in the prevention of deficiency diseases and the lower risk of contamination has contributed to the reduction in incidence of infantile gastro-enteritis. Dried milk is generally reconstituted by adding one scoop of milk powder to one fluid ounce of water and only in the first few days of life is it necessary to dilute further. Healthy mature infants will usually take full cream dried milk from the beginning, but a few may manifest symptoms suggestive of fat intolerance, such as abdominal colic, and some paediatricians there-

fore prefer to recommend half cream milk for the first few weeks, i.e. milk from which some of the fat has been removed before drying.

Evaporated milk is reconstituted by mixing one part of milk with two parts of water, though the proportions can be varied depending upon the age of the infant. Sugar should be added to both dried and evaporated milks when reconstituted, unless sugar has been added during manufacture as is the case with some dried milks.

Humanized milks are available in which the proportions of fat, carbohydrate and protein are adjusted to correspond with those in human milk. There is also a variety of special milks for special purposes, e.g. low-sodium milk for use in cardiac failure and hypernatraemia and milks with reduced phenylalanine content for feeding infants with phenylketonuria.

WEANING

This means accustoming the infant to new articles of diet and should be started not later than four to five months after birth. Infants will accept and digest a variety of solid foods well before this age and very early weaning has become popular in Britain, partly due to the convenience of tinned baby foods. While there appears to be no harm in this practice, apart from a possible tendency to fatten the infant too quickly, there is equally no great advantage and during the first four months most infants are satisfied on a purely milk diet. Nevertheless, there are a few who appear hungry even when offered as much milk as they will take and in such cases solids may have to be introduced earlier. These may consist of cereal with milk, minced meat, sieved vegetables and egg, or the mixtures of foods specially prepared in tins for infant feeding. A rusk or baked crust should be given for the infant to chew on when cutting teeth.

When the breast-fed infant has become accustomed to a variety of foods, he can gradually be weaned from the breast on to cow's milk. This process may be started at about 6 months and completed by 7 or 8 months, though some mothers prefer to continue breast-feeding longer. Cow's milk, preferably as reconstituted dried milk, can be given from a cup and will continue to form a large part of the diet well into childhood, for it constitutes an important source of calcium. It should be noted that in many parts of the world where safe cow's milk is not available, breast-feeding must be continued for two or more years, and early weaning is only recommended if an adequate and safe substitute for human milk can be provided.

The normal phase of handling and putting objects into the mouth facilitates the introduction of cup and spoon feeding, and as soon as the infant shows an inclination to hold his cup or to try and feed himself he should be encouraged to do so, even although he makes a mess at first and feeding time is prolonged. Many of the later feeding difficulties of childhood date from mismanagement of weaning and can be avoided if the infant is allowed to experiment with a liberal choice of tastes at this time and exercise some personal selection in what he eats.

DIFFICULTIES IN MANAGEMENT

Many of the difficulties met with in infant feeding are directly due to overanxiety or wrong management. It is important that both mother and infant should be comfortably at ease while feeding takes place. Tenseness in the mother will readily convey itself to the infant and it is generally true that a placid mother will be more successful in feeding her infants than one who is over-anxious. Insistence on 'feeding by the clock' without regard to the infant's hunger will often result in his being fed after a period of prolonged crying and frustration when he is no longer in a state to feed contentedly. If a more flexible approach is adopted, observation will soon show how long the infant can go between feeds without distress. This will usually prove to be about four hours after the first few weeks of life, but the need for a night feed will vary considerably. It need not be assumed that because an infant starts by requiring a night feed he will continue to do so and the stage at which the mother is able to have six to eight hours uninterrupted sleep may be reached more quickly if the infant is allowed to extend the night interval gradually. Babies of the same age differ widely in the amounts they require to satisfy their needs and the amount an individual infant takes may vary from one feed to the next and on successive days. Feeding behaviour also varies considerably. While one baby sucks steadily and contentedly throughout a feed, another may require short rests, or become exasperated immediately if the nipple slips from his mouth, or swallow excessive amounts of air and require to be held up repeatedly. Failure to recognize and make allowances for these individual behaviour differences and attempts to rear babies according to rigid rules are among the important causes of feeding difficulties in infancy. The active restless baby who fusses and tends to regurgitate instead of settling to feed quietly requires careful observation and examination to exclude intrinsic or extrinsic factors which may be interfering with feeding. When the behaviour appears to be essentially one manifestation of general overactivity, sedation with 100 mg of chloral hydrate 20 minutes before each feed is indicated and should be continued until a more normal feeding routine is established. The handling of such babies requires great patience, since obvious anxiety or exasperation tends to make matters worse.

Very occasionally a breast-fed infant persistently refuses to fix and suck, even when lactation is adequate and the nipple is normal. Such 'breast-shyness' may be due to early feeding difficulty, which has led the infant to associate the breast with discomfort or frustration, while occasionally an excessive draught reflex is responsible. In some instances no cause can be found: the difficulty may be overcome by expressing milk on to the infant's lips or by giving a sedative before feeding, but sometimes a change to artificial feeding is necessary. The rare infant who persistently refuses both breast and bottle for no apparent reason may later prove to be mentally subnormal.

Underfeeding

This is an important cause of difficulty in feeding both breast- and bottle-fed infants. When a breast-fed baby cries a lot and fails to gain weight, it is often found that lactation is inadequate, at least temporarily. He may then be given a *complementary feed*, i.e. an artificial feed given immediately after the breast, so that stimulation of the latter will continue. A *supplementary feed*, which is an artificial feed substituted for a breast feed, is sometimes given when lactation is inadequate at a particular time of day or when the mother has not leisure to breast-feed completely. While such measures will often serve to tide over a period of temporary inadequacy of lactation, during which the breast will be stimulated by the vigorously hungry baby, it is important not to persist too long with breast feeding to the detriment of the infant.

In the case of artificially fed infants, underfeeding is liable to occur either when the total quantity of feed is inadequate or when the feed has been diluted to too great an extent. The latter mistake is often made when an infant is fretful because the feed is already inadequate.

Causes of underfeeding other than inadequacy in quantity or quality of milk include abnormalities of nipple or teat; inability of the infant to suck owing to a blocked nasal airway or to being held in the wrong position; local causes in the infant's mouth, e.g. thrush, cleft palate; and failure to suck owing to illness or intracranial injury.

The early signs of underfeeding will be failure to gain weight and fretfulness. When underfeeding has continued for a longer period, the baby becomes apathetic and may refuse to feed altogether; the skin becomes inelastic and the stools small and green, containing little faecal matter ('hunger stools').

Overfeeding

If the healthy infant is offered abundant milk he will feed until satisfied and only exceptionally take more than he needs. Occasionally when lactation is copious the breast-fed infant will ingest an excessive amount of milk but will then usually reject some by possetting, i.e. bringing up small mouthfuls of milk. The difficulty can generally be overcome by reducing the time of feeding, by lengthening the intervals between feeds or by giving one breast at each feed. Overfeeding is otherwise only likely to occur in hot weather or if the infant has a fever, when thirst makes him take more than he needs. In these circumstances boiled water should be offered to drink between feeds, so that his fluid requirements can be met without increasing his caloric intake.

In bottle-fed infants, overfeeding with a single constituent of the diet is a possible danger. If carbohydrate is excessive, the infant becomes fat and flabby and is liable to develop fermentative diarrhoea. Overfeeding with fat may cause vomiting, abdominal discomfort and pale stools. Milk from Jersey cows, which may contain over 5 per cent of fat, is generally too rich for young infants. Very young infants may not tolerate the fat in full-cream dried milk and then do better on half-cream milk for a few weeks. Dried milk should never be reconstituted at greater than full strength, since the salt intake may be excessive and lead to hyperchloraemic brain damage. Overfeeding with protein is unlikely to occur.

When the infant is consistently overfed, weight gain may be unusually rapid, so that it is far above average by the age of 1 year. This is not necessarily undesirable if weight and length are in proportion and the child's general health is satisfactory, but gross obesity should be countered by some restriction of food intake, since it is liable to persist into later life.

Air swallowing

Small amounts of air are normally swallowed during feeding and the infant is held upright at intervals during the feed and at the end so that the air rises into the fundus of the stomach and is eructated. If the infant is laid supine before eructation has occurred, milk may be regurgitated later with the swallowed air. If, on the other hand, the air passes with the feed through the pylorus it is likely to cause colic (spasmodic abdominal pain).

Excessive air swallowing may occur if the milk flows with difficulty from breast or bottle, or if the infant cannot suck easily for mechanical reasons. In bottle feeding, the teat should be of suitable size for the infant's mouth and the hole large enough to allow milk to flow a drop at a time when the bottle is inverted.

Vomiting

Vomiting is a common complaint in infancy and the doctor must first satisfy himself that the infant really is vomiting and not merely possetting milk, which is sometimes described as 'being sick' by the inexperienced mother. Careful enquiry into the details of feeding, and watching the mother giving a feed if necessary, will often reveal one or more of the feeding difficulties discussed above. As in the newborn period, however, vomiting may be due to obstruction, infection or intracranial causes (see p. 69) and these possibilities must always be considered. Urinary infection in particular is a common cause of vomiting in infancy and there may be no other evidence of its presence, which is only revealed by examination of the urine. Minor degrees of pyloric stenosis can also be difficult to recognize and repeated examination during feeds may be necessary. If the history suggests the presence of a hiatus hernia, barium swallow will be indicated.

Should none of these relatively frequent causes of vomiting be disclosed by examination or investigation, less common conditions must be considered. The infant may have a disorder of metabolism, revealed by screening the urine for abnormal amino acids or reducing substances or by more specific biochemical tests. Persistent vomiting with dehydration and collapse suggest the possibility of congenital adrenal hyperplasia. Very occasionally an atopic infant manifests allergy to cow's milk by vomiting forcefully after a feed. This may be accompanied by abdominal colic and urticarial wealing round the mouth, so that the diagnosis is usually evident. Rumination is a rare disorder of behaviour in which the infant learns to regurgitate milk and swallow it repeatedly. Since a little is lost by overflow from the mouth each time, the infant fails to gain weight. The habit is best countered by thickening the feeds and giving a sedative if necessary.

Constipation

This should be judged not so much by the frequency of the stools as by their consistency. If the stools are soft and passed without discomfort, and the infant is thriving, there is no cause for concern if they are infrequent. When the stools are hard and dry and passed with difficulty, the following possible causes should be considered:

Underfeeding, which will be associated with failure to gain weight; here constipation will be corrected by increasing the diet.

Inadequate fluid intake. It may be found that, while the caloric value of the feeds is sufficient, the infant requires additional fluid and the stools become normal when it is given.

Change of feeding. A change from breast to artificial feeding may be accompanied by constipation which is usually temporary. If it persists, increasing the sugar in the feeds may give relief, since sucrose is slightly laxative.

Local causes. If the stool is hard and streaked with blood, there may be a tear or fissure in the region of the anus, which will tend to perpetuate constipation owing to the pain caused by defaecation. In such cases, a laxative such as milk of magnesia will keep the stools soft until healing has occurred and local application of anaesthetic ointment will give relief. Dilatation of the anus may be required if a fissure is persistent.

Abnormalities of the intestine, e.g. stenosis, redundant loop, or Hirschsprung's disease, may cause obstinate constipation from early infancy often with some abdominal distension. Pyloric stenosis and other types of high partial obstruction will cause secondary constipation, though vomiting is generally the presenting symptom.

Hypothyroidism leads to sluggish bowel action and constipation, which will sometimes be the first symptom to draw attention to the disorder.

TREATMENT is that of the primary cause. In cases of habitual constipation, in which no local or endocrine cause is found, it is always advisable to increase the fluid intake and to review the diet. Increasing the amount of fruit juice given or adding puréed fruit will sometimes relieve mild constipation. Milk of magnesia may be used as a temporary measure but should not be continued for long periods. An enema or suppository, repeated if necessary, may be required to clear the bowel of hard faeces, but again should not be relied upon for producing regular evacuation. The aim should be to establish regular bowel action by natural means rather than by intermittent stimulation with purgatives.

FAILURE TO THRIVE

An infant is said to be thriving when he gains weight at a normal rate and shows vigorous activity, with firm muscles and healthy skin. Failure to thrive thus implies unsatisfactory weight gain with soft musculature, scanty subcutaneous tissue, loose skin and lack of energy. Elucidation of the etiology in a particular infant may require exhaustive investigation in hospital and even after such studies a few infants are discharged without a diagnosis other than failure to thrive, though their number has steadily diminished as medical knowledge, especially of biochemical disorders, has increased.

In considering the diagnosis, attention is first directed to nutrition and feeding, since an infant may fail to thrive because he is not given enough food or is losing nutrients by vomiting or malabsorption. If there is no apparent fault in nutritional intake, the history or examination may reveal evidence of chronic infection, congenital malformation of a major organ or neoplastic disease. Failure to thrive is sometimes a feature of severe mental subnormality but this is usually obvious from the infant's behaviour.

If the cause is not clear, it may be advisable simply to observe the effect of careful feeding by experienced nurses; progressive weight gain over two or three weeks, with restoration of vigour and well-being, will suggest that there has been an element of mismanagement and render further diagnostic tests unnecessary. Should the infant not thrive despite skilled nursing, investigation will be required to exclude renal abnormalities, metabolic errors or endocrine disorders such as hypopituitarism. The possibility of chronic poisoning must be ruled out. Intracranial conditions such as craniopharyngioma or chronic subdural haematoma may occasionally account for failure to thrive, which is also a feature of the rare diencephalic syndrome associated with hypothalamic astrocytoma.

The necessary investigations should be completed as quickly as possible, for long sojourn in hospital may itself prevent an infant from thriving, due to deprivation of maternal care and stimulation. It must not be forgotten that more than one cause may be operative, e.g. chronic infection in a malnourished infant or maternal deprivation in a baby with congenital cardiac abnormality. Finally, some infants fail to thrive for no demonstrable reason and one can only postulate that there is some congenital inadequacy, comparable to that held accountable for the poor progress of infants with multiple congenital defects.

PROTEIN–CALORIE DEFICIENCY

This term describes severe malnutrition resulting from dietary inadequacy of protein or calories or both and indicates the interdependence of the two. In general, a diet predominantly deficient in calories will cause marasmus, while a deficiency mainly of protein will lead to kwashiorkor, but the two deficiencies usually occur together in varying degrees and may result in syndromes having some features of both marasmus and kwashiorkor. Moreover, children vary in their adaptive responses to diet and the clinical picture will vary correspondingly. In general, children less than 60 per cent of expected weight for age are considered to be marasmic if they are not oedematous and to have marasmic kwashiorkor if they show hypoproteinaemic oedema. The term kwashiorkor is applied to oedematous children between 60 and 80 per cent of expected weight. Lesser degrees of protein–calorie malnutrition result simply in reduced growth and low weight for age (nutritional growth failure). Protein–calorie deficiency syndromes must be regarded as an important index of nutritional standards in the developing areas of the world and their eradication depends on improving the staple diet and weaning habits in the areas where they are prevalent.

Marasmus

This is a condition of extreme and chronic malnutrition which may arise from gross underfeeding or a variety of diseases which in less severe degree simply cause failure to thrive. The infant with marasmus is not only far below his expected weight but is very small for his age, since both growth and nutrition are affected. There is almost complete loss of subcutaneous fat. As in dehydration, the skin is inelastic. Loss of orbital fat causes the eyes to appear deeply sunken, while the fontanelle, if patent, is likely to be depressed. Muscular development is very poor and activity greatly reduced. The abdomen is often distended or appears so in comparison with the rest of the body. Since the infant is largely living on his own tissues, the excessive metabolism of fat will lead to ketosis and destruction of protein to muscle-wasting.

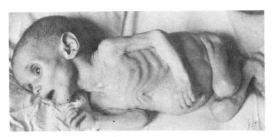

Fig. 6.1 Marasmus. Infant aged 4 months, showing sunken eyes and loss of subcutaneous fat.

While treatment will aim in the first instance at correction of the primary cause, the infant's general condition must be improved at the same time. Intravenous fluid and electrolyte may be required, with alkali to correct acidaemia and sometimes transfusion of small amounts of blood or plasma. Adequate feeding must be achieved slowly, by gastric tube if necessary, since the infant who has reached the marasmic stage takes a long time to respond and his digestive processes are easily overloaded. Many of these infants are in a state of vitamin deprivation, so that additional vitamins should be given in concentrated form.

Kwashiorkor (*Severe or malignant malnutrition*)

This clinical syndrome, which was first described in West Africa, has since been recognized in many tropical and subtropical areas where the staple diet is deficient in first-class protein. It represents a multiple deficiency of which methionine-deficiency is probably the most important element. Infants between 6 months and 5 years of age are most commonly affected, the symptoms appearing when a previously breast-fed infant is weaned on to an exclusively vegetarian diet, usually following the birth of a younger infant. The syndrome is characterized by growth failure; loss of lustre and depigmentation of the skin and hair (see Plate 11), which latter becomes sparse, silky, and grey or reddish in colour; oedema, affecting principally the limbs and face; gastro-intestinal upsets; and apathy, anorexia, and misery. A variety of dermatoses occur, of which a 'crazy-pavement' appearance of the legs and trunk is the most common (see Plates 12 and 13); less frequently the lesions are haemorrhagic or may assume the character of 'elephant' or 'lizard skin' (Fig. 6.2). The liver undergoes fatty change. Anaemia is commonly present, and may be macrocytic in type. Although the urine may show proteinuria and the albumin:globulin ratio of the blood may be reduced, the condition is otherwise distinguishable from the nephrotic syndrome. The clinical picture is usually complicated by the co-existence of infection or infestation.

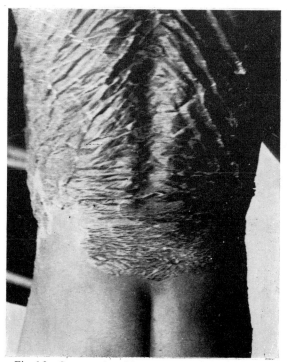

Fig. 6.2   Severe malnutrition with 'lizard skin' dermatosis.

If untreated, this type of malnutrition carries a very high mortality, but even severe cases may respond well to prolonged treatment. Initially, depletion of water and electrolytes may require correction, by intravenous infusion if necessary, though a high sodium intake must be avoided since it may precipitate cardiac failure. Antibiotic therapy is generally indicated for associated infection. Small frequent feeds of skimmed milk are given by mouth or gastric tube and, as the child begins to improve, the diet is gradually increased and supplements of vitamins and iron added. Adequate intake of sodium, potassium and magnesium must be assured. When kwashiorkor affects many children in famine conditions, the administration of a calorie-rich, vitamin-fortified mixture of skimmed milk, cereal and leguminous protein is the most appropriate and economical way of supplying their nutritional needs. Unfortunately, relapse is likely to occur after recovery unless the household diet can be improved and parasitic disease prevented.

DISEASES DUE TO VITAMIN DEFICIENCY

Of the many accessory food factors or vitamins which have been identified, a number are known to be essential for normal growth or for the maintenance of health. Deficiencies usually arise in one of two ways: either the diet may contain vitamins in inadequate amount (the most common finding), or a diet which would be adequate for a normal child may prove inadequate for a sick one owing to faulty assimilation. Very occasionally, the intake of a vitamin required to maintain health is much greater than normal. Such 'vitamin dependency' is probably genetically determined. As a simple deficiency of one vitamin alone seldom occurs except under experimental conditions, it is not always possible to attribute particular clinical syndromes to lack of a single food factor. This is particularly true of the manifestations of disease related to deficiency of vitamin B complex, where many vitamins are likely to be contained in the same food substances. The use of pure products for therapeutic trials, however, has led to a clearer understanding of their role in the prevention and cure of disease.

The only two major vitamin-deficiency diseases which were relatively common in Britain until the post-war era were rickets and infantile scurvy, though minor manifestations of vitamin

A deficiency were also more frequent than generally realized. It is significant that both rickets and scurvy occur typically in infancy, at an age when the infant has little opportunity of choosing his own diet; both are preventable, and since vitamin supplements are readily available in this country, rickets and scurvy must be regarded as an index of ignorance and neglect rather than of poverty. In some of those countries where rice forms the most important food substance, the introduction of polished rice or other interference with natural diet has led to serious increase in deficiency diseases due to lack of vitamin B complex. It has also been found that as a result of war conditions or severe economic depression, vitamin deficiencies amongst the infant and childhood population may assume alarming proportions unless adequate protection against them is provided. If the maternal diet during pregnancy or lactation is so deficient that the mother is suffering from a deficiency disease, it is possible for the infant to be affected *in utero* or during very early infancy.

Table 6.2 indicates the more important vitamins, their sources, and the clinical manifestations related to deficiency.

RICKETS

This is a disorder of calcium and phosphorus metabolism resulting from a deficiency of vitamin D. While the most characteristic manifestations occur in the skeleton, the effects of the disorder are widespread, and involve the musculature, gastro-intestinal tract, growth and

Table 6.2   The vitamins

Vitamin	Chemical product	Natural sources	Properties	Clinical deficiency
A	Retinol	Fish-liver oils, carrots and carotene-containing vegetables; sheep and ox liver	Fat-soluble. Resistant to 120°C and alkaline saponification, but destroyed by aeration at all temperatures and by exposure of fish oils to light	Xerophthalmia Keratomalacia Night-blindness (?) Defective growth (?) Infection
B complex (In addition to thiamine (B_1), riboflavine and nicotinic acid, the B complex contains folic acid, pantothenic acid, pyridoxine, cobalamin, biotin, etc.)	Thiamine (B_1)	Yeast, Marmite, wheat and rice germ, egg yolk, liver, roe, peas, and beans	Water-soluble. Moderately thermostable but destroyed by prolonged heating, by alkalis, and by ultraviolet irradiation	Beri-beri
	Riboflavine	Yeast, milk, egg white, liver, roe, leaf vegetables	Water-soluble. More thermostable than B_1. Destroyed by ultraviolet irradiation, in which it shows blue-green fluorescence	Angular stomatitis Seborrhoeic dermatitis Cheilosis Corneal vascularization
	Nicotinic acid	Yeast, meat, whole grain, peanuts, etc.	Soluble in hot water. More thermostable than thiamine and riboflavine, not destroyed by ordinary cooking, or on exposure to air, light or alkalis	Pellagra
C	Ascorbic acid	Orange, lemon, blackcurrant, tomato juice; swedes, spinach, watercress, cabbage; rose-hips	Water-soluble. Destroyed by aeration and rapidly by heat in presence of oxygen or alkalis	Scurvy
D (D_2 and D_3)	Calciferol (D_2)	Irradiation of pro-vitamin on or in skin (D_3) or of sterol-containing foods Fish-liver oils	Fat-soluble. Thermostable and resistant to aeration. Calciferol is destroyed by prolonged irradiation	Rickets Tetany
E	Alpha, beta, and gamma tocopherol	Wheat germ; green leaves	Fat-soluble. Heat, alkali, and acid resistant. Destroyed by ultraviolet irradiation	Infertility Abortion
K	Phylloquinone	Alfalfa, spinach, cauliflower, cabbage, soyabean, etc. (Possibly synthesized in gut by bacterial action)	Fat-soluble (some analogues are water-soluble). Destroyed by alkalis, oxidizing agents, and strong acids; inactivated by light. Moderately thermostable	Hypoprothrombinaemia Haemorrhagic disease of newborn
P	Citrin	Blackcurrant, grape, lemon, orange juice; rose-hips	Water-soluble	Increased capillary permeability

development. The disease typically occurs in infancy between 6 months and 2 years of age, but may appear earlier, e.g. in pre-term infants, or later if the etiological factors necessary for its production are present. Since the disease is closely related to growth, an infant whose growth is arrested, e.g. owing to coeliac disease, may remain in a potentially rickety state and only show active manifestations when growth is resumed. Cases of late rickets or juvenile osteomalacia may also occur when the diet is exceptionally poor and when the child is deprived of exposure to sunlight, e.g. in the case of African children living in a northern climate. 'Renal rickets' and vitamin D refractory rickets associated with amino aciduria have a different etiology from nutritional rickets, and are considered subsequently (pp. 202 and 190).

ETIOLOGY. Vitamin D is normally obtained from two sources, viz. preformed in the diet and by photosynthesis from its precursors (sterols) in the skin. The vitamin D content of both breast milk and fresh cow's milk may be very low, particularly during the winter months, but modern dried and evaporated milks used for infant feeding are fortified with vitamin D. Formation of the vitamin in the infant's skin is variable and depends on exposure to ultraviolet rays. The smoke-pall present over most industrial cities filters off a large proportion, while during the winter months the amount of ultraviolet light reaching the earth in northern climates is greatly reduced. At the same time, it should be remembered that 'sky-shine' as well as direct sunlight is an important source of ultraviolet light.

Experimentally, it has been shown that gross imbalance of calcium and phosphorus in the diet will produce or predispose to rickets, but where milk forms the major component of the infant's diet, excess or lack of calcium or phosphorus will not arise. In prophylaxis, therefore, attention is concentrated on vitamin D.

Infection predisposes to rickets and may precipitate tetany. Chronic infection may also be responsible for an infant failing to get normal exposure to sunlight.

PROPHYLAXIS. All infants should receive the equivalent of 400 international units of vitamin D daily. Fish-liver oils are widely used for this purpose, but where fortified dried milk is used, requirements will be partly covered from this source. Thus in Britain, dried milk generally contains about 100 i.u. of vitamin D per oz (25 g) of powder, i.e. per 8 fl oz (227 ml) of reconstituted milk. The recommended daily intake should not be exceeded, since calciferol (D_2) is toxic in large amounts. After the age of 5 years the intake may be reduced since requirements are less.

Regular exposure of the infant to sky-shine, if not to direct sunlight, is also important in prophylaxis. Since ordinary window-glass filters off ultraviolet rays, exposure should be out of doors.

PATHOGENESIS. The exact mechanism by which vitamin D aids the absorption of calcium and phosphorus from the bowel, and their deposition in the skeleton, is not clear. Absorption of calcium apparently takes place throughout the whole length of the small bowel, and the vitamin may act both by enhancing an active transport system and by increasing permeability to calcium ion. Vitamin D has a dual action on bone, sometimes promoting deposition of calcium and sometimes demineralizing, depending on the state of equilibrium at the time. The action on the kidney is complex. Directly or indirectly, renal tubular reabsorption of phosphorus is increased by the vitamin, which also helps to regulate acidification and amino acid reabsorption by the renal tubules. When vitamin D is deficient, there is a failure of absorption, a fall in the inorganic blood phosphorus, a rise in plasma alkaline phosphatase, and defective ossification. The serum calcium is usually maintained at normal levels, but this occurs at the expense of the calcium reservoirs in the skeleton. It is probable that compensatory overaction of the parathyroids results in withdrawal of calcium from the skeleton to maintain the blood-level, with consequent osteoporosis. When this mechanism breaks down, and the serum calcium falls below 6 mg per 100 ml, tetany is likely to occur.

PATHOLOGY. The characteristic changes seen in the skeleton consist of (a) general osteoporosis and softening, bending of the long bones, and deformities of the thorax and pelvis; (b) irregular proliferation and defective ossification of the epiphyseal cartilage columns, with resultant enlargement of the costochondral junctions, wrists, ankles, etc. Microscopically, it is found that the cartilage columns are not only extremely irregular but that the zone of differentiation between cartilage and bone becomes unrecognizable. This is illustrated radiologically by the cupped and feathery appearance of the growing ends of the long bones. Uncalcified osteoid tissue may be produced and show increased vascularity.

INCIDENCE. Formerly a disease of sunless northern cities, rickets is now most prevalent in large tropical cities, where diets are poor and social customs often prevent exposure to sunshine. Though now rare in Britain, it has reappeared recently in some large cities, especially amongst coloured immigrants. In this country, rickets is most liable to occur in winter and spring, when ultraviolet irradiation is minimal.

CLINICAL FEATURES. Depending to some extent on the age at which active rickets occurs, the presenting symptoms will often relate to the generalized hypotonicity and delayed development which are characteristic of the disease rather than to the bony deformities. It will be noticed that a young infant fails to raise his head or sit up at the normal time, that an older infant fails to crawl or walk, or that one who has already begun to walk 'goes off his legs'. The infant is commonly lethargic or fretful, often sweats profusely and may be pale due to associated nutritional anaemia. The general nutrition is sometimes deceptive; thus an infant with marasmus who has ceased to grow is unlikely to show active rickets, whereas a fat, flabby infant who has had a high carbohydrate diet and is overweight for age is particularly likely to do so. Examination confirms the general hypotonicity which is often shown by abnormal flexibility of the limbs. There is usually distension of the abdomen due partly to hypotonia of the abdominal muscles, partly to distension of the intestine with gas, and partly to downward displacement of the liver and spleen due to deformity of the thorax.

Gastro-intestinal symptoms are common, the infant showing alternating constipation and passage of undigested green stools, frequently associated with abdominal discomfort. Bronchial and nasal catarrh are also common, and recurrent attacks of bronchitis will tend to increase thoracic deformity. There may be disturbance of renal tubular function in nutritional rickets, causing glycosuria and aminoaciduria, though of lesser degree than in vitamin D refractory rickets with renal tubular defects (p. 190). Spasmus nutans (p. 389) is occasionally seen in association with rickets.

BONY MANIFESTATIONS. These will vary with the age of the infant.

Head. Failure of the anterior fontanelle to close is common when rickets develops during

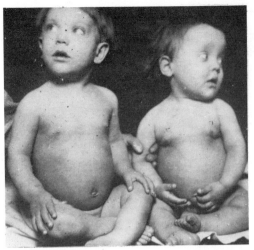

Fig. 6.3   Brother and sister with rickets. Boy on left shows bending of tibia and enlarged radial epiphyses; girl on right shows frontal bossing and Harrison's sulcus.

the first 15 months. A large fontanelle at the age of a year or more should always suggest the possibility of rickets in the absence of raised intracranial tension or cretinism.

Craniotabes, or localized softening of the skull, is not very common and not invariably due to rickets. Pressure over the softened area will give a sensation of egg-shell crackling. *Frontal bossing* may develop in severe rickets.

Spine. Kyphosis and scoliosis may occur as the result of rickets from osteoporosis of the spine associated with muscular hypotonicity.

Pelvis. Deformities of the pelvis, of which reduction of the inlet is clinically the most important, are often overlooked in infancy but may complicate delivery when the child-bearing age is reached.

Thorax. The most common deformities of the thorax consist of: (1) *Harrison's sulcus,* a horizontal groove lying just above the attachment of the diaphragm, developing as the result of respiratory embarrassment. (Although this deformity is particularly liable to occur in the softened thorax in rickets, it is not diagnostic, and may be seen in non-rickety children if severe respiratory embarrassment has occurred early.) (2) *Beading of the ribs* ('rickety rosary'), due to enlargement of the costochondral junctions. The enlargement is rounded and affects both the costal and chondral side of the junction, as distinct from scurvy-beading (see below) which represents expansion of the rib only. (3) *Deformities of the sternum,* which may be depressed, or

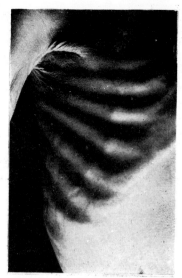

Fig. 6.4   Beading of ribs in rickets.

characteristic swelling at the wrists and ankles which is commonly described as enlargement of the epiphyses. The deformity may be very obvious when it is extreme, but it is often difficult to detect minor degrees of expansion in a fat baby.

Deformities of long bones. Weight-bearing on the softened long bones results in curvature, or more commonly angulation at the junction of the lower and middle thirds, of the forearms and lower legs. In an infant who has learnt to sit up but not to walk, the forearms are most likely to be affected, and in one who has begun to stand, the legs. The lower limbs may show genu valgum or varum deformities.

DIAGNOSIS. The clinical diagnosis can be made with confidence if the condition is severe, and a number of the above signs are present. It is more difficult in very mild or early rickets. Enlargement of the costochondral junctions is one of the earliest bony changes, but the ease with which the junctions can be palpated will vary considerably with the covering of the chest wall. The size of the anterior fontanelle is so variable in early infancy that this is seldom of diagnostic value before the normal age of closure is approached. The normal slight curve of the infant's anterior tibial margin should be distin-

prominent ('pigeon breast') with lateral depression of the ribs. (4) *Flaring*, or upward deflection, of the lower ribs.

Enlargement of epiphyses. Expansion of the growing ends of the long bones gives rise to a

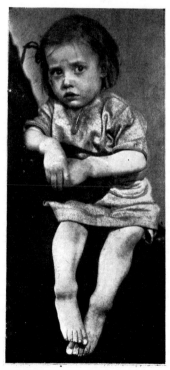

Fig. 6.5   Enlargement of epiphyses in rickets.

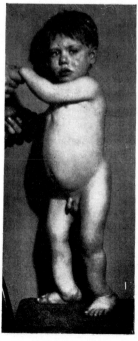

Fig. 6.6   Rickety deformity of legs.

guished from the characteristic angulation of rickets.

Radiological examination is very helpful in confirming the clinical diagnosis. The wrists are usually selected for examination although they are not necessarily the first areas to show changes. These consist of cupping and expansion of the lower end of the radius and ulna, with a feathery, indeterminate margin, the appearance being compared to that of a frothing champagne-glass (Fig. 6.7). As healing takes place, calcium is deposited within the affected area, which becomes denser than normal; the growth line assumes a more regular, sharply demarcated outline, and expansion becomes progressively less marked. Further radiological evidence of rickets is given by the general osteoporosis of the long bones.

The most sensitive test of active rickets is estimation of the plasma alkaline phosphatase, which is invariably raised; the inorganic blood phosphorus may be normal but in all but the slightest degrees of rickets is likely to be well below the average infantile value of $4 \cdot 5$ mg per 100 ml (e.g. 3 or $2 \cdot 5$ mg).

TREATMENT consists of administration of vitamin D, 1000 to 2000 i.u. daily, until healing is complete. This may be combined with exposure to sunlight or ultraviolet radiation. Calcium gluconate should be given orally in severe cases, and the milk requirements adequately covered. The infant should be prevented from standing or from weight-bearing on the arms while the condition is active, in order to prevent further deformity. It is important not to immobilize the infant more than absolutely necessary, however, since activity is essential when healing is established.

In cases where severe deformities have occurred and where the condition is no longer active, osteotomy or other surgical correction is likely to be required.

PROGNOSIS. The prognosis as regards life is good, death when it occurs being due to intercurrent infection, diarrhoea, or other complication. Early cases adequately treated make a complete recovery, but neglected cases are likely to show persistent deformities of greater or less severity.

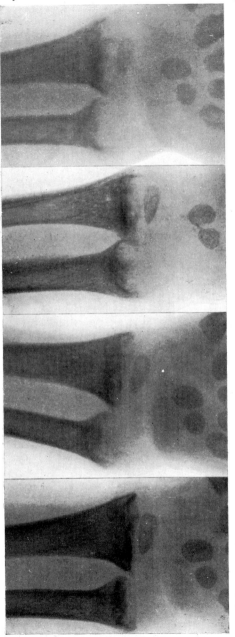

Fig. 6.7   Active rickets (above), showing progressive healing. First three films taken at weekly intervals; the last film, which shows that healing is well advanced, was taken five weeks after beginning treatment.

Infantile tetany (spasmophilia)

Tetany is a common manifestation of severe rickets and is due to neuromuscular hyperexcitability caused by reduction of ionizable calcium. This is reflected in the level of total serum calcium, which is found to be below 6 mg per 100 ml. The disorder may remain latent, or the onset may be fulminating. In the latter case, a generalized convulsion or series of convulsions may be the first indication, or spasm of the larynx may cause a high-pitched crowing sound with respiratory embarrassment (*laryngismus stridulus*). The infant may become cyanotic during such an attack, and appear about to suffocate, though death in an attack is fortunately rare.

The hands and feet assume a position known as *carpopedal spasm*, the fingers being flexed on the hands and the interphalangeal joints extended. The thumb is drawn across the palm. The feet are flexed on the ankle, and the toes directed downward. Carpopedal spasm may be elicited by

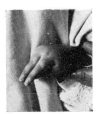

Fig. 6.8   Position of fingers and thumb in carpopedal spasm.

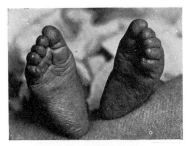

Fig. 6.9   Position of toes in carpopedal spasm.

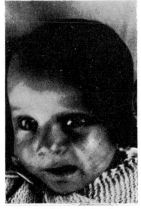

Fig. 6.10   Chvostek's sign in infantile tetany. Twitch of left angle of mouth on tapping over left facial nerve.

constriction of the arm or leg (*Trousseau's sign*).

The neuromuscular hyperexcitability is demonstrated by tapping the face over the facial nerve, when a twitch at the angle of the eye or mouth will be elicited (*Chvostek's sign*). The reactions of the muscles to galvanic stimulation may be characteristic (*Erb's sign*), a cathodal opening contraction obtained with less than 5 mA being diagnostic.

DIAGNOSIS. The clinical evidence of neuromuscular hyperexcitability or painful spasms of muscle associated with rickets will indicate the diagnosis, which can be confirmed by the finding of a low serum calcium. Tetany due to other causes, e.g. malabsorption, hypoparathyroidism, or alkalosis arising from persistent vomiting or hyperventilation can usually be excluded on the history and by the absence of rickets. Tetanus, after the newborn period, is only likely to occur following an injury, and the clinical picture is characteristic.

TREATMENT. The administration of calcium gluconate (10 to 20 ml of a 10 per cent solution intramuscularly or intravenously) and vitamin D is curative. Rapid relief of symptoms may be obtained by the administration of calcium chloride or ammonium chloride (1 to 2 g four-hourly by mouth), these drugs acting by producing an acidosis and so increasing the amount of ionizable calcium immediately available.

PROGNOSIS is good if the condition is recognized and treated promptly, but convulsions or laryngismus stridulus occasionally prove fatal.

SCURVY

The essential deficiency giving rise to scurvy is lack of vitamin C (ascorbic acid). The disease is characterized by haemorrhages and disturbances of ossification. It generally affects infants between 6 and 18 months of age, but may occur at any age.

ETIOLOGY. Scurvy is now seldom seen in infants in Britain but the disease occasionally occurs in severely disabled children, especially the mentally subnormal, who are liable to be undernourished because of difficulties in feeding them. Since the vitamin C content of human breast milk is usually 4 to 7 mg per 100 ml, it is rare for scurvy to occur in a breast-fed infant unless the mother is herself suffering from severe vitamin C deficiency. Most processed milks now used in artificial feeding are fortified with ascorbic acid but in the case of infants fed on fresh cow's milk, a rich source of vitamin C, e.g. orange juice, must be given routinely in addition to the feeds. Even when this is done, it will sometimes be found that the vitamin C has been partly inactivated by boiling or alkalinization in misguided attempts to render the orange juice 'sterile' or 'less acid'.

Probably only 5 to 10 mg of ascorbic acid is needed daily to prevent scurvy, but most infants receive 20 mg or more daily. This intake is assured by 50 to 100 ml of fresh orange juice; orange juice concentrate, which should be diluted, contains 60 mg ascorbic acid to the fluid ounce (28·5 ml).

After the age of 2 years, the infant's requirements are likely to be covered by a liberal mixed diet containing fruit and green vegetables; but since some of the vitamin C content of vegetables may be destroyed by improper cooking, it is advisable to continue giving orange juice up to the age of 4 or 5 years. Although most children take orange juice readily, black-currant purée or syrup of rose-hips may be substituted if desired.

PATHOLOGY. The primary pathological lesion is an increased permeability of the capillary-bed, due to failure of connective tissue formation. Blood leaks between the endothelial cells of the capillaries, resulting in haemorrhage. In addition, there is failure of osteoblastic function, and while deposition of calcium is uninterrupted, with the production of a wide area of calcified matrix at the growing ends of the long bones, this calcified matrix is not converted into bone. The shafts and epiphyses of the long bones become rarefied; fracture through the calcified matrix or through the line of rarefaction immediately adjacent may result in displacement of the epiphyses. Haemorrhage below the periosteum is responsible for stripping-up of the periosteum and pain; the haematoma subsequently becomes calcified.

Vitamin C deficiency is also liable to cause a specific anaemia which will only respond to vitamin C administration, while secondary anaemia will be present when the haemorrhages are sufficiently severe.

CLINICAL FEATURES. Latent scurvy may result in some general interference with nutrition and be associated with anaemia, but frequently the onset is abrupt in an infant who has previously appeared well. The first symptom is commonly severe pain referred to the lower extremities. The infant screams if picked up or moved, and when

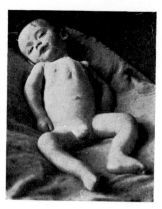

Fig. 6.11   'Frog position' in infantile scurvy, with swelling of left thigh.

at rest assumes a 'frog position' with the thighs abducted and the lower legs partially flexed. There may be obvious swellings of the legs, which are acutely tender. The temperature may be raised during the acute phase, but unless there is intercurrent infection, the white blood count is not significantly increased.

Haemorrhages may occur at any site, but are common in the gums of infants who are cutting teeth. Haematuria, haemorrhage from the bowel, and spontaneous ecchymoses into the skin or orbits are liable to occur in severe cases; red blood cells can almost invariably be demonstrated microscopically in the urine.

Scurvy-beading is a most valuable diagnostic sign. The ribs are expanded at the costochondral junction, giving rise to a sharp ridge immediately

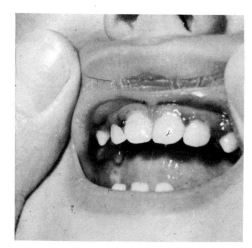

Fig. 6.12   Infantile scurvy. Swelling and haemorrhage of gums.

adjacent to the costal cartilage. This can best be appreciated by running the finger from the lateral aspect of the rib towards the sternum, when the expansion or beading of the rib will first be felt, followed by the abrupt 'step down' as the cartilage is reached.

DIAGNOSIS. The occurrence of severe pain and tenderness of both lower limbs, associated with evidence of haemorrhage elsewhere and red blood cells in the urine, strongly suggests the diagnosis, which is confirmed clinically if scurvy-beading is present. In osteomyelitis the lesions are less likely to be bilateral, and the temperature and white blood count are typically higher than in scurvy.

Radiological changes in scurvy are diagnostic, and depend partly on the occurrence of sub-periosteal haemorrhages, and partly on failure of osteoblastic function.

The earliest changes are usually seen at the wrist or ankle, and consist of a small wedge-shaped area of rarefaction immediately proximal to the lower end of a long bone. As the disease progresses, this area of rarefaction extends across the width of the bone to form the zone of rarefaction, and fracture may occur through it. Lipping of the distal corner of the radius occurs early, and subsequently dense lines of calcified matrix form distally to the zones of rarefaction in the affected long bones, extending laterally beyond the normal contour of the shafts. This calcified matrix fragments readily and parts of it are frequently displaced.

Osteoporosis of both the shaft and epiphyses

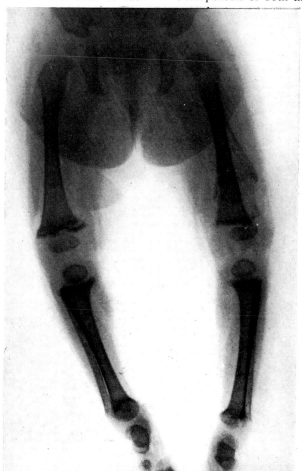

Fig. 6.13 Infantile scurvy. Right femur shows densely calcified matrix and zone of rarefaction. Left femur shows calcifying subperiosteal haemorrhage, fracture through rarefied zone, and displacement of epiphyses.

gives them a ground-glass appearance, the epiphyses being outlined so that they may resemble signet-rings. When subperiosteal haemorrhages have occurred along the shaft, the stripped-up periosteum may be recognizable by a thin line of new bone deposited beneath it. As the subperiosteal haematoma calcifies, it becomes increasingly obvious radiologically. The contour of the shaft will be altered by the surrounding calcification for many months after healing has occurred, but ultimately the normal contour becomes re-established and no permanent deformity is left.

Biochemical tests are seldom necessary to establish the diagnosis in manifest scurvy, but in early or latent cases measurement of ascorbic acid concentration in leucocytes is the most reliable index. A saturation test with a measured amount of vitamin C will demonstrate delay in the appearance of vitamin C in the urine.

TREATMENT AND PROGNOSIS. Response to the administration of 100 ml of fresh orange juice or 100 mg of ascorbic acid daily is dramatic, improvement being noticeable within 24 to 48 hours, and all pain usually being relieved within a week. In all except the most long-standing cases and those complicated by intercurrent infection, complete and rapid recovery is the rule.

VITAMIN A DEFICIENCY

Although vitamins A and D are both fat-soluble and occur in some of the same natural products, e.g. fish-liver oils, vitamin A deficiency is not necessarily associated with rickets. The vitamin A content of both human and cow's milk varies considerably with maternal diet. Vitamin A can also be formed in the body from carotenoid pigments in carrots and a number of other vegetables. The principal disturbances caused by vitamin A deficiency are keratinization of epithelium and a failure of production of visual purple. It has been claimed that vitamin A has a specific anti-infective property, but it is probable that the hyperkeratinization of epithelium predisposes to infection particularly of the respiratory tract.

The complete clinical picture of vitamin A deficiency is seldom seen in older children except under conditions of semi-starvation. Subclinical states are probably not very uncommon during the first year of life, however, and in parts of Asia infantile xerophthalmia (see below) is an important cause of blindness. Secondary effects include atrophy of muscles and lymphoid tissue and anaemia.

Night-blindness

Defective dark adaptation is directly due to failure of formation of visual purple. The incidence of this in the childhood population is thought to be high, though it is frequently overlooked in infancy. Children sometimes come under observation on account of the specific complaint that they are less able to see clearly in the evening than in the morning. Response to treatment with vitamin A serves as a therapeutic test of etiology.

Xerophthalmia

The earliest sign of this condition consists of dryness (xerosis) and lack of lustre of the eye, which may be associated with wrinkling of the conjunctiva and photophobia. Subsequently, *Bitot's patches*, which have been compared to frost on window-panes, appear on the scleral conjunctivae. In advanced cases the cornea becomes softened and oedematous (*keratomalacia*), and finally ulcerates.

Response to treatment with vitamin A is good in the early stages, but if clouding or ulceration of the cornea has occurred, permanent blindness may result.

DIAGNOSIS. Apart from the clinical picture and estimation of dark adaptation, vitamin A deficiency can be diagnosed by scrapings of epithelial surfaces and demonstration of keratinized cells. The urine should be examined for the presence of epithelial cells.

TREATMENT. The addition of vitamin A to the diet in the form of cod-liver oil, butter, fresh milk, and vegetables, will result in rapid relief of symptoms.

DEFICIENCY OF VITAMIN B COMPLEX

Although deficiencies of the components of the vitamin B complex are likely to be multiple, it is possible to distinguish several specific syndromes related to deficiency of particular substances. Certain stigmata, such as glossitis, have been attributed to a variety of constituents of the B complex, including riboflavine, nicotinic acid, pyridoxine, and biotin. Folic acid is effective in the treatment of megaloblastic anaemia which is rare in childhood but occasionally complicates

due to primary invasion by the virus of herpes simplex is accompanied by fever, headache and malaise. Symptoms persist for 10 to 14 days and then subside spontaneously.

Angular stomatitis, while characteristic of riboflavine deficiency, may also occur in conditions of debility, and disappear with improvement in the general health.

Gangrenous stomatitis (*Cancrum oris, noma*)

This is now extremely rare in Britain, but is relatively common and often lethal in countries where malnutrition and oral sepsis are widespread. The initial lesion commonly starts as an area of ulceration of the gum, which rapidly

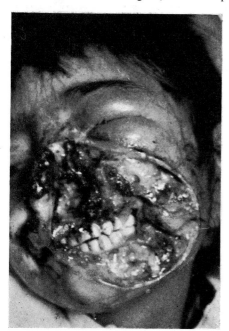

Fig. 6.16   Cancrum oris, with extensive destruction of face.

becomes gangrenous and may destroy the greater part of the cheek. While the prognosis has greatly improved with antibiotic therapy followed by plastic surgery, it is still poor in infancy.

Sublingual ulcer occurs most commonly during an attack of pertussis and usually responds rapidly to local treatment.

Gingivitis

Inflammation of the gums commonly occurs in the types of stomatitis described above. When the gums alone are affected, the condition may be due to teething, a localized Vincent's infection, scurvy, or dental sepsis. Occasionally lead poisoning is responsible, but the 'lead line' is unlikely to occur if the gums are otherwise healthy. In some older children the gums are found to bleed abnormally easily in the absence of vitamin C deficiency or haemorrhagic diathesis. In most of these cases the condition is due to a low-grade infection and to neglect of the toothbrush. The gums should be rubbed with a strong solution of table salt, and the use of a soft tooth-brush introduced when it can be tolerated. It may be found that the teeth require scaling, while any local dental infection will require appropriate treatment.

Teething

Many minor disorders of infancy are attributed to teething without any very adequate reason. However, the eruption of the deciduous teeth may cause local swelling and redness of the gums, with some general disturbance including irritability and slight fever. Pain may necessitate an analgesic such as paracetamol and an adequate fluid intake should be ensured.

Glossitis

The tongue is likely to be involved in all types of stomatitis. In addition, the 'strawberry tongue' seen during the second week of scarlet fever, and the various types of glossitis associated with vitamin B deficiency, are more or less characteristic. A smooth, atrophic tongue is sometimes seen in cases of coeliac disease and of severe nutritional anaemia. In '*geographical tongue*', which is not very uncommon in childhood, sharply demarcated areas which are bright red in colour and abnormally smooth are surrounded by a whitish margin. The condition, which is of little clinical importance, may appear in the course of a febrile illness, or arise and disappear without obvious cause. *Furring* of the tongue, which varies in colour from white to dark brown, may occur with any digestive disturbance or severe febrile illness. It calls for special care in the hygiene of the mouth, but otherwise requires no special treatment.

The teeth

The causes of *dental caries* are still a matter of controversy but cariogenic bacteria and dietary sucrose are believed to be important in etiology, while fluoride in the tooth enamel helps to resist decay. Experimentally, it has been found that the addition of milk to the diet of school children has significantly reduced the incidence of caries. The fluorine content of the drinking water has been shown to be of great importance. In areas where the fluorine content is low the incidence of caries is abnormally high; the raising of the fluorine content to 1 part per million brings about a significant reduction in caries. On the other hand, when fluorine is present in the water in excessive amount *dental fluorosis* (pitting and discoloration) is liable to occur. Fluoride may also be administered topically in mouth rinses or toothpastes. The fall in incidence of caries observed during periods of severe dietetic deprivation has been attributed to the reduction in the refined foods eaten, and in particular to the lack of refined sugars. Neglect of dental hygiene and the lodgement and decomposition of starchy foods between the teeth are contributory causes of dental caries which can be avoided. Care of the first dentition should never be omitted on the grounds that 'the teeth will come out anyway', since the proper development of the permanent teeth is closely related to the integrity of the first.

Malocclusion and displacement of the permanent dentition may arise from deformities of the jaws or palate, infection, premature removal of the deciduous teeth, or prolonged retention of the latter. Thumb-sucking, which is frequently blamed, is probably quite unimportant during the first two years of life, though it may be responsible for dental displacement if continued into middle childhood. Malocclusion should receive orthodontic treatment.

Delayed dentition

While the central incisors commonly erupt at about the age of 6 months, there is considerable variation in the time of eruption of both the first and permanent dentitions. Pathological delay is observed in active rickets, and in certain endocrine disorders, particularly cretinism, hypopituitarism, and hypogonadism. In some cases, absence of one or more of the permanent teeth is a hereditary disorder.

Salivary glands

With the exception of epidemic parotitis (mumps), diseases of the salivary glands are rare in childhood. Chronic or recurrent pyogenic infection of the parotid or submaxillary glands will occasionally lead to sialectasis of the ducts and abscess formation; during the periods of recurrent swelling, pus can be massaged from the ducts. The infection usually proves to be an ascending one from the mouth. A more acute form of suppurative parotitis is occasionally observed in newborn infants, and usually responds to antibiotic therapy.

The term '*Mikulicz syndrome*' is given to a condition of symmetrical and painless swelling of the parotid, submaxillary, and lachrymal glands which is liable to be associated with failure of secretion of saliva and tears. The condition may be malignant, tuberculous, or of unknown etiology.

MALABSORPTION SYNDROME

Under this title are included a number of digestive and absorptive disorders of infancy and childhood which are characterized by wasting, failure of growth, distension of the abdomen and the passage of loose bulky stools. The term 'coeliac disease' should be confined to those cases in which there is intolerance of gliadin in wheat and rye gluten, associated with impaired fat absorption. Other causes of the malabsorption syndrome include cystic fibrosis (p. 310), rare forms of familial pancreatic insufficiency, parasitic and bacterial intestinal infections, and anatomical abnormalities of the bowel, such as congenital malrotation or surgical excision of small intestine. The clinical picture of malabsorption is occasionally seen in other congenital and nutritional disorders. Sugar intolerance is generally secondary to other conditions but occasionally occurs as a primary disorder, when it causes fermentative diarrhoea with excess sugar in the stools, which have a pH of less than 6·0.

DIAGNOSIS. When the malabsorption syndrome is suspected from the history and clinical features, the presence of malabsorption should be established before steps are taken to identify the cause. A useful screening procedure is the xylose excretion test, in which 5 g of D-xylose is given by mouth and the urine collected for the following five hours. Normally more than 25 per cent of the oral dose appears in the urine whereas when malabsorption is present, less than 20 per cent is so excreted. It should be noted, however, that in cystic fibrosis the xylose excretion test is generally normal. The rise in blood or urine levels after oral administration of various other substances, such as glucose or iodine preparations, may also be used as indices of malabsorption but are not so simple and informative as the xylose test.

The stools in malabsorption may appear pale and bulky, with an offensive smell, but a normal appearance does not exclude malabsorption. On a normal diet, a healthy child excretes no more than 4 g of fat in the stools per day, and generally much less. In the fat excretion test, stools are collected for at least three days and their fat content determined. An average daily fat excretion of more than 5 g is definite evidence of malabsorption and over 4 g is suggestive. A single normal result, however, does not absolutely exclude the diagnosis of malabsorption, since continuous steatorrhoea is not invariable.

A barium meal may provide supporting radiological evidence, for in malabsorption the barium flocculates in the intestine in a characteristic way.

Coeliac disease

The *etiology* of this condition is not completely understood, though it is now generally regarded as a constitutional intolerance of gluten (a constituent of wheat flour), which damages the

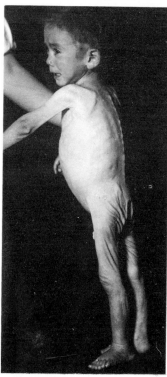

Fig. 6.17   Coeliac disease, showing wasting of buttocks.

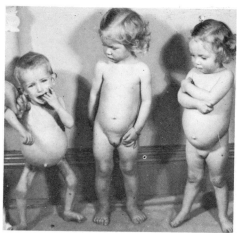

Fig. 6.18   Coeliac disease. Boy on left untreated, showing dwarfing, extreme wasting, and large abdomen. Girl on right, a mild case after a year's treatment; good general nutrition but abdomen still enlarged and genu valgum present. Normal girl of the same age in centre.

intestinal cells and results in a disturbance of fat-absorption and steatorrhoea. Evidence that failure of fat-absorption is not the primary defect is given by the improvement in fat-absorption which occurs when gluten is removed from the diet.

The disease occurs in both sexes, and the familial incidence is higher than would be expected in random occurrence. The disease is seldom manifest before the sixth month of life, in which it differs from cystic fibrosis of the pancreas, although in recent years the earlier introduction of cereals in the diet has tended to lower the age of onset of symptoms.

CLINICAL FEATURES. The history typically shows that the infant has progressed normally until shortly after the introduction of cereals, usually at about 4 months of age. During the next few months, failure to thrive and loss of weight and appetite are associated with the passage of large, pale, and offensive stools, which often appear greasy. The stools are not necessarily frequent, but the bulk of faecal matter passed daily is considerably more than normal.

The first digestive upset may be of short duration and followed by a period of partial remission, but further attacks occur at progressively shorter intervals, often precipitated by infections. The infant's general condition and nutritional status deteriorate, and he becomes extremely miserable and irritable. In severe untreated cases a state is reached in which sub-

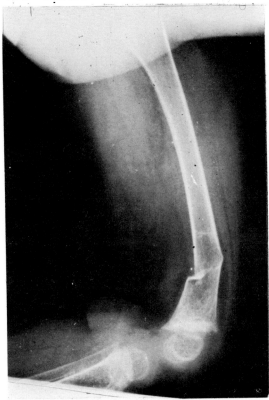

Fig. 6.19   Coeliac rickets. Osteoporosis of femur with spontaneous fracture.

development if the condition is still active when the normal age of puberty is reached (Fig. 8.12).

Vitamin deficiencies. Unless particular care is taken to cover the vitamin D and calcium requirements of coeliac patients, they will develop latent rickets which will become active when growth resumes under treatment. Tetany is observed in a small proportion of cases. Scurvy will occur if the vitamin C intake has been inadequate. Some degree of shifting oedema, which partly accounts for the large and sudden variations in weight, is not uncommon. This is possibly due to vitamin B deficiency, though hypoproteinaemia may be responsible in some cases.

Anaemia is a very common finding, the anaemia usually being of hypochromic microcytic type. Very much more rarely the anaemia is megaloblastic, and these cases are the only ones likely to benefit from folic acid.

DIAGNOSIS. In establishing the diagnosis of coeliac disease as a cause of the malabsorption syndrome, it is necessary to exclude infection of the gastro-intestinal tract, and also cystic fibrosis, which is done by measuring the sweat electrolytes and by demonstrating trypsin in the duodenal juice. The stools must be examined for ova and parasites, including *Giardia lamblia*. Tuberculosis should also be excluded by the tuberculin test. Intestinal biopsy by the peroral route shows microscopical changes in the villi of the proximal jejunum which are characteristic of coeliac disease. This flattening of the jejunal mucosa, in conjunction with the other clinical findings and the response to treatment, confirm the diagnosis.

The presence of disaccharidase deficiencies, whether of lactase, sucrase, maltase or a combination of these, may be established by demonstrating a rise of blood glucose after oral administration of glucose and an absence of such rise after administering the suspect disaccharide. When the glucose tolerance curve is flat, as it often is in coeliac disease, excess disaccharide may be demonstrable in the stools.

TREATMENT. A diet from which all wheat gluten has been removed, but which is otherwise normal, is the accepted treatment for coeliac disease, but in severely affected patients first coming under treatment it is advisable to build up the diet gradually from skimmed milk with added protein until it is clear that fat-absorption has improved.

cutaneous fat is almost entirely lost, growth ceases, and there is generalized muscular wasting. This is well seen in the gluteal region, where the normal contour of the buttocks is lost. At the same time the abdomen becomes increasingly distended, owing to intestinal fermentation. Ladder patterning, splashing, or borborygmi may be observed, while X-ray will demonstrate fluid levels and gaseous distension of the bowel.

This classical presentation of the disease is not difficult to recognize but it must be emphasized that coeliac disease can also present in less obvious ways, such as failure to thrive, chronic diarrhoea, or deficiency syndromes with apparently normal stools.

Children with severe coeliac disease may show *infantilism*, which represents the late result of retarded growth and development, and becomes more obvious in untreated cases with advancing age. The small size and immaturity of the patient is reflected in the radiological picture, which shows a corresponding delay in ossification. Older children may show delay in sexual

It is essential to cover the vitamin require-ments of the patient, and for this purpose vita-mins A and D should be prescribed in con-centrated water-soluble form and in rather larger dosage than that normally required. Orange juice or ascorbic acid and vitamin B preparations (yeast, Marmite) should be included in the diet. An adequate calcium and phosphorus intake is also necessary. When there is associated sugar intolerance, it will be necessary to exclude the offending disaccharide (usually lactose) from the diet, otherwise the response to removal of gluten will be unsatisfactory.

Treatment must be prolonged, since inclusion of even small amounts of gluten in the diet may result in relapse, and in most, if not all cases, a gluten-free diet should be continued into adult life.

COURSE AND PROGNOSIS. Individual cases vary greatly in severity and duration. Some patients undergo symptomatic improvement in middle childhood, while others pass into the adult sprue syndrome. Probably some degree of mucosal flattening persists in all patients who have not received gluten-free diet. The inter-ference with growth which occurs in all except the very mildest untreated cases will result in some permanent reduction of adult stature.

The mortality in coeliac disease is low if the patient can have prolonged and careful treat-ment, but death from malnutrition or intercurrent infection may occur if the condition is neglected.

DISEASES OF THE LIVER

The functions of the liver include glycogen stor-age and release (glycogenesis and glycogeno-lysis), haematopoiesis, formation of prothrombin and fibrinogen, the intermediary metabolism of fat, the metabolism of protein, detoxication and excretion of bile. Disease processes affecting the organ may therefore give rise to widely different symptoms, depending on the function principally disturbed. There are numerous tests of isolated functions of the liver, but each one is necessarily of limited clinical value, especially in infancy. Of the tests of excretory function, the brom-sulphalein test is one of the more useful. Very high values of serum glutamic oxalo-acetic trans-aminase (SGOT) are found in severe hepato-cellular damage. In chronic hepatitis the electro-phoretic pattern of plasma proteins may be abnormal, with low albumin and raised beta and gamma globulins.

Jaundice

Jaundice, i.e. yellow staining of the skin or sclerotics by circulating bile pigments, does not necessarily imply hepatic disease. The genesis of jaundice is complex and often more than one etiological factor is involved. No classification is therefore wholly satisfactory, and the conven-tional divisions into obstructive, toxic or infec-tive, and haemolytic types or into pre-hepatic, hepatic and post-hepatic causes are an over-simplification. When cholestasis is present, the plasma bilirubin is nearly all conjugated, since the bilirubin has passed through the liver cells and has been reabsorbed (p. 60). Serial estima-tion of unconjugated and conjugated serum bili-rubin is useful in following the course of jaundice.

In infancy and childhood, the response of the liver to disease processes will be affected (1) by its immaturity and (2) by its capacity for re-generation. The child's liver is less likely than that of the adult to be subjected to the action of toxins such as alcohol, but is more liable to suffer from the effects of malnutrition and infection. In some tropical countries, however, childhood cir-rhosis has been attributed to plant and fungal toxins, while veno-occlusive disease in Jamaica is thought to be caused by a hepato-toxic agent in 'bush tea'.

Infiltrations

Glycogen disease, the lipidoses, and amyloid disease are considered in Chapter 7. *Fatty in-filtration* of the liver occurs readily in infancy as a result of starvation, infection and the action of toxins. It is a common post-mortem finding in fatal cases of infantile diarrhoea and in chronic infection. The liver cells are filled to a greater or less extent with globules of neutral fat. While the condition is often symptomless during life, the liver may be enlarged and tender. Treatment is that of the primary cause, though a high pro-tein–carbohydrate diet will usually be indicated.

Cirrhosis of the liver

Hepatic fibrosis with nodule formation may follow chronic fatty infiltration, or arise from infection (e.g. viral hepatitis), biliary or venous obstruction (e.g. biliary atresia or veno-occlusive disease), immunological disturbance (e.g. active chronic hepatitis) or disorders of storage (e.g. glycogenosis). It may occur in hepato-lenticular degeneration, cystic fibrosis, galactosaemia, or without associated disease ('idiopathic'). The condition is therefore the end product of a variety of factors causing repeated or chronic liver damage, and not a disease *sui generis*. The following clinical types, in addition to those occurring as complications of specific diseases, are recognized:

Infantile hepatic cirrhosis. This condition is rare in temperate climates, but is liable to affect children under 4 years of age in parts of India and elsewhere. The etiology is still obscure, and it is uncertain whether nutritional, toxic or infective factors are primarily responsible. There is destruction of liver cells, intercellular fibrosis, and proliferation of pseudo-bile canaliculi. Jaundice is gradually progressive, and is associated with marasmus and increasing oedema preceding death.

Biliary cirrhosis. This results from prolonged cholestasis, due to cholangitis or to mechanical obstruction of the biliary passages, e.g. in atresia of the bile-ducts. Jaundice appears early and slowly deepens, the urine contains bile, and the stools are either normal or pale in colour. The liver is likely to be enlarged, hard, and smooth, with a sharp lower margin. Evidence of portal obstruction, haemorrhages, and oedema only appear late. Symptoms may be slight or absent at first but later include headache, pyrexia, abdominal pain, and loss of appetite. The course may be prolonged for several years, depending on the cause, but the outcome is ultimately fatal if the cirrhosis is progressive.

Portal (micronodular) cirrhosis. This type of cirrhosis, in which evidence of portal obstruction occurs early and jaundice appears late, is rare in childhood as compared with adult life. In many cases no causative factor can be identified; in others there is evidence that nutritional factors are responsible, and that the condition has followed fatty infiltration. Occlusion of the hepatic veins is a rare cause except in Jamaica, although it may be commoner than is realized in countries where children's diets may contain plant toxins. Congestive cardiac failure or obstruction of the inferior vena cava will have a similar effect. Portal hypertension, in which hypersplenism, gastric haemorrhage, and leucopenia are associated with hepatic cirrhosis, is considered on p. 242. Viral hepatitis may be

the cause of some cases of cirrhosis, although the relationship has not yet been proven.

Premonitory symptoms usually include loss of appetite and some general failure to thrive before portal obstruction occurs, but the onset may be very insidious and growth is not usually retarded. Portal obstruction is evidenced by the occurrence of ascites, and by dilatation of veins over the abdominal wall forming a 'caput medusae'. The

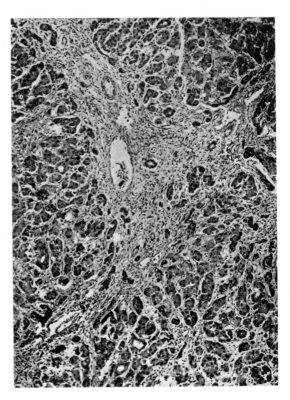

Fig. 6.20   Multilobular cirrhosis of liver of unknown etiology. Boy aged 8 years.

liver is hard, and may either be enlarged or reduced in size. Abdominal pain is a common symptom in this stage. Spider naevi are highly suggestive of the diagnosis. Spontaneous haemorrhage, usually from an oesophageal varix, is often an early sign, and may later be so severe as to prove fatal. The presence of oesophageal varices may be demonstrated radiologically.

Jaundice, generalized oedema, and cardiac failure occur in the final stages of the disease,

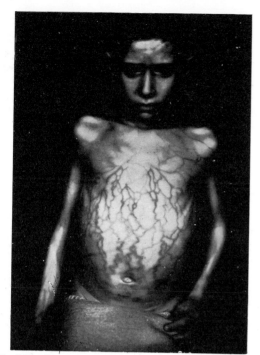

Fig. 6.21   Venous engorgement in caval obstruction associated with hepatic cirrhosis and chronic tuberculous mesenteric adenitis. Lower margin of liver shown by transverse mark in right loin. Boy aged 11 years.

unless the child succumbs early to haemorrhage or infection.

Hepatolenticular degeneration (Wilson's disease) is a rare autosomal recessive genetic defect, in which portal cirrhosis is associated with degeneration of the basal ganglia. There is failure of formation of caeruloplasmin and increased deposition of copper in the tissues. The hepatic condition often gives rise to little disability, the neurological symptoms being most in evidence. These include torsion spasm, tremor, dysarthria and mental deterioration. A pigmented ring may be present in the cornea.

TREATMENT OF CIRRHOSIS. Any existing obstruction should be relieved surgically if possible. In some selected cases it may be possible to relieve portal hypertension by lienorenal anastomosis. The diet should be rich in protein and carbohydrate, since reduction of serum proteins and hypoglycaemia are likely to occur with advanced cirrhosis. Vitamin supplements, including vitamins K and B complex, should be given. Transfusion may be necessary when haemorrhages occur. With a few exceptions such as Wilson's disease, which responds to

treatment with penicillamine, advanced cirrhosis represents an irreversible and progressive change, so that treatment in these cases is largely palliative.

Infectious hepatitis (*Catarrhal jaundice*)

A virus infection involving the liver and causing diffuse hepatitis and focal necrosis of liver cells, this condition is common in childhood, though not in early infancy. It frequently occurs in small epidemics, most commonly in the autumn. Infection almost certainly occurs by way of the alimentary tract, and excreta should be regarded as infective. The incubation period has been estimated as 14 to 40 days, whereas in the much more severe condition of *serum hepatitis*, which is probably due to a different virus, the incubation period is considerably longer (60 to 135 days). Serum hepatitis is usually transmitted by human serum, e.g. via improperly sterilized syringes or during haemodialysis, but it may occasionally be conveyed by personal contact. The virus has not been isolated but an apparently

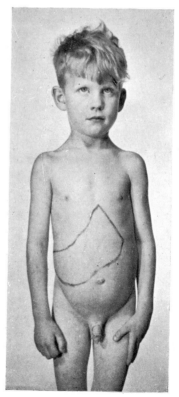

Fig. 6.22   Infective hepatitis, showing enlargement of liver. Boy aged 5 years.

specific antigen (Australia antigen) has been found in the serum of a high proportion of patients in the early stages of serum hepatitis.

CLINICAL FEATURES. The appearance of jaundice is preceded by a pre-icteric phase lasting up to a week which may cause difficulty in diagnosis in the absence of an epidemic. The temperature is raised, usually to 38·5°C (101°F) but occasionally higher, the child complains of headache, anorexia, and vomiting, and abdominal pain may be sufficiently severe to suggest the possibility of appendicitis. Examination, however, will show that the pain is upper abdominal, and the liver may be enlarged and tender.

Daily examination of the urine will show the presence of bile immediately preceding or coincident with the appearance of jaundice. The stools at this time become pale. The jaundice may be associated with itching of the skin or urticaria, bradycardia, and abdominal distension. In the great majority of cases, however, the symptoms improve dramatically when the jaundice has appeared and the early anorexia is followed by increased appetite. The jaundice gradually fades, usually within a period of two to three weeks. The liver, which may be enlarged during the acute phase, rapidly returns to its normal size. Splenomegaly occurs more frequently in childhood than in adult cases.

The disease is typically benign in childhood, and recovery rapid and complete. It is exceptional for relapses to occur and very rare for the condition to progress to chronic hepatitis (see below). Subclinical cases, in which jaundice is absent, may occur during the course of an epidemic.

TREATMENT. The child should be kept in bed until the acute symptoms have subsided. The diet should include liberal amounts of protein and carbohydrate, particularly during the period when appetite is regained. The child is likely to refuse foods during the period of anorexia, but subsequently exclusion of fat is unnecessary. Vitamin supplements should be given. If vomiting is very severe, intravenous therapy will be necessary until food can be taken by mouth. Gamma globulin has been used in prophylaxis during an epidemic, but is valueless in treatment where infection has already occurred.

Chronic hepatitis

Infectious hepatitis may rarely be followed by *chronic persistent hepatitis*, characterized by

vague malaise, tender enlargement of the liver and minimal or absent jaundice. Histological changes in the liver are slight, the condition seldom progresses to cirrhosis and the ultimate prognosis is good. In *active chronic hepatitis*, which is believed to be due to an antigen–antibody reaction, the patient is jaundiced and liver necrosis is extensive, with disturbance of the lobular pattern. There is biochemical evidence of continuing hepatocellular damage and the condition usually progresses to liver failure or cirrhosis. In the early stages, corticosteroids or immunosuppressive drugs may be of value.

Weil's disease

This is a type of jaundice due to infection with *Leptospira icterohaemorrhagiae*, characterized by multiple haemorrhages, which may prove fatal, pyrexia, abdominal pain, haemorrhagic herpes, rigors or convulsions, and the presence of albumin and red blood cells in the urine. It is transmitted by rats and is rare in childhood, though children may be affected in the course of an epidemic. Tetracycline is the treatment of choice, though the specific antiserum is effective if given very early. The prognosis is considerably less good than that of infectious hepatitis, though complete recovery may occur.

Acute liver failure

This is fortunately rare in childhood, but may occur as the result of poisoning with phosphorus, chloroform, or arsenic, or very occasionally follow viral hepatitis. It is sometimes impossible to determine the primary cause. After a variable period of malaise and nausea, the child passes into a state of intractable vomiting, pyrexia, mental confusion and coma. Convulsions and haemorrhages may occur. Jaundice is usually deep, but death may occur so rapidly that jaundice is sometimes barely detectable. The liver may be at first enlarged, but is ultimately greatly reduced in size. The urine contains albumin, casts and crystals of leucine and tyrosine. Although temporary remissions may occur, the condition is always fatal, the course varying from a few days to two or three weeks.

A very acute form of liver failure, with fatty degeneration of viscera and acute encephalopathy, is characterized by rapid onset of coma without jaundice, often after a transient febrile illness. Severe vomiting, hypoglycaemia and convulsions are usually followed by death within two or three days.

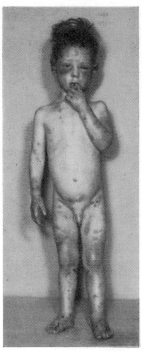

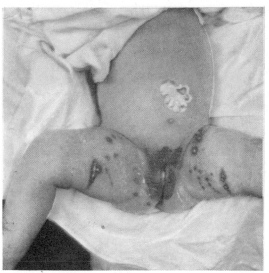

PLATE 2 Staphylococcal pustules in skin folds of infant of a diabetic mother.

PLATE 1 Battered child syndrome.

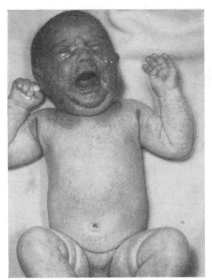

PLATE 3 Exfoliative dermatitis of face of an infant aged 3 weeks.

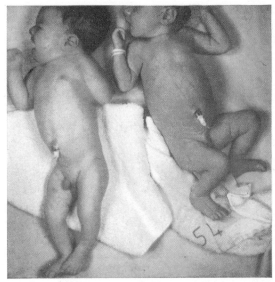

PLATE 4 Icterus gravis neonatorum (right) with normal infant.

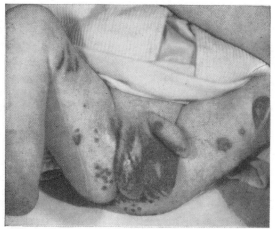

PLATE 5 Napkin rash involving buttocks, scrotum and thighs.

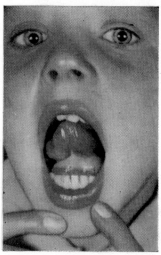

PLATE 6 Ranula lying below tongue.

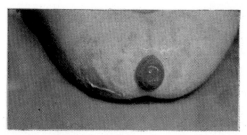

PLATE 7 Prolapse of rectum.

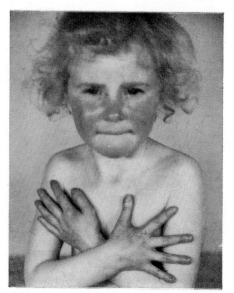

PLATE 8 Clubbing of fingers and cyanosis in child with Fallot's tetralogy.

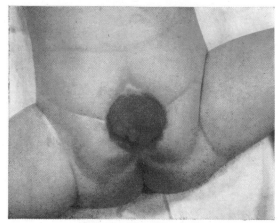

PLATE 9 Ectopia vesicae.

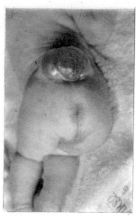

PLATE 10 Lumbar mye-
lomeningocele in a newborn
infant, showing defect of
over-lying skin and patulous
anus.

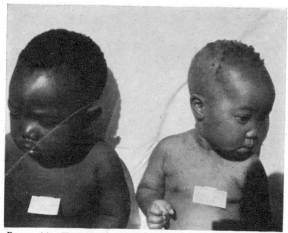

PLATE 11   Kwashiorkor (severe malnutrition), right, showing
loss of pigmentation of skin and hair, compared with normal
control, left.

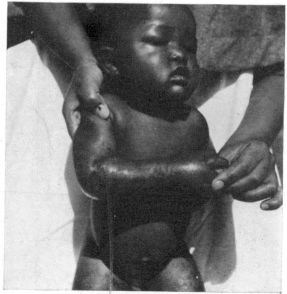

PLATE 12   Kwashiorkor, showing oedema and dermatosis of
arm and oedema of face.

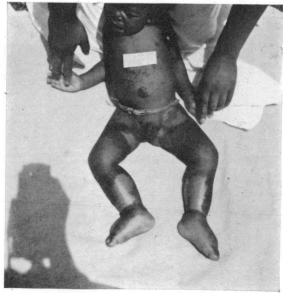

PLATE 13   Kwashiorkor, showing oedema and dermatosis of
legs and haemorrhagic lesions on abdomen.

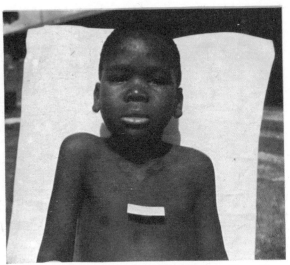

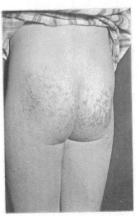

PLATE 15 Lesions of anaphylactoid purpura on the buttocks.

PLATE 14 Pellagrin aged 7 years, showing Casál's necklace and lesions on cheeks and forehead. Hair colour normal. (Courtesy of Dr S. Wayburne.)

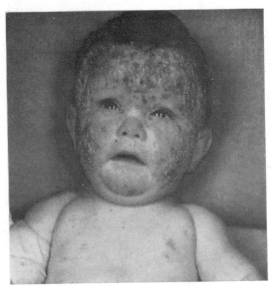

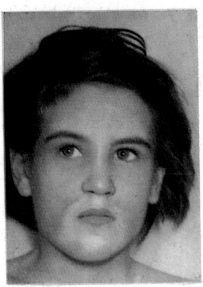

PLATE 16 Infantile eczema.

PLATE 17 Dermatomyositis, showing violet erythematous rash on the face, brow and eyelids, with circumoral pallor.

Liver abscess

Multiple abscesses of the liver occasionally occur as a complication of pyaemia in infancy, or of ascending infection from the umbilicus in the newborn. Solitary abscesses are very rare in childhood. Symptoms include pyrexia, upper abdominal pain, and vomiting. Surgical drainage is required. The prognosis is poor.

DIARRHOEAL DISORDERS

The diarrhoeal disorders of infancy and childhood have no common etiology but may broadly be divided into the acute infective diarrhoeas and the non-infective diarrhoeas, which are usually subacute or chronic. Infective diarrhoea may occur at any age but when it affects infants under the age of 2 years it is generally called infantile gastro-enteritis.

INFANTILE GASTRO-ENTERITIS

This important condition is highly infectious and outbreaks occur especially in hospitals, residential homes and other institutions in which numbers of infants are housed together. Severe epidemics carrying a high mortality were formerly common in the summer months but gastro-enteritis now occurs throughout the year in Britain, and indeed may be more common in winter in association with outbreaks of respiratory infection. The environmental conditions associated with a high incidence of infantile gastro-enteritis in the community are those favouring the spread of infection, viz. poor housing, overcrowding, large families and the poverty and ignorance that often go with these. The death rate from gastro-enteritis has fallen steeply in the past 20 years but there has been an appreciable mortality in recent epidemics, mainly among malformed infants and those of low birth-weight.

Infection of the gastro-intestinal tract is now considered to be the principal cause of infantile gastro-enteritis, even although a pathogenic organism can be demonstrated in only a minority of cases. Faulty diet and parenteral infection, once considered to be important primary causes, are now believed to be of secondary importance in predisposing to infection of the bowel.

Diet

The incidence of gastro-enteritis is significantly lower in breast-fed than in artificially fed infants. This may be attributed partly to the risk of contamination of milk or feeding utensils in artificial feeding and partly to the composition of cow's milk, which results in an intestinal flora consisting almost exclusively of *Bacillus bifidus* and in greater acidity of the intestinal contents. By contrast, the stools of the infant fed on cow's milk are alkaline and show a mixed flora.

Although the composition of an artificial feed is blamed for causing diarrhoea more often than is justified, when it is too dilute the stools may become small and green (see p. 146), while if it contains excess carbohydrate the stools may be frothy and unformed, causing excoriation of the buttocks. In either case, infection readily supervenes.

Parenteral infection

Parenteral infection is an important precipitating cause of diarrhoea, particularly in the absence of an epidemic. Infections of the respiratory tract, middle ear and urinary tract may be accompanied by vomiting and some looseness of the stools but when fulminating diarrhoea develops, it usually signifies the onset of intestinal infection in an infant whose resistance has been lowered by the parenteral infection.

Enteral infection

Infection of the gastro-intestinal tract with organisms of known pathogenicity can be demonstrated in some cases of infantile gastro-enteritis, the type of infection affecting the severity of the disease and its epidemiology.

Dysentery group. The presence of blood and mucus in the stools should always be regarded as suggestive of dysenteric infection, which is likely to be associated with a rise of temperature, or even a convulsion, at onset. Macroscopic blood may only be found in one or two stools, but mucus, pus, and microscopic amounts of blood are likely to persist for a considerably longer period. The commonest and mildest type of dysenteric infection in Britain is *Shigella sonnei*, but Flexner and Shiga infections also occur. Since older children are often very mildly affected by *Sh. sonnei* but may remain carriers for many weeks, it is often difficult to eradicate an outbreak in an overcrowded area or institution.

Typhoid-paratyphoid group. Salmonella typhosa itself is seldom responsible for infantile diarrhoea, though no age group is wholly immune during a typhoid epidemic. Various paratyphoid organisms, however, have been found from time to time in diarrhoeal epidemics confined to infants, though their pathogenicity has not always been established.

Other Salmonella infections are a comparatively rare cause of infantile diarrhoea in Britain, but epidemics have been caused by *S. typhimurium* and in some localities the organism is isolated comparatively frequently. In these cases also, blood and mucus may be found in the stools.

Escherichia coli group. Enteropathogenic strains of *E. coli*, particularly serotypes 0.26, 0.55, 0.111, 0.119 and 0.128, are at present the most important of the demonstrable causes of infantile gastro-enteritis and have been responsible for a number of small outbreaks in the past few years, e.g. on Teesside in 1968 (0.119 and 0.128) and in Manchester in 1969 (0.114).

Other enteral infections. Viruses are sometimes grown from the stools in infantile gastro-enteritis but their role in pathogenesis is not clear. Other occasional causes of diarrhoea in infancy are protozoal infections and intestinal thrush. Appendicitis is very rare during the first year of life, but peritonitis is a possible cause of diarrhoea in this age period.

CLINICAL FEATURES. While these will vary to some extent with the etiology, the clinical picture of severe infantile gastro-enteritis is generally characteristic. Infants under 6 months of age are likely to be those most severely affected.

Premonitory symptoms such as refusal of feeds and weight-loss may precede the onset of frank diarrhoea by one or more days, but frequently the onset is fulminating. In these cases the infant passes within a few hours from a condition of apparent well-being to one of severe prostration and shock. The stools become green, watery, offensive, and extremely frequent, finally containing only minimal quantities of faecal matter.

Feeds are refused, or if taken are vomited immediately, until not even glucose-saline can be retained. In younger infants particularly, the vomitus may become of 'coffee-ground' appearance, due to the presence of altered blood. This latter sign is of bad prognosis. Urinary output is reduced and may cease entirely. The pulse becomes rapid and feeble, and the infant may show air-hunger. The temperature varies, depending on the nature of such infection as may be present. When there is parenteral infection, e.g. otitis media or urinary infection, the temperature is

likely to be high at onset, and the disease may even be ushered in by a convulsion, but in very severe gastro-enteritis the temperature is often subnormal.

Owing to the loss of fluid in the stools and vomitus, the infant rapidly becomes dehydrated. This is shown clinically by rapid loss of weight and loss of elasticity of the skin, which lies in folds in the axillae and groins. A fold of skin lifted between the fingers will only slowly return to its normal contour. The fontanelle and eyes become sunken, and the lips and mouth dry. In the severest cases there is cyanosis of the lips and extremities, and greyish pallor of the face. Hypertonic dehydration is sometimes seen (p. 181) and occasionally there is jaundice, but this is exceptional and appears to be confined to particular epidemics. Hypernatraemia due to dehydration during the acute stage is an important cause of permanent brain damage in survivors. Terminal pneumonia is a relatively common complication in fatal cases.

The series of metabolic disturbances brought about by severe diarrhoea comprise: (1) fluid loss, with consequent haemoconcentration; (2) loss of alkali in the stools; (3) retention of acid products of metabolism due to suppression of urine; (4) ketosis; (5) accumulation of lactic acid, due to circulatory failure and anoxaemia (see p. 182). If urine is passed, it is concentrated and strongly acid. Ketone bodies and albumin may be present.

In addition to the changes affecting the extracellular fluids, there is a loss of intracellular potassium, which is in excess of that which would be expected from the nitrogen loss. In some cases at least, this loss of intracellular potassium appears to result in a replacement of intracellular potassium by sodium which must be corrected during treatment (p. 183).

PATHOLOGY. Necropsy will frequently demonstrate the presence of parenteral infection, though the terminal bronchopneumonia or otitis media which often occurs shortly before death should be distinguished from a primary infection precipitating the diarrhoea.

The condition of the gastro-intestinal tract will vary with the type of enteral infection. In dysenteric infections the intestinal mucosa may be acutely inflamed or ulcerated, but in the majority of cases of infantile diarrhoea of other types there are often only catarrhal and atrophic changes in the small bowel, in marked contrast to the severity of the symptoms. The term gastro-enteritis, which implies inflammation of the stomach and intestines, is therefore inappropriate as a general description, although it has come to be widely used.

The liver often shows some degree of fatty degeneration, which may be very extensive; more rarely, areas of actual necrosis are found. The kidneys commonly show cloudy swelling of the tubules.

PREVENTION. Breast-feeding is a partial safeguard against diarrhoeal disorders of infancy, although breast-fed infants are not immune. In the case of artificial feeding, the feeding utensils must be kept scrupulously clean, and contamination of the feeds by flies or dirty hands avoided. This is particularly important in institutions, where strict control of cross-infections must be maintained. The routine of making up feeds in the milk kitchen must be meticulous and frequently inspected: the personnel should not be responsible for changing napkins. Every case of diarrhoea should be regarded as highly infectious and be nursed in isolation.

TREATMENT. This will include specific treatment of infection, both enteral and parenteral, whenever this is possible; treatment of shock; correction of dehydration; replacement of electrolytes; correction of ketosis and acidosis; and re-establishment of urinary excretion (see p. 182).

Infection. When the primary infection can be determined, the appropriate antibiotic should be used in full dosage; sulphonamides should only be used with caution in dehydrated patients and never in young infants. In 'non-specific' enteral infection, including cases in which a pathogenic *E. coli* has been isolated, antibiotics are seldom helpful, but gentamicin, colistin or neomycin may be of limited value. The treatment of bacillary dysentery is considered on p. 348.

Shock must be combated by warmth, a minimum of handling, and the administration of fluids. Adrenaline hydrochloride is sometimes effective when there is severe collapse. The infant should be nursed in continuous oxygen if cyanosis is present.

Correction of dehydration is an essential of early treatment. In the milder cases, when diarrhoea is not associated with vomiting, it may be possible to cover the normal fluid requirements and to replace the fluid lost in the stools by oral administration of 5 per cent glucose in $\frac{1}{2}$ isotonic saline. All other food should be withheld

for at least 24 hours, and the glucose and saline mixture should be given at hourly intervals (subsequently increasing to two-hourly). The volume given will depend on the infant's weight, degree of tolerance, and dehydration, but an intake of 150 ml/kg body weight per 24 hours should be the minimum.

In severe cases vomiting is likely to preclude oral administration of fluid, which must then be given by the intravenous route until oral feeding can be tolerated (see p. 183).

Subsequent management. Every case must be judged on its own merits in deciding when to recommence oral feeding. With careful regulation of fluid and electrolytes, infants can be maintained for two or more days on intravenous therapy alone. Oral feeding should be recommenced cautiously with small amounts, e.g. 4 to 10 ml of saline and glucose, the amounts and time-interval being gradually increased. When fluids are satisfactorily retained without vomiting, dilute milk feeds should be introduced, and a gradual return to normal feeding effected over a period of a week or more. If diarrhoea persists, it may indicate a transient intolerance of lactose and a low-lactose feed should be substituted.

NON-INFECTIVE DIARRHOEA

Non-infective diarrhoea is usually subacute or chronic, although it may start acutely, especially when it is a manifestation of an underlying metabolic disorder. An allergic reaction may occasionally account for explosive diarrhoea following the ingestion of cow's milk by an infant.

Chronic diarrhoea is a common and troublesome complaint and often no satisfactory explanation can be found. The diet should be carefully reviewed and infection excluded by bacteriological investigation. The possibility of malabsorption due to coeliac disease, cystic fibrosis or sugar intolerance must be considered. Increased intestinal motility can be due to emotional disturbance but frequently there is no evidence of this. In the majority of cases no cause can be demonstrated and it must be assumed that there is a functional disturbance of the bowel. This has been called the 'irritable colon syndrome' and tends to be familial.

A bland diet with a minimum of roughage, fruit and other constituents liable to increase bowel motility is advisable and all laxatives and purgatives should be avoided. During exacerbations, symptomatic relief may be obtained by mixtures containing kaolin or chalk, or by antispasmodics such as propantheline. The prognosis is generally good and the bowel gradually becomes less active, although it may remain rather easily stimulated.

ABDOMINAL PAIN

Pain referred to the abdomen is one of the commonest and often one of the most baffling symptoms in infancy and childhood. It is also one where accurate and early diagnosis may be of the highest importance. While the general principles of examination are the same as in adult life, much of the history in the case of infants has to be reached by inference, and even in older children localization and description of pain may be vague and unsatisfactory.

The first point to determine is whether the pain really is arising from a lesion within the abdomen. Careful examination of the hips, spine, chest, and groins may demonstrate a bony lesion, basal pneumonia, painful inguinal nodes, ectopic testis, or strangulated inguinal hernia. Of these, pneumonia is perhaps the commonest cause of pain referred to the abdomen, and here the raised respiration rate, temperature, and free movement of the abdomen on respiration may serve to distinguish a lesion above the diaphragm before signs of consolidation in the lung are demonstrable.

The age of the patient will often be extremely helpful in reaching a diagnosis. Thus evidence of obstruction occurring within the newborn period will almost invariably be due to a congenital abnormality; during the first year of life, colic, pyelonephritis and intussusception are the most important causes of severe abdominal pain; while after the age of 2 years, appendicitis becomes increasingly frequent. It must also be remembered that accidental injuries, particularly falls, are common during early childhood and that the rupture of a viscus, e.g. the spleen, may result. In such cases the pain is likely to be accompanied by severe shock, pallor, and evidence of blood in the abdomen, but these signs are sometimes surprisingly slight.

Recurrent abdominal pain

The consequences of misdiagnosing abdominal pain due to a serious organic disease are so grave that first consideration must be given to the possibility of such a cause. It should be realized, however, that in the majority of cases of recurrent abdominal pain in childhood, no physical disease is present and the pain is a manifestation of emotional stress. Many perfectly healthy children complain of abdominal pain in the morning before some unpleasant experience, especially if they have been anxiously anticipating it for several days. Similarly, the excitement of going to a party, perhaps tinged with vague apprehension, will often induce an attack. Such symptoms, though caused by emotional tension, are very real and must not be considered as deliberately contrived by the child. Judgement and experience are required in deciding how far to carry investigation of such children, balancing the risk of overlooking an organic cause against possible psychological trauma and the undesirability of emphasizing the symptom unduly. If investigation is undertaken, it will generally include urinary examination, intravenous pyelography, a tuberculin test and blood count, barium studies of the gastro-intestinal tract and possibly electroencephalography. The stools should be examined for bacteria, ova and parasites. Other special investigations may be indicated by the history.

If no organic cause of the symptoms is found, the parents and the child must be strongly reassured that there is no disease requiring treatment and time must be spent in explaining the nature of recurrent abdominal pains in childhood. The parents should be advised to handle the child sympathetically but firmly, for it is important not to allow the symptom to dominate the child's life or to be used as an excuse for evading potentially stressful situations.

Colic

Apart from abdominal pain having a clearly defined cause such as intussusception or renal stone, the term 'colic' is used to describe the type of abdominal pain thought to be related to irregular contraction of the intestine. In the young infant, it is frequently due to air-swallowing and occurs about 20 minutes after a feed. These cases are relieved by the eructation of wind. Some otherwise healthy infants, however, appear to suffer from more or less regular attacks of colic, usually occurring in the evening and during the first three months of life, when there is no evidence of excessive air-swallowing and no cause can be found. This recurrent colic, which results in prolonged bouts of screaming, is extremely distressing to the infant and his parents. A double-blind trial of dicyclomine hydrochloride, 5 mg before the 6 p.m. feed, showed that this drug was effective in relieving the symptoms (Illingworth, 1959).

In the child, colic may be precipitated by dietetic indiscretion, e.g. a surfeit of raw apples, or by the abuse of purgatives. The pain, though often sufficient to cause crying and drawing-up of the legs, is unassociated with acute tenderness or rigidity of the abdomen. Borborygmi may be heard, or gurgling of the caecum elicited on palpation. The pain is frequently followed and relieved by diarrhoea. If appendicitis and obstruction can be excluded with confidence, and the colic is clearly dietetic in origin, a laxative may be given; but in cases in which there is any doubt as to the diagnosis, it is preferable that the bowels should be opened by the use of an enema.

OBSTRUCTION

The passage of intestinal contents will be interfered with by mechanical factors, or by nervous and vascular disturbances which result in failure of peristalsis, e.g. paralytic ileus. *Strangulation* of the intestine, in which the vascular supply is cut off and necrosis rapidly follows, is the most dangerous complication or association of obstruction.

Blockage of the lumen of the bowel may arise from the presence of a foreign body or impacted faeces within the lumen; from thickening or scarring of the bowel wall due to tuberculosis or chronic regional ileitis; from congenital atresia or stenosis; from invagination of one portion of the bowel within another (intussusception); from rotation of a loop of bowel upon itself (volvulus) or nipping of a portion of bowel within a hernial orifice; from the presence of bands or adhesions, of congenital origin or resulting from infection; from kinking of the bowel over some abnormal structure such as a Meckel's diverticulum; and from external pressure by neoplasms or cysts.

Obstruction may be acute or chronic, and either partial or complete, but in every case constitutes a serious risk to life. The prospect of survival depends very largely on early recognition and prompt relief.

CLINICAL FEATURES. The cardinal signs and symptoms of obstruction are severe abdominal pain; vomiting, which may become faecal if unrelieved; abdominal distension and later ladder-patterning; and constipation after the bowel below the obstruction has been emptied. In some types of obstruction, e.g. intussusception, a mass may be felt. In acute cases a rising pulse-rate is commonly observed. The facies is often characteristic, appearing pale, toxic, and anxious. Prolonged vomiting will cause dehydration and ketosis, and alkalosis may result from high obstruction. When strangulation has occurred, there is profound shock, and blood may be passed per rectum; peritonitis complicating strangulation is indicated by abdominal rigidity and increased toxicity. Strangulation occurs most rapidly in volvulus and strangulated hernia (which is uncommon in childhood), and over a period of one to three days in cases of intussusception.

DIAGNOSIS. The clinical picture is sufficiently characteristic in acute cases to indicate that obstruction is present, though not necessarily to establish the cause. Straight X-rays, taken in several positions, will often confirm the diagnosis or establish the site of obstruction, the bowel above the obstruction containing air and that below being collapsed. Contrast media, with the possible exception of gastrografin in the newborn period, should not be used in acute cases, though a barium follow-through may be necessary in chronic or incomplete obstruction.

Occasionally cerebral tumour or diabetes mellitus may have to be excluded in differential diagnosis. In cyclical vomiting the retching and vomiting precede the abdominal pain, for which they are responsible, and the pain is seldom severe.

TREATMENT. If hernia has been excluded, a laparotomy and relief of the obstruction will be required. While pre-operative treatment with intravenous fluids or blood transfusion is advisable, and should always include the passage of a stomach tube, operation should be delayed as little as possible in the acute case, since the ease with which acute obstruction can be relieved will depend very largely on how long it has been present. The necessity for resecting strangulated bowel which is no longer viable adds very greatly to the operative risk. Post-operative treatment will include gastric suction if vomiting persists, and the administration of intravenous fluids.

Congenital abnormalities causing obstruction

These include intestinal atresia and stenosis, malrotation of the bowel, Meckel's diverticulum,

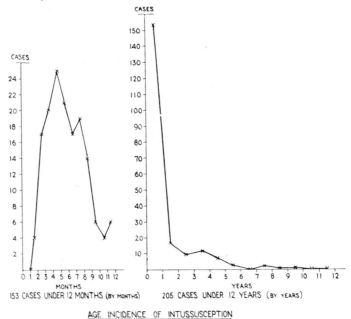

AGE INCIDENCE OF INTUSSUSCEPTION

Fig. 6.23   Age incidence of 205 cases of intussusception admitted to the Royal Hospital for Sick Children, Edinburgh.

imperforate anus, and hernia, either external or internal. Pyloric stenosis, though a type of partial obstruction, presents a somewhat different picture from that described above. Volvulus may be either congenital or acquired, causing acute or recurrent obstruction at any period of childhood. It very rarely affects any part of the bowel other than the small intestine. Acquired cases are those in which an adhesion or band has caused a loop of bowel to become fixed at one point, when it is liable to rotate and become strangulated.

Intussusception

The invagination of one portion of intestine into that immediately distal to it occurs most frequently in the region of the ileo-caecal valve. Here the ileum may either be invaginated through the valve into the caecum and thence into the colon (ileo-colic type), or the valve itself may form the apex of the intussusceptum (ileo-caecal type). An ileal intussusception, in which ileum is invaginated into ileum, and a colic intussusception, in which the colon only is affected, are much less common. In the great majority of cases the intussusception passes in the same direction as the intestinal contents, but occasionally an intussusception occurs in the reverse direction. More than one intussusception may occur at the same time.

ETIOLOGY. The etiology of intussusception is usually obscure, though in some cases the presence of a polyp, Meckel's diverticulum, or enlarged lymph node in the invaginated portion suggests that this may have initiated the process. It is probably significant that the great majority of cases occur at about the time that soft solids are being introduced into the diet. Thus the condition is typically seen during the first year of life, and most commonly during the fourth to seventh month (Fig. 6.23). The infants have usually been in good health previously, and are of good nutrition. Preceding constipation is more common than diarrhoea. Males are affected twice as frequently as females.

CLINICAL FEATURES. The history is usually so typical that it immediately suggests the diagnosis. An infant who has previously been well, suddenly screams with pain, draws up his legs and turns ashen white. The attack lasts for a matter of seconds, and is followed by remission of pain and return of colour. Further attacks occur, often at about 20 minute intervals. As these become more severe, each one is accompanied by evidence of shock which may be so severe as to cause transient fainting (an extremely rare phenomenon in infancy). In the early stages, however, the infant quickly appears normal again after the attack has passed. Vomiting usually occurs early, and the infant becomes rapidly dehydrated.

One or more normal stools may be passed after the onset of pain, representing the faecal matter already in the lower bowel below the intussusception. Subsequently, a small amount of blood or blood-stained serum and mucus, with little or no faecal matter, is passed. This is an important diagnostic sign, though it should be possible to make the diagnosis before blood appears either on the napkin or on the finger during rectal examination.

On examination of the abdomen there is often no rigidity or tenderness between the spasms of pain if the infant is seen early, and it is then usually possible to feel a mass, which may harden and soften during palpation. Its position will depend on the site of the intussusception, but when the latter is ileo-caecal the mass will usually lie in the right upper quadrant, sometimes concealed under the edge of the liver. In such cases the right iliac fossa may feel abnormally empty, but this sign is unreliable. Where no mass is felt, the examination should be repeated under an anaesthetic, with preparations made to proceed to immediate operation. Rectal examination should always be carried out, and though the head of the intussusception is only likely to be felt when it is nearing the anus, the examination will often confirm the presence of blood in the lower bowel.

DIAGNOSIS. It is of the utmost importance to make the diagnosis within 24 hours of the onset of symptoms, since the prospects of successful operation during this time are extremely good. The longer operation is delayed, the greater is the likelihood of strangulation and the mortality in cases of more than two days duration rises very rapidly. In doubtful cases a straight X-ray or barium enema will usually confirm the diagnosis.

With a typical history and age-incidence there should be little doubt as to the diagnosis, but occasionally anaphylactoid purpura or dysentery, both of which give rise to blood in the stools, may simulate intussusception. In dysentery the temperature is high and a rectal swab will show the presence of dysentery organisms. Anaphylactoid purpura usually occurs in older children and shows the typical distribution of purpuric lesions, sometimes with painful joints. In neither case will there be evidence of a mass or of obstruction, but very occasionally anaphylactoid purpura may be complicated by intussusception.

TREATMENT. Preparation for operative reduction of the intussusception should be made in all cases, including the pre-operative passage of a stomach tube and administration of intravenous fluids as required. Although in a proportion of selected cases (babies over 6 months of age seen within 24 hours of onset) it may be possible to reduce the intussusception by skilled barium enema under fluoroscopy, attempts at conservative treatment should never unduly delay laparotomy and surgical reduction when this proves necessary, or when there is any doubt as to the success of reduction by enema. Unless resection of bowel is necessary owing to the intussusception having become so adherent to the containing portion of bowel that it is irreducible, or a portion of the bowel being nonviable, simple reduction only is required. Recurrence may be expected in less than 2 per cent of cases.

CHRONIC OR RECURRENT INTUSSUSCEPTION. This type of intussusception, in which there is incomplete obstruction, is commoner in older children but may occur at any age in childhood. Pain is much less severe and characteristic, and vomiting is transient or minimal. The stools are likely to be smaller than normal, and to contain traces of blood intermittently. The child is irritable and fails to thrive. A barium enema will usually be necessary to confirm the diagnosis. Surgical reduction is required when the diagnosis is established.

Regional ileitis

In this rare condition a sharply demarcated portion of the small bowel is affected. In acute cases the bowel is distended, bright red in colour, and paralytic. There may be associated haemorrhage into the skin or elsewhere. The condition, which is transient, should be treated conservatively, using gastric suction and intravenous therapy. In chronic regional ilietis (*Crohn's disease*), which is probably of different etiology from the above, a portion of lower ileum becomes greatly thickened and the lumen reduced in size. A mass is sometimes palpable. Treatment is by resection.

Paralytic ileus

Paralysis of a portion of small bowel may occur in cases of generalized peritonitis, e.g.

following rupture of an inflamed appendix. Obstruction is due to failure of peristalsis in the affected area. In the great majority of cases it is transient, and the patient can be successfully treated with gastric suction and intravenous fluids.

Foreign bodies

It is extremely common for young children to swallow small toys and other objects. The great majority of these are passed spontaneously without ill effect, and it is quite exceptional for even sharp or pointed objects to cause perforation once they have negotiated the oesophagus. The sites at which there is a risk of hold-up are the oesophagus, pylorus, duodenum, and, less frequently, the ileo-caecal valve. Radio-opaque objects should be followed by X-ray examination, and unless they are causing symptoms, may safely be left alone for three or more weeks. If there is then no evidence of progress, operative removal may be necessary. In the case of objects which cannot be visualized radiologically, the stools should be examined daily until they are passed.

A peculiar type of foreign body, the *hair-ball* or *trichobezoar*, is occasionally encountered in children with perverted appetite who are continually pulling out and eating their hair. The stomach becomes filled with a solid mass of hair, which gives rise to indigestion, foetor of the breath, vomiting, and failure to gain weight. When the ball has reached too large a size to be vomited, operative removal may be necessary.

Impacted faeces

It should be remembered that faeces represent the commonest abdominal 'tumour' encountered in childhood, and that the masses may reach great size without apparent effect on the general health. The nature of the mass is generally obvious from palpation, when it is found that it can readily be indented. Such masses may either become tunnelled, when the passage of fluid faeces may cause the constipation to be overlooked, or cause obstruction. Removal of the faecal masses can usually be effected over a period of several days by the use of oil-retention enemata. Strong purgatives should not be used. When the faeces have been removed, it will be possible to determine whether their accumulation has been due to an organic lesion or to faulty bowel habit (see p. 83).

INFECTION
Appendicitis

Inflammation of the appendix is the commonest surgical emergency of childhood, and one which is still responsible for many preventable deaths. As in the case of intussusception, early operation carries a very low mortality, but this rises rapidly the longer treatment is delayed. The pernicious practice of giving a purgative for abdominal pain before a diagnosis has been made is undoubtedly responsible for rupture of an inflamed appendix in some cases.

ETIOLOGY. Although a number of etiological factors are recognized, it is probable that obstruction and stagnation of contents are the most important. Complications are more likely to occur in infants and young children than in adults, since the appendix is relatively thin-walled and the omentum provides less protection. The sexes are equally affected. The disease is rare during the first year, after which the incidence rapidly increases (Fig. 6.24).

PATHOLOGY. The changes, which are at first described as catarrhal, begin in the mucosa and spread outward through the wall of the appendix. They include infiltration with leucocytes, oedema, vascular engorgement, and ultimately thrombosis, ulceration, and gangrene. Serous exudate occurs around the appendix, and may become purulent. Subsequent events will depend on the success of the peritoneal defences. If the lesion becomes walled off, a localized abscess is formed, but if the infection is widely disseminated, general peritonitis occurs, which may in turn be followed by paralytic ileus.

CLINICAL FEATURES. The presenting symptoms are abdominal pain, beginning centrally and later referred to the right iliac fossa but sometimes poorly localized; vomiting; and low-grade pyrexia, which is seldom above 38·5°C (101·3°F) unless peritonitis has occurred. Constipation is an unreliable symptom since bowel action may be normal, or diarrhoea occasionally occur.

The great majority of cases seen in childhood have an acute onset, and though repeated attacks may occur in a child if the condition remains untreated, a 'grumbling' appendix seldom if ever occurs.

Examination of the child will sometimes show that he is apprehensive and in pain, though disturbance may be minimal if the appendix is pelvic or retrocaecal. If the child is lying with the

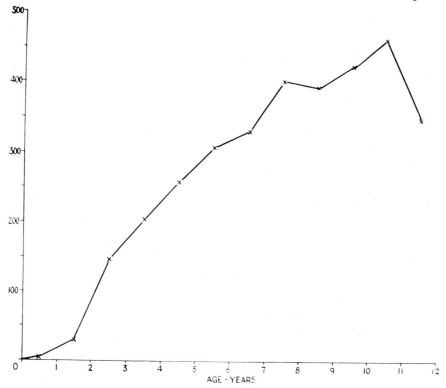

Fig. 6.24   Age incidence of 3308 cases of appendicitis under 12 years. (Royal Hospital for Sick Children, Edinburgh, 1900–48.)

right thigh flexed, it is suggestive that pain is relieved in this position by relaxation of the psoas. The respiration and pulse-rate and movement of the abdomen (which will be restricted on respiration) should be noted. The pulse-rate is likely to be raised to a greater extent than the respiration-rate, and the rise tends to continue as the disease progresses. If vomiting has continued for more than twelve hours, the tongue is likely to be furred, the breath offensive or smelling of acetone, and evidence of dehydration and toxicity beginning to appear.

Very light palpation of the abdomen is quite adequate to demonstrate local rigidity and tenderness, usually in the right iliac fossa. In retrocaecal appendix, tenderness may be in the right loin. In the case of a pelvic appendix, tenderness may only be demonstrated by rectal examination, which should be left until the end of the abdominal examination. A localized abscess may be detected on palpation of the abdomen, or by bimanual examination.

Urinary examination may show a few pus cells

if an inflamed appendix is lying adjacent to the ureter but pus in large amount indicates that the pain is renal in origin.

The leucocyte count may be raised, but a normal count does not exclude the diagnosis. Higher counts occur if rupture of the appendix has resulted in peritonitis.

DIFFERENTIAL DIAGNOSIS. Pneumonia and urinary infection must be excluded. In young children, acute abdominal pain may be due to tonsillitis; the diagnosis of non-specific mesenteric lymphadenitis is considered below. Infectious hepatitis in the pre-icteric phase may also enter the differential diagnosis of appendicitis, but here such abdominal tenderness as may be present will be in the upper abdomen rather than the right lower quadrant.

Peritonitis

Infection of the peritoneum may be: (1) *acute primary peritonitis*—pneumococcal, streptococcal, staphylococcal, gonococcal; (2) *acute secondary peritonitis*—due to rupture of an inflamed appendix, Meckel's diverticulum, or ulcerated colon, the peritoneal fluid showing *E. coli* and other faecal organisms on culture; (3) *tuberculous* (see p. 336); (4) *chronic non-tuberculous*.

Acute peritonitis

Peritonitis is most commonly secondary to a ruptured appendix. The relative incidence of pneumococcal and streptococcal peritonitis, both of which are rare, is evidently different in different clinics. Pneumococcal peritonitis is more likely to occur in ill-nourished patients in late infancy or early childhood coming from poor homes. Most series of cases of pneumococcal peritonitis show a higher incidence in girls. There is still considerable difference of opinion as to whether the infection is haematogenous in these cases, or whether the portal of entry of the pneumococcus is by way of the female genital tract. Probably both modes of origin are possible. Pneumococcal peritonitis is an occasional complication of the nephrotic syndrome with ascites. The onset of secondary peritonitis will be preceded by a history usually indicating acute appendicitis, or more rarely chronic ulcerative colitis or ulceration of a Meckel's diverticulum. Primary cases have a more fulminating onset which may be preceded by a respiratory infection. There is generalized abdominal pain, fever, and vomiting; diarrhoea, at least at onset, is more common than constipation and there is a danger of fatal delay in treatment if a wrong diagnosis of acute infantile gastro-enteritis is made.

On examination, the child appears acutely ill, with high fever, rapid pulse, prostration, and toxaemia. The abdomen typically shows generalized tenderness and rigidity with some distension, though in some cases (particularly in young infants) rigidity may not be present, and free fluid may be detectable. The leucocyte count is likely to be over 20,000 per mm³.

TREATMENT. In cases of general peritonitis secondary to appendicitis, the abdomen should be opened and drained, the appendix being removed either at the time of the original operation or subsequently.

In acute primary peritonitis, it is usually possible to identify the causative organism by blood culture or by examination of peritoneal fluid, and its sensitivity will determine the choice of antibiotic. Supportive treatment (gastric suc-

tion, intravenous fluids, and oxygen) should be given as necessary.

PROGNOSIS. Though acute primary peritonitis remains a serious risk, the mortality has improved remarkably of recent years, and in some clinics has fallen from over 60 per cent to under 20 per cent for all cases. The prognosis is somewhat less favourable in streptococcal than in pneumococcal primary peritonitis.

Chronic non-tuberculous peritonitis. This is rare at all ages, except as a residuum of acute peritonitis. A condition known as polyserositis is occasionally seen, in which chronic inflammatory changes of unknown etiology occur in the peritoneum and pericardium. It may be indistinguishable from chronic constrictive pericarditis associated with a peculiar thickening resembling 'sugar-icing' over the abdominal viscera (Pick's syndrome).

Mesenteric lymphadenitis

The association of an upper respiratory infection with acute abdominal pain due to *mesenteric lymphadenitis* is a not uncommon syndrome which enters into the differential diagnosis of acute appendicitis. The infecting organism in the upper respiratory tract is commonly a haemolytic streptococcus. The temperature may be raised, vomiting is slight or absent, and tenderness is usually more diffuse than in appendicitis. In doubtful cases the pulse-rate should be taken half-hourly and the abdomen re-examined, when it will be found that the condition does not progress in the manner to be expected in appendicitis. The condition is likely to subside without requiring surgical treatment, but if the diagnosis is in doubt it is safer to carry out a laparotomy.

Iliac adenitis

Most commonly this arises from an infection in the groin, perineum, lower limb, or region of the hip. The primary lesion will usually indicate the diagnosis, which may be confirmed by enlargement of the inguinal nodes. In approximately half the cases the nodes subside spontaneously; when suppuration occurs it will require retroperitoneal drainage.

Pancreatitis

This is rare in childhood, and acute suppurative or haemorrhagic pancreatitis very seldom constitutes a surgical emergency. Upper abdominal pain due to non-suppurative pancreatitis may, however, occur as a complication of mumps, and be associated with vomiting, fatty stools, and tenderness of the upper abdomen. The condition almost always subsides spontaneously without treatment.

Chronic ulcerative colitis

Ulceration of the large bowel, giving rise to blood and mucus in the stools, and not due to infection by dysentery bacilli or amoebae, occasionally occurs in older children, and is responsible for a variable degree of abdominal pain. It commonly starts with an acute febrile attack of enteritis, which is followed by tenesmus and the passage of small, frequent stools, which are semi-formed or liquid and contain small amounts of blood. The persistent loss of blood leads to severe secondary anaemia. Diagnosis will be confirmed by sigmoidoscopy. Barium enema should only be given with caution, and may show loss of haustration. The sudden occurrence of severe abdominal pain, tenderness and rigidity, should suggest perforation which is likely to result in generalized peritonitis.

The treatment of chronic ulcerative colitis is unsatisfactory. Rest and a low-roughage diet are essential. Antibiotic therapy should be tried, but is seldom very effective when the causative organism is unknown. Steroids, systemically or in enemata, may provide temporary relief but are not curative. Sulphasalazine may sometimes be of value. Blood transfusion is likely to be required for anaemia. Surgical treatment, in long-standing cases which have failed to respond to medical treatment, usually consists of ileostomy, but colectomy has been carried out when all other treatment has failed. Since there is commonly emotional disturbance in addition to the physical symptoms, psychotherapy may be indicated.

OTHER CAUSES OF ABDOMINAL PAIN

Many other conditions may cause abdominal pain of greater or less severity, including diseases of the liver and spleen, perinephric abscess, renal disorders, and neoplasms. As a general rule, neoplasms seldom cause severe pain at least until the disease is far advanced. Splenomegaly is also usually painless, and perisplenitis considerably less common than in adult life; a very large spleen, however, may cause dragging pain and abdominal discomfort, while in the case of splenic infarction the pain is more acute.

Cholecystitis and *cholelithiasis* are both very rare causes of abdominal pain in childhood, at least in temperate climates. In most patients in whom gall-stones have been found, e.g. in cases of familial acholuric jaundice, they have been symptomless.

Torsion of a cyst (arising from the mesentery or ovary), accessory lobe of the liver, or other congenitally abnormal structure, occasionally gives rise to acute abdominal pain and tenderness, requiring laparotomy.

Puberty

The onset of puberty in girls will not uncommonly cause rather vague abdominal pain preceding the first menstruation; the presence of early breast-development will usually indicate the diagnosis, and the subsequent establishment of menstruation confirm it. It must be remembered that menstruation sometimes occurs at 9 or 10 years of age or even earlier. When there is vaginal atresia or an imperforate hymen, the first symptoms may occur at the onset of menstruation. *Haematocolpos*, i.e. the retention of menstrual fluid, will result from such obstruction and will require surgical relief.

In boys, the onset of puberty may cause the rapid enlargement of an ectopic testis which sometimes becomes acutely painful if it is nipped in the inguinal canal or subject to trauma elsewhere. Although pain may be referred to the abdomen, examination should make clear the real cause.

Peptic ulcer

Although a less frequent cause of abdominal pain in childhood than in adult life, peptic ulcers are more common than is generally recognized and occur even in infancy, when they may result in haematemesis. Most infantile ulcers are associated with severe systemic disease or are discovered at necropsy in infants dying from other causes. In later childhood, peptic ulcers of either stomach or duodenum give rise to a clinical picture similar to, but less definite than, that in adult life, and require similar treatment. Special diets are unnecessary and the child should be encouraged to drink milk and take frequent normal meals. Transfusion may be necessary for haemorrhage. The association of hunger pain relieved by food, nocturnal pain referred to the upper abdomen, haematemesis, or melaena should suggest the possibility of peptic ulcer, and the need for radiological investigation.

Ectopic gastric mucosa in a Meckel's diverticulum is a possible site of peptic ulceration. The pain is commonly referred to the umbilical region, and the diagnosis may be suspected when melaena or massive haemorrhage occurs. Perforation occasionally occurs in these cases. It is rarely possible to confirm the presence of a Meckel's diverticulum by radiography, and if the diagnosis is suspected, laparotomy should be performed and the diverticulum removed surgically.

BIBLIOGRAPHY AND REFERENCES

ACHAR, S. T. (1955). Childhood hepatic cirrhosis in India. *Indian Journal of Child Health*, 3, 291.

ANDERSON, C. M. (1966). Intestinal malabsorption in childhood. *Archives of Disease in Childhood*, 41, 571.

ANDERSON, C. M., GRACEY, M. & BURKE, V. (1972). Coeliac disease. *Archives of Disease in Childhood*, 47, 292.

APLEY, J. (1959). *The Child with Abdominal Pains*. Oxford: Blackwell.

BLATTNER, R. J. (1969). Acute mesenteric lymphadenitis. *Journal of Pediatrics*, 74, 479.

BROWN, J. J. M. (1962). *Surgery of Childhood*. London: Arnold.

CULLITY, G. J. & KAKULAS, B. A. (1970). Encephalopathy and fatty degeneration of the viscera. *Brain*, 93, 77.

DARROW, D. C. (1946). The retention of electrolyte during recovery from severe dehydration due to diarrhoea. *Journal of Pediatrics*, 28, 515.

DAVIDSON, Sir S., PASSMORE, R. & BROCK, J. F. (1972). *Human Nutrition and Dietetics*, 5th edn. Edinburgh: Livingstone.

DEAN, R. F. A. (1965). Kwashiorkor. In *Recent Advances in Paediatrics*, 3rd edn. Edited by D. Gairdner. London: Churchill.

GOPALAN, C. (1967). Malnutrition in childhood in the tropics. *British Medical Journal*, iv, 603.

HOLZEL, A. (1970). Prevention and treatment of gastro-enteritis in infancy. *Practitioner*, 204, 46.

ILLINGWORTH, R. S. (1959). Evening colic in infants. *Lancet*, ii, 1119.

JELLIFFE, D. B. (1968). *Child Health in the Tropics*, 3rd edn. London: Arnold.

LANCET (1970). Classification of infantile malnutrition. *Lancet*, ii, 302.

MACAULAY, D. & MOORE, T. (1955). Subacute and chronic intussusception in infants and children. *Archives of Disease in Childhood*, 30, 180.

MACKEITH, R. & WOOD, C. (1970). *Infant Feeding and Feeding Difficulties*, 4th edn. London: Churchill.

MCNICHOLL, B. (1970). Childhood coeliac disease. *Journal of the Irish Medical Association*, 63, 1.

MITCHELL, R. G. (1967). Modern views on rickets and hypercalcaemia in infancy. *World Review of Nutrition and Dietetics*, 8, 207.

SCRIVER, C. R. (1970). Vitamin B_{12} dependency. *Pediatrics, Springfield*, 46, 493.

SHERLOCK, S. (1968). *Diseases of the Liver and Biliary System*, 4th edn. Oxford: Blackwell.

SHINER, M. (1957). Duodenal and jejunal biopsies. *Gastroenterology*, 33, 64.

SPENCE, J. C. (1931). Nutritional xerophthalmia and night-blindness. *Archives of Disease in Childhood*, 6, 17.

TAYLOR, J. (1970). Infectious infantile enteritis. *Proceedings of the Royal Society of Medicine*, 63, 1297.

TURNER, G. C. (1971). Infectious and serum hepatitis. *British Journal of Hospital Medicine*, 5, 296.

WEIJERS, H. A., VAN DE KAMER, J. H. & DICKIE, W. K. (1957). Celiac disease. In *Advances in Pediatrics*, vol. 9. London: Year Book Publishers.

ZACHARY, R. B. (1955). Acute intussusception in childhood. *Archives of Disease in Childhood*, 30, 32.

ZACHARY, R. B. (1965). Diagnosis of the acute abdomen in childhood. *British Medical Journal*, i, 635.

7 Disorders of Metabolism and Storage

The metabolic processes of infants and young children are more labile than in later life, due to the relatively larger content of body water, the more variable appetite and activity and the immaturity of compensatory mechanisms. Genetically determined metabolic defects usually come to notice in infancy or early childhood and are thus of greater importance in paediatrics than in adult medicine. Moreover, it is at this time that action can most easily be taken to correct metabolic disorders or to establish regimens which will lessen the disability caused by disorders of metabolism or storage in later life.

DISORDERS OF FLUID AND ELECTROLYTE METABOLISM

SALT AND WATER METABOLISM

The infant's body contains proportionately more water than the child's, the extracellular fluid compartment is relatively larger, and the daily intake and output of fluid are greater in comparison to the total body content. Infants therefore become dehydrated rapidly if water is withheld or if there is excessive loss from the body, as in vomiting, diarrhoea, excessive sweating or polyuria. In hypotonic and isotonic dehydration, the skin loses its turgor, so that if pinched up it remains elevated, subsiding slowly instead of returning immediately to its previous state. The fontanelle becomes depressed and the urine output progressively diminishes. The eyes lose their lustre, sinking back into the orbits. As dehydration increases, the infant becomes apathetic, with cold, grey, inelastic skin. If the loss of water is disproportionately greater than the loss of electrolyte, hypertonic dehydration ensues. Thirst is then intense, the infant is restless and fevered, and the skin feels thick and rubbery, so that the inexperienced examiner may not realize that the infant is dehydrated. The hyperosmolality of body fluids may affect the brain, causing convulsions and haemorrhages which can result in permanent cerebral damage. A similar sequence of events occurs when excess solutes are given to a healthy infant, e.g. dried milk feeds at more than full strength or accidental addition of salt instead of sugar to a feed. In such circumstances hypernatraemia develops and cerebral signs are likely to appear at levels of serum sodium exceeding 160 mEq per litre.

ACID/BASE REGULATION

The pH of plasma can be determined by direct measurement and is normally 7·30 to 7·45. A lower pH implies increased hydrogen ion concentration and is called acidaemia. Similarly decrease in hydrogen ion concentration, i.e. an elevated pH, is alkalaemia. A deviation in pH may be partly or wholly corrected by the buffering effect of bicarbonate, haemoglobin and other buffers in the plasma, by the action of the kidneys in altering the concentration of buffers, and by pulmonary regulation of the carbon dioxide tension in the blood. Diminution in the total concentration of buffer base in the plasma is called acidosis, while increase is alkalosis. The plasma standard bicarbonate, normally 21 to 25 mEq per litre, gives an indirect indication of the buffering capacity of the blood but is not completely reliable as an index of acidosis or alkalosis, since the total concentration of buffers may be unchanged when the bicarbonate is lowered, due to an increase of other buffers.

Disorders in which acid metabolites are produced, such as diabetes, starvation, severe infection and conditions resulting in loss of alkali, e.g. diarrhoea, tend to produce acidosis, since the buffer base is diminished by combination with the acid. Whether acidaemia develops or not depends on whether pH can be maintained within normal limits by renal and other mechanisms, which counter the fall in buffer, and by increased breathing, which removes carbon dioxide. Similarly, alkalosis may be produced by excessive vomiting or by ingestion of alkali and whether alkalaemia develops or not depends on the efficiency of bicarbonate excretion by the kidneys and carbon dioxide retention by the lung.

Hyperventilation due to emotional disturbance or primary respiratory disorders causes alkalaemia directly by removing carbon dioxide. Reduction in plasma bicarbonate by renal action follows and would create acidosis were it not that increase in other buffer bases tends to maintain the total concentration, so that neither acidosis nor alkalosis develops. Only when compensation fails does the total buffer base decrease, i.e. acidosis appears. It is obviously wrong to call this state 'respiratory alkalosis', as has been the custom in the past, since in fact it is alkalaemia with acidosis. By the same token, hypoventilation may lead to acidaemia with alkalosis.

In respiratory distress syndrome of the newborn infant, however, the acidaemia caused by retention of carbon dioxide is largely uncompensated by alkalosis because the immature kidneys are unable to increase the concentration of buffer base sufficiently. Indeed, the associated hypoxaemia leads to overproduction of organic acids with resultant acidosis and intensification of the acidaemia, the pH falling to 7·0 or less.

In salicylate poisoning, the initial overbreathing causes alkalaemia but the later metabolic disturbance produces such excessive quantities of acid that the reaction swings over to acidaemia with acidosis (see p. 21).

Ketosis

The ketone bodies (acetone, diacetic acid and β-hydroxybutyric acid) are intermediary products in the metabolism of fat and their accumulation in the body (ketosis) implies that the liver is unable to metabolize fat completely. This may occur either when the amount of fat ingested is excessive and the carbohydrate minimal (ketogenic diet) or when liver function is deranged as in starvation or diabetes. Children develop ketosis much more readily than do adults and ketone bodies can frequently be detected in the urine during acute infections, gastro-intestinal disturbances and metabolic disorders. Acetone can also be smelt on the breath though observers vary widely in their ability to detect the odour. The appearance of ketonuria or the smell of acetone on the breath may thus be early signs of disturbed metabolism and indicate the possibility that infection or some other disease is present.

FLUID AND ELECTROLYTE THERAPY

Replacement therapy aims at restoring lost water and electrolyte and acid/base equilibrium, while maintenance therapy supplies the daily requirements normally taken in the diet.

Initial assessment of the severity of dehydration is made on clinical grounds from the history and physical examination. Acid/base status and the levels of urea and electrolytes in venous or capillary blood should be determined by laboratory methods but haemo-concentration may result in deceptively high plasma electrolyte levels, which do not reflect total body losses and are therefore of limited value in calculating needs at this stage. Only after the infant has been re-hydrated can their significance be assessed and the loss of electrolyte estimated.

Mild degrees of dehydration may be corrected by administration of fluids orally, if the infant can retain them, or subcutaneously with hyaluronidase but moderate or severe degrees necessitate intravenous infusion, given by needle into a scalp vein or by cannula inserted into a limb vein (see p. 404). Fluid is run in quickly at first and then at a slower rate, with the general aim of restoring the fluid lost (about 5 to 20 per cent of body weight depending on severity) within the first 8 to 24 hours. Replacement may be achieved more quickly than this if necessary, but care should be taken since too rapid replacement may overwhelm the infant's homeostatic mechanisms, with consequent overexpansion of the extra-cellular fluid compartment.

The nature of the fluid infused will depend on the clinical state but is essentially a solution of sodium chloride in water. In young infants, the electrolyte content should be at less than physiological levels, in order to supply surplus water, the solution being made isotonic with glucose. Half-normal saline with glucose is commonly used (i.e. sodium chloride 0.45 per cent, glucose 4.3 per cent): some prefer to give a calculated amount of normal saline initially, but this carries the risk of producing hyperelectrolytaemia if dehydration is severe. If hypertonic dehydration is suspected clinically or has been diagnosed by finding hypernatraemia as well (plasma sodium over 150 mEq per litre), the repair fluid should not contain more than 50 mEq sodium per litre and the calculated fluid loss should be replaced slowly over 24 hours.

When there is proven acidaemia with acidosis, sodium bicarbonate or lactate may be added to the repair fluid. The plasma bicarbonate level will be raised approximately 1 mEq per litre by 0.5 ml of a molar (8.4 per cent) solution of sodium bicarbonate or 4 ml of a sixth-molar solution of sodium lactate per kg body weight. The alkalinizing effect of lactate depends on its oxidation with subsequent formation of bicarbonate, so that bicarbonate itself seems the therapeutic agent of choice. Indeed, lactate is theoretically contraindicated in severe illness, when hypoxia may impair oxidation and lead to lactic acidosis.

However, in practice lactate therapy is usually effective, possibly by restoring peripheral circulation and so increasing tissue oxygenation.

A standard repair solution containing sodium chloride, lactate and glucose, such as Ringer-lactate solution, is sometimes used, especially in emergency or while awaiting the results of bio-chemical tests.

When dehydration has been largely corrected, maintenance therapy is instituted, a suitable fluid being fifth-normal saline with glucose. The amount will vary from 150 ml per kg body weight per day for an infant under 1 year of age, to 70 ml per kg per day for a child over 7 years. At this stage it is important to give potassium chloride by mouth or intravenously to restore intracellular potassium. If this is not done, an infant who is apparently recovering may become weak and listless instead of regaining strength and vitality and may die from potassium depletion. Low plasma proteins are an indication for infusion of half-strength plasma, while low levels of haemoglobin may be corrected by blood transfusion.

As an example, an infant with moderately severe dehydration due to acute gastro-enteritis, whose expected body weight is 8 kg, requires about 800 ml of fluid (i.e. 10 per cent of his weight) in the first 8 to 12 hours to restore lost fluid. This is given as half-strength saline with glucose, with bicarbonate added as necessary, or as Ringer-lactate solution, since it may generally be assumed that diarrhoea is accompanied by acidaemia. In the next 12 hours, fifth-normal saline with glucose and 30 mEq per litre of added potassium is given as maintenance therapy, the quantity based on a daily requirement of 1200 ml (i.e. 150 ml per kg). This is continued during the following day and, if recovery is rapid, oral feeding may be started towards the end of the period, allowing the intravenous infusion to be slowed and finally stopped after 48 to 72 hours.

When there has been a prolonged period of preceding dehydration, so that fluid and electrolyte regulation is grossly disturbed, or when the condition which caused the dehydration persists, continuing intravenous therapy may be indicated. In that case requirements must be determined more precisely, based on estimated loss and on frequent measurement of plasma electrolytes, acid/base status, and plasma proteins, and calculated in terms of quantities per unit of surface area. Requirements of calcium, magnesium, and vitamins must also be considered. When prolonged intravenous therapy is necessary, the caloric intake may be increased by the infusion of fat emulsions, amino acids, sorbitol or fructose.

Newborn infants, especially those of very low birth-weight, pose special problems of intravenous therapy because of their small size and the immaturity of their homeostatic mechanisms. There is a real risk of overhydration unless the quantity of fluid administered is very carefully controlled.

DIABETES MELLITUS

While this metabolic disorder is characterized by a failure of utilization of carbohydrate and incomplete combustion of fat, and is corrected by the administration of insulin, the etiology is poorly understood. Statural overgrowth precedes the onset of symptoms in some cases, suggesting the importance of the diabetogenic action of pituitary growth hormone. It is not yet clear whether insulin antagonists are important in childhood diabetes. Infection frequently precedes the onset of symptoms, but it is probable that it serves to precipitate these in an early diabetic state and not to cause the condition. The familial incidence of the disease is consistent with its being inherited usually as a polygenically determined predisposition with variable clinical expression.

The disease occurs in both sexes, with little sex discrimination. It is rare during the first two years of life, but after that age the incidence rises. Very rarely, transient diabetes occurs in the newborn infant.

PATHOLOGY. The changes found in the pancreas at necropsy are frequently slight, and may not suggest that the islets of Langerhans are primarily at fault. In about half the childhood cases, however, the islets are reduced in number and show hydropic degeneration or atrophy. In cases which have been inadequately stabilized, the liver may be enlarged and show fatty infiltration, and evidence of malnutrition is present. Degenerative changes may be found when the diabetes is of long standing.

BIOCHEMICAL FINDINGS. Carbohydrate is absorbed into the blood-stream of the diabetic child but cannot be stored as glycogen or utilized normally in the tissues. This results in a high fasting blood-sugar level in established cases, and

a characteristic glucose-tolerance curve, viz. after a loading dose of glucose is given (e.g. 1·5 g per kg body weight), the blood sugar rises to hyperglycaemic levels over a period of one to two hours; it falls abnormally slowly to reach the previous fasting level.

The glucose-tolerance curve, or the estimation of fasting blood sugar when this is grossly raised, will usually establish the diagnosis but in very early cases, or where the glucose-tolerance curve is anomalous, there may be difficulty. It is often stated that the fasting blood sugar should be over 130 mg per 100 ml for the diagnosis to be made. This is misleading, since it will occasionally be found that the fasting blood sugar is below this level, but that the high rise and delayed fall following glucose administration indicate the diagnosis, which is subsequently confirmed with the progress of the disease. A *lag curve*, in which there is a normal fasting level, a rapid rise above the threshold, and an equally rapid fall, i.e. to fasting level within one and a half hours, is not necessarily an indication of diabetes; however, children with latent diabetes, characterized by a lag curve and transient glycosuria at times of illness or stress, may become overtly diabetic, sometimes years later.

Glycosuria

The excretion of sugar by the kidney will occur whenever the blood sugar rises above the renal threshold level (normally 180 mg per 100 ml). This level may occasionally be exceeded in a normal child by the taking of very large amounts of carbohydrate by mouth, when *alimentary*

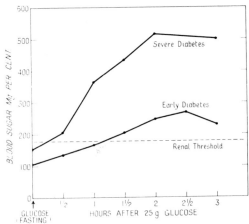

Fig. 7.1   Blood-sugar curves in two cases of childhood diabetes mellitus.

glycosuria occurs, or when carbohydrate is first given following starvation. It may be exceeded when the liver is severely damaged or its glycogen-storage mechanism interfered with from any cause. Concentrated solutions of glucose given intravenously are also likely to cause excretion of excess glucose in the urine.

The commonest cause of glycosuria of non-diabetic origin, however, is lowering of the renal threshold (*renal glycosuria*). In such cases, glucose is excreted while the blood sugar is still within the normal range and carbohydrate metabolism is unaffected. It is of no clinical significance, but is apt to cause much confusion in diagnosis unless the level of sugar excretion is checked by a glucose-tolerance test. In those rare cases of childhood diabetes in which there is also renal glycosuria, the difficulties of management are greatly increased, since glycosuria is no indication that the proper range of blood-sugar level has been exceeded.

When a reducing substance is detected in the urine of a child, it is first necessary to establish that it is in fact glucose. If glucose is present without any trace of ketone bodies, it is unlikely that the condition will prove to be diabetes (except possibly in very early infancy), but a glucose-tolerance test is indicated to establish the diagnosis. *Pentosuria*, *fructosuria*, and *galactosuria* (p. 189) are all rare congenital metabolic disorders, and are unlikely to simulate diabetes.

Keto-acidosis

The incomplete metabolism of fat with the appearance of ketone bodies in the blood and urine is an integral part of the diabetic picture and results in metabolic acidosis, which cannot be fully corrected by the kidneys (see p. 182).

Dehydration. A raised blood sugar and also ketonaemia will cause diuresis, and this in turn will result in water and electrolyte loss. An attempt is made by the body to correct this by increased fluid intake, as evidenced by the excessive thirst which is an early symptom, but, as the disease progresses, dehydration becomes increasingly pronounced.

Hyperlipidaemia

This is commonly found at the onset of childhood diabetes and predisposes to later vascular disease. The level of serum lipids is lower when control of diabetes is good and can be reduced even further by a diet rich in polyunsaturated fat (e.g. corn oil), but such a diet is not readily accepted by children.

CLINICAL FEATURES. The height and weight of diabetic children are usually average or above average at the onset of symptoms, but there is no tendency to obesity as in adult diabetes. Early symptoms are loss of weight, malaise, anorexia, thirst, and polyuria. The last of these may attract attention by causing enuresis. Excessive hunger is exceptional. Constipation is common, particularly if the symptoms are precipitated by infection. Upper abdominal pain is complained of in a small proportion of cases. The urine will contain sugar and usually ketone bodies at this stage.

The progress of the disease is in general considerably more rapid in childhood, and particularly in infancy, than in adult life, and frequently the child will have reached a stage of coma or pre-coma and severe dehydration before he comes under observation. At this stage, drowsiness, an odour of acetone in the breath, air-hunger, and wasting will be present, and the picture may be complicated by vomiting. The skin is inelastic and the intraocular tension reduced. Urine examination and a single blood-sugar examination (which is likely to show a value of over 200 mg per 100 ml) will confirm the diagnosis. Treatment should not be delayed for a complete glucose-tolerance test if the stage of coma or pre-coma has been reached.

TREATMENT. This consists of (1) immediate treatment, (2) stabilization, and (3) subsequent management. It is preferable for the first two to be undertaken in hospital if practicable, after which the subsequent management is essentially a matter for the home.

Immediate treatment. The correction of the ketosis, acidosis, and dehydration must be regarded as an emergency, whereas there is no immediate necessity to reduce the blood sugar below the renal threshold. Indeed, since the full action of insulin is delayed in the presence of severe ketosis, it is considerably safer to maintain a moderate hyperglycaemia until the acute symptoms have been relieved.

Soluble insulin should be given intramuscularly immediately the diagnosis has been made, the amount being judged by the age of the child, the severity of symptoms, and the blood-sugar level. When there is severe circulatory failure, it is necessary to give half the initial dose intravenously. In the case of infants 10 to 20 units and in older children 20 to 40 units or more will usually be suitable as an initial dose; insulin may have to be repeated two-hourly at first and subsequently four- to six-hourly until ketosis and air hunger have been relieved, the dosage depending on the blood-sugar levels. Unless the blood sugar is over 300 mg at onset, insulin should, after the first dose, be 'covered' by glucose (1 g per unit) to prevent sudden hypoglycaemia from cumulative insulin action.

If fluids cannot be retained by mouth, they must be given intravenously, using saline with lactate or bicarbonate (see p. 183). In comatose patients it is always advisable to have glucose immediately available for intravenous use to correct hypoglycaemia should it occur.

The stomach should be emptied initially by gavage: this is an essential part of emergency treatment. The patient should be carefully investigated for evidence of infection, and appropriate treatment given. All comatose patients are likely to be in a state of shock, and should be kept warm. Circulatory stimulants and oxygen may be needed. As recovery takes place, potassium will be required to restore that lost in the urine. Potassium chloride 2 g daily may be given by mouth, or a repair solution containing potassium given intravenously.

Stabilization. When the immediate symptoms and ketosis have been relieved, there is often a period during which appetite is increased; since the child will have lost weight, often very considerably, before coming under treatment, it is advisable not to limit the diet during this time, but to allow liberal carbohydrate for a week or more, giving soluble insulin three times a day in sufficient amount to bring the blood sugar within approximately normal limits, viz. 100 to 180 mg per 100 ml. The aim will then be to adjust the diet to a suitable one for maintenance, and to find the optimum insulin dosage. This can be regulated by urine testing and frequent blood-sugar estimations are not usually necessary at this stage. It will be found that even under close supervision there is great individual variation between children with diabetes of similar severity, one stabilizing readily and quickly, another showing day-to-day variations which cannot always be accounted for by infection, irregular appetite, or activity.

During the period of stabilization the child should be given his principal meals at the same time that he will get them at home, and it is most desirable that he should have exercise. Children who are stabilized in bed will very commonly develop hypoglycaemia soon after getting home, since increased exercise will tend to reduce their insulin requirements.

Insulin injections should be reduced during the period of stabilization to the minimum number that will keep the blood sugar as nearly as possible within normal limits. With the newer preparations of insulin, it is possible to combine short-acting and long-acting insulin, and to reduce injections to one before breakfast. Insulin zinc suspension (I.Z.S.), consisting of a 3/7 mixture of I.Z.S. (amorphous)/I.Z.S. (crystalline), is satisfactory for some children but more commonly a larger proportion of the shorter-acting amorphous preparation is required and the proportions should be adjusted to suit the individual child. Alternatively, a mixture of soluble and isophane insulins can be injected twice daily. Older children should be taught how to look after the syringe and needles and how to measure and inject the insulin themselves; the mothers of younger children should learn the technique during the period of stabilization. The site of injection must be constantly changed to minimize induration and 'insulin atrophy': both mother and child must be impressed with the importance of this rotation.

Oral hypoglycaemic agents have no place in the management of established childhood diabetes but chlorpropamide given daily for several years may prevent latent diabetes from becoming overt.

It is advisable for older children to be allowed at least one mild hypoglycaemic attack while in hospital so that the symptoms may immediately be recognized and combated. Parents must be warned about their possible occurrence, and the need for treatment with carbohydrate.

Maintenance and management. There is still considerable difference of opinion as to the type of diet which should be recommended for the child diabetic. Some clinicians advocate a strictly weighed and rigid regimen, while others go to the opposite extreme and claim good results on a completely 'free' diet. The first has the disadvantage that it is apt to be broken or to prove too great a burden for the average home; the second carries the risk that, although the immediate results may appear satisfactory, frequent and irregular hyperglycaemia may result in early degenerative changes.

However, with the co-operation of the mother

it is usually possible to strike a satisfactory compromise between these two extremes. The aim should be to provide a good mixed diet with ample protein, vitamins and calories, and sufficient carbohydrate to satisfy the child's appetite, i.e. to correspond with his normal intake, so that there will be less risk of the amount being exceeded, but to ensure that approximately the same amount is taken each day and at the same times of day. The intervals between taking carbohydrate during the daytime should be not more than four hours, and when active exercise is taken, a shorter interval is advisable to avoid hypoglycaemia. There is no necessity to eliminate all soluble carbohydrates (sweets, sugar, jam, etc.), but the daily amount of these should be constant. It has been found that, with the use of relatively high carbohydrate diets (e.g. 150 g daily for a child of 5 years and 200 g at 10 years), the insulin requirements are often little higher than on a low carbohydrate diet, while the prospect of the diet being adhered to is greater. It is advisable for the portions of carbohydrate to be weighed at first, so that a working knowledge of the weight of 'a slice of bread' and 'a helping' of potato can be acquired, and parents and child should learn the items of diet which are equivalent to 10 g of carbohydrate.

The child and his mother should be taught to test the urine for sugar and for ketones and to keep accurate records of the testing. While a trace of sugar in the first morning specimen may be ignored, a sudden increase of glycosuria or the presence of ketones should call for medical advice. It should also be impressed on the mother that intercurrent infection is an indication for more rather than less insulin, and that if the normal diet is refused during an infection, soluble carbohydrate must be given liberally in its place. Infection represents the main danger to the diabetic child, and even minor infections call for careful supervision. Because of the increased risk of tuberculosis, B.C.G. vaccination should be carried out in tuberculin-negative reactors.

The aims of management are to ensure normal growth and to help the child to live as normal a life as possible within the limitations imposed by diabetes. Good control is indicated by normal growth and activity, no more than occasional slight glycosuria, no ketonuria, random blood sugar always less than 150 mg per 100 ml and only slight occasional hypoglycaemic symptoms.

Insulin requirements may gradually increase during childhood; this is not necessarily a sign of increasing severity. The child should be weighed and measured regularly. In patients who are unsatisfactorily controlled, growth is likely to be retarded, and occasionally diabetic infantilism with gross hepatomegaly occurs.

Hypoglycaemia

Insulin overdosage and sometimes extreme exertion lead to a fall in blood sugar which causes headache, inco-ordination, sweating, pallor, and ultimately convulsions or coma. Symptoms are more liable to occur when the fall in blood sugar is rapid, and while levels below 60 mg per 100 ml are commonly associated with symptoms, there is no absolute 'hypoglycaemic level'. The child and his parents must be made aware of the significance of the symptoms, and that they must be promptly treated by the administration of soluble carbohydrate. It is advisable for older children who may be away from home for many hours to carry glucose sweets routinely. If a diabetic child under treatment is found in coma and there is any doubt as to whether the coma is due to hypoglycaemia or there is delay in carrying out a blood-sugar estimation, intravenous glucose should be given; sugar found in the urine does not exclude hypoglycaemia, since the urine may have been in the bladder before hypoglycaemia occurred.

Frequent attacks are an indication that the dosage of insulin should be reduced, or the intake of carbohydrate more carefully related to the time of injection. Difficulty in stabilizing a child may be due to the effect of hypoglycaemia in inducing hyperglycaemia, the resulting 'see-saw' effect causing the unwary physician to give larger and larger doses of insulin.

PROGNOSIS

With good control, there is every prospect of the diabetic child not only reaching adult life, but enjoying almost normal health and activity during childhood and adolescence. The prognosis is considerably less good for children coming from homes where they cannot receive intelligent supervision, since degenerative changes such as retinopathy and nephropathy may occur early. The overall incidence of arterial degeneration in patients surviving 20 years from the onset of the disease is high.

INBORN ERRORS OF METABOLISM

Individuals may inherit abnormalities of bio-chemical structure giving rise to deviations from normal metabolism, which may appear in more than one member of a family. In most instances there is inactivity or lack of an enzyme, the result of a change in the sequence of bases on one of its polypeptide chains, due to a mutation of the corresponding gene. The enzyme deficiency interrupts normal metabolism at the point at which the enzyme should operate. This interruption may result (1) in the accumulation of a primary material or intermediary product of metabolism in the blood or tissues; (2) in a deficiency of the normal end-product of the metabolic sequence; (3) in the abnormal production of toxic metabolites.

The number of identified inborn errors is now very large and growing as new ones are discovered, known diseases are shown to have a metabolic basis and recognized metabolic disorders are found to have more than one variant, due to slight differences in allelic genes. Some examples of inborn errors of metabolism known or thought to be due to enzyme deficiency are given in Table 7.1.

Inborn errors may be associated with failures of renal tubular reabsorption, e.g. de Toni-Fanconi syndrome; with failure of synthesis of a constituent of the blood, e.g. gamma globulin, fibrinogen, antihaemophilic globulin; or with the synthesis of an abnormal haemoglobin. In Wilson's disease there is defective synthesis of caeruloplasmin, resulting in a generalized disturbance of copper metabolism. In certain inborn errors, early diagnosis and treatment may save life, e.g. galactosaemia, or prevent disability, e.g. phenylketonuria. A few defects have been detected before birth by demonstrating that cultured fetal cells from amniotic fluid do not contain a specific enzyme, but usually diagnosis must wait until after birth, when some abnormalities can be detected by screening techniques, such as the Guthrie test for phenylketonuria. In addition, investigation for metabolic disease should be undertaken in any infant who shows developmental retardation, failure to thrive, hepatosplenomegaly, ocular opacities or abnormal neurological signs, and in all infants with a family history suggestive of metabolic disease. Appropriate tests would include examination of the urine for unusual odours, crystals or reducing substances and chromatography of blood and urine for amino acids. Further information may be obtained by oral loading tests or enzyme assays.

Treatment of certain of these inborn errors of metabolism has been attempted on one or other of the following lines.

Replacement of deficiency, e.g. familial goitrous cretinism (thyroxine); agammaglobulinaemia (gamma globulin); haemophilia (antihaemophilic globulin); afibrinogenaemia (fibrinogen); Hartnup disease (nicotinamide).

Removal or alteration of the toxic factor, e.g. Wilson's disease (penicillamine); hyperbilirubinaemia (exchange transfusion); infantile renal tubular acidosis (alkalis).

Excluding diet, e.g. phenylketonuria (low phenylalanine diet); galactosaemia (galactose-free diet); maple syrup urine disease (synthetic diet low in leucine, isoleucine, and valine); hypercalcaemia (low calcium diet).

In a considerable number of these disorders, e.g. alkaptonuria, albinism, the glycogen diseases, the haemoglobinopathies, oxalosis, sucrosuria, etc., no effective treatment is at present available.

Table 7.1 Inborn errors of metabolism due to enzyme deficiency

Character	Missing enzyme
Albinism	Tyrosinase
Alkaptonuria	Homogentisic acid oxidase
Argininosuccinic aciduria	Arginino succinase
Fructosaemia	Fructose-1-phosphate aldolase
Galactosaemia	Galactose-1-phosphate uridyl transferase
Glycogenosis	
(i) Hepatic	Glucose-6-phosphatase
(ii) Cardiac	α-1,4-Glucosidase
(iii) Limit dextrinosis	Amylo-1,6-glucosidase (debranching enzyme)
Goitrous cretinism (one form)	Dehalogenase
Haemolytic anaemia (drug-induced)	Glucose-6-phosphate dehydrogenase
Histidinaemia	Histidase
Homocystinuria	Cystathionine synthetase
Hypophosphatasia	Alkaline phosphatase
Methaemoglobinaemia (one form)	Methaemoglobin reductase
Neonatal hyperbilirubinaemia	Glucuronyl transferase
Phenylketonuria	Phenylalanine hydroxylase
Tyrosinosis	Parahydroxyphenylpyruvic acid oxidase

Phenylketonuria

This is characterized by a failure of hydroxylation of phenylalanine to tyrosine in the liver. The disease is inherited as a mendelian recessive, and occurs about once in every 10,000 to 20,000 births. Since the majority of untreated cases develop severe mental defect, whereas some at least of those diagnosed and treated in early infancy may develop normally, the condition is of great interest in providing a biochemical approach to the prevention of one type of mental retardation. The primary defect results in the excretion of phenylpyruvic acid and other metabolites in the urine, and in the accumulation of phenylalanine in the blood. Although the latter cannot be regarded as the direct cause of the mental deterioration (which is possibly related to an associated deficiency of 5-hydroxytryptamine or of glutamine) it has been found that continued treatment with a diet low in phenylalanine content may prevent or arrest mental deterioration, though it cannot reverse the brain damage when this has already occurred.

Clinically, patients appear normal at birth, though phenylketonuria may be detected within the first week of life. There is a tendency to vomit and an eczematous skin condition in infancy; mental deterioration occurs gradually during the first three years. The great majority of patients show a deficiency of pigmentation of the hair and have blue eyes. When severe mental defect has already developed, there are frequently repetitive movements of the fingers, restlessness, clumsiness of gait, and minor or major epileptic attacks.

DIAGNOSIS. Phenylketonuria is demonstrated by the addition of 10 drops of 10 per cent ferric chloride to 5 ml of acidified urine, when a deep green colour appears rapidly: hyperphenylalaninaemia confirms the diagnosis, the level rising to 30 mg per 100 ml or more in the second week of life. Tests of blood and urine suitable for mass screening of populations for phenylketonuria are now available and all newborn infants should be tested by these methods. Screening may also be carried out for other metabolic defects. Care must be taken in the diagnosis of phenylketonuria, since the majority of positive tests in screening programmes are due to transient hyperphenylalaninaemia and tyrosinaemia. A positive ferric chloride test is also found in the rare metabolic disorder, histidinaemia.

TREATMENT should be started in earliest infancy and is of little value if delayed to 2 or more years of age. The basis of the low phenyl-

alanine diet is a protein hydrolysate preparation, the phenylalanine content of the diet being adjusted to maintain the blood level at 2 to 5 mg per 100 ml.

Tyrosinosis

Tyrosinosis is a disorder of tyrosine metabolism in which deficiency of parahydroxyphenylpyruvic acid oxidase has been demonstrated. Tyrosine and its metabolites are found in the urine of patients, who show hepatosplenomegaly and refractory rickets. High blood tyrosine levels can be reduced by a tyrosine-restricted diet, which may cause clinical improvement. Tyrosinaemia with tyrosyluria and sometimes hyperphenylalaninaemia may occur as a transient symptomless disorder of immature newborn infants. The abnormalities disappear spontaneously or after the administration of ascorbic acid. The ferric chloride test is often positive.

Homocystinuria

This occurs almost as often as phenylketonuria. It is characterized by a malar flush, dislocated lens of the eye and shuffling gait. Affected children are generally but not invariably mentally subnormal. Thromboembolic phenomena may cause early death. There is homocystine in the urine, increased methionine in the blood and deficiency of cystathionine synthetase, an enzyme necessary for the breakdown of methionine to cystine. A diet low in methionine with added cystine is indicated.

Galactosaemia

In this rare disease, failure of conversion of galactose into glucose results from a deficiency of galactose-l-phosphate uridyl transferase. When milk feeding is started, accumulation of galactose-l-phosphate in the tissues results in failure to thrive, vomiting, hepatosplenomegaly, cataracts, and renal tubular damage with aminoaciduria. The urine contains galactose, which reduces Benedict's solution but does not react to tests specific for glucose. Untreated cases are likely to be mentally subnormal. Response to a galactose-free diet is good unless irreversible damage to the brain has already occurred.

Maple syrup urine disease

The characteristic odour of the urine gives the name to this condition. Vomiting, failure to thrive, and evidence of mental deterioration appear early. The metabolism of leucine, isoleucine, and valine is disordered and treatment with a diet low in these amino acids may be effective if started early.

Defects of renal tubular function

A number of syndromes have been described in which disturbance of renal tubular reabsorption is thought to occur, often associated with other metabolic defects. They may result in failure to thrive, dwarfing and sometimes rickets. The failure of reabsorption may be limited to one substance, as in renal glycosuria (glucose), nephrogenic diabetes insipidus (water) or vitamin D-resistant rickets (phosphate), or may affect several, as in the de Toni-Fanconi syndrome (amino acids, glucose, phosphate). Aminoaciduria, glycosuria, and hypophosphataemia associated with deposition of cystine in the reticuloendothelial system is believed by some to be a distinct disease (cystinosis, Lignac's syndrome) while others consider it to be a form of the de Toni-Fanconi syndrome. The condition is characterized by polyuria, vomiting, constipation, retardation of growth, rickets and ultimately renal failure.

Aminoaciduria may occur with mental subnormality, muscular hypotonia, ocular defects and renal acidosis (Lowe's syndrome) or with disturbed tryptophane metabolism (Hartnup disease). In Hartnup disease, named after the first affected family, the patient has pellagra and develops cerebellar ataxia. Many other combinations of renal tubular and metabolic defects have now been reported. These disorders are frequently accompanied by defects in the transport of amino acids across the intestinal wall, which may be specific for one or more amino acids, e.g. in Hartnup disease, or may affect transport mechanisms in general, as in Lowe's syndrome.

A distinction must be made between aminoaciduria due to failure of renal tubular reabsorption (renal aminoaciduria) and overflow aminoaciduria, where amino acids which have accumulated in the blood appear in the urine, as occurs in the metabolic defects described above. The detection of abnormal aminoaciduria by chromatographic methods is an essential step in the elucidation of the cause of mental subnormality or other abnormal neurological finding.

DISORDERS OF STORAGE

Although the conditions which follow have no common etiology they can conveniently be considered together since they are characterized by abnormal deposition or storage of particular products of metabolism. Local deposition within tumours or infective granulomata, e.g. cholesterol within certain neoplasms or calcification of tuberculous lesions, are not regarded as general disorders of storage while fatty degeneration of individual tissues is also arbitrarily excluded.

OBESITY

While no hard and fast distinction can be drawn between normal and abnormal amounts of subcutaneous fat, many children can be distinguished on clinical grounds alone as being obviously obese. In the grosser cases there is likely to be a disturbance of salt and water retention as well as fat deposition. For statistical purposes, various arbitrary standards have been suggested, e.g. an excess of 20 per cent over the mean weight for height in each age group. It is obviously essential that height should be taken into consideration in applying such standards, and even then it will be found that no rule of thumb is completely satisfactory. A more elaborate standard includes body width (as indicated by the breadth of the pelvis), and attempts to allow for skeletal differences which are not included in simple height and weight measurements. It must be remembered that each phase of maturity has its characteristic growth pattern, and that maturity is not accurately assessed by chronological age. This applies particularly to the onset of puberty, which is commonly associated in both sexes with changes in fat deposition and distribution. Thus a girdle distribution of fat may appear in boys as one of the earlier manifestations of puberty; in such cases it is likely to disappear as adolescence is reached.

ETIOLOGY

The erroneous belief that obesity in childhood is evidence of endocrine disease is deep-rooted and it cannot be too strongly emphasized that the great majority of fat children have no demonstrable endocrine disorder. A common mistake is to diagnose 'hypogenitalism' when there is nothing to justify the description. The age of onset of puberty varies widely and in boys the genitalia may be small or infantile at the age of 15 or 16 and yet subsequently develop perfectly normally. Most obese children are above average height and are normal or advanced in skeletal maturation for their age. This simple type of childhood obesity is generally the result of a number of interacting etiological factors.

The child's dietary habits are obviously important and a dietetic history should always be obtained initially. This is unlikely to be reliable unless actual details of meals can be supplied, since parents' ideas of what constitutes 'normal' intake vary widely. Sometimes it will be found that the whole family is inclined to overeat and that in the family or individual diet, carbohydrate predominates. A family history of obesity may be obtained but should not necessarily be taken as evidence of hereditary obesity, since the family pattern of overeating and lack of exercise may be responsible for the same condition occurring in the various members affected. It is nevertheless true that there is a genetically determined predisposition to obesity in many cases.

In other children, overeating may be of psychogenic origin, the child seeking solace and escape from anxieties and emotional stress by self-indulgence in the larder. Often, however, the obese child does not eat more than the average child of his age and it must be assumed that his intake, though modest, is yet excessive for his expenditure of energy. This may be low because his physical activity is low and many fat children do take little exercise, move slowly and tend to sit a great deal. In some cases with no family history, it may be found that the condition dated from an illness, surgical operation or prolonged period of inactivity, suggesting that some physiological mechanism may have been altered by the event.

EXAMINATION

In examining the individual child in whom it is considered that weight is excessive for height, a careful note should be made of the distribution of the obesity and of any associated abnormalities. The obesity may be generalized, i.e. affecting the extremities and trunk to a corresponding extent; central, i.e. affecting the trunk most, the upper arms and thighs to a less extent, and the peripheral parts of the limbs not at all; or of girdle distribution, with the fat almost entirely localized to the hips and lower abdomen. (In most cases where the obesity is generalized, there is still a

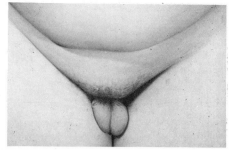

Fig. 7.2   Obesity in a boy aged 13½ years, showing retraction of penis into suprapubic fat. (Puberty normally established within six months.)

tendency for it to be most marked around the hips and across the chest and shoulders.)

The skin should be examined for reddish-purple striae which are most likely to appear at the sites of maximum fat distribution. Any evidence of hirsuties should be noted. In cases of extreme obesity, the surface of the skin will often show multiple small flattened areas, giving it a dappled appearance in certain lights. This is probably related to excessive water retention.

If the testicles lie above the scrotum but below the external inguinal ring and are covered by

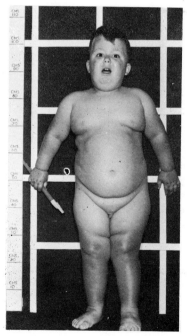

Fig. 7.3   Childhood obesity with generalized distribution; plethoric facies and genu valgum; advanced skeletal development. Boy aged 3 years.

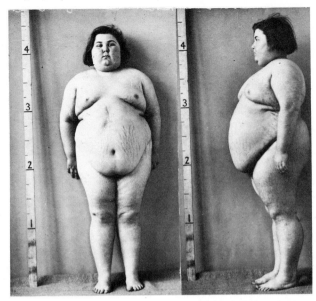

Fig. 7.4 Cushing's syndrome in a girl aged 12 years. Plethoric facies, obesity, and striae on abdomen and shoulders. Patient also showed hirsuties and hyperpiesis. (Previous laparotomy.)

suprapubic fat, they may be thought to be intra-abdominal unless the child is carefully examined. Retraction of the penis into the suprapubic fat (Fig. 7.2) may give an erroneous impression of underdevelopment.

Skeletal development should be assessed clinically and radiologically. Knock-knee is frequently observed when the obesity is very marked and represents a secondary mechanical deformity due to the weight. Osteoporosis may occur in cases of steroid-induced obesity.

The systolic blood pressure is commonly raised during periods of activity, but tends to return to normal when the child is put at rest. If it remains consistently raised, and there is associated hirsuties, adrenal cortical hyperplasia or tumour should be suspected.

When the patient is investigated in hospital, the daily fluid intake and urinary and salt output should be estimated over a three-day period before the ingestion of 10 g of salt, and for three days subsequently. This may serve to demonstrate abnormal salt and water retention. The blood-sugar curve may show either increased or decreased sugar tolerance.

There are so many difficulties in the interpretation of the basal metabolic rate in obese children that its estimation is not usually undertaken as a routine.

OTHER TYPES OF OBESITY

Although the great majority of cases of obesity in children are of the simple childhood type, occasionally obesity of endocrine or other evident pathological origin is encountered, generally in children who are below average in stature. It may be possible to incriminate a particular endocrine gland or to suspect a local lesion affecting the hypothalamus or neighbouring structures. Although it is common to hear references to 'hypopituitary obesity', there is little evidence that dysfunction of the pituitary itself is directly responsible for excessive fat deposition (see Cushing's syndrome, Fröhlich's syndrome).

Lesions of the central nervous system

Obesity occasionally occurs following infections of the nervous system, such as encephalitis and meningitis. While such infections are likely to be followed also by decreased activity, it appears probable that centres in the mid-brain controlling fat deposition may be directly affected. Cerebral degeneration, neoplasms, and haemorrhage may also result in secondary obesity.

Hypothyroid obesity

This should be suspected when there is associated evidence of hypothyroidism (p. 209), including sluggish mental and physical reactions, slow pulse, or the stigmata of juvenile myxoedema. Although thyroxine is sometimes prescribed in the treatment of adult obesity of various types, its use should be restricted in childhood to those cases in which there is evidence of hypothyroidism.

Cushing's syndrome

Obesity associated with striae atrophicae, plethoric facies, hirsuties, hyperpiesis, and osteoporosis occasionally occurs in childhood as the result of hyperfunction or tumour of the adrenal cortex, or more frequently following excessive treatment with corticosteroids. The obesity most commonly involves the upper part of the body including the face, neck, and shoulders but may be generalized. In older girls, amenorrhoea, hypertrophy of the clitoris and other signs of androgen activity such as acne are usually present. Although the adult cases originally described by Cushing were thought to be due to a minute basophil adenoma of the anterior pituitary, primary changes in the pituitary are now regarded as less commonly responsible for the syndrome than adrenal dysfunction.

Obesity associated with hypopituitarism

The name *Fröhlich's syndrome* is sometimes applied to the combination of infantilism with obesity; the description is much abused and often wrongly given to cases of obesity in which there is neither hypogenitalism nor statural infantilism. The true syndrome is extremely rare; when it does occur an intracranial cyst or tumour should be excluded.

The *Laurence-Moon-Biedl syndrome* is a very rare familial condition in which infantilism, obesity, mental subnormality, and polydactyly are associated with a peculiar type of retinitis pigmentosa.

Hypogonadal obesity

Failure of development or destruction of the gonads before puberty is rarely associated with gross obesity, though males are likely to show a degree of fat deposition around the hips and buttocks giving them a pseudofeminine contour. Usually growth in height continues at a slower rate but for a longer period than in those individuals in whom puberty occurs normally, so that the adult height (due to delayed fusion of the epiphyses) is finally above the normal.

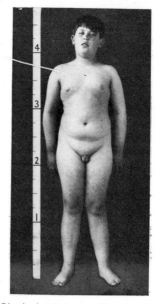

Fig. 7.5   Obesity in a boy aged 10½ years. Pseudofeminine contour due to fat deposition over chest, abdomen, and hips, genu valgum and pes planus. Puberty normally established during fourteenth year.

An uncommon syndrome has been described in which a hypotonic infant subsequently shows obesity, cryptorchidism, dwarfism and mental subnormality. Scoliosis is often present and there may be diabetes in later life (Prader-Willi syndrome).

TREATMENT

Obesity in childhood usually responds well to dietetic restriction if the co-operation of both parents and child can be obtained. In designing an anti-obesity diet for a child, it must be remembered that requirements for growth must be covered and that the diet must be sufficiently bulky to prevent hunger if adherence to the diet is to be maintained. In the milder cases it is best to aim at keeping the weight stationary while growth continues, so that the child 'grows up to his weight' rather than losing weight rapidly.

The general principle followed in constructing the diet will be the restriction of fat, carbohydrate, and starch, while allowing ample protein. The bulk of the diet is increased with green vegetables and fruit. Where there is evidence of abnormal salt and water retention, salt intake should also be restricted. The total calorie value should not exceed 1000. Exercise should be increased at the same time. In the more severe cases, admission to hospital and a carefully controlled low-calorie diet (600 calories or less) for three or more weeks may bring about a rapid loss of weight; in some cases a subsequent anti-obesity diet will prevent the weight loss being regained.

Although initial response to treatment is often encouraging, it is all too often found that the enthusiasm of both mother and child flags and the weight begins to increase again. The intelligence of the mother, her will to co-operate and her influence over the child will be the main factors determining the success or failure of treatment. Some parents, while expressing the desire to co-operate, are really reluctant to do so, for they take the view that a 'well-nourished' child is a healthy one and that children ought to eat heartily: hence they have no real belief in the rationale of dieting. Others are too careless or indulgent to exert the prolonged discipline necessary. Few young children have sufficient incentive to adhere to a diet without constant supervision, even although they dislike being fat and resent being teased at school. Not until adolescence is there likely to be a strong desire to lose weight. Regular attendance at the clinic for weighing, advice and exhortation is necessary if the initial weight loss is to be maintained, but despite this the physician often feels that he is fighting a losing battle.

Appetite-suppressant drugs have little or no part to play in the management of obese children, for their use is undesirable in growing children and those who most need such aids are the least likely to take them regularly. When there is evidence that emotional disturbance is important in the genesis of obesity, psychotherapy may be necessary.

PROGNOSIS

While a considerable number of otherwise normal children show some degree of transient obesity at puberty, which disappears during adolescence without treatment, gross obesity occurring either during childhood or at puberty is both a physical and a psychological disability for the patient and a danger in later life. From the histories of obese adults, it is often clear that the condition dates from childhood. Moreover, many fat infants become fat children and most fat children will be obese adults. Treatment should therefore be undertaken as early as possible and sustained throughout childhood, taking care that growth is not interfered with and that the child is not made unnecessarily anxious about his condition. Such long-continued effort is justified because obesity at adolescence may cause serious emotional and orthopaedic problems and afterwards may affect both health and length of life.

FAILURE OF FAT DEPOSITION

Just as overeating and reduced activity will produce obesity, an inadequate caloric intake, failure of absorption, or an increased metabolic rate will tend to result in failure of fat deposition, e.g. in infantile marasmus, coeliac disease and thyrotoxicosis. *Anorexia nervosa*, producing what is essentially the picture of starvation, is occasionally seen in older children. Most infections of long standing will interfere with nutrition or metabolism sufficiently to cause obvious loss of subcutaneous fat, while diarrhoea and vomiting in infancy will result not only in loss of fat but severe dehydration also. Fat deposition in the pre-term infant is less advanced than in the infant born at term, and is responsible for the characteristic thin appearance of the former. In addition to these secondary failures of fat deposition, there are endogenous conditions which are more properly classified as disorders of storage and occasionally occur in childhood.

Pituitary cachexia (*Simmonds' disease*)

Although this condition is very rare before adolescence, cases have been observed in infancy and childhood. Symptoms of hypopituitarism including infantilism are associated with severe generalized cachexia, muscle wasting and a low basal metabolic rate. If the condition arises after puberty, there is loss of secondary sexual characters and atrophy of the gonads. The syndrome has been described in association with dysontogenetic pituitary cysts and other lesions causing dysfunction of the anterior lobe of the pituitary. Since hypotension and pigmentation may occur as associated symptoms, the diagnosis of Addison's disease (though also rare in childhood) must be considered. Cases of pituitary cachexia, however, do not respond to the administration of desoxycorticosterone. When the diagnosis of a cyst or tumour can be established, surgical removal offers the only hope of recovery.

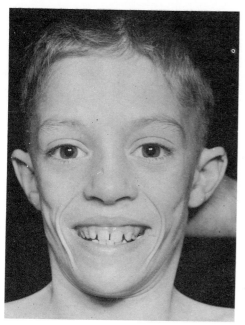

Fig. 7.6 Lipodystrophia progressiva, showing loss of subcutaneous fat over face. The neck, arms, and upper thorax were affected, with normal fat distribution over abdomen and legs.

Lipodystrophia progressiva

In this condition, which occurs rarely in middle or later childhood, there is a segmental loss of subcutaneous fat, affecting first the face and upper extremities, and either descending gradually to the level of the iliac crests or becoming arrested at any point above them. The buttocks and lower extremities are typically unaffected. The condition is symptomless, and the general health and muscle power are unaffected. The extreme emaciation of the face (Fig. 7.6) commonly arouses a suspicion of some wasting disease, but the plumpness of the lower extremities is in striking contrast to the appearance of the affected areas.

Although a pituitary origin has been suggested, the etiology of the condition is unknown. No treatment has been found effective. Apart from the cosmetic disability, the condition is harmless and does not affect the expectation of life.

LIPIDS, MUCOPOLYSACCHARIDES, AND GLYCOGEN

The lipidoses

These include a number of conditions in which various types of lipid are stored in abnormal amount in the cells of the reticulo-endothelial system and histiocytes. With the exception of those types of xanthomatosis associated with a high blood cholesterol, it is probable that in each instance the abnormality is due to an abnormal production of lipid within the cell rather than to the taking-up·of lipid by the cell from the bloodstream. All the types described below are rare, but since they are most likely to be observed in infancy or childhood require special consideration in this age group. In several types there is a familial incidence. Gaucher's disease, Niemann-Pick disease, the gangliosidoses and metachromatic leukodystrophy are grouped as the sphingolipidoses, since they are characterized by storage of compounds related to sphingolipids. These compounds are all derived from ceramide and differ in the composition of added side chains.

Gaucher's disease

The stored lipids are cerebrosides, which accumulate in the cells of the lymphohaemopoietic system; these are transformed into the diagnostic Gaucher cells which measure 20 to 80 μm, are pale and waxy-looking, and have from one to 12 nuclei. Acid phosphatase is increased in both cells and plasma.

The disease is a rare familial condition, occurring most frequently (but not exclusively) in those of Jewish race, and more commonly in females than males. It is believed to be due to absence of the enzyme glucocerebrosidase: two main clinical forms of the disease are recognized.

In the *infantile type*, the manifestations are fulminating, occurring during the first year of life, and the disease is fatal before the end of the second year. The infant shows great splenomegaly, which is more marked than hepatomegaly. Neurological signs include hypertonia, laryngeal spasm, and strabismus, and the patient shows progressive mental deterioration. The fundi appear normal. Blood examination usually shows a leucopenia, but Gaucher cells are not observed in the peripheral blood. The blood cholesterol is not raised. Diagnosis depends on biopsy or splenic puncture, with demonstration of the typical Gaucher cells, and on biochemical analysis of biopsy specimens from liver or spleen.

The *chronic form* of the disease is observed in childhood and adult life. Abdominal distension due to splenic enlargement is commonly the first manifestation. The liver is often enlarged also, but to a less extent than the spleen. Patchy

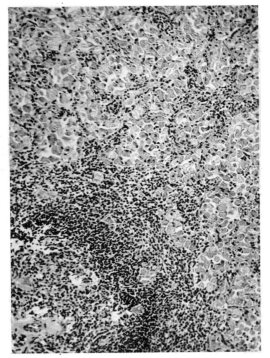

Fig. 7.7   Gaucher's disease. Section of spleen from an infant aged 15 months, showing contrast between large lipid-containing Gaucher cells and the remaining lymphocytic cells. × 80.

pigmentation of the skin, probably the result of haemochromatosis, and pingueculae of the conjunctivae occur later in these chronic cases. Gaucher deposits in the long bones result in a flask-shaped expansion of the bone, spontaneous fractures, a characteristic X-ray picture, and

ultimately in haemorrhage due to thrombocytopenia.

The prognosis as regards expectation of life is variable, and although the disease is ultimately fatal, patients frequently survive many years without serious disability. Splenectomy may be performed for the relief of symptoms directly due to splenomegaly.

Niemann-Pick disease

This condition differs from Gaucher's disease in that there is a more widespread involvement of the reticular cells and histiocytes, and that the lipid stored is a phosphatide, sphingomyelin. The Niemann-Pick cells ('foam cells') are vacuolated and smaller than Gaucher cells, rarely contain more than three nuclei, appear in the peripheral blood, and may also be distinguished from Gaucher cells by their staining reactions.

The disease is predominantly one of infancy, the manifestations appearing during the first year of life and proving rapidly fatal. The spleen and liver are greatly enlarged and ascites is often present. The infant usually shows muscular hypotonia or hypertonia and progressive mental deterioration; blindness and deafness may occur. In a number of instances a cherry-red spot is seen at the macula. Radiological examination of the chest may show widespread opacities, due to deposits in the lung tissue. The blood cholesterol shows a high normal or increased value.

DIAGNOSIS. This will be suggested by gross hepatosplenomegaly and the clinical picture described. The appearance of large vacuolated cells in the peripheral blood is highly suggestive.

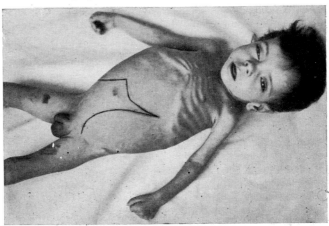

Fig. 7.8   Niemann-Pick disease. Male infant aged 27 months, showing wasting and hepatosplenomegaly, the spleen reaching the pelvis. Akinesia with marked hypertonia.

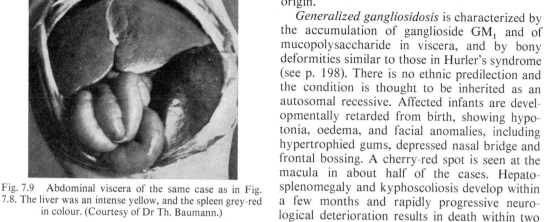

Fig. 7.9 Abdominal viscera of the same case as in Fig. 7.8. The liver was an intense yellow, and the spleen grey-red in colour. (Courtesy of Dr Th. Baumann.)

Chemical analysis of biopsy tissues showing a total phospholipid content which is double, or more than double, the normal is regarded as diagnostic of Niemann-Pick disease, although a more detailed analysis should demonstrate that the lipid is sphingomyelin.

Gangliosidoses

These constitute a group of diseases characterized by storage of a ganglioside, e.g. ganglioside GM_2 in Tay-Sachs disease and GM_1 in generalized gangliosidosis. The term *amaurotic family idiocy* is often applied to these disorders, but this is not a biochemical entity and not always a gangliosidosis.

Tay-Sachs disease is inherited as an autosomal recessive and, though biochemically distinct, has many clinical similarities to Niemann-Pick disease.

Thus both occur predominantly in Jewish infants, the manifestations appearing during the first year of life and usually proving fatal before the end of the second year. Both are characterized by progressive mental defect, lipid deposits in the brain, and the appearance of a cherry-red spot at the macula. In both conditions the infants are likely to become blind and deaf, though in Tay-Sachs disease there is perhaps more consistent evidence of optic atrophy and often an enhanced startle response to noise. The liver and spleen are not necessarily enlarged in classical cases of Tay-Sachs disease.

At necropsy the most characteristic finding is swelling of the ganglion cells (due to the presence of lipid) throughout the nervous system, and

ballooning of the dendrites close to their point of origin.

Generalized gangliosidosis is characterized by the accumulation of ganglioside GM_1 and of mucopolysaccharide in viscera, and by bony deformities similar to those in Hurler's syndrome (see p. 198). There is no ethnic predilection and the condition is thought to be inherited as an autosomal recessive. Affected infants are developmentally retarded from birth, showing hypotonia, oedema, and facial anomalies, including hypertrophied gums, depressed nasal bridge and frontal bossing. A cherry-red spot is seen at the macula in about half of the cases. Hepatosplenomegaly and kyphoscoliosis develop within a few months and rapidly progressive neurological deterioration results in death within two years. Pathologically, there are vacuolated cells in bone marrow and liver, and neuronal lipidosis.

Other clinical and biochemical varieties of gangliosidosis have been reported in older children.

Metachromatic leukodystrophy

This is primarily a disorder of sulphatide storage, with secondary demyelination in cerebral hemispheres, spinal tracts and peripheral nerves. Granular cells containing metachromatic granules appear in the demyelinated areas. In infants, the condition is commonly manifest as difficulty in walking due to muscular hypotonia and inco-ordination, followed successively by weakness, spasticity, visual and bulbar symptoms and progressive dementia. The protein of the cerebro-spinal fluid is usually elevated and sulphatide is excreted in the urine. There is decreased conduction time in the peripheral nerves. The infantile form of the disease generally causes death within two or three years but juvenile types pursue a less rapid course, presenting initially as ataxia in middle childhood.

Other disorders of lipid metabolism

A number of rare conditions have been recognized in which there is excess or deficiency of a normal lipid constituent of plasma. In the familial hyperlipidaemias, there is a primary excess of triglyceride or of cholesterol in the blood: both may be associated with xanthomas in skin, tendons or bones.

Absence of beta-lipoprotein is characterized by steatorrhoea, acanthocytosis (spiny appearance of red cells) and ataxia. Absence of alpha-lipoprotein has also been reported as a rare cause of hepatosplenomegaly.

The mucopolysaccharidoses

Disorders of mucopolysaccharide storage were formerly described as a single entity (gargoylism) but it is now clear that there are several clinically and biochemically distinct varieties. Moreover, Morquio's chondro-osteodystrophy, hitherto regarded as a different disease, should now be considered under the same general title. These disorders are characterized by intracellular storage and urinary excretion of glycosaminoglycans (sulphated mucopolysaccharides).

Hurler's syndrome affects both sexes and is inherited as an autosomal recessive. The clinical features develop insidiously during the first two years, with progressive mental retardation. The face becomes peculiarly gross and unchildlike, with thick lips, wide nostrils and heavy nasolabial folds. The eyes are set wide apart (hypertelorism) and the corneae may be cloudy due to deposits within them. The head is large and square or scaphocephalic, the ears are set low and deafness may develop. The majority of patients have dark, coarse eyebrows with finer, fairer hair. Thick purulent nasal discharge causes troublesome obstruction to breathing. The abdomen is distended due to firm enlargement of

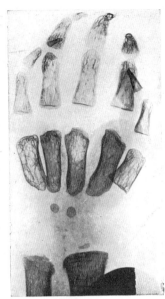

Fig. 7.11   Hurler's syndrome. Hand, showing extreme irregularity of metacarpals and phalanges.

liver and spleen and herniae are common. The heart is often affected, a systolic murmur being evident, and left ventricular hypertrophy may be followed by cardiac failure.

Failure of development of the upper and anterior portions gives the lumbar vertebral bodies a sabot-shaped or hooked appearance (Fig. 7.10) and causes kyphosis, which together with flexion deformities of knees and hips, results in dwarfing. Irregular thickening of metacarpal bones and phalanges produces claw hands, while elbows and shoulders may develop flexion deformities. The sternum is not usually affected.

Many of the clinical features of *Hunter's syndrome*, which is inherited as a sex-linked recessive, are similar though less pronounced. There is little or no kyphosis, the corneae are not cloudy and intellect is usually less impaired. Survival is generally longer, even into adult life. In both conditions, dermatan and heparan sulphates are excreted in excess in the urine.

In *Morquio's chondro-osteodystrophy* there is dwarfism, with variable deformities of sternum, vertebrae and joints, and fragmentation of the epiphyses and metaphyses of the long bones. The neck is short and the head appears telescoped on to the deformed trunk. The femora show coxa vara or valga deformities and the acetabulum is often defective. There may be slight coarsening of the features and corneal clouding after some

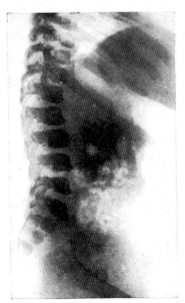

Fig. 7.10   Hurler's syndrome, showing deformity of lumbar vertebrae, two of which appear to have an anterior hook-shaped process.

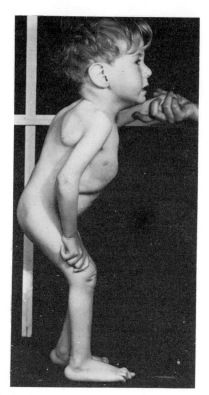

Fig. 7.12   Chondro-osteodystrophy (Morquio's disease).

years. Unlike Hurler's syndrome, the skull is not deformed and the intelligence is normal. Abnormal amounts of keratan sulphate are excreted in the urine. The condition is inherited as an autosomal recessive.

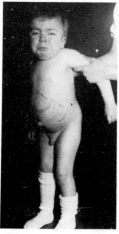

Fig. 7.13   Hurler's syndrome, showing facies, hepatosplenomegaly, umbilical hernia, and flexion deformities of knees, hips, and phalanges. Boy aged 3½ years.

Other varieties of mucopolysaccharidosis are the *Sanfilippo, Scheie* and *Maroteaux-Lamy syndromes*, all inherited as autosomal recessives and differing in the degree of neurological and corneal involvement and in the proportions and types of glycosaminoglycans excreted in the urine.

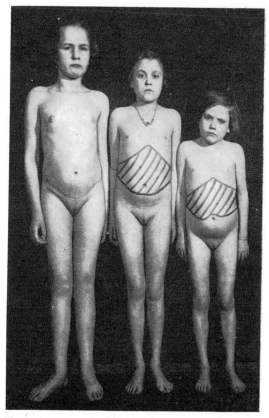

Fig. 7.14   Glycogen disease in two sisters aged 14 years and 11 years 10 months, with normal control aged 12 years, showing hepatomegaly and infantilism.

The glycogenoses (*Glycogen storage diseases*)

These include a number of congenital disorders of glycogen metabolism, mostly inherited as autosomal recessives and often showing a familial incidence. They ocur in both sexes and many different nationalities. They are characterized by accumulation of glycogen in one or more organs. At least seven forms with known or presumed specific enzyme deficiencies have been identified.

Hepato-renal glycogenosis (*von Gierke's disease*). In this condition the liver and sometimes the kidneys are grossly and painlessly

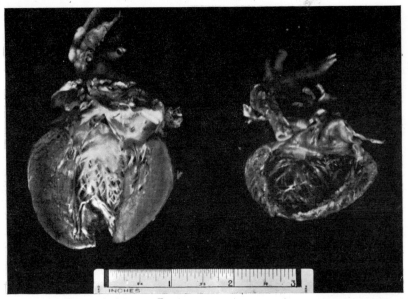

Fig. 7.15   Generalized glycogenosis. Heart of infant aged 4 months on left, compared with
normal control of same age on right.

enlarged, often from birth. The spleen is not enlarged, though enlargement of the left lobe of the liver may be mistaken for splenomegaly. The fasting blood sugar is low, and ketonuria occurs readily. Occasionally hypoglycaemic manifestations such as convulsions occur, but usually there is comparatively little disturbance of general well-being. Growth, however, is markedly affected, and with increasing age these children show a striking degree of infantilism (Fig. 7.14).

The condition is due to a deficiency of glucose-6-phosphatase, the enzyme responsible for hepatic conversion of glucose-6-phosphate to glucose; glycogen thus accumulates in the liver owing to failure of mobilization.

BIOCHEMICAL EXAMINATION. While the fasting blood sugar is low (less than 50 mg per 100 ml), the administration of glucose is likely to result in a prolonged rise and slow fall in blood sugar. Injection of glucagon or adrenaline, however, which in the normal child produces a rise in blood sugar of more than 30 mg, results in little or no rise, demonstrating the inability of the liver to convert glycogen to glucose. The blood levels of lactic acid, glycogen, and lipids are commonly raised.

COURSE AND PROGNOSIS. Affected patients appear to have an increased susceptibility to infection, including hepatitis, but in many instances have survived into adult life. Indeed, the condition may undergo spontaneous remission in

late adolescence, although adult stature is likely to be permanently dwarfed.

TREATMENT. It is doubtful whether any form of treatment which has been attempted has been effective, but it has been recommended that glucose should be given in divided doses throughout the day if any symptoms of hypoglycaemia have occurred, and that the diet should contain a liberal allowance of protein.

DIAGNOSIS. The occurrence of hepatomegaly without splenomegaly, associated with ketonuria, hypoglycaemia, and failure of response to glucagon injection, forms the criterion of diagnosis. Liver biopsy shows cells packed with glycogen which is abnormally stable. When the clinical disorder is mild and the response to glucagon is normal after a short fast but becomes abnormal after prolonged fasting, glycogen disease due to deficiency of the debranching enzyme, amylo-1,6-glucosidase (limit dextrinosis) may be suspected. A similar clinical picture may also be due to deficiency of hepatic phosphorylase. Cirrhosis and hepatic failure in early infancy occur in the rare amylopectinosis, due to diminished brancher enzyme activity.

Generalized glycogenosis (*cardiomegalia glycogenica*). Accumulation of glycogen within the cardiac muscle, giving rise to great enlargement of the heart, occurs in association with glycogen storage in tissues throughout the body,

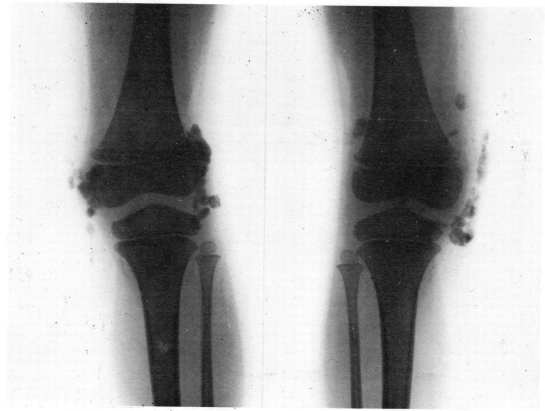

Fig. 7.16 Calcinosis universalis. Calcium deposits around both knees; a number of superficial deposits had ulcerated through the skin. Girl aged 6 years.

especially skeletal muscle and the central nervous system. A specific deficiency of the enzyme α-1,4-glucosidase has been demonstrated in this type. The condition should be kept in mind as a possible cause of so-called 'idiopathic hypertrophy of the heart' in infancy. Neuromuscular glycogenosis involving the respiratory muscles is likely to result in respiratory failure.

The glucagon and glucose tolerance tests in this type are normal. In many instances the cardiac condition has resulted in sudden death, and has only been recognized at necropsy.

Glycogenosis of skeletal muscle. Deficiency of muscle phosphorylase is a rare cause of muscle weakness and cramps, simulating muscular dystrophy. The muscles may also be involved in other forms of glycogenosis.

DISORDERS OF CALCIUM STORAGE

The normal processes of calcium absorption and metabolism, including ossification, may be-come deranged at any point. The result may be abnormal calcium deposition in tissues other than bone, e.g. calcinosis universalis, renal calcinosis, myositis ossificans; or abnormal calcium deposition within the skeleton itself, e.g. osteopetrosis. Deficiency of intake or failure of absorption will result in defective calcification of the skeleton, while depression of osteoblastic activity (as in scurvy) will lead to a similar osteoporosis from failure to convert available calcium into bone. Osteoporosis will also result from an excessive mobilization of calcium from the skeleton, as occurs in hyperparathyroidism and rickets. Finally, the skeleton may be excessively fragile from a congenital abnormality of bone formation (osteogenesis imperfecta).

Calcinosis universalis

Widespread deposition of calcium in the subcutaneous tissues, particularly around the larger joints, and more rarely in the viscera, is occasionally observed in childhood. The con-

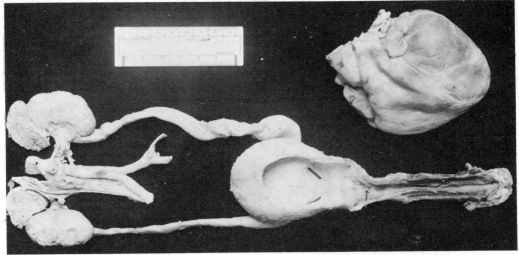

Fig. 7.17   Specimen from a case of renal rickets (boy aged 9 years), showing small sclerotic kidneys, dilated ureters, and hypertrophied bladder. The site of a posterior urethral valve is indicated by an arrow. Symptoms included dribbling incontinence, thirst, polyuria, and enuresis. The blood urea was never less than 95 mg per 100 ml on repeated examination over a period of 5 years, and reached 244 mg 15 months before death. The blood pressure was not consistently raised until shortly before death, but there was some hypertrophy of the left ventricle.

dition may follow an infection or dermatomyositis or arise without obvious cause. Where the calcium deposits are superficial, they tend to ulcerate through the skin, leaving areas of scarring. ACTH has occasionally proved effective in treatment.

Idiopathic hypercalcaemia

Although this condition was only recognized in 1952, a considerable number of cases have been reported of infants who, after a period of four to five months' well-being, fail to thrive and show anorexia, vomiting, constipation, and hypotonia associated with raised serum calcium levels (12 to 18 mg per 100 ml), raised blood urea, and sometimes hypercholesterolaemia. While some infants recover completely, there are others, representing a severer variant of the syndrome, who show in addition osteosclerosis, a harsh systolic murmur, developmental retardation and hypertension. In fatal cases there is nephrocalcinosis at necropsy. Survivors later show a typical facies with mental subnormality and aortic stenosis. Since the clinical picture may closely resemble that of renal acidosis (p. 290), and nephrocalcinosis may occur in both, the diagnosis during life rests on the biochemical findings, viz. hypercalcaemia and raised blood urea without a consistently alkaline urine. The etiology is uncertain but hypersensitivity to vitamin D is a probable factor. A calcium-free milk has been used successfully in treatment and corticosteroids are sometimes of value in the acute stage.

Renal rickets

Rickets, which in some cases is characterized by generalized osteoporosis, may occur in association with severe impairment of renal function. At least two types of renal rickets are distinguishable radiologically, one in which the appearances are similar to those of nutritional (vitamin D deficiency) rickets, and one in which a woolly or stippled appearance is seen in long bones and skull, with areas simulating subperiosteal erosion. Since renal impairment has generally been of long standing before the bony lesions occur, most cases first come under observation in middle or later childhood. Deformities are often severe and retardation of growth and infantilism are commonly associated.

The metabolic disturbance in renal rickets is complex. There is phosphorus retention due to glomerular inadequacy and reduced intestinal absorption of calcium. The associated acidosis helps to maintain the blood calcium level and tetany seldom occurs. The blood urea is increased and the cholesterol may also be high. The

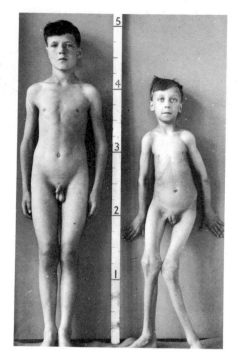

Fig. 7.18 Hyperparathyroidism. Boy aged 12 years with normal control, showing dwarfing and deformities due to osteoporosis.

blood pressure is seldom raised until the terminal stages.

The condition is usually chronic and there may be periods of remission or partial healing. The final outcome, however, is fatal. If there is any evidence of obstruction or urinary infection, appropriate treatment should be instituted; but by the time bony lesions have appeared it is probable that the renal lesion will be far advanced. Large doses of vitamin D will produce temporary improvement in the rickets.

Disturbance of renal tubular reabsorption (p. 190) may result in a form of 'renal rickets', though this term is usually restricted to rickets secondary to severe impairment of glomerular function.

Hyperparathyroidism

Primary hyperparathyroidism, though rare in childhood, occasionally occurs as the result of an adenoma. Secondary hypertrophy of the parathyroids is seen in chronic renal insufficiency. Since an excess of parathormone causes mobilization of calcium from the skeleton, it results in osteoporosis or, in extreme cases, osteitis fibrosa cystica; in the latter condition, the cancellous tissue of the long bones is replaced by cystic areas. In primary hyperparathyroidism, the serum calcium is raised, e.g. to 12 or 15 mg per 100 ml, the serum phosphorus reduced, and the serum phosphatase raised. Clinically, the extreme softening of the long bones results in gross deformities and spontaneous fractures may occur. When a parathyroid adenoma is present, surgical removal will be required.

Hypoparathyroidism

Idiopathic hypoparathyroidism is a rare condition characterized by convulsions, painful muscular cramps, laryngeal stridor, and dry skin with sparse hair. The blood calcium is low and the phosphate high. Such children have sometimes been treated as epileptics for years before the true nature of the disease has been recognized. In long-standing cases, mental retardation is likely to occur.

A familial syndrome with similar symptoms arises not from deficiency of parathyroid hormone but from failure of the organism to respond to the hormone (pseudo-hypoparathyroidism). The patients are short and obese, with characteristic deformity of the hands, the index finger being longer than the other fingers.

Treatment for both conditions consists of large doses of calciferol (50,000 units or more daily).

Hypoparathyroidism may also be secondary to thyroidectomy or may occur as a transient phenomenon in the newborn infant.

Myositis ossificans

This rare condition should probably be considered a congenital abnormality of metabolism, since it is usually associated with characteristic shortening of the thumbs and great toes, and occasionally with other congenital abnormalities. Localized areas of what appears at first to be inflammatory swelling arise within the muscles, and progress to ossification. Although the site of these lesions may at first be conditioned by local trauma, the condition commonly becomes widespread. No treatment is known, and the condition, though chronic, is ultimately fatal.

OTHER DISORDERS OF DEPOSITION AND STORAGE

Amyloid disease

This is essentially a degenerative condition occurring as the result of rheumatoid arthritis or chronic suppurative diseases. The liver and spleen become gradually enlarged until they attain very great size. They are firm and smooth, and at necropsy are found to have a lard-like consistency. Since the kidneys also undergo amyloid degeneration (*amyloid nephrosis*), proteinuria is almost always present. The diagnosis can be confirmed by rectal or, if necessary, renal biopsy.

Treatment consists in elimination of the primary cause, but when amyloid degeneration of the viscera is far advanced, it is likely to be irreversible and fatal.

Hyperuricaemia

Gout is rare in childhood, and does not differ materially from the condition in adult life. It is characterized by hyperuricaemia and deposition of uric acid in the tissues, giving rise to pain and swelling of joints. Hyperuricaemia also occurs in acute leukaemia, in hepatic glycogenosis and in association with microencephaly, mental retardation, choreo-athetosis and self-mutilation in the Lesch-Nyhan syndrome, which is inherited as a sex-linked recessive.

Serum uric acid levels may be reduced by increasing urinary excretion with probenecid and diminishing production with allopurinol. In acute gout, pain may be relieved by rest and colchicine.

BIBLIOGRAPHY AND REFERENCES

AMERICAN ACADEMY OF PEDIATRICS (1967). Obesity. *Pediatrics, Springfield*, **40**, 455.

BICKEL, H. & SMELLIE, J. M. (1952). Cystine storage disease with amino-aciduria. *Lancet*, i, 1093.

BLATTNER, R. J. (1966). Hurler's syndrome. *Journal of Pediatrics*, **69**, 313.

CARSON, N. A. J. (1970). Homocystinuria. *Proceedings of the Royal Society of Medicine*, **63**, 41.

DRASH, A. (1971). Diabetes mellitus in childhood. *Journal of Pediatrics*, **78**, 919.

EFRON, M. L. & AMPOLA, M. G. (1967). The aminoacidurias. *Pediatric Clinics of North America*, **14**, 881.

ELLIS, R. W. B., SHELDON, W. & CAPON, N. B. (1936). Gargoylism. *Quarterly Journal of Medicine*, **5**, 119.

FANCONI, G. (1954). Tubular insufficiency and renal dwarfism. *Archives of Disease in Childhood*, **29**, 1.

FORFAR, J. O. & TOMPSETT, S. L. (1959). Idiopathic hypercalcemia of infancy. *Advances in Clinical Chemistry*, vol. 2. New York: Academic Press.

GARROD, A. E. (1923). *Inborn Errors of Metabolism*, 2nd edn. London: Oxford University Press.

HARRIS, H. (1970). Genetical theory and inborn errors of metabolism. *British Medical Journal*, i, 321.

HSIA, D. Y.-Y. (1966). *Inborn Errors of Metabolism*, 2nd edn. Chicago: Year Book Medical Publishers.

HSIA, D. Y.-Y. (1967). Phenylketonuria. *Developmental Medicine and Child Neurology*, **9**, 531.

HUTCHISON, J. H. & MACDONALD, A. M. (1951). Chronic acidosis in infants due to renal tubular deficiency. *Acta paediatrica, Stockholm*, **40**, 371.

KOMROWER, G. M. & LEE, D. H. (1970). Long-term follow-up of galactosaemia. *Archives of Disease in Childhood*, **45**, 367.

KUO, P. T. & BASSETT, D. R. (1963). Primary hyperlipidemias and their management. *Annals of Internal Medicine*, **59**, 495.

LLOYD, J. K. (1968). Diabetes mellitus in childhood. *Hospital Medicine*, **2**, 426.

MCBEAN, M. S. & STEPHENSON, J. B. P. (1968). Treatment of classical phenylketonuria. *Archives of Disease in Childhood*, **43**, 1.

MAHLER, R. (1968). Glycogen storage diseases. *Journal of Clinical Pathology*, **22**, suppl. 2, 32.

MANLEY, G. & HAWKSWORTH, J. (1966). Diagnosis of Hurler's syndrome. *Archives of Disease in Childhood*, **41**, 91.

MITCHELL, R. G. (1960). The prognosis in idiopathic hypercalcaemia of infants. *Archives of Disease in Childhood*, **35**, 383.

MONTGOMERY, D. A., WELBOURN, R. B., MCCAUGHEY, W. T. & GLEADHILL, C. A. (1959). Pituitary tumours manifested after adrenalectomy for Cushing's syndrome. *Lancet*, ii, 707.

ØSTERGAARD, L. (1954). On psychogenic obesity in childhood. *Acta paediatrica, Stockholm*, **43**, 507.

PILZ, H. (1970). Clinical, morphological and biochemical aspects of sphingolipidoses. *Neuropädiatrie*, **1**, 383.

RAINE, D. N. (1972). Management of inherited metabolic disease. *British Medical Journal*, ii, 329.

ROTHSTEIN, J. L. & WELT, S. (1936). Calcinosis universalis and circumscripta in infancy and childhood. *American Journal of Diseases in Children*, **52**, 368.

SALT, H. B. and 5 others (1960). On having no beta-lipoprotein. *Lancet*, ii, 325.

SPENCER-PEET, J., NORMAN, M. E., LAKE, B. D., MCNAMARA, J. & PATRICK, A. D. (1971). Hepatic glycogen storage disease. *Quarterly Journal of Medicine*, **40**, 95.

STRAUSS, R. G., SCHUBERT, W. K. & MCADAMS, A. J. (1969). Amyloidosis in childhood. *Journal of Pediatrics*, **74**, 272.

WOLFF, O. H. (1965). Obesity in childhood. In *Recent Advances in Paediatrics*, 3rd edn. Edited by D. Gairdner. London: Churchill.

8 Disorders of Growth and Development

Growth and development are two of the characters which distinguish the infant and child most sharply from the adult. It has already been pointed out that each successive phase of development has its characteristic degree of maturity reflected in dentition, ossification, relative physical proportions, and behaviour, and to some extent in the functional efficiency of individual organs. The stage of development reached will normally show considerable variation amongst children of the same chronological age; the latter point is illustrated by the age-range of onset of puberty, with which childhood may be said to end.

When allowance for these physiological variations is made, however, it will be found that with regard to height, weight, and development there are children who lie outside the normal distribution curve for age, and whose retardation or precocity of development must be regarded as pathological. Since normal growth and development are dependent on a large number of interacting factors, it is understandable that either endocrine disturbance or gross disease of any essential organ acting over a sufficiently long time is likely to upset the normal balance and to affect development as a whole. Even short-term illnesses may be recognizable radiologically in the long bones, where they give rise to transverse lines of increased density representing periods of arrested growth. In addition, local lesions may interfere with the growth of a single organ resulting in local dwarfism or gigantism.

The term 'dwarfism' is used to indicate small stature (2·5 s.d. or more below mean height for age) or small size in the case of a single organ; 'infantilism' implies general retardation of development. 'Gigantism', whether general or local, indicates large size, and 'precocity' advanced development for age.

Disorders of growth and development may be classified as follows:

I. DWARFISM WITHOUT INFANTILISM

1. *Simple hereditary dwarfism* (racial and familial)

2. *Congenital dwarfism.* Trisomic syndromes, Silver's syndrome.

3. *Dwarfism due to developmental skeletal disease*
Achondroplasia, mucopolysaccharidoses, fragilitas ossium, etc.

4. *Dwarfism due to acquired skeletal disease*
Rickets. Spinal deformities, e.g. spina bifida, poliomyelitis, osteomyelitis. Hyperparathyroidism.

5. *Dwarfism following precocity*
Premature fusion of epiphyses following precocious puberty.

II. DWARFISM ASSOCIATED WITH INFANTILISM

1. *Endocrine*
Hypothyroid—cretinism and juvenile myxoedema.
Hypopituitary—panhypopituitarism, isolated growth hormone deficiency.
Hypogonadal—eunuchoid infantilism. Turner's syndrome.
(?) Multiple—progeria.

2. *Metabolic*
Glycogenoses

3. *Infective*
Tuberculosis, malaria, Leishmaniasis, hook-worm, congenital syphilis.

4. *Systemic disease*
Renal—renal infantilism and rickets.
Intestinal—coeliac infantilism and rickets.
Cardiac—congenital malformation of the heart.
Cerebral—microcephaly and primary mental defect.
Pulmonary—cystic fibrosis, tuberculosis, bronchiectasis.

5. *Pre-term birth*

III. LOCAL DWARFISM

1. *Congenital*
Failure of development of individual organs.

2. *Acquired*
For example—destruction of epiphyses, atrophy due to disease or constriction.

IV. GIGANTISM WITHOUT PRECOCITY

1. *Simple hereditary gigantism* (racial and familial)
2. *Gigantism due to developmental skeletal disease*
Arachnodactyly.
3. *Metabolic gigantism*
Infants of diabetic mothers.
4. *Endocrine gigantism*
Eunuchoidism with delayed fusion of epiphyses.
5. *Cerebral gigantism*

V. PRECOCITY (WITH VARIABLE DEGREE OF GIGANTISM)

1. *Endocrine*
Hypergonadal—tumours of testis or ovary.
Hyperpituitary—juvenile acromegaly; secondary hyperfunction.
Hyperadrenal—congenital adrenal hyperplasia.
Hyperthyroid—thyrotoxicosis.

2. *Systemic disease*
Cerebral—tumours of hypothalamic region; hydrocephalus; cerebral degeneration; meningo-encephalitis.

3. *Constitutional*

VI. LOCAL GIGANTISM

1. *Congenital*
Macrodactyly, macromelia, macroglossia, etc.

2. *Acquired*
Overgrowth due to vascular anomalies, e.g. haemangioma.
Elephantiasis.
Hypertrophy due to overuse.
Neoplasms.
Disorders of storage, e.g. glycogen hepatomegaly and cardiomegaly.

It will be seen from the above that a number of pathological conditions appear under different headings. Thus precocious puberty, due to any cause, is likely to be associated with statural overgrowth and advanced skeletal development in its early stages, while if the child survives, premature fusion of the epiphyses will result in premature discontinuance of growth and ultimately in dwarfism. Conversely, the child with hypogonadism is likely to grow less rapidly than

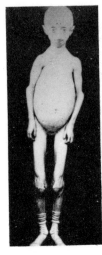

Fig. 8.1 Progeria. Girl aged 12 years, showing premature senile changes (facies, alopecia, wrinkled skin) associated with infantilism.

his normal contemporaries throughout later childhood, but since fusion of the epiphyses is delayed, growth may continue longer and his final height be actually greater than normal. (This does not apply to those cases of hypopituitary infantilism in which the growth factor is itself deficient.) *Progeria* stands in a somewhat peculiar position, since the syndrome combines features of infantilism, e.g. failure of sexual development, and of premature senility, e.g. baldness, wrinkled skin, senile facies and atherosclerosis (Fig. 8.1).   Birth before term is usually associated with small stature and retarded development and, although many children eventually catch up with their contemporaries, in extreme cases dwarfism is likely to be permanent. Growth-retarded children are often disproportionately small at birth, so that low-birth-weight dwarfism is a feature of many syndromes of congenital dwarfism and not a distinct clinical entity.

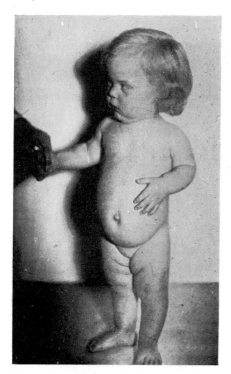

Fig. 8.2   Achondroplasia,   showing   disproportionate dwarfism due to shortness of legs.

Since many of the conditions included above are considered in more detail elsewhere, the present chapter is concerned primarily with illustrating the ways in which interference with growth and development may occur.

DWARFISM WITHOUT INFANTILISM

An excellent illustration of this is furnished by achondroplasia, in which small stature results from the extreme shortness of the legs and to a lesser extent from the lordosis by which it is accompanied. Development, apart from growth of the extremities, is normal or even advanced for

age, and sexual maturation occurs. In severe spinal disease with kyphosis, dwarfing is due principally to shortening of the trunk, though there may also be some general interference with growth. In the mucopolysaccharidoses and diastrophic dwarfism, dwarfing results from deformities of both spine and lower limbs, while this also applies to a varying extent to cases of severe nutritional rickets and fragilitas ossium with multiple fractures.

Dwarfism due to the late effects of precocious puberty is rare, though it is generally true that 'normal' individuals who reach puberty early will be larger than their contemporaries at this phase of their development and will subsequently be exceeded in height by those who mature later and in whom growth continues longer.

Congenital dwarfism is seen in chromosomal anomalies and in Russell's syndrome of low birth weight, triangular face small in relation to the head and other congenital abnormalities such as short incurved fifth finger, syndactyly and hypomandibulosis. Silver's syndrome is similar but with asymmetry in addition (p. 131).

Simple hereditary dwarfism requires no special consideration, since it cannot be regarded as pathological in the ordinary sense. It should be

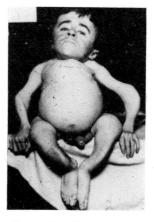

Fig. 8.3   Fragilitas ossium. Gross dwarfing due to multiple deformities without sexual infantilism. Boy aged 17 years.

distinguished, however, from those examples of racial or familial dwarfism in which the growth of a whole community or family is affected by the sharing of a common disease, e.g. parasitic infestation or malnutrition.

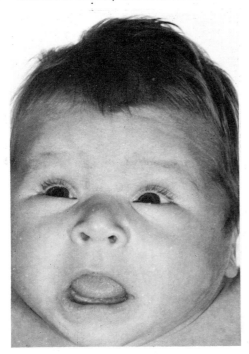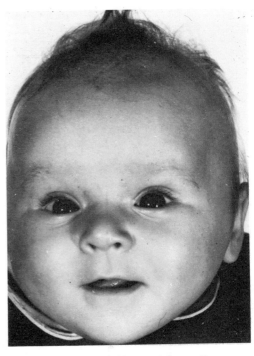

Fig. 8.4   Cretinism: (a) five-month-old female infant before treatment; (b) same infant at 7 months, after treatment.

DWARFISM ASSOCIATED WITH INFANTILISM

While all dwarfs are not examples of infantilism, all patients showing generalized infantilism, i.e. uniform delay in development, are necessarily dwarfed. (The example quoted of hypogonadal infantilism in which adult stature may be greater than normal represents a type of incomplete infantilism.) In 'perfect' infantilism the patient would show the exact physical, mental, and emotional development of a normal child of younger age. In practice, such uniform retardation is seldom seen. Thus in hypopituitary infantilism, in some examples of which a man of 50 may pass for a boy of 11 across the footlights, closer examination of the skin, fat-distribution, etc., will clearly show that the resemblance is only superficial. Mental development is often such as might be expected for age, whereas emotional development (which depends more on physical maturity) is likely to be retarded.

An example in which both physical and mental development are retarded is cretinism, though here again the cretin can readily be distinguished from a normal child of younger age.

Cretinism

The disease is endemic in those parts of the world in which there is widespread iodine deficiency with a high incidence of goitre, and where prophylaxis has not been effectively undertaken.

Endemic cretinism is commonly associated with *congenital goitre* and not infrequently with deaf-mutism, though congenital goitre may occur in endemic areas without the manifestations of cretinism being present. These goitres may be ectopic and cause pressure symptoms.

Non-endemic goitrous cretinism. Failure of synthesis of thyroxine may occur as a genetic defect, in some instances inherited as a mendelian recessive character. These cases are rare, and probably include at least four types of metabolic failure of synthesis, unrelated to iodine deficiency or thyroid aplasia. Goitre occurs as the result of increased production of thyrotropin, due in turn to deficiency of thyroxine.

Sporadic cretinism, which is the type most commonly seen in Britain, is the direct result of aplasia or hypoplasia of the thyroid gland. In most cases of sporadic cretinism there is no obvious cause for the thyroid hypoplasia, and a cretin may be born between two normal children.

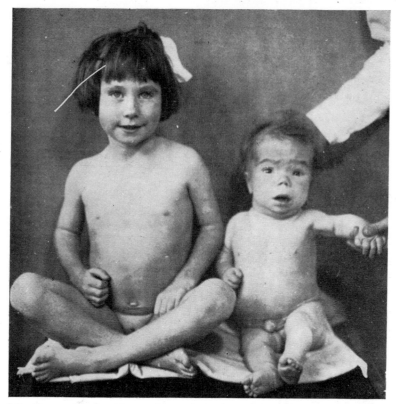

Fig. 8.5   Untreated cretin with normal control, showing facies, infantilism, and large umbilical hernia.

It is very rare for the mother herself to show evidence of hypothyroidism or other endocrine deficiency.

A distinction has been made between congenital and acquired aplasia or hypoplasia of the thyroid, but while it is possible for a thyroid which is normal at birth to be damaged by disease, e.g. autoimmune thyroiditis, the great majority of cretins must be classified as examples of congenital thyroid deficiency, differing in degree and the rapidity with which clinical manifestations become obvious. The term *juvenile myxoedema* is used when evidence of hypothyroidism only appears after a considerable period of normal development.

CLINICAL FEATURES. In sporadic cretinism, the manifestations of thyroid insufficiency are very seldom recognizable in the neonatal period and frequently the condition is not obvious until the sixth week of life or later.

The most striking features of severe cretinism are the retardation of growth, associated with delay in ossification, and a general slowing-down of metabolism, manifested by sluggish mental and physical reactions, constipation and slow pulse.

The facies shows a heavy, lethargic expression, yellowish pallor, wrinkled forehead, flat nose, and large protruding tongue. The hair-line is low on the forehead, and the eyelashes and outer third of the eyebrows may be sparse or absent. The hair may be luxuriant in the newborn period but typically becomes thin, dry, and lustreless. Palpation of the neck will usually demonstrate that the thyroid is hypoplastic or absent.

The abdomen is distended and an umbilical hernia is almost always present. The skin is dry, sallow, mottled and cold; perspiration is minimal. There are frequently myxoedematous pads above the clavicles.

In untreated patients developmental progress is delayed and in severe cases mental retardation is profound. The child shows delayed dentition and retains the infantile body proportions. The extremities are short, the head relatively large and the hands spatulate. There is failure of sexual development, or such development as occurs is very late in appearance and is incomplete (sexual infantilism). Amenorrhoea or lack of spermatogenesis is the rule in older patients.

Radiological examination will show dysgenesis of the epiphyses, and general delay in ossification, and in some cases will demonstrate deformity of the first or second lumbar vertebra giving rise to kyphosis.

Anaemia is almost constant, and is only likely to respond to thyroid therapy. The yellowish discoloration of the skin which may be present is due to an increase of carotene in the blood.

DIAGNOSIS. The fully developed condition is obvious, but early cretinism should be suspected if an infant is lethargic, feeds slowly, is constipated or has a hoarse cry. In addition to the clinical findings, radiology of the skeleton will confirm the retardation of development, e.g. delayed appearance of centres of ossification.

The blood cholesterol is often normal in early infancy but increases in the majority of untreated cases and may reach high levels, e.g. 400 to 600 mg per 100 ml. This falls under treatment.

A low level of protein-bound iodine (generally less than 2 μg per 100 ml) is the most sensitive indication of sporadic cretinism, but is of no value in the diagnosis of goitrous hypothyroidism. The latter may require investigation with radioactive iodine, ^{132}I having a limited value in determining the site of thyroid tissue when operation is contemplated and carrying little risk. ^{131}I is a more valuable research tool but should only be used under strictest control, and not for routine diagnosis, owing to the possible risk of future carcinogenesis.

TREATMENT. This consists essentially of replacement therapy with thyroxine which must be continued throughout life. Increase in the pulse-rate and symptoms of overdosage (irritability, loss of weight, and diarrhoea) on the one hand, and return of symptoms on the other, will usually serve to determine the optimum maintenance dosage and progress may be followed by plotting height periodically on a growth chart. Estimations of protein-bound iodine (normal 4 to 8 μg per 100 ml) and blood cholesterol may be used as a check if required.

The initial dosage of thyroxine necessary to correct symptoms will be greater than that required for maintenance. It is usually best in infants to start with a small dose, e.g. 0·025 mg

daily, increasing every two weeks by 0·025 mg until intolerance is indicated by tachycardia. The dosage is then reduced until the maintenance dose is reached. Since individual cases vary considerably in the amount of thyroxine required, dosage is necessarily determined by trial and error, but it is usually unnecessary to exceed 0·2 mg daily in simple hypothyroidism without primary mental subnormality.

PROGNOSIS. This depends on two factors: (1) the age at which treatment is commenced, and (2) the extent to which thyroid insufficiency retarded prenatal brain development. When the whole picture is dependent solely on postnatal hypothyroidism, the mental response is likely to be reasonably good. When there is mental defect of prenatal origin, however, the difference between the physical and mental response is very striking. Results, as regards both mental and physical development, are likely to be best when treatment is started early and continued without remission. Even under the most favourable circumstances, however, when the child's physical status virtually becomes normal, it is rather exceptional for the intelligence quotient to reach 100, while many children remain mentally subnormal.

Hypopituitary infantilism

True hypopituitary infantilism of any type is rare. Isolated deficiency of a hormone or any combination of deficiencies may occur. In panhypopituitarism all the hormones of the anterior pituitary will be deficient, including the growth hormone and the gonadotropic, thyrotropic and corticotropic hormones. The condition may be primary, dating from birth, occurring mainly in boys and occasionally showing a familial incidence; or secondary to tumour, infection, haemorrhage, or malnutrition. Some of the 'primary' cases may in fact be secondary to unrecognized perinatal anoxia. Isolated growth hormone deficiency may occur sporadically or may be inherited as an autosomal recessive.

Deficiency of growth hormone causes growth retardation, commonly though not invariably associated with failure of sexual development. Body length is usually normal at birth, since fetal growth is largely independent of growth hormone, but the slow rate of postnatal growth results in progressive divergence from the mean, the height eventually falling well below the normal range. The child is small and plump, with

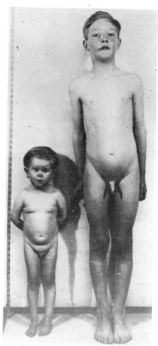

Fig. 8.6   Hypopituitary infantilism. Boy aged 7 years with normal control. Hypogenitalism and girdle distribution of fat.

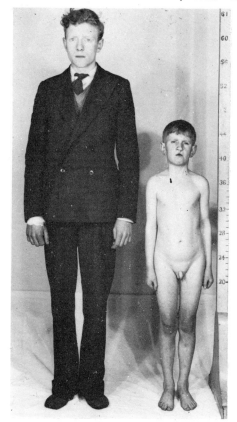

Fig. 8.7   Lorain infantilism. Boy aged 16 years with normal control.

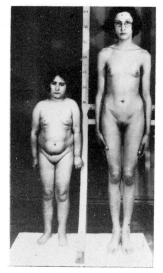

Fig. 8.8   Laurence-Moon-Biedl syndrome (forme fruste). Girl aged 13 years, showing obesity and infantilism, with normal control. Retinitis pigmentosa was present.

a round 'baby-like' face. Delayed appearance of centres of ossification and delayed fusion of epiphyses are the rule. Spontaneous attacks of hypoglycaemia may occur in early childhood. There is commonly some degree of associated thyrotropic hormone deficiency, with low levels of protein-bound iodine and in some cases clinical evidence of hypothyroidism. Obesity, when it occurs, is related to disturbance of the hypothalamus. The diagnosis of growth hormone deficiency depends on demonstrating low plasma levels by radioimmunoassay and by assessing the response to insulin-induced hypoglycaemia, when there is absence of the normal increase in plasma growth hormone. Rare cases have been reported of pituitary dwarfism with normal plasma levels of growth hormone, believed to be due to lack of end-organ response, although biological inactivity of the hormone is a possibility.

Various other clinical types of infantilism presumed to be due to hypopituitarism have been described in the past. In the Lorain type, the patient retains the slender habitus of childhood into adult life. The Laurence-Moon-Biedl syndrome is another rare clinical picture (p. 193).

Severe emotional and physical deprivation can sometimes simulate hypopituitarism.

Diabetes insipidus is occasionally associated with hypopituitary infantilism; in this condition the fluid intake and output of urine are grossly in excess of the normal but can be controlled by daily injections of pitressin.

TREATMENT. The treatment of hypopituitary infantilism has been extremely disappointing in the past, but human growth hormone (HGH) is now giving promising results, although it is unfortunately still in short supply. HGH produces a striking acceleration of growth, e.g. increasing from 3 up to 10 or more cm per year. In isolated growth hormone deficiency, hypogonadism is corrected by HGH, producing pubertal development and so distinguishing the hypogonadism from that due to gonadotropic hormone deficiency, which does not respond to HGH. Sexual maturation may occur spontaneously in isolated growth hormone deficiency, however, and it is therefore important to start treatment before puberty, so that a growth response is achieved before epiphyseal fusion occurs. Treatment should be continued until the end of childhood in order to achieve maximum height. The response to HGH may be reduced by the development of antibodies to the hormone.

When the condition is due to an intracranial tumour, surgical relief is sometimes possible, while in cases secondary to malnutrition the primary disturbance should be treated. In some idiopathic cases the deficiency is relative, and growth and sexual development occur spontaneously at a later stage than normal.

The treatment of gonadotropic hormone deficiency in the male by testosterone, and in the female by stilboestrol, will result in the appearance of secondary sexual characters and enlargement of the penis although not the testicles in the male, but will not correct the functional deficiency. Such treatment should not be undertaken until it is reasonably certain that sexual development will not occur spontaneously; fusion of the epiphyses under hormone treatment will prevent further growth in stature, although testosterone may cause a temporary acceleration of growth before fusion occurs.

Hypogonadal infantilism

Since the gonads have relatively little direct effect on growth until the onset of puberty, patients with primary hypogonadism (failure of development, atrophy or destruction from infection or trauma) may show little if any retardation of growth during infancy and childhood. The normal pubertal spurt of growth, however, will fail to occur and during the early teen ages patients are likely to be of smaller stature than their contemporaries, and show retarded ossification, and absence or incomplete development of secondary sexual characters. The terminal height of the male eunuch, however, may be greater than normal since growth continues longer; there is frequently associated deposition of fat around the hips. One type of primary ovarian agenesis is associated with webbing of the neck and increased carrying-angle at the elbow (*Turner's syndrome*). These patients have been shown to carry a single X chromosome instead of the XX of a normal female (XO). In boys, testicular hypoplasia may be associated with gynaecomastia, aspermatogenesis without a-Leydigism, and increased excretion of follicle-stimulating hormone (*Klinefelter's syndrome*). Some of these cases show a female chromatin pattern on

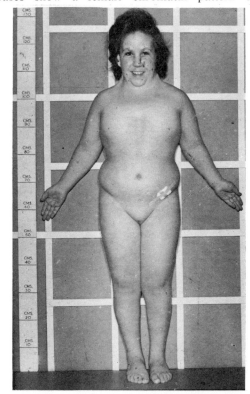

Fig. 8.9   Turner's syndrome showing webbing of neck, increased carrying-angle at elbow, absence of secondary sexual characters and dwarfism. (Patient aged 14 years.)

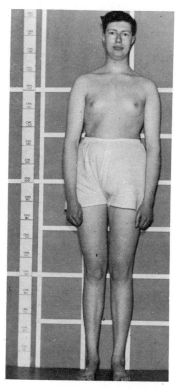

Fig. 8.10 Klinefelter's syndrome. Breast development in a youth aged 18 years with eunuchoid habitus and testicular failure. External genitalia were those of a male.

nuclear sexing, and carry XXY chromosomes, with a total of 47 chromosomes.

Infantilism due to other causes

Generalized infection will only cause infantilism when it acts over a sufficiently long period for retardation of growth to become manifest, e.g. malaria acquired in infancy or early childhood is liable to produce infantilism in which general physical development and onset of puberty are delayed, and adult stature affected.

Chronic disease of any essential organ sufficiently severe to impair function and acting over a sufficiently long period is liable to result in infantilism. The classical examples are *coeliac* (Fig. 8.12) and *renal infantilism* (Fig. 8.13). In untreated coeliac disease, delayed growth and development are constant features of the disease. Renal infantilism occurs in those cases of chronic nephritis or pyelonephritis in which there is severely impaired renal function with nitrogen retention, and also in cases of renal tubular insufficiency. The dwarfing of both coeliac and renal infantilism is often increased by the association of skeletal deformities (*coeliac* or *renal rickets*).

Other examples of infantilism due to disease of a single system are cardiac, cerebral, and pul-

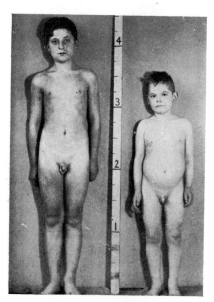

Fig. 8.11 Syphilitic infantilism. Patient on right aged 10½ years with normal control of same age on left. Proportions are those of early childhood.

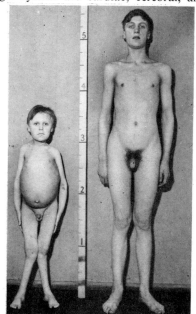

Fig. 8.12 Coeliac infantilism. Boy aged 16 years with normal control, showing dwarfing, immature facies and genitalia, large abdomen, and genu valgum.

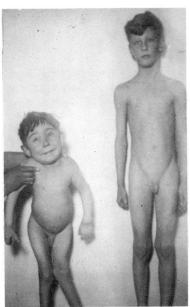

Fig. 8.13   Renal rickets and infantilism. Boy aged $9\frac{3}{4}$ years with normal control.

ary infantilism, though in none of these is the picture as well defined as in coeliac and renal disease. Congenital heart lesions, when sufficient to cause severe impairment of function, are very commonly responsible for failure of growth and development. True *hepatic infantilism* is extremely rare, since the regenerative capacity of the liver is such that hepatic function is seldom sufficiently impaired over a long period in childhood for retardation of growth to become manifest. Infantilism may be marked in hepatic glycogenosis, though here other factors than retention of glycogen in the liver and hypoglycaemia may be contributory.

Cerebral infantilism is often seen in cases of severe primary mental defect, microcephaly, etc., and although in some cases of extensive cerebral defect secondary sexual characters appear early rather than late, stature is usually significantly below the average and sexual function incompletely established.

LOCAL DWARFISM AND GIGANTISM

Various examples of failures of development and of local overgrowth occurring as congenital malformations have been considered in Chapter 5. Local dwarfism occurring as the result of birth injury is exemplified by hemiplegia; after birth,

paralysis, e.g. due to poliomyelitis, may result in defective development of the whole or part of a limb, and trauma or infection of epiphyses or growing bone is liable to have a similar effect.

Local gigantism developing after birth is considerably rarer than dwarfism. Progressive gigantism of a limb or other organ may result from anomalies of vascular supply, e.g. secondary to an extensive haemangioma, or from blockage of lymphatics in elephantiasis. Infections and neoplasms are rare causes.

The importance of both local dwarfism and gigantism lies in their interference with function. This is clearly seen when the lower limbs are of unequal length. Although minor degrees of congenital hemihypertrophy or atrophy may be successfully compensated for by tilting the pelvis without functional disability, gross shortening of one leg will require orthopaedic compensation if deformities of the spine are to be avoided.

GIGANTISM, PRECOCITY, AND VIRILISM

Statural overgrowth occurs as a racial or familial character, or as the result of endocrine dysfunction. In the latter event, it may be due to tumour and hypersecretion of a single gland; to

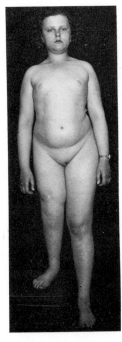

Fig. 8.14   Local dwarfism of right leg.

secondary effects on the pituitary from cerebral lesions (tumour or hydrocephalus); or to hyperplasia and hyperfunction of one or more glands without clear evidence of the primary cause. When over-secretion of the pituitary growth factor is primarily responsible, other hormones of the anterior pituitary group are frequently affected. The close interrelationship of the endocrine system is illustrated by the changes which occur at puberty, when endocrine balance is normally readjusted and when many of the symptoms of major endocrine disorders appear in miniature. Thus a rapid increase in growth, and enlargement of the nose, mandible, and extremities (pituitary growth factor), are associated with increased secretion of gonadotropic hormone, stimulating genital development; transient thyroid enlargement and tachycardia commonly occur (thyrotropic hormone); while the appearance of secondary sexual characters is evidence of increased activity of the adrenal cortex and gonads. In addition, obesity of girdle distribution is of common occurrence in both sexes, and breast-development in the female is often paralleled by some degree of gynaecomastia in boys.

Hyperpituitary gigantism

While the classical picture of acromegaly is essentially one of adult life, some of the features of the condition (e.g. enlargement of extremities, nose, and jaw) normally occur at puberty. When these physiological changes of puberty are exaggerated, and the rapid spurt of growth by which they are accompanied does not show the normal slowing-down during adolescence, a state of gigantism will result. The adult 'acromegalic giants' are those in whom the disorder has been operative before fusion of the epiphyses has made further growth in height impossible. It should be emphasized, however, that gigantism due to adenoma of the eosinophil cells of the anterior pituitary occurring during adolescence is very rare, and that in the great majority of cases in which rapid growth occurs during puberty the condition is self-limited by early fusion of the epiphyses.

Hypogonadal gigantism

While patients with primary hypogonadism will fail to show the normal spurt of growth associated with onset of puberty, growth will in some cases continue for a longer period than normal, owing to failure of fusion of the epiphyses.

Cerebral gigantism (*Sotos' syndrome*)

In this rare syndrome there is excessively rapid growth from infancy with moderate mental retardation, clumsy motor behaviour and sometimes epilepsy. The head is large and dolichocephalic, the palate high and arched and the eyes widely spaced. Bone age is usually advanced, with increased urinary excretion of 17-ketosteroids. There may be mildly acromegalic features but pituitary dysfunction has not been demonstrated. The disorder is possibly due to a congenital hypothalamic anomaly.

Precocious puberty (*Pubertas praecox; macrogenitosoma*)

It is often difficult to determine arbitrarily at how early an age onset of puberty should be considered pathological, since, particularly in girls, cases are encountered in which pubic hair followed by sexual development appears at 8 years or even earlier without other evidence of abnormality. In boys, examples of familial precocity have been described, e.g. at 5 or 8 years, which appeared to be genetically determined. Before the age of 8, however, onset of puberty may generally be considered pathological in either sex.

Precocious puberty is almost invariably associated with statural overgrowth and pre-

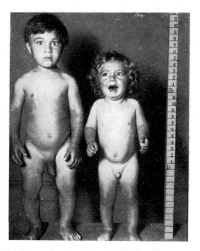

Fig. 8.15 Precocious puberty ('infant Hercules' type). Male infant aged 20 months, showing statural and genital overdevelopment and presence of pubic hair; with control of same age.

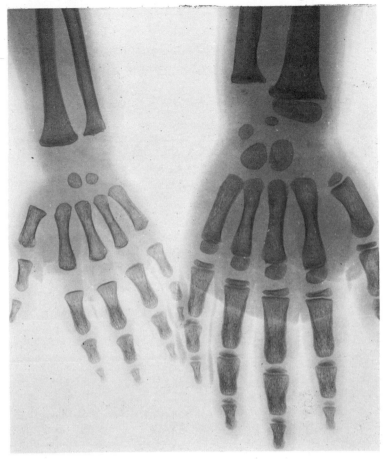

Fig. 8.16   Precocious puberty. Hand on right is that of patient shown in Fig. 8.15, with normal control of same age (18 months). Large size and advanced ossification.

cocious ossification. Cases may be divided clinically into those in which development is advanced but orderly, and the patient has the general appearance of a much older child; and those (males) in whom the precocity is associated with a remarkable degree of muscular development ('Infant Hercules' syndrome). These clinical types do not, however, correspond with a uniform pathology.

True precocious puberty, due to premature activation of the hypothalamic–pituitary–gonadal axis, is characterized by ovulation or spermatogenesis as well as the appearance of secondary sexual changes. The condition usually occurs sporadically, girls being affected more often than boys. In the majority of cases, especially in girls, no primary cause is demonstrable. Occasionally,

true precocious puberty is familial, when boys are more likely to be affected. In those cases in which it is possible to incriminate a primary lesion, a common cause is a glioma in the hypothalamic region. Hydrocephalus, encephalitis and tuberous sclerosis may all be accompanied by true precocity, presumably also by involvement of the hypothalamus. Destructive lesions of the pineal gland may cause sexual precocity, whereas the rare pinealoma is more likely to be associated with hypogonadism.

In pseudo-precocity, pubertal changes appear early but spermatogenesis or ovulation does not occur, and in the male the testes do not enlarge. The following causes may be recognized: (1) Hyperplasia or neoplasia of the adrenal cortex. In boys, these lesions will give rise to hirsuties

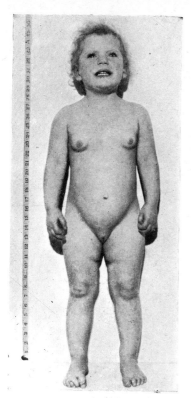

Fig. 8.17 Precocious puberty (menstruation and breast development in a girl aged 20 months). Ovary showed multiple small granulosa-cell cysts but no primary lesion.

treatment of precocious puberty are unsatisfactory.

Hermaphroditism, pseudohermaphroditism and virilism

In true *hermaphroditism*, testicular and ovarian tissues co-exist in the same individual (gonadal intersex). The infant usually has ambiguous external genital organs, while in the abdomen there will be a uterus and ovotestes or separate ovarian and testicular gonads. In the majority of cases, the karyotype is that of a normal female, though mosaicism is not uncommon.

Pseudohermaphroditism is much more frequently seen than true hermaphroditism and is generally due to congenital adrenal hyperplasia. Female pseudohermaphroditism is characterized by hypertrophy of the clitoris, which has the appearance of a hypospadic penis, and by fusion and rugosity of the labia majora which resemble a scrotum (virilism). The vaginal orifice may be patent or represented only by a dimple in the

and enlargement of the penis, while in girls they cause virilism (masculine changes). Congenital adrenal hyperplasia is the most frequent finding: carcinoma and adenoma of the adrenal cortex are rare at all ages. (2) Tumours of the gonads. Granulosa-cell tumours or dysgerminoma of the ovary and tumours of the Leydig cells of the testis are rare though possible causes of pseudo-precocity. Surgical removal may be followed by regression of signs.

Careful clinical examination, with estimation of urinary 17-ketosteroids and other laboratory tests as indicated, will generally serve to elucidate the etiology of sexual precocity. When no remediable cause is found, as will be the case in the majority of patients, management will be aimed at avoiding undesirable psychological effects of early pubertal changes, though these are often less troublesome than might be expected. In true precocity, there may be difficulties if spermatogenesis or ovulation is associated with corresponding libido, and there is a risk of pregnancy occurring. The results of hormonal

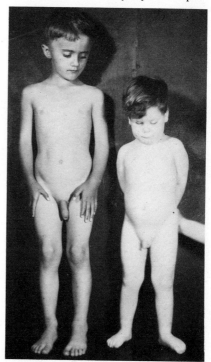

Fig. 8.18 Precocious puberty and statural overgrowth associated with hydrocephalus in a boy aged $3\frac{1}{2}$ years (with normal control). At 6 years pubic and axillary hair were present, and genital development was that of late adolescence.

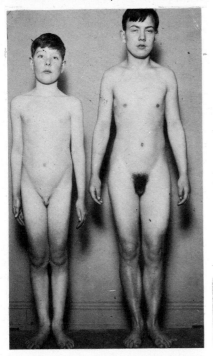

Fig. 8.19   Female pseudohermaphrodite (on right) aged 9 years with normal boy of same age. Masculine habitus and statural overgrowth; pubic hair had been present since age of 5 years. Patient had been brought up as a boy.

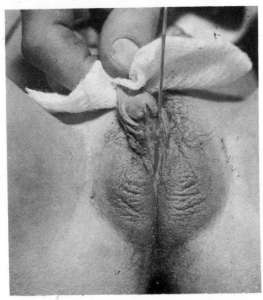

Fig. 8.20   Pseudohermaphroditism. Genitalia of patient shown in Fig. 8.19. The labia have fused to form a rugose 'scrotum' and the hypertrophied clitoris has the appearance of a penis with scrotal hypospadias. (Probe passed into urethra.)

perineum. The upper part of the vagina, uterus, and ovaries are normally present. The nuclear sex of female pseudohermaphrodites is female.

Male pseudohermaphroditism occurs in the syndrome of testicular feminization. This affects chromosomally normal males who develop as females because they are insensitive to androgenic hormones. The condition may be recognized in childhood when a testis is found during operation for inguinal hernia in a girl. In the complete form, the patient appears like a normal female and remains so after puberty. In the incomplete form, there may be partial response to androgens, causing enlargement of the clitoris during childhood. The testicular production of testosterone increases at puberty and may cause masculinization, with consequent psychological disturbance. It is therefore best to remove the gonads before puberty, giving replacement oestrogen therapy after adult height has been reached.

Congenital adrenal hyperplasia

This is due to deficiency of one of the enzymes (most commonly 21-hydroxylase) necessary for the synthesis of hydrocortisone. This results in excessive secretion of ACTH, hypertrophy of the adrenal cortex, and overproduction of adrenal androgens. The condition is an autosomal recessive and the sex incidence is equal. In mild cases, the male infant appears normal while the female shows virilism. More severely affected infants also develop *adrenal failure* during the neonatal period, characterized by salt loss, dehydration, hyperkalaemia, vomiting, and diarrhoea. While masculinization will indicate the diagnosis in the female, the condition may be unsuspected in the male until collapse occurs. Unless it is recognized and promptly treated with corticosteroid hormones, fluid and electrolytes, it is likely to be rapidly fatal. Maintenance therapy consists of giving cortisone to suppress abnormal adrenocortical function and to supply glucocorticoid, and desoxycorticosterone acetate or fludrocortisone to correct mineralocorticoid deficiency.

Patients who survive infancy are likely to show statural overgrowth, advanced skeletal development and an incomplete type of 'precocious puberty', i.e. growth of the penis without corresponding development of the testes in boys, and the appearance of body hair in both sexes. Excretion of 17-ketosteroids is raised to a greater extent than in true precocious puberty. Hypoaldosteronism, which occurs in salt-losing cases, is not found in the simple virilizing form. Rarely, adrenal hyperplasia is accompanied by hyperaldosteronism and consequent hypokalaemia.

When signs of virilism, which may include Cushing's syndrome, first appear in childhood, tumour of the adrenal cortex should be suspected. If this diagnosis is confirmed, operative removal is indicated.

Thyrotoxicosis (*Graves' disease*)

This condition occurs comparatively rarely before puberty, but has been described in early infancy and even at birth. Girls are affected

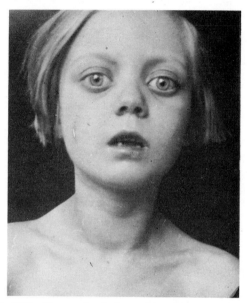

Fig. 8.21 Thyrotoxicosis in a girl aged 10 years. The patient is tall and thin and shows exophthalmos and thyroid enlargement.

considerably more frequently than boys. The condition is occasionally familial. Long-acting thyroid stimulating immunoglobulin (LATS) is frequently found in the plasma and thyroglobulin antibodies may also be present, suggesting that an autoimmune reaction may be involved. Various other contributory factors, physical, emotional and infective, have been suggested. The fact that many of these children are considerably above the average height for age and show advanced ossification suggests that the anterior pituitary may play a contributory role. Transient neonatal thyrotoxicosis in babies born to thyrotoxic mothers is probably due to passage

of LATS across the placenta. The symptoms of thyrotoxicosis are due to an excess of thyroid hormone.

CLINICAL FEATURES. Early symptoms include loss of weight despite increased appetite, tachycardia, sweating, irritability, and emotional lability. The appearance of thyroid enlargement and exophthalmos establishes the diagnosis. Evidence of tonsillar or other infection is frequently found. In advanced cases the wasting, fine tremor of the hands, and nervous symptoms, are very obvious. The pulse rate and systolic blood pressure are consistently raised, and the skin is hot and moist. Cardiac enlargement and murmurs may be present. Decreased glucose tolerance may cause glycosuria. The serum content of protein-bound iodine is above 8 μg per 100 ml.

DIFFERENTIAL DIAGNOSIS. Exophthalmos from other causes, e.g. acrocephaly, haemorrhage, sinus thrombosis, neoplasms, or xanthomatosis, is unlikely to be mistaken for thyrotoxicosis in the absence of thyroid enlargement and tachycardia.

TREATMENT. Patients should be given preliminary treatment with sedatives and bed-rest. Lugol's iodine may be given before subtotal thyroidectomy, if this is contemplated; in expert hands the operation has given good results, with low recurrence rates. Many authorities prefer to treat the condition with propyl thiouracil, e.g. 150 to 300 mg daily for a child of 10 years for three to four weeks, reducing the dosage as the pulse rate falls. A maintenance dose, or repeated courses, may have to be given for 12 or more months. As an alternative, carbimazole, 10 to 40 mg reducing to a daily maintenance dose of 5 to 15 mg, may be used. A proportion of cases relapse after one or more courses of therapy and surgery is then indicated.

Goitre

Thyroid enlargement at puberty is common, and is frequently associated with transient tachycardia and nervous symptoms. Since this does represent a temporary endocrine imbalance, the distinction from thyrotoxicosis is one of degree. The absence of exophthalmos and wasting, and the fact that the condition is closely associated with other pubertal changes, will confirm its physiological character.

Enlargement of the thyroid gland without evidence of thyrotoxicosis is not very uncommon during childhood, and is most often due to *Hashimoto's lymphocytic thyroiditis*. This auto-immune disorder develops insidiously at any age and predominantly affects girls. The thyroid is at first diffusely enlarged but later may become nodular and cause pressure symptoms. *Endemic goitre* (p. 160) has now been almost abolished in most temperate regions by iodine prophylaxis. *Carcinoma of the thyroid* is very rare in childhood and gives rise to a hard nodular tumour.

BIBLIOGRAPHY AND REFERENCES

ANDERSEN, H. J. (1961). Studies of hypothyroidism in children. *Acta paediatrica, Stockholm*, 50, suppl. 125.

BUTLER, L. J., SNODGRASS, G., FRANCE, N., RUSSELL, A. & SWAIN, V. (1969). True hermaphroditism or gonadal intersexuality. *Archives of Disease in Childhood*, 44, 666.

CLAYTON, B. E., EDWARDS, R. W. H. & RENWICK, A. G. C. (1963). Adrenal function in children. *Archives of Disease in Childhood*, 38, 49.

CLOUTIER, M. D. & HAYLES, A. B. (1970). Precocious puberty. *Advances in Pediatrics*, vol. 17. Chicago: Year Book Medical Publishers.

GILFORD, H. (1911). *The Disorders of Post-natal Growth and Development*. London: Adlard.

GROSS, R. E. (1940). Neoplasms producing endocrine disturbances in childhood. *American Journal of Diseases in Children*, 59, 579.

HAMILTON, W. (1972). *Clinical Paediatric Endocrinology*. London: Butterworths.

HAYLES, A. B., CARBALLO, E. C. & McCONAHEY, W. M. (1967). The treatment of hyperthyroidism in children. *Mayo Clinic Proceedings*, 42, 218.

HUBBLE, D. V. (1967). Growth hormone deficiencies in childhood. *Canadian Medical Association Journal*, 97, 1144.

HUTCHISON, J. H. & McGIRR, E. M. (1954). Hypothyroidism as an inborn error of metabolism. *Journal of Clinical Endocrinology*, 14, 869.

JOLLY, H. (1955). *Sexual Precocity*. Oxford: Blackwell.

KEAY, A. J., OLIVER, M. F. & BOYD, G. S. (1955). Progeria and atherosclerosis. *Archives of Disease in Childhood*, 30, 410.

KLINEFELTER, H. F., REIFENSTEIN, E. C. & ALBRIGHT, F. (1942). Syndrome characterized by gynecomastia, aspermato-genesis, etc. *Journal of Clinical Endocrinology*, 2, 615.

LAWSON, D. (1955). On the prognosis of cretinism. *Archives of Disease in Childhood*, 30, 75.

McKENDRICK, T. & NEWNS, G. H. (1965). Thyrotoxicosis in children: a follow-up study. *Archives of Disease in Childhood*, 40, 71.

NEW, M. I. (1968). Congenital adrenal hyperplasia. *Pediatric Clinics of North America*, 15, 395.

NEW, M. I. & PETERSON, R. E. (1968). Aldosterone in childhood, in *Advances in pediatrics*, vol. 15. Chicago: Year Book Medical Publishers.

RAITI, S. (1970). Testicular feminization syndrome. *British Journal of Hospital Medicine*, 3, 728.

SILVER, H. K. & FINKELSTEIN, M. (1967). Deprivation dwarfism. *Journal of Pediatrics*, 70, 317.

SMITH, D. W. (1967). Compendium on shortness of stature. *Journal of Pediatrics*, 70, 463.

SOYKA, L. F., BODE, H. H., CRAWFORD, J. D. & FLYNN, F. J. (1970). Long-term HGH therapy for short stature in children with growth hormone deficiency. *Journal of Clinical Endocrinology and Metabolism*, 30, 1.

TALBOT, N. B., SOBEL, E. H., McARTHUR, J. W. & CRAWFORD, J. D. (1952). *Functional Endocrinology from Birth through Adolescence*. Cambridge: Harvard University Press.

TANNER, J. M. & HAM, T. J. (1969). Low birth weight dwarfism with asymmetry (Silver's syndrome). *Archives of Disease in Childhood*, 44, 231.

TANNER, J. M., WHITEHOUSE, R. H., HUGHES, P. C. R. & VINCE, F. P. (1971). Effect of human growth hormone treatment. *Archives of Disease in Childhood*, 46, 745.

TURNER, H. H. (1938). A syndrome of infantilism, congenital webbed neck, and cubitus valgus. *Endocrinology*, 23, 566.

WILKINS, L. (1948). Abnormalities and variations of sexual development during childhood and adolescence, in *Advances in Pediatrics*, vol. 3. New York and London: Interscience Publishers.

WILKINS, L. (1965). *The Diagnosis and Treatment of Endocrine Disorders in Childhood and Adolescence*, 3rd edn. Springfield: Thomas.

WILKINS, L. (1962). Adrenal disorders. *Archives of Disease in Childhood*, 37, 1, 231.

9 Neoplastic Disease

The importance of neoplastic disease in infancy and childhood may be judged by the fact that this and accidents now represent the two major causes of death in Britain in the age-group 2 to 15 years. The proportion of children with neoplastic disease who survive has increased in recent years, owing to earlier diagnosis, more effective chemotherapy and improved surgical and radiotherapeutic techniques, but despite this the deaths from malignant disease are actually increasing in number. This cannot be attributed solely to improved diagnosis, e.g. of leukaemia, and the causes are not certainly understood. The hazards of increased irradiation, particularly that resulting from radiological techniques, are at present under review, and the need for reducing unnecessary exposure to a minimum has been emphasized.

The terms 'benign' and 'malignant' are used for convenience, and the distinction is not absolute. Thus pigmented naevi of the skin or polyposis of the rectum (both of which may be classified as congenital malformations) are commonly benign during early life, but may. in some cases become malignant later; papillomata and juvenile nasopharyngeal angiofibromata may be locally invasive but show little tendency to metastasize; while teratomata may behave as benign or malignant tumours in different instances. A number of the commoner benign tumours are considered elsewhere (see congenital malformation), and this chapter is primarily concerned with malignant or potentially malignant lesions.

Teratomata

A clear distinction can be made between the appendages which represent a second twin, and *teratomata* in which a variety of differentiated tissues or organs are found, but in which the arrangement of the tissues is less orderly and cannot be regarded as making up a second individual in miniature. Teratomata may occur in any site, but are most commonly seen in the sacral region (*sacrococcygeal tumour*, Fig. 9.1), testis, ovary, abdomen and cranium. They may be predominantly cystic or solid. X-ray will sometimes demonstrate the presence of enamel or bone within them. They are usually benign in

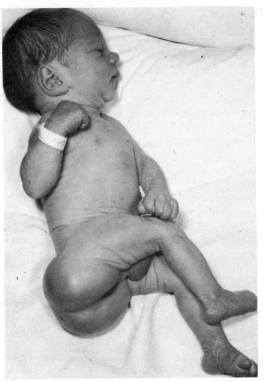

Fig. 9.1   Sacrococcygeal tumour in a newborn infant.

childhood, but may produce daughter tumours or undergo malignant change. Teratomata of the testis and ovary are particularly liable to do so, and it is thought that displacement of sex cells may account for the appearance of at least some teratomata occurring elsewhere. In the absence of malignant change, teratomata may be symptomless or cause local pressure symptoms, e.g. when they arise within the mediastinum. The nomenclature has been confused by the use of the term 'teratoid' to describe tumours arising from less differentiated fetal rests, and 'dermoid' to describe a variety of tumours and cysts in which ectodermal elements predominate. While some of the so-called dermoids are true teratomata, others are due to a disorder of fusion, e.g. dermoid cysts occurring at the margin of the eye, and others again to trauma, e.g. implantation dermoids.

MALIGNANT NEOPLASMS

Statistics relating to the incidence of malignant disease in infancy and childhood are not altogether satisfactory, owing to the different method of classification employed and the difficulties of accurate diagnosis in the absence of post-mortem examination or biopsy. With the exception of leukaemia and tumours of the central nervous system, any one type of malignant growth must be regarded as rare under the age of 15. But if all malignant neoplasms, including those of the haemopoietic and lymphatic tissues, are grouped together, an indication is given of the relative importance of neoplastic disease as a cause of death in childhood by comparing the deaths from this cause between 5 and 14 years with those due to certain other diseases in the same age period (Fig. 9.2). Despite the relatively low *incidence* of neoplastic disease in early life, it will be seen that the *mortality* from this cause is actually very much higher than from many other commoner diseases. This is attributable to the high malignancy, rapid dissemination, and poor response to treatment of many of the neoplasms encountered in childhood, and also possibly to the delay which often occurs in the recognition of growths which might prove amenable to treatment in their early stages.

TYPE

While malignant disease may affect any organ in childhood, the emphasis is quite different from that in adult life. Thus primary involvement of

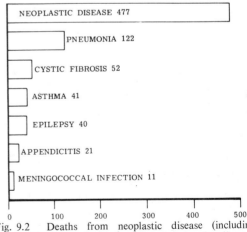

Fig. 9.2   Deaths from neoplastic disease (including leukaemia) compared with those from certain other diseases in children aged 5 to 14 years. England and Wales, 1969.

the lungs, gastrointestinal tract, breast, bladder, prostate or female genital tract is extremely rare in childhood, and carcinoma represents no more than 5 to 10 per cent of all cases. Many of the tumours are in fact embryonal neoplasms (as indicated by the term blastoma), and it is understandable that these will appear in early life.

In a series of 1580 malignant tumours in children collected by the Manchester Children's Tumour Registry (1971), representing all cases in a child population of about a million during a 15-year period, 464 (29 per cent) were leukaemia, 282 (17·8 per cent) were gliomas, 187 (11·8 per cent) were connective tissue tumours (including sarcomas), 115 (7·3 per cent) were sympathetic nervous tumours and 87 (5·5 per cent) were renal tumours. These proportions are typical of Britain but in other countries the pattern may be different. Thus in parts of Africa primary hepatoma and Burkitt's lymphoma are the common tumours of childhood. The latter is a malignant neoplasm commonly involving the jaw or orbit. It is endemic in certain areas of Africa, suggesting an environmental cause, possibly an arthropod-borne virus.

CONGENITAL NEOPLASTIC DISEASE

In addition to the sometimes-malignant teratomata referred to above, examples of malignant tumours of many organs (brain, kidney, retina, liver, bones, etc.) have been described as being present at birth, and in some cases metastases have occurred during intrauterine life. Three types of malignant tumour which characteristically occur in infancy may be regarded as 'congenital' in the sense that they arise from aberrant embryonal tissue which is already potentially malignant at birth. These three types are retinoblastoma, neuroblastoma and nephroblastoma.

Retinoblastoma

This is the only malignant tumour showing the association of a relatively high familial incidence, hereditary transmission, and over 5 per cent of cases recognizable at birth (by the characteristic light reflex). Approximately 80 per cent of cases are seen within the first four years of life. The tumour is thought to be due, in at least some cases, to an incompletely dominant mutant gene. The disease is liable to be bilateral, though clinical manifestations are often present in one

eye before the other is obviously affected. The characteristic early appearance is described as the 'amaurotic cat's eye'. Since the tumour grows forward into the vitreous, it gives rise to a creamy-yellow light reflex, while vision is obstructed and the pupil appears white and

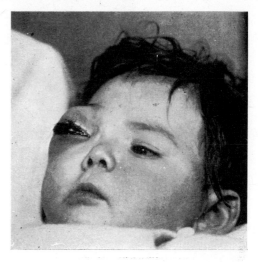

Fig. 9.3   Retinoblastoma. The globe has ruptured and the orbit is filled with fungating growth. Infant aged 7 months.

dilated. The tumour subsequently destroys the globe, producing a fungating mass filling the orbit, and grows backward, involving the optic nerve.

External radiation with the cobalt beam or early enucleation of the eye followed by radiation may save life, but it must be realized that the second eye may already be involved, or may become affected subsequently. Since the tumour is familial and heritable, the eyes of siblings of affected children and of the progeny of survivors should be examined repeatedly in early infancy. Appropriate genetic counselling should be given.

Neuroblastoma

These tumours of the adrenal medulla and sympathetic nervous tissue are also characteristically seen within the first four years of life, about one-third being recognized within the first six months. Metastasis occurs early and widely, especially to lymph nodes, liver and bones. Unfortunately, this has usually happened before the infant first comes under observation, and occasionally during intrauterine life. Frequently both adrenals are involved (Fig. 9.4), though it is sometimes impossible to determine whether this

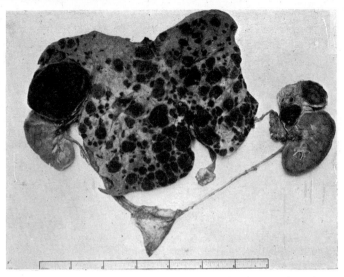

Fig. 9.4   Adrenal neuroblastoma, showing involvement of both adrenals and metastases in liver.

represents metastasis or whether the tumours are originally bilateral.

The original tumour may be small at the time of death or reach a very large size; it is highly vascular and histologically shows 'rosettes' which may be reproduced in the metastases. Occasionally calcification occurs in the tumour, which may be recognized radiologically.

Although the tumour is usually highly malignant, there is occasional regression under treatment even when widespread metastasis has occurred. Recovery after surgical removal followed by irradiation has been increasingly reported (principally in infants under one year of age, over half of whom may survive). The value of drug therapy (e.g. vincristine, cyclophosphamide) in addition is uncertain. Occasionally a malignant neuroblastoma will regress spontaneously to a more benign ganglioneuroma.

The features of neuroblastoma arising outside the adrenal medulla are essentially similar, though when they are extra-abdominal in origin, e.g. cervical or mediastinal, the local signs and symptoms will be influenced by their site.

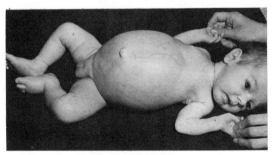

Fig. 9.6   Neuroblastoma presenting as a large intra-abdominal mass in early infancy.

The diagnosis should be suggested by the presence of a rapidly enlarging abdominal tumour in a young infant, and is too often confirmed by the presence of metastasis causing great enlargement of the liver or appearing clinically or radiologically in the bones or lungs. It is finally established by biopsy or aspiration of bone marrow. Since some of these tumours secrete catecholamines, the estimation of these in the urine may be helpful in diagnosis and in the assessment of treatment.

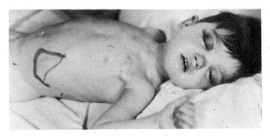

Fig. 9.5   Neuroblastoma in left loin, with exophthalmos and periorbital haemorrhage due to metastases in the skull. Child aged 2 years.

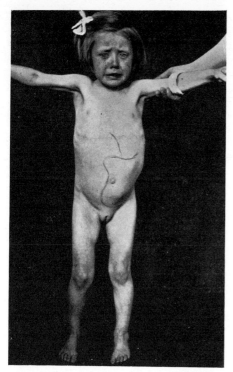

Fig. 9.7 Wilms' tumour filling left side of abdomen.

Nephroblastoma (*Wilms' tumour; embryoma of the kidney*)

This is the commonest kidney tumour occurring in infancy, the majority of cases appearing during the first three years of life and tumours having been observed at birth. It is rare for the first symptoms to occur after middle childhood. The tumours are commonly unilateral but may involve both kidneys simultaneously. Girls are affected twice as commonly as boys.

The tumour structure shows great variation, but the predominance of undifferentiated renal tissue is usually obvious. In many instances there will be areas of haemorrhage and cyst formation. The tumour often appears superficially to be encapsulated with the unaffected portion of the kidney stretched over part of its circumference.

A characteristic feature is the rapid growth and large size attained by the tumour before the general health of the infant is seriously impaired. It is common for the presenting sign to be the increasing size of the abdomen, or for the tumour to be felt by the mother or nurse. In other cases, haematuria or abdominal pain will be the first symptom noted, or the child may present with listlessness, failure to thrive and pyrexia.

The diagnosis will be suggested by the presence of a large, firm tumour in the kidney area, which may sometimes show radiological evidence of calcification. Intravenous pyelography will demonstrate the displacement and distortion of the renal pelvis, and while some dilatation of pelvis and calyces may be seen it will usually be obvious that the main tumour is not a hydronephrosis. The lungs should be X-rayed, since they are the most common site for metastases; the bones, liver, and lymph nodes may also be involved, or the tumour may spread via the renal veins.

Treatment consists of transperitoneal nephrectomy followed by irradiation, care being taken to reduce the risk of spread via the renal veins or ureter. The abdominal nodes should be examined at operation for evidence of metastasis, and dissected out if necessary. Although the likelihood of recurrence is still high, the prognosis has been considerably improved recently by earlier diagnosis, by more effective therapeutic techniques, and by reducing preoperative palpation of the tumour to a minimum. The administration of actinomycin D appears to render the tumour cells more sensitive to radiation: it may be given in combination with vincristine.

Hepatoblastoma (*Embryoma of the liver*)

This is rare, but is occasionally seen at birth or in early infancy. Like the other types of embryoma, it is highly malignant. Diagnosis from secondary metastasis, e.g. of a neuroblastoma, or from haemangioendothelioma, may only be possible on biopsy.

LEUKAEMIA, LYMPHOSARCOMA, AND HODGKIN'S DISEASE

Leukaemia

Although the cause of leukaemia is still unknown, the condition is regarded as neoplastic with proliferation of lymphatic cells giving rise to lymphosarcoma and lymphoblastic leukaemia, and myeloid cells producing myeloblastic leukaemia. It is a form of malignant disease with a definite and disturbing increase in incidence in infancy and childhood. In mongolism, the risk of leukaemia is increased twentyfold.

The disease may occur at any age, and has been described at birth and within the first two months, though it is seen most frequently between 2 and 5 years: it is more common in

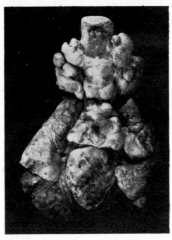

Fig. 9.8   Acute lymphoblastic leukaemia (boy aged 6 years), showing enlarged paratracheal nodes and thymus, and petechial haemorrhages over pericardium.

boys than in girls. The process may run an acute course characterized by the excessive production of primitive cells in the leucopoietic tissues (acute leukaemia), or a more chronic one with large numbers of more mature forms in the blood and blood-forming tissues. Acute lymphoblastic leukaemia is by far the commonest variety in childhood, with lymphoblastic proliferation in the marrow and immature lymphocytes in the peripheral blood. Anaemia and thrombocytopenia reflect the extent of marrow involvement, occurring almost invariably as the disease progresses. There is increased liability to infection as normal granulocytes are suppressed. Acute myeloblastic and monocytic leukaemia occur much less frequently in children, except in the first year of life: chronic leukaemia of any type is rare. In the undifferentiated form of acute leukaemia, the proliferating cells are so primitive as to make differentiation of cell type difficult, while the term aleukaemic is used in any variety when the total leucocyte count in the peripheral blood is not significantly raised.

SYMPTOMS. The presenting signs and symptoms vary widely, and the onset may be insidious or abrupt. Commonly the child will show well-marked pallor by the time he comes under observation, but the history will often indicate a preceding period of lassitude, dyspnoea, and anorexia. A history of preceding infection is also frequently given. Pains in the limbs or joints may be severe. In other cases, epistaxis or spontaneous haemorrhage from mucous membranes, stomatitis, spontaneous bruising or purpuric lesions may be the first indication of the disease. Occasionally enlargement of lymph nodes will be the first abnormality noticed.

SIGNS. In addition to pallor, ecchymoses, haemorrhage, and purpura, the patient will sooner or later show enlargement of the spleen and usually hepatic enlargement also. In the majority of cases, superficial lymph nodes are found to be enlarged, discrete, rubbery, and non-tender; in others, an X-ray of the chest will show enlargement of the mediastinal nodes before the superficial nodes are obviously affected. Dyspnoea from this cause may be marked.

X-rays of the long bones, especially in those cases where pains in the limbs have been a presenting symptom, may show rarefaction, particularly of the metaphyses; irregular osteosclerosis; or stripping-up of the periosteum due to leukaemic deposits beneath it.

During drug-induced remission, leukaemic meningeal infiltration may continue, giving rise to headache, vomiting, papilloedema and cranial nerve palsies, with numbers of primitive cells in the cerebrospinal fluid.

DIAGNOSIS. This can usually be made from examination of the peripheral blood, but should be confirmed by examination of the bone-marrow, obtained by iliac, vertebral or tibial puncture.

DIFFERENTIAL DIAGNOSIS. In infancy a large variety of noxious stimuli may produce very high leucocyte counts and the appearance of primitive cells in the peripheral circulation. The leukaemoid reaction to infection sometimes shown by infants can be distinguished from leukaemia by the variety of types of leucocyte present in the peripheral blood, and by marrow puncture.

In the early stage, pains in the limbs may simulate rheumatism or osteomyelitis, or haemorrhage may suggest thrombocytopenic purpura. Again the diagnosis will rest on blood and marrow examination. Occasionally it is necessary to examine the bone-marrow repeatedly in order to distinguish leukaemia from aplastic anaemia.

Glandular fever and infectious lymphocytosis, both virus infections producing lymph node enlargement, pyrexia and an abnormal blood picture, are very important in differential diagnosis.

The absence of anaemia and immature cells in the marrow and blood are reassuring findings in these conditions.

COURSE AND PROGNOSIS. Before modern chemotherapy became available, the average time from onset of symptoms to death was approximately three months in patients under 12 years of age. Chronic cases were exceptional and, although spontaneous remissions of short duration occasionally occurred even in acute cases, the outcome was invariably fatal.

Treatment has profoundly altered the duration of the disease, especially of acute lymphoblastic leukaemia, and survival for three or more years may be expected in a substantial proportion of cases. It is now believed that, in a small number of patients, complete cure may be possible by the eradication of all leukaemic cells.

TREATMENT. Before the child is subjected to treatment, the parents should clearly understand that the disease is a grave one which is likely to cause death and that the treatment carries the risk of serious side-effects. The aim of chemotherapy is first to induce a remission of the disease and then to prevent relapse. Drugs used to induce a remission are prednisone and vincristine, with the more toxic daunorubicin, cytosine arabinoside and L-asparaginase in reserve. For maintenance therapy, mercaptopurine, methotrexate and cyclophosphamide are commonly used. Drugs should be given in combination, usually at least three simultaneously, to induce remission and singly thereafter for maintenance treatment, during which there may be some advantage in changing the drug every two to three months.

As an example of a suitable regimen for acute lymphoblastic leukaemia, prednisone 2·5 mg per kg daily by mouth, vincristine 0·05 mg per kg weekly intravenously, and mercaptopurine 2·5 mg per kg daily by mouth may be used to induce a remission, which will usually occur within four weeks. Then mercaptopurine 2·5 mg per kg daily by mouth, alternating every two months with methotrexate 1·0 mg per kg twice weekly by mouth, is continued as long as the patient remains in remission. When relapse occurs, the drug in use is unlikely to be effective again but, after a further remission, a different drug may be used for maintenance. In this way, several remissions lasting for many months may be achieved, during which the child is well and shows no signs of leukaemia. Eventually, however, chemotherapy will fail to induce a remission and death then ensues.

During early induction, there is a risk of nephropathy from the massive release of uric acid from destroyed leukaemic cells. Fluids should therefore be given freely, the urine kept alkaline, and the serum uric acid level watched in order to institute treatment if necessary (see p. 204). Because there is a serious risk of infiltration of the central nervous system, some like to give a course of radiotherapy to the brain and spinal cord as soon as remission has been achieved; during the course, chemotherapy should be suspended. If signs of meningeal leukaemia develop later, methotrexate 0·5 mg per kg should be injected intrathecally at weekly intervals for three doses. This usually results in dramatic improvement for a while but recurrence is common.

At any time during treatment, infection may necessitate giving the appropriate antibiotic, blood transfusion may be required to correct anaemia, or haemorrhage may indicate the need for transfusion of fresh platelets to prevent further bleeding. Such supportive therapy has materially contributed to the improved prognosis in childhood leukaemia. In order to achieve the best results and to avoid the more serious toxic effects of chemotherapy, the treatment of leukaemia should normally be undertaken in centres having the requisite resources and experience.

Lymphosarcoma

Most authorities now recognize that lymphosarcoma and lymphoblastic leukaemia represent different manifestations of a lymphoproliferative process in which involvement of the marrow is reflected by a leukaemic picture in the peripheral blood. Histologically the lymph nodes are identical, and cases will be encountered which show at

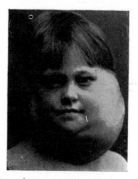

Fig. 9.9   Lymphosarcoma involving cervical nodes.

first the clinical picture of lymphosarcoma, with apparently normal peripheral blood, and subsequently show the typical leukaemic blood picture.

Any group or combination of lymph nodes may be involved, the cervical, mediastinal, and abdominal groups being the most commonly affected; however, it is often impossible to determine the original site of the sarcomatous process. As the disease progresses, the involvement of lymph nodes is likely to become generalized, and other organs (liver, heart, kidneys, skin, marrow, etc.) will be invaded.

Symptoms will depend on the principal site or sites of the disease. Pressure symptoms from mediastinal involvement will cause cardiac embarrassment or dyspnoea which is increased if pleural effusion occurs. Abdominal node involvement will result in palpable abdominal masses, which may simulate faecal scybala: later there will be intestinal obstruction, distension of the abdomen, and other local symptoms.

The child will suffer from rapidly increasing weakness, fatigue, and wasting, while enlargement of superficial lymph nodes, e.g. above the clavicle or in the axillae and groins, and hepato-splenomegaly, will become obvious.

PROGNOSIS AND TREATMENT. As in the case of leukaemia, the condition is ultimately fatal. Shrinkage of lymph nodes may be induced by therapy with corticosteroids and vincristine. Radiotherapy will sometimes be required for relief of mediastinal pressure and for reduction of splenic enlargement.

Hodgkin's disease (*Lymphadenoma*)

This disease is considerably less common than leukaemia in childhood, and is rare before the age of 5 years. Boys are affected approximately three times as frequently as girls, and there is a familial tendency. The lymphoid tissue shows a loss of normal structure and the presence of multinucleated giant cells and, later, an increasing degree of fibrosis. The liver, spleen, and bone marrow become involved and, finally, the lungs may show extensive deposits.

Clinically, the affected lymph nodes remain discrete and non-tender even when they have reached great size. The spleen is usually palpable relatively early in childhood cases, and may become enormously enlarged.

A characteristic temperature reaction (Pel-Ebstein) is sometimes seen, periodic high rises of temperature lasting one to three weeks being followed by periods of complete remission.

SYMPTOMS may be minimal in the early stages, and subsequently will depend on the pressure effects of the groups of nodes involved. Cachexia and haemorrhage are likely to occur in the later stages of the disease.

DIAGNOSIS rests on biopsy of an enlarged lymph node. The blood picture is not characteristic, though eosinophilia and polymorph leucocytosis are commonly present, and when there is extensive marrow involvement pancytopenia results. Tuberculosis must be excluded in making the diagnosis, and other causes of adenopathy (pyogenic infection, glandular fever, etc.) considered. The chest should always be X-rayed in view of the likelihood of mediastinal involvement.

PROGNOSIS AND TREATMENT. The disease is usually fatal, but the course is often prolonged and older children may survive two or more years after the diagnosis has been established. In the very early stages local irradiation of enlarged lymph nodes may effect a cure in a proportion of cases. In the later generalized stages chemotherapy with cyclophosphamide or nitrogen mustard may give temporary relief of symptoms.

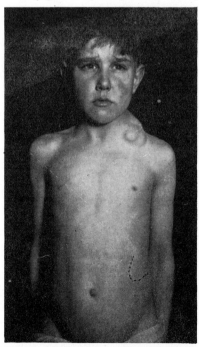

Fig. 9.10   Hodgkin's disease, showing enlargement of lymph nodes and spleen.

INTRACRANIAL TUMOURS

The great majority of intracranial tumours are gliomata, and of these the commonest types are the cerebellar astrocytoma and medulloblastoma, and ependymoblastoma of the fore-brain. Many other varieties of glioma, blood-vessel tumours, pinealomata, etc., are observed occasionally in young children. Of the intracranial neoplasms which are less common in childhood, the craniopharyngioma is perhaps the most frequently encountered.

SEX AND AGE INCIDENCE

While the sex incidence of intracranial tumours in general is approximately equal, medulloblastoma is three times more frequent in boys than in girls. Intracranial tumours occur at all ages of childhood but show a peak of incidence at the age of 4 to 5 years, largely owing to the frequency of medulloblastoma in boys of this age.

MALIGNANCY

Gliomata vary greatly in malignancy, from the most rapidly growing highly vascular type of medulloblastoma to the slow-growing astrocytoma. Medulloblastoma of rapid growth soon becomes disseminated by way of the cerebrospinal fluid, and metastases within the thecal, ventricular, and subarachnoid spaces are common; it should be noted, however, that the tumour is highly radiosensitive. The astrocytoma of childhood is a relatively benign, well-demarcated tumour of slow growth, though its mechanical effects may be accelerated by cyst formation. Complete surgical removal may be possible.

The ependymoblastoma is of much less rapid growth than the medulloblastoma, but it also tends to dissemination through cerebrospinal fluid spaces. It, too, is radiosensitive.

SITE

Approximately two-thirds of the intracranial tumours observed in childhood are subtentorial. The astrocytoma and medulloblastoma, and also the ependymoblastoma of the cerebellum, tend to occur in or near the vermis. The ependymoblastomata of the fore-brain are widely distributed, though an origin near the wall of one of the ventricular spaces is commonly observed. Of all intracranial tumours occurring in children,

less than 20 per cent are likely to be found in the cerebral hemisphere.

CLINICAL SIGNS AND SYMPTOMS. The clinical picture presented by a space-occupying lesion within the skull is modified in infancy by the readiness with which the sutures separate in response to raised intracranial pressure. Thus a tumour may have attained large size before either cerebral vomiting or papilloedema becomes manifest, and unless the gradual enlargement of the skull or bulging of the fontanelle has been recognized, the history in infancy is disproportionately short.

In older children, although the sutures will still separate more readily than in adult life, evidence of raised intracranial pressure and localizing signs are likely to appear earlier. Since the majority of tumours are subtentorial, papilloedema is usually an early sign, though it may be necessary to examine the discs at intervals to detect the earliest changes. The association of headache and vomiting unrelated to meals should always raise the suspicion of intracranial tumour, while the occurrence of fits without other cause, particularly in a child over 18 months of age, is another suggestive sign.

In the case of cerebellar tumours, the early appearance of ataxia, unsteadiness of posture, and nystagmus will be valuable evidence of subtentorial tumour, but it must be remembered that these signs may be produced by raised intracranial pressure alone if this has been sufficient to cause herniation of the cerebellum into the foramen magnum. The order of appearance of symptoms (e.g. whether ataxia appears before or after headache and vomiting) is therefore likely to be significant.

In young children, and particularly in those who are still learning to walk securely, the interpretation of ataxia may be a matter of considerable difficulty. Since there is a wide variation in the normal age of walking and running, and in physical dexterity generally during early childhood, careful observation and enquiry are necessary to elicit the onset of ataxia when this occurs before the age of 5. The child may simply have been regarded as backward or clumsy if a normal skill has not been attained. When, however, the child has definitely regressed and a skill has been lost, it is usually easier to determine the time of onset. The gradual appearance of a hemiparesis is also liable to be masked in early childhood, and at first confused with right- or left-handedness or clumsiness; it will become more obvious, however, when dragging of the affected leg is recognizable. Similarly the attribution of such symptoms to trauma should be accepted with caution, since either ataxia or hemiparesis are themselves likely to result in frequent falls. It is obviously necessary to distinguish a disability that has been present from birth and represents a congenital cerebral palsy from one that has appeared later and may indicate the growth of a tumour.

Homonymous hemianopia again is much more readily detected in older children, but may sometimes be recognized in younger children and even in infants; the nurse may, for instance, find that the infant consistently fails to notice her approach when she reaches the cot from one particular side.

It is often found that the clinical picture changes rapidly, either due to obstruction of the ventricular system with rapid production of internal hydrocephalus, or in the case of rapidly invasive tumours, owing to haemorrhage within the tumour.

Cranial nerve palsies may be of localizing value, but here again they may be produced by raised intracranial pressure without indicating local disease; this is particularly true of sixth nerve palsies.

Raised intracranial pressure will also sometimes cause a general expansion of the sella turcica, or evidence of dysfunction of the pituitary or hypothalamus, without necessarily indicating a local lesion in these areas. Radiological evidence of erosion of the clinoid processes is more valuable in this respect. As intracranial pressure increases, it will be associated with increasing papilloedema or optic atrophy, stupor, and cranial enlargement. The temperature may be irregularly raised, particularly when the mid-brain and medulla are affected. The pulse is likely to become slow, and respiration irregular. A bruit over the sinuses may be heard, but is not of diagnostic significance in infancy.

Pituitary tumours, usually cystic, are liable to produce infantilism, obesity or cachexia, diabetes insipidus, and bitemporal hemianopia from pressure on the optic chiasma. As already indicated, however, some at least of these symptoms may occur in the absence of pituitary tumour, due to ventricular distension and particularly to distension of the third ventricle from any cause.

While the history and clinical examination alone will sometimes give a strong indication of the nature and site of an intracranial tumour (e.g. whether the tumour is likely to prove a slow-growing astrocytoma or a highly malignant medulloblastoma), ancillary aids to diagnosis will always be required in order to attain such accuracy in diagnosis as to permit effective treatment.

RADIOGRAPHIC EXAMINATION of the skull, using stereoscopic technique, may reveal separation of the sutures, areas of local erosion (e.g. of the clinoids), pressure markings, or increased vascularity, though the last two must be interpreted with great caution. It is rare to see calcification of a tumour in childhood, though this occasionally occurs in ependymoblastoma of the fore-brain at this age. The much rarer craniopharyngioma, however, shows recognizable calcified structures in about 50 per cent of cases. The pineal becomes calcified in a small proportion of normal children, without the calcification being of pathological significance.

VENTRICULOGRAPHY. Direct filling of the ventricles with air, and subsequent radiography, is of great value in the localization of tumours, but should only be carried out in a neurosurgical clinic. Ventriculography is only used as an immediate preliminary to operation for effective relief of pressure. In other circumstances it is dangerous.

AIR-ENCEPHALOGRAPHY. This is used in the investigation of children who show cerebral symptoms in the absence of increased intracranial pressure and in whom it may be desirable to investigate the gross anatomy of the brain, e.g. for general or local atrophic changes, or porencephalic cysts. Air is introduced by the lumbar route, and the patient then X-rayed.

CEREBRAL ANGIOGRAPHY. The injection of radio-opaque substances into the carotid artery, followed by immediate radiography, may show distortion or abnormality of the vessels in the area of the tumour, and confirm its localization, while congenital aneurysms and cirsoid formations may be demonstrated by this means.

ELECTROENCEPHALOGRAPHY is mainly useful in confirming and defining varieties of epilepsy, in assessing the effectiveness of varieties and dosage of antiepileptic drugs, and in the localization of pathologically affected areas in the brain.

LUMBAR PUNCTURE is necessary in doubtful cases to exclude infective processes such as meningitis or encephalitis, but must be undertaken with the utmost caution, using a fine needle and withdrawing fluid very slowly and in small amount. The danger of producing a pressure cone and respiratory failure is a very real one, and if a subtentorial tumour is suspected it is best to wait until fluid has been withdrawn from the ventricles and intracranial pressure relieved. In cases of cerebral tumour, the cerebrospinal fluid may be normal, or show a raised protein content; the more malignant tumours may show some lymphocytosis, e.g. 10 to 40 cells per mm³.

DIFFERENTIAL DIAGNOSIS. A great variety of conditions may simulate intracranial tumour in childhood, and only those which cannot be readily distinguished by examination of the cerebrospinal fluid will be mentioned.

Hydrocephalus

Hydrocephalus due to other causes than tumour can usually be demonstrated by ventriculography, while a careful history may point to the primary cause, e.g. previous meningitis or cerebral haemorrhage.

Cerebral abscess

Unless cerebral abscess is the result of cyanotic heart disease, there is likely to be a history of previous infection, e.g. an aural discharge which has dried up before the onset of symptoms, or existing bronchiectasis. Since the type of cerebral abscess likely to be confused with tumour is the chronic encapsulated abscess, both temperature and blood examination are normal and are of little help in differential diagnosis. The cerebrospinal fluid may show an increase in protein and cell content, though it will be sterile unless meningeal involvement has occurred.

Vascular lesions

Cerebral haemorrhage may derive from such various causes as birth injury, sinus thrombosis, septicaemia, and pertussis, but in all these instances the onset is more abrupt than that of tumours. Chronic subdural haematoma is most likely to be seen in early infancy, as the result of birth injury, when tumours are of great rarity. When it occurs in later childhood, there is usually a clear history of trauma. Exploratory aspiration may be necessary to establish the diagnosis. In cases of recent subarachnoid haemorrhage, the cerebrospinal fluid will be blood-stained or xanthochromic. Spontaneous subarachnoid haemorrhage in children occurs occasionally from the more malignant tumours, and rarely from the rupture of congenital aneurysm or congenital arteriovenous varices.

Heredo-degenerative cerebral conditions

With or without epilepsy as a symptom, these will not be associated with the clinical picture of raised intracranial pressure, though optic atrophy may occur.

Tuberculoma

The differential diagnosis of tuberculoma from neoplasm is based largely on evidence of tuberculous lesions elsewhere in the body, and on examination of the cerebrospinal fluid, which is apt to show a higher protein content and cell count than are associated with neoplastic tumours. The tuberculin test will be of the same value as in the case of tuberculous lesions elsewhere.

TREATMENT AND PROGNOSIS. Both will obviously depend on the nature and site of the tumour. The cerebellar astrocytoma is one of the most favourable of all intracranial tumours for surgical treatment, provided that this is undertaken before vision has been permanently damaged. Cure without any residual defects is the rule, since, being subtentorial, the tumour removal carries little risk of postoperative epilepsy, while in young patients it is exceptional for any recognizable cerebellar dysfunction to persist.

The prognosis in cerebellar medulloblastoma is very much less favourable, but is not necessarily hopeless. Recent treatment has included decompression, securing material for biopsy or carrying out a partial removal, and treating the whole cerebrospinal axis in a single course with X-ray. Some patients have already survived for four or five years without further symptoms. Ependymoblastoma is treated in the same manner as medulloblastoma, with a somewhat more secure prognosis.

SPINAL CORD TUMOURS

With the exception of metastases from intracranial medulloblastomata and secondary involvement of the cord in Hodgkin's disease or mediastinal growth, tumours of the spinal cord are rare in childhood. Occasionally primary gliomata arise in the cord, and when they do so, are usually highly malignant. Extradural tumours involving the cord or causing spinal blocking include sarcomata, neurofibromata, and lipomata. Cysts within the spinal canal may also be responsible for pressure symptoms.

SYMPTOMS AND SIGNS. These will depend on the site of the lesion, but when the tumour is extramedullary, pain is likely to be an early and severe symptom from involvement of nerve roots. Later symptoms include weakness or spasticity of the lower limbs, anaesthesia, and, finally, incontinence of urine.

DIAGNOSIS. Radiological examination may show local bony changes in the vertebrae, while injection of radio-opaque substances into the canal will help to confirm the exact location of the tumour. Lumbar puncture in cases in which there is spinal blocking often reveals xanthochromic cerebrospinal fluid under reduced pressure, having a very high protein content.

TREATMENT is surgical if there is no evidence of metastasis, the subsequent employment of radiotherapy depending on whether the tumour is radiosensitive.

INTRATHORACIC TUMOURS

With the exception of lymphosarcoma and Hodgkin's disease, both of which may arise in the mediastinal lymph nodes, primary intrathoracic tumours are seldom highly malignant.

Bronchogenic carcinoma

This is extremely rare in childhood.

Sarcomata

Sarcomata arising from the lung or pleura occur only occasionally. In the latter case, the diagnosis may be indicated by the finding of malignant cells in the pleural exudate (Fig. 9.11).

Neurogenic tumours

Neurogenic tumours of the mediastinum (ganglioneuroma, neurofibroma, etc.) are usually of slow growth, though highly malignant neuroblastomata may also occur in this area. Since the prospects of successful surgical removal of slowgrowing tumours are reasonably good if the diagnosis is made early, they should be borne in mind as possible causes of intrathoracic pressure

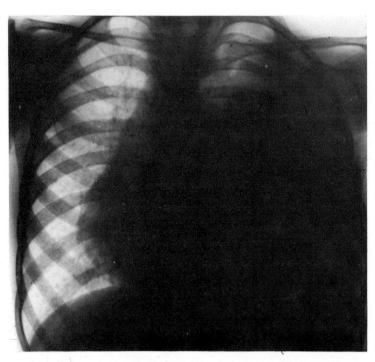

Fig. 9.11   Small spindle-celled sarcoma of lung. Boy aged 3½ years. The tumour presented in the interlobar fissure and was associated with a blood-stained pleural effusion containing tumour cells. Patient was in good general health 18 months after surgical removal followed by irradiation.

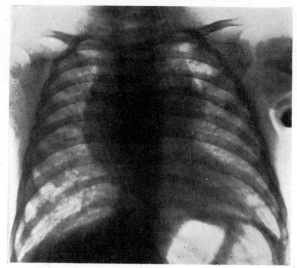

Fig. 9.12   Lymphosarcoma of thymus in an infant aged 9 months. Acute dyspnoea occurred four days before death, the infant having previously appeared well.

symptoms. Radiologically the tumours have a well-demarcated, rounded outline. Their nature may be suspected if they lie in the posterior mediastinum or posterior part of the upper mediastinum, since thymic tumours are situated anteriorly and mediastinal cysts are likely to lie in close proximity to the trachea (usually in the angle between the trachea and the right main bronchus). Although relatively benign, they are ultimately likely to prove fatal unless completely removed.

Teratomata

These may also occur within the mediastinum, but are usually situated anteriorly. They may remain unchanged for long periods or undergo malignant change at any age.

Thymic tumours

Thymic enlargement is frequently mis-diagnosed in infancy, partly owing to failure to recognize the normal radiological variations in size of the upper mediastinal shadow which may occur during crying, and partly to misconceptions as to the normal size of the thymus in infants dying suddenly from any cause. The gland is occasionally involved in lymphatic leukaemia, lymphosarcoma, and Hodgkin's disease, and may attain very large size. Primary malignant tumours of the thymus (thymoma) are rare, but may be associated with myasthenia gravis.

Metastases

Neuroblastoma occasionally metastasizes in the lung, and should be suspected as the primary tumour in infancy when the bones and liver are also involved. Wilms' tumours, osteogenic neoplasms, etc., also give rise to pulmonary metastases, which appear as rounded solid opacities. The presence of a primary tumour elsewhere will indicate the nature of the metastasis.

TUMOURS OF THE UPPER RESPIRATORY TRACT

Nasopharyngeal fibroma

This condition, which affects boys usually about the time of puberty, is not a true tumour according to pathological definition, but can be described as locally malignant; it does not metastasize, but constantly recurs after surgical removal. It gives rise to unilateral nasal obstruction, frequently associated with haemorrhage. It is radiosensitive, and tends to regress spontaneously in late adolescence.

Larynx

Various types of tumour of the larynx have been described, any one of which may give rise to hoarseness or stridor. *Papilloma* of the larynx, though rare, is of some importance, as it is locally malignant and tends to recur after removal.

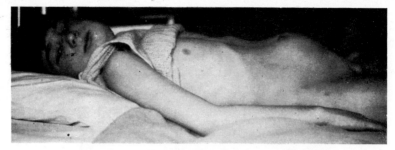

Fig. 9.13   Lymphosarcoma arising from ileo-caecal region, showing deformity of abdomen,
Symptoms were minimal until tumour had attained large size. Boy aged 9 years.

ABDOMINAL AND GONADAL TUMOURS

The most common malignant abdominal tumours in infancy and early childhood are neuroblastoma and Wilms' tumour. The abdominal lymph nodes are likely to be involved in lymphosarcoma, leukaemia, and Hodgkin's disease. Since retroperitoneal and other lymphosarcomata are likely to have extended widely before the diagnosis is made, it is not always easy to define the site of origin, which is usually from the retroperitoneal nodes and more rarely from the intestine (Fig. 9.13). The patient often comes under observation on account of the tumour mass, which is readily palpable and may distort the contour of the abdomen. Pain is not usually an early symptom, though it will occur sooner or later and be associated with cachexia.

Phaeochromocytoma (*Paraganglioneuroma*)

This is a rare tumour arising from chromaffin tissue, either of the adrenal medulla or elsewhere. It gives rise to hypertension, which may be paroxysmal or steadily progressive, associated with headache, fatigue, and, in some cases, convulsions. Since there is abnormal production of adrenaline and noradrenaline, the effect of phentolamine in temporarily lowering the blood pressure should be used as a diagnostic test. It may be possible to localize the tumour by radiological techniques and the diagnosis should be confirmed by measuring the metabolites of adrenaline and noradrenaline in the urine.

Although these tumours are rare in childhood, they should be remembered as a possible cause of unexplained hypertension. They can be removed surgically, though operation carries a considerable risk.

Adrenal cortex

Tumours of the adrenal cortex, e.g. carcinoma, are a rare cause of the adrenogenital syndrome, in which hirsuties, hypertension, and virilism may be associated with obesity (p. 217).

Pancreas

Malignant tumours of the pancreas are extremely rare in childhood. Benign adenomata of the islets of Langerhans occasionally occur even in infancy, giving rise to spontaneous hypoglycaemic attacks from overproduction of insulin. Surgical removal results in relief of symptoms.

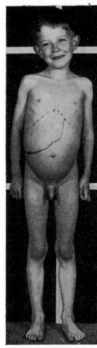

Fig. 9.14   Malignant hepatoma, filling right upper quadrant of abdomen. Diagnosis confirmed by biopsy. Boy aged 8 years.

Liver and spleen

The liver and spleen are rarely the site of primary malignant disease, but both are frequently involved secondarily, e.g. in lymphosarcoma, leukaemia, Hodgkin's disease, neuroblastoma. Carcinoma of the liver is extremely rare before puberty in Great Britain, but has a higher incidence in some countries where there is widespread malnutrition. In the case of malignant hepatoma illustrated in Figure 9.14, the tumour had given rise to no symptoms other than abdominal enlargement and transient abdominal discomfort occurring a week before the date of examination, at which time the tumour mass filled the right upper quadrant of the abdomen.

Testes

The most important malignant growth of the testis is the seminoma, a type of carcinoma which may affect an undescended testis and present as an intra-abdominal tumour, or arise within the scrotum. There is slow and usually painless enlargement of the affected testis and, while the inguinal nodes are not enlarged, metastases in the abdominal lymph nodes, lungs, or elsewhere occur early. Treatment is by surgical removal and radiotherapy. If the diagnosis is made early, there is a good prospect of recovery.

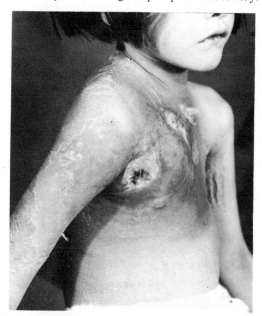

Fig. 9.15   Liposarcoma arising in axilla. The swelling had at first been thought to be inflammatory and had been incised before child's admission to hospital.

Teratoma of the testis is usually of slow growth and should be regarded as potentially malignant, though the prognosis following early removal is better in infancy and childhood than in adult life.

Tumours of the Leydig cells of the testis are likely to produce signs of virilization which usually regress after surgical removal of the tumour.

Ovaries

Tumours of the ovary are rare in infancy and childhood. They include teratoma (p. 221); dysgerminoma, occasionally associated with signs of precocious puberty, which is malignant but which may in some cases be successfully removed; lymphosarcoma; carcinoma; and granulosa-cell tumour, which also produces signs of precocious puberty. Ovarian tumours commonly present when torsion causes abdominal pain and a palpable mass.

Vagina

A rare tumour, sarcoma botryoides, occasionally arises from the vaginal wall in female infants, protruding as grape-like clusters of cysts from the vulva and invading the bladder. Response to surgical treatment and radiotherapy is poor.

TUMOURS OF SOFT SOMATIC TISSUES

Since no single type of tumour except the benign lipoma is at all common in the soft tissues, it will suffice that the possibility of malignant growth should be kept in mind in the differential diagnosis of any swelling for which no satisfactory explanation can be found. This is particularly the case when the swelling tends to spread or disseminate. Examples are liposarcoma, myxosarcoma, and rhabdomyosarcoma.

The superficial *neurofibromata* occurring in association with *café-au-lait* spots in von Recklinghausen's disease are sometimes classified as congenital malformations, but may become malignant at any age.

Keloid

It is relatively common for the skin of children who have suffered from extensive burns, trauma, or operation, to form an excessive amount of scar tissue. Excision is apt to be followed by recurrence. The condition is unsightly and sometimes painful, but is self-limited. Keloid should not be regarded as a true neoplasm, though it has some neoplastic characters. There appears to be an individual tendency to its development.

TUMOURS OF BONE

Exostoses and enchondromata

Exostoses and enchondromata, which may be single or multiple, have been considered as congenital malformations, though it should be emphasized that they may continue to enlarge during childhood and cause increasing disability. Both are typically benign, though occasionally malignant changes occur.

Osteogenic sarcoma

Since this is the most highly malignant of bone tumours, early diagnosis is essential in preventing a fatal outcome. The presenting symptoms are commonly severe pain and swelling, and it will often be found that patients have been treated for rheumatism, the effects of trauma, or osteomyelitis, before the true nature of the condition is recognized. The commonest sites of the tumour are the lower end of the femur or upper end of the tibia, usually the metaphysis.

X-ray examination will show expansion, sclerosis, or radiating spicules of bone at the site of the swelling; the appearance may be diagnostic, but it is sometimes difficult to distinguish from a localized low-grade osteomyelitis. Aspiration or biopsy should always be used to confirm the diagnosis. Since these tumours are radio-insensitive, early amputation will be necessary. If metastases have occurred, the condition will prove fatal.

Chondrosarcoma

Also highly malignant, the diagnosis and treatment are carried out in the same manner as in the case of osteogenic sarcoma. These tumours, which are rare, occur in the pelvis and at the ends of the long bones.

Ewing's tumour

This tumour, which arises from the reticulo-endothelial system, occurs characteristically in childhood and adolescence, and usually affects the shaft of the femur or tibia. It may remain localized for many months, but metastases occur in the later stages.

The presenting symptoms are local pain,

tenderness and swelling; the temperature may be elevated and the leucocyte count raised, though the elevation is less than in cases of osteomyelitis. The characteristic X-ray picture shows expansion with successive depositions of subperiosteal bone, giving an 'onion-peel' appearance.

Although these tumours are radiosensitive, irradiation cannot be relied on for cure; the results of amputation, or irradiation followed by resection and chemotherapy with vincristine and cyclophosphamide, are disappointing and survival rates are only about 10 per cent.

Multiple myeloma

Arising in the marrow and affecting any of the bones, including the skull, it is rare in childhood. The radiological picture is characteristic and shows widespread areas of rarefaction. Spontaneous fractures may occur. The condition is fatal, although irradiation may cause temporary remission of symptoms.

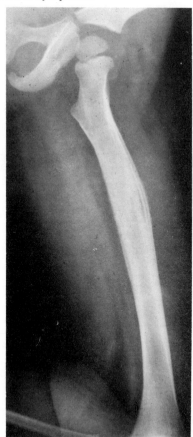

Fig. 9.16   Ewing's tumour of femur showing 'onion-peel' appearance.

Secondary metastases in bone

Of the tumours occurring in infancy and child-hood, neuroblastoma is the one which most commonly metastasizes in the skeleton. Since the metastases are radiosensitive, they may be mistaken for Ewing's sarcoma unless the primary tumour is recognized. Hodgkin's disease, leukaemia, and lymphosarcoma may also involve the skeleton.

DIFFERENTIAL DIAGNOSIS. The conditions most likely to simulate a malignant bony tumour are osteomyelitis and tuberculosis. Gaucher's disease or xanthomatosis, both of which may affect the skeleton, can usually be distinguished on the X-ray appearance and other evidences of lipidosis. Syphilis should always be excluded in any atypical case. *Haemangioma* of bone gives a peculiar radiating 'sun-ray' appearance radiologically, which is usually diagnostic. *Osteitis fibrosa cystica* (in which single or multiple bone cysts occur) may, in its disseminated form, result in spontaneous fractures, though it does not show the generalized osteoporosis which is associated with hyperparathyroidism. Single cysts are usually symptomless. The benign *osteomata* arising from membrane bones are very slow-growing and of extremely dense consistency. Benign giant-cell tumours, which probably arise as the result of trauma and haemorrhage, are usually found at the ends of the long bones; they may be present for years before they give rise to symptoms, e.g. spontaneous fracture.

Whenever the diagnosis is in doubt, aspiration or biopsy should be performed promptly. Delay in establishing the diagnosis of a malignant tumour will often render treatment hopeless.

RETICULO-ENDOTHELIAL GRANULOMA (HISTIOCYTOSIS X)

This is probably not a true neoplastic disease but is included here because it has some of the features of a malignant process, with infiltration of tissues by proliferating histiocytes and, in the more severe forms, a rapidly fatal outcome. It includes three clinical syndromes, *Schüller-Christian disease*, *Letterer-Siwe disease* and *eosinophilic granuloma* of bone, but many cases show features of more than one syndrome and cannot be readily classified in this way. In general, widely disseminated histiocytic proliferation occurs in the younger age group, whereas in older children the lesions tend to be

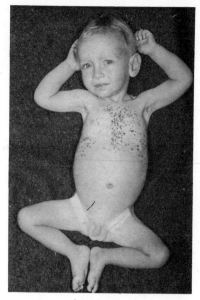

Fig. 9.17 Letterer-Siwe disease, showing characteristic rash. The infant had hepatosplenomegaly and lymphadenopathy.

more localized. The disease occurs at any age but predominantly in the first four years of life; it affects males nearly twice as often as females.

Eosinophilic granuloma

In eosinophilic granuloma the signs are related to local involvement of bone only: the most common presenting feature is a tender mass overlying the osseous lesion. The condition responds to radiotherapy and the prognosis is good.

The more generalized forms of the disease cause progressive wasting and weakness and, as the skeleton becomes increasingly infiltrated, anaemia, thrombocytopenia and haemorrhage.

Letterer-Siwe disease

In this syndrome there is visceral involvement with enlargement of liver, spleen and lymph nodes, and a characteristic raised petechial rash over the anterior aspect of the thorax (Fig. 9.17). Pulmonary infiltration commonly occurs but may not give rise to symptoms. In these rapidly progressive cases, there is generally no deposition of cholesterol in the cells, as occurs in the more slowly developing Schüller-Christian syndrome.

Schüller-Christian syndrome

This consists of exophthalmos, defects in the membranous bones, and diabetes insipidus. To this triad has been added infantilism, which is likely to become obvious when the condition occurs in early childhood and the patient survives sufficiently long for retardation of growth and development to be recognizable. The exophthalmos, diabetes insipidus, and infantilism are secondary to cholesterol deposits in the base of the skull. Similar deposits in the vault are easily recognizable on radiological examination, the irregular punched-out areas having been given the name of *geographical skull*. Deposits may also be seen in the bones of the pelvis, in the skin, in the alveolar margin (causing falling-out of teeth), liver, spleen, lungs, etc. The blood cholesterol may be raised or within normal limits.

In generalized reticulo-endothelial granuloma, no treatment has been found to be curative. The diabetes insipidus may be temporarily controlled in some cases by the use of pitressin. Limitation of fat in the diet may reduce cholesterolaemia, but has little effect on the progress of the disease. Corticosteroid hormones or chlorambucil may

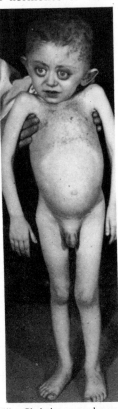

Fig. 9.18 Schüller-Christian syndrome, showing exophthalmos, wasting and xanthomatous lesions on chest.

induce temporary remission. Irradiation has been tried in some cases with apparent improvement, but owing to the generalized character of the disease there is little prospect of its effecting any permanent relief.

CARE OF THE CHILD WITH MALIGNANT DISEASE

The diagnosis of malignant disease must be established beyond doubt before the parents are informed, because the implications are so grave. The manner in which they are told depends on the doctor's assessment of their personality and ability to understand. Some parents should be given a full and frank explanation with as accurate an appraisal of the prognosis as possible. In other cases the seriousness of the disease can only be conveyed gradually and even then the parents may not be able to or may not wish to grasp its full significance.

Although cancer research and new therapeutic measures have not yet achieved a major reduction in mortality from juvenile malignant disease generally, some small advances have been made and the future is in some respects more hopeful. Thus multiple chemotherapy has prolonged the remission period in leukaemia and has even effected permanent remission in a small number of cases, though in the great majority death is inevitable sooner or later. Earlier diagnosis, surgery and irradiation have improved the prognosis in Wilms' tumour and to a lesser extent in neuroblastoma, though the mortality rate is still high. Where there is any hope at all, the parents must be given the full benefit of it, for too pessimistic a view will cause them distress which may be unwarranted.

If a fatal outcome is anticipated, their attitude towards the child must be discussed at an early stage, since parents require advice and help in their attempts to avoid betraying their extreme anguish by word or look. It is particularly difficult in the case of leukaemia, since many children today know that the word signifies a fatal disease. Every precaution must be taken to ensure that such revealing words are not used within the hearing of the child or of other children or parents in the ward, and the doctor should give a simple explanation of the illness to the young patient which will satisfy his curiosity without arousing apprehension.

When the inevitability of early death becomes

clear, it is sometimes kinder to allow the child to die at home and the parents may prefer this. In most cases, however, death takes place in hospital, where the child can be kept sedated and free from pain. While infants and toddlers have little or no understanding of what death means, older children have the same dread of it as adults, though this is not always realized. Children need to discuss their illness and vocalize their anxieties and should not be subjected to a conspiracy of silence. On the other hand, few children can accept the idea of dying with equanimity and they should always be given hope of recovery, even if this means a deliberately untruthful answer to direct questioning. Although we know that children of earlier generations could and did face the reality of early death, and although some physicians have advocated the careful preparation of children for their own deaths, it is generally kinder to keep them in ignorance of their fate. When a child dies in a hospital ward, however, there is no point in trying to hide the fact from the other children, who will certainly know what has happened or learn it from one another, even if they affect unawareness. A simple explanation of the truth is best, and ill children in the ward may need specific reassurance that they themselves are going to get well.

REFERENCES

GENERAL

BODIAN, M. & OCKENDEN, B. G. (1965). Aspects of cancer in childhood. In *Recent Advances in Paediatrics*, 3rd edn. Edited by D. Gairdner. London: Churchill.

CAMPBELL, A. C. P., GAISFORD, W., PATERSON, E. & STEWARD, J. K. (1961). Tumours in children. *British Medical Journal*, i, 448.

CASE, R. A. M., STEWARD, J. K. & WILLIAMS, I. G. (1965). Symposium on malignant disease in childhood. *Proceedings of the Royal Society of Medicine*, 58, 607.

STEWART, A., WEBB, J. & HEWITT, D. (1958). A survey of childhood malignancies. *British Medical Journal*, i, 1945.

WELLS, H. G. (1940). Congenital malignant disease. *Archives of Pathology*, 30, 535.

WILLIS, R. A. (1967). *Pathology of Tumours*, 4th edn. London: Butterworth.

WILLIS, R. A. (1962). *The Borderland of Embryology and Pathology*, 2nd edn. London: Butterworth.

LEUKAEMIA, LYMPHOSARCOMA AND HODGKIN'S DISEASE

FURTH, F. (1957). Recent studies on the etiology and nature of leukaemia. *Blood*, 6, 964.

HARDISTY, R. M. & NORMAN, P. M. (1967). Meningeal leukaemia. *Archives of Disease in Childhood*, 42, 441.

HARDISTY, R. M. (1970). The treatment of acute leukaemia. *Practitioner*, 204, 127.

JONES, B. & KLINGBERG, W. G. (1963). Lymphosarcoma in children. *Journal of Pediatrics*, 63, 11.

NEVILLE, B. G. R. (1972). Central nervous system involvement in leukaemia. *Developmental Medicine and Child Neurology*, 14, 75.

SMITH, C. H. (1960). Leukemia. *Blood diseases of Infancy and Childhood*. St Louis: Mosby.

SMITHERS, D. W. (1967). Hodgkin's disease. *British Medical Journal*, ii, 263, 337.

STEWART, A. (1961). Etiology of childhood malignancies: congenitally determined leukaemias. *British Medical Journal*, i, 452.

INTRACRANIAL AND INTRASPINAL TUMOURS

ANDERSON, F. M. & CARSON, M. J. (1953). Spinal cord tumours in children. *Pediatrics, Springfield*, 43, 190.

BAAR, H. S. (1947). Dysontogenic pituitary cysts. *Archives of Disease in Childhood*, 22, 118.

BAILEY, P., BUCHANAN, D. N. & BUCY, P. C. (1939). *Intracranial Tumours of Infancy and Childhood*. Chicago: University Press.

RUSSELL, D. S. (1939). The pathology of intracranial tumours. *Post-Graduate Medical Journal*, 15, 150.

OTHER TUMOURS

BRAILSFORD, J. F. (1953). *Radiology of the Bones and Joints*, 5th edn. London: Churchill.

DAHLIN, D. C. (1967). *Bone Tumours*, 2nd edn. Springfield: Thomas.

deLORIMER, A. A., BRAGG, K. U. & LINDEN, G. (1969). Neuroblastoma in childhood. *American Journal of Diseases in Children*, 118, 441.

ENRIQUES, P., DAHLIN, D. C., HAYLES, A. B. & HENDERSON, E. D. (1967). Histiocytosis X. *Proceedings of Staff Meetings of the Mayo Clinic*, 42, 88.

LEDLIE, E. M., MYNORS, L. S., DRAPER, G. J. & GORBACH, P. D. (1970). Natural history and treatment of Wilms' tumour. *British Medical Journal*, iv, 195.

McWHORTER, H. E. & WOOLNER, L. B. (1954). Pigmented nevi, juvenile melanomas, etc. *Cancer*, 7, 564.

10 Disorders of the Blood

(See also cretinism, p. 208; haemolytic disease of newborn, p. 61; haemorrhagic disease of newborn, p. 66; infant feeding, p. 143; leukaemia, p. 225; low birth weight, p. 50; and scurvy, p. 155.)

PHYSIOLOGICAL CHANGES

Haematological examinations during early infancy and childhood are apt to be misinterpreted unless it is clearly realized that the physiological variations in the blood findings in early life are very much greater than in the adult, and also that there are changes characteristic of each phase of growth and development. The postnatal fall in prothrombin level and the reduction of fetal haemoglobin which occur during the neonatal period, have been referred to in connection with haemorrhagic disease of the newborn and neonatal jaundice. Many authors have attempted to establish 'normal' values for red cells, haemoglobin, and white cells at birth and during the neonatal period, but from a comparison of their figures it is obvious that there are wide differences, e.g. from 4 to 9 million red blood cells at birth, and that such factors as the site and time of sampling, early or late clamping of the cord (the latter providing a transfusion of over 100 ml of placental blood) and weight-loss will influence the findings during the newborn period. The concentration of haemoglobin in umbilical venous blood averages about 17 g per 100 ml but ranges from 14 to 20 g in normal infants. The haemoglobin concentration rises during the first 12 hours of life but by 14 days has returned to the level at birth and thereafter falls until about 3 months of age when it is approximately 11·5 g per 100 ml and the red cells number 4·1 million. The fall during this period is due partly to slow adaptation of the marrow to major responsibility for red-cell formation, the fetal erythropoietic centres in the liver, spleen, kidneys, thymus, and adrenals ceasing to function. The fall is normally uninfluenced by the administration of iron. Throughout childhood the haemoglobin commonly lies between approximately 75 and 90 per cent (12·0 g per 100 ml at 1 year and 14·0 g at 10 years), tending to rise with age (14·8 g represents 100 per cent). The blood at birth shows relative macrocytosis and immature red cells (normoblasts) are often seen but these rapidly disappear from the circulation.

The white blood cells during the neonatal period vary greatly in number, not only in different infants but in the same infant when counts are made at short intervals. Counts of 20,000 to 25,000 per mm³ within the first 48 hours after birth are not uncommon, polymorphonuclear cells predominating at this time, and immature forms often being present. The total number of polymorphs soon falls to adult levels, and shows little change subsequently. The lymphocytes, however, continue to show more variation in number, and during infancy exceed the polymorphs. At about 4 years of age, the lymphocytes and polymorphs each represent approximately 45 per cent of the white cells in the circulation, after which the proportions gradually assume the adult ratio; in some normal children, however, the infantile ratio is maintained for several years longer. The total number of leucocytes normally exceeds 10,000 per mm³ until 4 or 5 years of age, when it gradually falls to approximately 6,000 at puberty.

GENERAL CONSIDERATIONS

The response of the haemopoietic tissues to pathological stimuli is more erratic than in the case of the mature adult, and the manifestations, e.g. leucocytosis or lymphocytosis, are often exaggerated. Thus enlargement of the liver, spleen, and lymphatic tissues occurs readily; primitive cells of either the red- or white-cell series may reach the circulation in a wide variety of disorders, e.g. infection or malnutrition, and the resulting peripheral blood picture does not represent a disease entity; and the bone marrow is easily affected by abnormal conditions, although it also has a great capacity for rapid and complete regeneration.

In so far as the red cells and haemoglobin are concerned, the great majority of disorders seen in infancy and childhood are anaemias. It is rare for polycythaemia to occur at this age except as the result of cyanosis due to chronic pulmonary or cardiac disease; the rare familial condition of *polycythaemia vera* is unlikely to cause symptoms in childhood.

THE ANAEMIAS

Anaemia represents a reduction in the red-cell and haemoglobin content of the blood below the values considered 'normal' for age. Since the range of normality is not sharply defined and absolute, there will be some cases in which the diagnosis of anaemia must be made somewhat arbitrarily. In most instances, however, the severer grades of anaemia can be classified according to etiology. Clinically, examination of the mucous membranes is likely to give a better indication of anaemia than the colour of the face, which may be influenced by neuro-circulatory disturbances or complexion; pallor is often misleading in the case of a child who is overtired or one who is exceptionally fair-skinned. Common symptoms of severe anaemia are fatigue, breathlessness, and slight oedema, though these often do not become obvious until the haemoglobin has fallen below 50 per cent. In the interpretation of haemoglobin estimations, allowance must be made for changes in blood volume. Thus dehydration from diarrhoea or loss of serum from extensive burns will cause haemo-concentration and tend to mask anaemia, while hydraemia will result in haemodilution and have the opposite effect.

In examining the peripheral blood it is usual to classify the red cells according to their average size as macrocytic, normocytic, or microcytic, and according to the haemoglobin concentration within the cells as normochromic, or hypochromic, i.e. with a lower concentration than normal. As a general rule, anaemia due to sudden severe haemorrhage will at first be normocytic and normochromic. Anaemia due to iron deficiency will be microcytic and hypochromic. *Macrocytic anaemia* is uncommon in childhood, though it occasionally occurs in coeliac disease and is a feature of some haemolytic anaemias. True pernicious anaemia is very rare. Some at least of the infantile macrocytic anaemias with megaloblastic marrow are associated with dietary deficiency of vitamin C or B_{12} or folic acid. Interference with absorption of folic acid, resulting in megaloblastic anaemia, may also occur as the result of prolonged oral antibiotic therapy and certain anticonvulsant drugs may produce the same effect by interfering with the utilization of folic acid (p. 378).

The presence of reticulocytes in the peripheral circulation is an indication that the bone marrow is attempting to overcome the anaemia by increased production of red cells. Although reticulocytes are commonly seen in the blood of the normal newborn infant, they disappear shortly after birth, and subsequently a reticulocyte response is often of prognostic value. Reticulocytes are absent in aplastic anaemia.

The following classification of anaemias is based on etiology, though it will often be found that more than one factor is operative. Thus infection and nutritional deficiency, which together account for the great majority of cases of anaemia in infancy and childhood, are very frequently associated.

ANAEMIA DUE TO LOSS OF BLOOD BY HAEMORRHAGE

1. Post-traumatic haemorrhage
2. Haemorrhage due to ulceration
   Chronic ulcerative colitis
   Peptic ulceration
3. Haemorrhage due to mechanical obstruction
   Splenic thrombosis with haemorrhage from varices
4. Haemorrhagic diseases
   Haemorrhagic disease of newborn
   Haemophilia
   The purpuras
5. Haemorrhagic nephritis
6. Haemorrhage from fetal into maternal circulation or from one fetus into its twin.

ANAEMIA DUE TO BLOOD-DESTRUCTION (HAEMOLYTIC ANAEMIA)

1. Primary haemolytic anaemias due to abnormality of red cells
   Hereditary spherocytosis
   Sickle-cell anaemia
   Thalassaemia
   Glucose-6-phosphate dehydrogenase deficiency
2. Haemolysis due to presence of antibodies
   Haemolytic disease of newborn
   Transfusion of incompatible blood
   Autoimmune haemolytic anaemia
   (including Lederer's anaemia)
   (?) Paroxysmal haemoglobinuria
3. Haemolysis due to toxins
   Infection
   Lead poisoning.

ANAEMIA DUE TO DISTURBANCE OF BLOOD-FORMATION (*Dyshaemopoietic anaemia*)

1. *Mechanical interference with marrow-function (myelophthisic anaemia)*
   Osteosclerotic anaemia (osteopetrosis)
   Leukaemia
   Neoplastic metastases
   Lipidoses
2. Toxic dyshaemopoietic anaemias
   Anaemia due to bacterial and chemical toxins
   Anaemia associated with chronic nephritis
   Some cases of aplastic anaemia
3. Primary aplastic and hypoplastic anaemia
   Acquired idiopathic aplastic anaemia
   Familial aplastic anaemia
   Congenital hypoplastic anaemia
4. Deficiency anaemias
   (a) Iron-deficiency anaemia
       Anaemia of low birth weight
       Nutritional anaemia
       Congenital iron-deficiency anaemia
   (b) Vitamin-deficiency anaemia
       Anaemia of scurvy
       Vitamin B_{12} deficiency
       Deficiency or defective utilization of folic acid
   (c) Endocrine-deficiency anaemia
       Cretinism.

ANAEMIA DUE TO LOSS OF BLOOD BY HAEMORRHAGE

In those cases in which loss of blood has occurred over a short period, regeneration will normally occur rapidly once the haemorrhage has been arrested. Infants and young children, however, withstand haemorrhage badly, and a transfusion should generally be given when the haemoglobin has been reduced below 50 per cent. Transfusion is a routine procedure when any considerable loss of blood is expected at operation.

The continual loss of small amounts of blood occurring over a long period is likely to produce profound anaemia with exhaustion of bone-marrow. This is well illustrated by the condition of chronic ulcerative colitis, in which anaemia is likely to be one of the most severe and intractable symptoms.

The haemorrhagic diseases are considered below.

Anaemia due to transplacental bleeding

Transplacental bleeding from the fetal into the maternal circulation occasionally results in the infant being born with profound anaemia and shock. It may be recognized by the presence of fetal red cells or haemoglobin in the maternal circulation. Infants who are born alive will require immediate transfusion.

Gastric haemorrhage with splenomegaly

Confusion has arisen from the use of the term *Banti's syndrome* to include a variety of different conditions characterized by splenomegaly, leucopenia, and gastric haemorrhage, with or without hepatic cirrhosis. Extrahepatic portal obstruction with hypertension occurring in childhood is a distinct entity in which splenomegaly and gastric or oesophageal haemorrhages are caused by thrombosis or other obstruction of the splenic or portal vein. Profuse haematemesis is commonly the first symptom and is found to be associated with splenomegaly. Radiological examination may demonstrate varices of the oesophagus, and trans-splenic venography show the site of obstruction. At operation, the splenic or portal vein is found to be occluded and clusters of varices are present around the stomach and lower end of the oesophagus. Treatment consists of splenectomy in those few cases in which only the splenic vein is thrombosed. When there is more extensive portal obstruction, a spleno-renal or other shunting procedure may be indicated.

HAEMOLYTIC ANAEMIAS

Haemolysis of red cells may be due to the presence of antibodies (haemolytic disease of the newborn, incompatible transfusion, etc.); to the presence of circulating toxins, as may occur in severe infections; to deficiency of the enzyme glucose-6-phosphate dehydrogenase (on exposure to certain drugs); or to a primary abnormality of the red cells themselves or of the haemoglobin they contain. When the haemolysis is sufficiently severe, it will produce jaundice. Unless the haemolysis is due to the presence of toxins which also serve to depress the bone-marrow, it is likely to be associated with reticulocytosis and erythroblastosis. The destruction of red cells by malarial parasites will cause anaemia comparable to that resulting from toxic haemolysis.

Hereditary spherocytosis (*Familial acholuric jaundice*)

This type of anaemia is congenital, affects both males and females, and may be inherited from either parent as a mendelian dominant. It is characterized by the presence of jaundice and by the absence of bile pigment in the urine. The red cells are more globular than normal, and have a smaller mean diameter (microspherocytes); they are excessively fragile, and haemolyse in concentrations of salt solution which would be withstood by normal red cells, e.g. haemolysis may begin at 0.7 per cent in hereditary spherocytosis and not until 0.45 per cent in the normal. The cells are metabolically as well as structurally abnormal and are destroyed in excessive number by the spleen. This continual haemolysis gives rise to an increase in unconjugated bilirubin in the plasma, a varying degree of anaemia, and enlargement of the spleen, which is due mainly to sequestration of red cells in the splenic pulp.

Reticulocytes are present in large numbers in the circulation.

From time to time aplastic crises occur, in which for no obvious reason the marrow suddenly ceases production and severe anaemia ensues. Such crises are seldom seen during infancy, but may occur at any time during childhood, or may be delayed until later life. Haemolytic crises with increase of jaundice may also occur. Though the crises are usually self-limited, any one of them may prove fatal if untreated.

In infancy the slight yellow tint may attract attention, particularly if other members of the family have been affected. In childhood the patients are likely to be slightly paler and less active than their normal contemporaries, although in some cases no symptoms are noted until the first crisis occurs. Then the haemoglobin falls rapidly, and the patient develops a peculiar lemon-yellow pallor; complaint is made of fatigue, breathlessness, and prostration, and the spleen, which is always enlarged, increases considerably in size. The stools remain coloured, but traces of bile pigments may appear at these times in the urine. The condition may be complicated by the formation of gall-stones, though these rarely give rise to symptoms.

TREATMENT. No form of treatment will permanently correct the abnormal fragility of the red cells, but since the spleen is principally responsible for their destruction, splenectomy will prevent excessive haemolysis and hence the anaemia. It has also been shown that splenectomy may cause a temporary return of the red cells towards the normal. The operation may have to be performed in early childhood if there are frequent crises or gross splenomegaly but it is preferable to postpone it until after 5 years, owing to the risk of infection in the young child after splenectomy.

Thalassaemia (*Cooley's anaemia*)

This is a genetically determined type of haemolytic anaemia occurring principally in patients of Greek or Italian extraction. Members of affected families who are heterozygous for the gene show abnormalities of the red cells but usually little or no anaemia (thalassaemia minor), while those who are homozygous present the full clinical picture (thalassaemia major). In cases of thalassaemia major there is persistence of fetal haemoglobin (Hb-F) with suppression of forma-

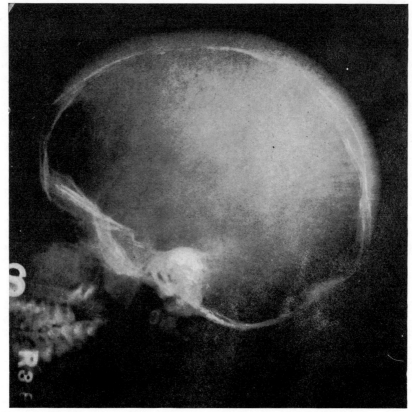

Fig. 10.1   Thalassaemia (Cooley's anaemia). Skull showing radiating spicules due to hyperplasia of bone marrow.

tion of adult haemoglobin (Hb-A); in the minor form there is little or no excess of Hb-F but Hb-A$_2$ is increased. The abnormality is congenital, and anaemia is usually observed in infancy or early childhood. Irregular, fragmented, and nucleated red cells are present in the peripheral blood, and 'target cells' may be seen in which the haemoglobin is concentrated centrally and peripherally with a paler area between. The occurrence of slight discoloration of the skin, due to the presence of pigment, and the thickening of the malar bones give these children a somewhat mongolian appearance. The skull shows well-marked radiological changes due to hyperplasia of the bone-marrow (Fig. 10.1). which is reflected in the erythroblastaemia. The liver and spleen are generally enlarged due to extramedullary haemopoiesis. The anaemia in thalassaemia major is severe and likely to prove fatal, but life can be prolonged for many years by repeated blood transfusion, splenectomy when transfusion is re-quired too frequently, e.g. monthly, and good general care. In longstanding cases, haemosiderosis is a danger which may be countered by the use of chelating agents.

Sickle-cell anaemia

This condition is a congenital abnormality comparable to thalassaemia. Examination of the red cells in the reduced state shows a peculiar sickle shape, due to the presence of haemoglobin S. These cells tend to be haemolysed in excess, though in heterozygous individuals carrying the trait, sicklaemia may exist without anaemia. The condition occurs almost exclusively in the African races. It is characterized by chronic anaemia, with acute episodes of splenic enlargement and circulatory collapse (sequestration crises). Accumulation of sickle cells in small vessels may cause thrombosis, with infarction and painful swelling of the tissues distally, e.g. of the digits in the 'hand–foot' syndrome. The consequent bone destruction may resemble osteomyelitis radiologically. The combination of Hb-S with Hb-C (see below) is not very uncommon.

Other hereditary haemoglobinopathies

An increasing number of abnormal haemoglobins, which have been described as Hb-C to Q, have recently been identified. These are genetically determined, and the individual may be a symptomless heterozygote, e.g. Hb-C and Hb-A; homozygous, e.g. with 100 per cent Hb-C giving rise to a chronic haemolytic process; or a double heterozygote, possessing the Cooley or sickle-cell gene together with the gene for another abnormal haemoglobin. Thus the gene for Hb-E, which is common in Thailand, will result in a modified form of Cooley's anaemia when it occurs in association with the Cooley gene.

Glucose-6-phosphate dehydrogenase deficiency

This inborn error of metabolism is of several distinct types which differ in incidence, degree, clinical significance, and probably in mode of inheritance in different ethnic groups, e.g. Mediterranean, African, southern Chinese, and non-Ashkenazic Jews. It is rare in northern European stock. In some areas, e.g. Greece, Thailand, but not Israel, it is an important cause of severe haemolytic disease of the newborn with deep jaundice, though it is probable that some other factor (possibly genetic) is also involved in affected patients. Children with G-6-PD deficiency are liable to develop haemolytic anaemia following ingestion of certain drugs, e.g. primaquine, sulphanilamide, P.A.S., or fava beans. This deficiency should be remembered as a possible cause of severe haemolytic disease of the newborn not due to Rhesus immunization or ABO incompatibility, or of unexplained haemolytic disease in childhood. (See also p. 61.)

Acute haemolytic naemia

In the type described by Lederer there is probably a close relationship to infection, the condition having a sudden onset associated with pyrexia and jaundice. Haemoglobinuria may occur, and the anaemia is accompanied by leucocytosis. Other acute haemolytic anaemias of infancy and childhood are associated with the presence of auto-agglutinins, which usually give a positive Coombs' test. Transfusion will be required when the anaemia is of severe degree.

Steroid treatment is indicated. In the majority of cases the disease is self-limited and does not recur once the initial haemolysis has been overcome. Haemolytic anaemia of the newborn due to maternal immunization resulting from Rhesus or ABO incompatibility has been described on pp. 61–65. In haemolytic anaemia of early infancy due to toxins, e.g. excessive dosage of vitamin K analogue, Heinz bodies (round or oval granules) may be seen adjacent to the surface of the erythrocytes.

Lead poisoning

This is probably commoner in Britain than previously suspected and is likely to be increasingly recognized as facilities for estimating lead in blood and urine become more generally available. It is most likely to occur in infants between 1 and 3 years of age who have chewed lead-containing paint off cots or window ledges, but may also be due to drinking water from contaminated supplies, inhaling fumes from burning batteries and swallowing lead toys. A history of pica, abdominal pain, behaviour disorder, or mental deterioration associated with refractory haemolytic anaemia suggests the possible diagnosis. Deposition of lead in the long bones as a 'lead line', coproporphyrinuria and punctate basophilia of the red cells are not always found in milder cases. Treatment includes eliminating the source of intake and removing lead from the body by a chelating agent. Oral penicillamine (150 mg b.d. for children under 5 years, and 450 mg b.d. for children over 10) may be effective in mild cases, but in more severe poisoning sodium calcium edetate (50 mg per kg daily i.m.) with or without dimercaprol (4·0 mg per kg 4-hourly i.m.) is indicated. Repeated transfusions may be necessary. While the anaemia is likely to respond to treatment, mental defect and optic atrophy are permanent once they have occurred. In severe poisoning, encephalopathy with convulsions and coma may precede death.

DYSHAEMOPOIETIC ANAEMIAS

Myelophthisic anaemias

Any condition which interferes mechanically with the functional activity of the bone marrow will ultimately cause anaemia. In osteopetrosis, the marrow cavity is gradually encroached on by bone and, although an attempt is made to compensate for this by enlargement of the liver, spleen and lymph nodes, severe and fatal anaemia finally occurs in a proportion of cases. Similarly, when lipid is deposited in the skeleton in the lipidoses, the marrow may become sufficiently compressed for anaemia and haemorrhage to result.

More familiar examples of this type of anaemia are provided by the leukaemias and by widespread bony metastases from malignant tumours. Although primitive white cells are commonly present in abundance in the peripheral blood in leukaemia, the red cells and platelets are grossly reduced owing to mechanical interference with the marrow. In the later stages the clinical picture of thrombocytopenic purpura is added to that of anaemia.

Toxic dyshaemopoietic anaemias

Here the anaemia, which is normocytic and normochromic, is due to depression of the haemopoietic tissues by toxins, either bacterial or chemical; there is also failure of iron utilization. In the severest cases this results in *aplastic anaemia* (see below). *Granulocytopenia*, in which there is selective reduction of granulocytes, is rare in childhood, either as a primary disease or as the result of drug hypersensitivity or radiation. Familial and cyclical neutropenias have been described. In other cases, neutropenia is due to increased destruction of cells.

INFECTION is probably the most important single factor in the causation of anaemia in infancy and childhood, and its action is predominantly toxic, preventing the incorporation of iron into haemoglobin. Treatment in such cases consists in removal of the primary cause, for iron is ineffective as long as infection persists.

PARASITIC INFESTATION may be responsible for anaemia of more than one type, e.g. malaria resulting in depression of marrow function and also in destruction of red cells, while intestinal parasites such as hookworm may be responsible for both blood loss and exacerbation of any existing nutritional anaemia.

CHEMICAL TOXINS. These are comparatively rare causes of anaemia in infancy and childhood, though overdosage with sulphonamide or hydantoin preparations or antibiotics (especially chloramphenicol) is occasionally responsible. Most cases respond to withdrawal of the drug and to transfusion.

Primary aplastic and hypoplastic anaemias

In aplastic anaemia there is complete failure of red-cell formation, an absence of reticulocytes,

and frequently leucopenia and thrombocytopenia also. While some cases are secondary to physical or chemical injury of the bone-marrow (see above), many cases occur in which no cause can be found. The diagnosis of primary aplastic anaemia is only made by exclusion of the various causes of dyshaemopoiesis, including radiation injury. Association with multiple congenital anomalies will suggest the diagnosis of familial aplastic anaemia (Fanconi syndrome). Transfusion will prolong life and oxymetholone or combined testosterone-corticosteroid therapy is sometimes beneficial. Unless there is spontaneous reactivation of marrow, however, the ultimate prognosis is fatal.

Congenital hypoplastic anaemia (*Erythrogenesis imperfecta*)

This is a rare type of congenital anaemia characterized by failure of maturation of erythroblasts, depression of the red cell count without abnormality of leucocytes or platelets, and absence of reticulocytes. The etiology is unknown. Affected infants require repeated transfusion to sustain life. Remission occasionally occurs spontaneously or with corticosteroid therapy.

Deficiency anaemias

Numerous factors are necessary for blood formation, including iron, vitamin B_{12} folic acid, thyroxine, and vitamin C. A deficiency of any one will result in anaemia, but in infancy and childhood a deficiency of iron is much the most common. The infant is born with only small stores of iron in the tissues but a relatively large red cell mass (the available iron totals approximately 74 mg per kg body weight). Breakdown of red cells provides sufficient haemoglobin iron for normal requirements during the first few months. In this period, iron absorbed from the intestinal tract does not make a major contribution but thereafter it assumes increasing importance, the level of body iron stores influencing the amount of iron absorbed. Iron deficiency anaemia is common later in the first year, because the infant's rate of growth exceeds his ability to absorb iron. An iron-deficient diet and occult blood loss from the intestine accentuate the deficit.

Infants of low birth weight are liable to develop severe anaemia because their red cell mass at birth is small and postnatal rate of growth disproportionately rapid. Additional factors are deprivation of blood by early tying of the umbilical cord, inadequate tissue store of iron and low erythropoietic activity of the immature marrow. Very small infants are also prone to develop anaemia from folic acid deficiency.

Congenital iron deficiency anaemia is occasionally seen when the mother has been severely anaemic during pregnancy, though usually the fetus will store iron even at the expense of an anaemic mother. The condition should be prevented by adequate treatment of severe maternal anaemia in pregnancy.

During the latter part of the first year, minor degrees of nutritional anaemia are relatively common in both breast- and bottle-fed infants. This is understandable when it is realized that milk alone is an inadequate source of iron for the infant's basic requirements, and that a grossly deficient maternal diet or a dilute cow's milk formula will result in an even smaller iron intake. The condition is usually seen during the second six months of life, but may extend into the second year or later. Anaemia develops particularly readily when the infant has suffered from repeated infections. A similar condition may be seen in older children who have been kept on a predominantly carbohydrate diet, with a minimum of meat, eggs and green vegetables.

It is probable that, in addition to iron, minute quantities of copper and other elements are required for normal blood formation. Vitamin C deficiency may cause anaemia which does not respond to iron alone. The anaemia of rickets is generally regarded as due to iron deficiency. The anaemias of cretinism and malabsorption have already been considered.

CLINICAL FEATURES. Even with moderate anaemia, some infants have no symptoms and retain their colour. With more severe degrees, the infants have a peculiar greyish pallor. They tend to be hypotonic, while older infants tire readily and may suffer from breathlessness or show slight oedema of the hands and feet. Respiratory infections and gastro-intestinal upsets are common, and there may be associated evidence of rickets. The spleen is enlarged in the more severe cases, and a blowing systolic murmur is sometimes heard over the precordium and veins of the neck. The anaemia is of hypochromic microcytic type, and the haemoglobin may fall to less than 5 g per 100 ml. There is commonly hypochlorhydria. Some of the features of iron deficiency, e.g. the oral and intestinal lesions, may be due to

the effects of deprivation of iron on the tissues, rather than to the anaemia.

COURSE AND PROGNOSIS. Untreated, the condition is likely to persist until the infant is put on to a mixed diet, and may cause prolonged debility and ill health. As these patients are particularly susceptible to infection of all kinds, death may occur from intercurrent infection. However, if the condition is recognized and treated promptly, recovery is rapid and the prognosis wholly good.

DIAGNOSIS. The occurrence of hypochromic microcytic anaemia in an infant whose diet is deficient in iron, in the absence of jaundice, will point to the diagnosis, which is confirmed by the response to iron administration in adequate amount. Estimation of plasma iron and iron-binding capacity and examination of the marrow are indicated if the diagnosis is in doubt or if the anaemia fails to respond to treatment with iron. A careful search should always be made for evidence of occult blood loss in the stools.

TREATMENT. In the case of breast-fed infants, the diet of the mother must be corrected and maternal anaemia treated with iron. Iron-rich foods such as minced meat, eggs and fortified cereals should be added to the infant's diet by the age of 4 months. The artificially fed baby should be given a relatively concentrated cow's milk formula: some dried milks are now fortified with iron. As with the breast-fed infant, iron-rich food should be introduced early.

Iron can be prescribed as ferrous sulphate mixture or as a more palatable elixir of chelated iron. All infants of low birth weight or known to have a low haemoglobin concentration at birth should receive additional iron from the first few weeks of life. While this will not prevent the later fall in the haemoglobin level it will minimize the degree of anaemia. Iron must be given in large doses to cure an already existing anaemia, and, theoretically, is best prescribed between feeds rather than with the feeds. Most commercial preparations of iron contain sufficient copper to remedy possible deficiency in this element. In addition to iron therapy, it is important to make good any vitamin or protein deficiency in the diet; cod-liver oil or other source of vitamin D and orange juice should be prescribed routinely.

Blood transfusion is a valuable form of therapy in the more severe cases, and will often expedite recovery. In milder cases, however, which are uncomplicated by infection, the response to iron administration and correction of diet is dramatic. A reticulocyte response will provide early evidence that the haemopoietic system is responding to treatment.

THE HAEMORRHAGIC DISEASES

In addition to those cases in which haemorrhage is the direct result of trauma, mechanical factors, e.g. pertussis, thrombosis, ulceration, or local defects of blood vessels (varices or aneurysms), there are a number of conditions which are characterized by an abnormal tendency to bleed. The causes of such haemorrhage are to be sought in the blood itself (haemophilia, haemorrhagic disease of the newborn), in the permeability of the capillary-bed (scurvy), or in a combination of factors (thrombocytopenic purpura).

Investigations should include the estimation of the bleeding and coagulation times of the blood, carried out by standard techniques for which the normal values at different ages are known; platelet count; examination of pressure points for purpuric spots or ecchymoses; and an estimation of capillary fragility. The tourniquet test will serve to demonstrate the production of purpuric lesions by minor pressure. The test is carried out on the arm using a sphygmomanometer, pressure being maintained midway between the systolic and diastolic values for five minutes. The arm beneath and below the band is then examined for purpuric spots. Estimations of prothrombin level, fibrinogen, calcium, or antihaemophilic factor will be required in appropriate cases. The presence of jaundice will suggest that the haemorrhagic tendency is associated with liver damage.

Haemophilia

Classical haemophilia (type A) is an inherited tendency to bleed from minor injuries, due to deficiency of antihaemophilic factor (AHF, factor VIII). In Christmas disease (haemophilia B) the inheritance is similar but the deficiency is one of a plasma thromboplastin component (PTC, factor IX) and in haemophilia C, a third factor (plasma thromboplastin antecedent, PTA, factor XI) is deficient.

SEX AND INHERITANCE. The disease virtually occurs only in males, and is inherited through the female. While extremely few cases have been described in females, it is theoretically possible

that the daughter of a haemophilic male and a 'transmitting' female should be a manifest haemophilic. It is also not uncommon to find transmitting females, i.e. the mothers of haemophilic boys, showing some abnormal tendency to bleed, though the AHF concentration of transmitting females may be normal or only very slightly reduced.

Approximately half the sons of a transmitting female may be expected to manifest the disease, and half the daughters to be capable of transmitting it to their sons.

Sporadic cases of haemophilia occasionally occur, though these should not be accepted as such in the absence of a detailed family history, since the disease may sometimes miss a generation.

PATHOLOGY. The coagulation-time of the blood in haemophilia is greatly prolonged (often 10 or 20 times the normal) and the plasma is abnormally stable. This stability is due to a failure of production (or possibly in some cases to an inhibitor) of antihaemophilic factor which is necessary for the formation of thromboplastin, and is normally present in the fibrinogen fraction (Cohn's fraction I) of the plasma. There is considerable periodicity in the delay in coagulation and consequently in the tendency to bleed, and this must be taken into account in assessing the effect of any form of treatment. The disease differs from idiopathic thrombocytopenic purpura in that the bleeding time (as measured by

Table 10.1

	Idiopathic thrombocytopenic purpura	Haemophilia
Hereditary tendency	Rare	Present
Sex	Male and female	Male, transmitted by female
Haemorrhage	Frequently spontaneous	Following injury
Petechiae	Present	Absent
Spleen	May be enlarged	Not enlarged
Joints	May show serous exudate and swelling	Haemarthrosis liable to be followed by chronic arthritic changes
Tourniquet test	Positive	Negative
Platelets	Reduced	Normal number
Bleeding-time	Prolonged	Normal
Clotting-time	Normal	Prolonged
Clot	Retraction defective	Fragile
AHF	Normal	Reduced

needle-puncture method) is normal, an apparent anomaly explained by the different mechanism of control of haemorrhage from a needle puncture and from a cut. Other differences are shown in Table 10.1. The serum calcium, the platelet count and the prothrombin time are normal in haemophilia.

CLINICAL FEATURES. About one in every 3500 liveborn males has haemophilia, but the condition is seldom manifest during the neonatal period, the first haemorrhage usually occurring during the second or third year. Occasionally the child escapes without symptoms until later childhood. The eruption or extraction of a tooth, circumcision, or some minor injury such as a scratch or biting the tongue is likely to draw attention to the disease. The haemorrhage does not alarm by its severity at onset, but by its continuance despite all efforts to stop it. The child will often lose sufficient blood from a small wound to cause profound anaemia and collapse.

Haematomata may occur in any site, and often reach alarming proportions. Haemorrhage into joints (haemarthrosis) is one of the commonest and potentially most disabling features. Swelling of the joint is associated with limitation of movement and very gradual resorption. The same joints, most commonly the knees, are liable to be repeatedly affected, and while there may be little permanent damage if treatment of each episode is prompt and effective, there is a risk of ultimate subluxation and deformity.

Haemorrhages from mucous membranes or large ecchymoses of the skin frequently occur from very minor injury, but spontaneous haemorrhage is unlikely to occur in the absence of any trauma. Bleeding from the urinary tract is quite common, however. Intracranial haemorrhage rarely occurs but may be indicated by persistent severe headache.

PROGNOSIS. This depends to a considerable extent on the measure of protection the patient can receive, the lack of necessity for operation, and the availability of effective treatment when the condition is in a bad phase and haemorrhages occur. Since almost all the normal activities of childhood are fraught with danger, it is not surprising that many patients suffer repeated haemorrhage which may lead to complete invalidism before puberty. Death may occur from intracranial haemorrhage, often apparently spontaneous; or from sublingual haemorrhage causing respiratory obstruction. In patients who survive to adult life, the haemorrhagic tendency shows some inclination to decrease.

DIAGNOSIS. The sex and familial incidence of the disease, the history of repeated haemorrhages from trivial injuries, and the age onset of symptoms in early childhood will indicate the diagnosis of haemophilia. It should be confirmed by estimation of the clotting-time of the blood and of the concentration of antihaemophilic factor. The distinction between haemophilia A, which accounts for 85 per cent of clinical haemophilia, and other coagulation factor deficiencies can only be made by specialized laboratory technique.

TREATMENT. There is no known cure for the disease. The females of haemophilic families should be given appropriate genetic counselling. Haemophilic children must as far as possible be guarded against trauma without instituting a life of complete invalidism. Special arrangements for education may have to be made and the boy's future career must be considered early.

Haemorrhage, when it occurs, is extremely difficult to control. The usual styptics have little effect, though the local application of blood from a normal individual, thrombin foam, or a 1 in 10,000 dilution of Russell viper venom may aid clotting.

Prompt treatment of episodes of bleeding, especially those into muscles or joints, is essential if chronic disability is to be avoided. The aim of therapy is to increase circulating AHF activity to a haemostatic level (15 to 30 per cent of normal or higher in serious haemorrhage). For

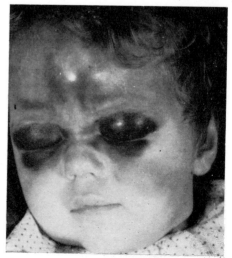

Fig. 10.2   Haemophilia showing haemorrhage into eyelids and brow following a fall. Boy aged 14 months.

minor bleeding, fresh-frozen plasma may be used but for more severe episodes human anti-haemophilic factor (factor VIII concentrate) or cryoprecipitate should be given in adequate amounts as judged by the severity of the bleeding and the clinical response, AHF assay or partial thromboplastin time and whole-blood clotting time. The latter must not be depended on alone, since it may be normal when the AHF level is less than 5 per cent of normal. Cryoprecipitate has the advantages that it is in relatively small volume and that it is fairly easily obtained from fresh blood. Animal products should not be used except in emergency and, usually, in the presence of circulating inhibitors of AHF. Whole blood should be avoided unless there has been a severe fall in haemoglobin level, because of the risks of sensitization. Affected joints should be splinted under orthopaedic supervision, though the use of corticosteroids in addition to the specific factor replacement may reduce the need for immobilization. Physiotherapy will be required for the un-affected muscles and occasionally joint aspiration may be indicated.

In coagulation factor deficiencies other than classical haemophilia, fresh-frozen plasma, fresh blood or cryoprecipitate may be used.

Pseudohaemophilia (*von Willebrand's disease*)

In this rare disorder, which clinically resembles haemophilia but is transmitted as a mendelian dominant to both males and females, the bleeding time is prolonged and the clotting time normal. There is defective contractility of superficial capillaries which may occur alone or with deficiency of AHF or one of the other coagulation factors. Transfusion is required for severe haemorrhage.

The purpuras

Although not all types of purpura are haemorrhagic in the sense of giving rise to free bleeding and anaemia, the group of conditions in which purpuric lesions occur in the skin and elsewhere can conveniently be considered here. The following classification is modified from that of Whitby and Britton:

A. PURPURAS SHOWING QUANTITATIVE
    DEFICIENCY OF PLATELETS
1. Idiopathic thrombocytopenia (capillary defect also)
2. Symptomatic purpura
   (a) Bone-marrow replacement or depression, e.g. leukaemia, acute infection
   (b) Hypersplenism.

B. PURPURAS WITH SLIGHT OR NO
    DEFICIENCY IN PLATELETS
    (vascular factor usually involved)
1. Anaphylactoid purpura
2. Purpura fulminans and purpura necrotica
3. Simple symptomatic purpura
   (a) Infections (platelets often diminished in acute stages), e.g. typhoid, meningococcal meningitis
   (b) Toxic, e.g. snake venom, drugs such as bella-donna
   (c) Miscellaneous (mechanical constriction, avita-minosis, convulsions).

There appear to be two factors which may be concerned in the production of purpura, viz. reduction of platelets and vascular defect. While capillary haemorrhage can occur without any quantitative reduction in platelets, it is less certain that thrombocytopenia alone, in the absence of abnormality of the capillaries, will result in purpura. In many cases, e.g. toxic and infective conditions, both factors are operative.

The platelets normally number 200,000 to 500,000 per mm^3, the numbers recorded depending to some extent on the method of counting employed and on individual factors such as activity and temperature; the number is lower in the immature newborn infant. Platelets may be reduced in number by suppression of formation in the bone marrow (e.g. by toxins or the presence of malignant deposits) or by excessive destruction in the spleen or rarely in an enlarging haemangioma. Vascular damage, rendering the capillaries abnormally permeable, may arise from the presence of circulating toxins, or from avitaminosis (scurvy). In anaphylactoid purpura, the changes in the vessels may be closely similar to those in polyarteritis nodosa.

Idiopathic thrombocytopenic purpura
(*Purpura haemorrhagica*)

In this type of purpura, spontaneous haemor-rhages from mucous membranes, purpuric lesions of the skin, and excessive bruising are the outstanding features (Fig. 10.4). The spleen is slightly enlarged in a minority of cases, but gross splenomegaly would suggest an alternative diag-nosis. The platelets are greatly reduced and the bleeding time prolonged. (Very roughly, it may be said that haemorrhages are liable to occur when the circulating platelets fall below 40,000 per mm^3, though this is by no means invariably true.) A circulating platelet antibody is demon-strable in some cases, but less commonly in children than in adults. The megakaryocytes are present in the bone marrow in normal or increased numbers, but the platelets produced may be quantitatively or qualitatively deficient. Constriction of the arm with a tourniquet causes the prompt appearance of a crop of purpuric lesions below the site of the constriction, there being a defect of capillary contractility in addition to platelet deficiency. If venepuncture is required, it is likely to cause a large haematoma, and needle puncture will sometimes result in prolonged haemorrhage.

Every case coming under observation should be carefully investigated for evidence of infection.

AGE AND SEX INCIDENCE. The condition may occur at any age, but is most frequently seen in middle childhood. Girls are rather more commonly affected than boys. Typically, the condition is not inherited, but *congenital thrombocytopenic purpura*, which is commonly mild and transient, may occur in infants of mothers in whom the disease is active at the time of delivery, or rarely of mothers with normal platelet counts.

DIAGNOSIS. The association of purpuric skin lesions, spontaneous haemorrhage and bruising, positive tourniquet test, prolonged bleeding time and thrombocytopenia indicates the diagnosis in the absence of other primary disease. Leukaemia must be excluded by bone marrow examination. The distinguishing features of idiopathic thrombocytopenic purpura and haemophilia are summarized in Table 10.1.

PROGNOSIS AND TREATMENT. The prognosis is on the whole good if the patient survives the first month. Many of the acute cases run a relatively short course, and improve spontaneously if they can be tided over the initial haemorrhagic phase, during which death may occur from bleeding into a vital organ. In others, repeated purpura and haemorrhages occur at irregular intervals, often over a period of years. The chronic cases will sometimes improve at puberty.

The immediate treatment required for severe haemorrhage is blood transfusion, which may have to be repeated. Steroid therapy will cause remission in approximately 50 per cent of cases and should be instituted at once if the patient is seen early, since it may lessen the risk of serious haemorrhage. Splenectomy carries a considerable risk during the acute phase, and should be reserved for those cases which have failed to respond to steroid therapy and in which chronic

or recurrent severe haemorrhage is proving a danger to life.

Symptomatic purpura

As already indicated, the clinical picture of thrombocytopenic purpura may be seen as part of the symptomatology of other diseases in which either platelet formation is depressed by damage to the bone marrow, or platelet destruction is excessive owing to splenic abnormality. In the former case, toxins acting on the bone marrow, and the presence of leukaemic deposits within the long bones and elsewhere, are examples. Symptomatic purpura with or without platelet deficiency may occur in specific fevers, particularly typhoid fever and meningococcaemia. In fulminating meningococcaemia and occasionally in other infections the purpuric rash may become confluent

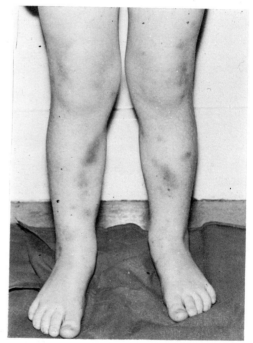

Fig. 10.3   Thrombocytopenic purpura with spontaneous bruising.

or necrotic (*purpura necrotica*, Fig. 10.4). Rarely purpura extends so rapidly and widely as to prove fatal (*purpura fulminans*).

Anaphylactoid purpura (*Henoch-Schönlein purpura*)

This is a vasculitis affecting primarily the arterioles and venules. The skin lesion is a brownish maculo-papular eruption which quickly becomes purpuric (Plate 15). It is largely confined to the extensor surfaces, especially the knees and ankles, the buttocks and the elbows. Crops of purpuric spots appear at intervals and may be the only features, though malaise and slight fever are usual. In other cases, the purpura may be associated with abdominal pain and haemorrhage from the bowel (Henoch's purpura) or with joint pains and swelling (Schönlein's purpura); either of these may precede the appearance of purpura and lead to the mistaken diagnosis of intussusception or acute rheumatism respectively. Occasionally all these features occur together and the child may be seriously ill.

Anaphylactoid purpura is often preceded by a throat infection, suggesting affinities with rheumatism and nephritis, but there is evidence that group A streptococcal infection is not an important precipitating factor.

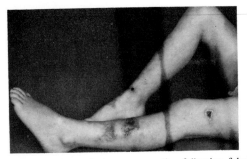

Fig. 10.4   Lesions of purpura necrotica following fulminating meningococcal meningitis.

Haemorrhage from the bowel is thought to be due to the presence of purpuric lesions in the intestinal wall and is frequently associated with colicky abdominal pain and vomiting. When the rash appears the diagnosis should not be in doubt, and if there is no evidence of intussusception (an occasional complication of anaphylactoid purpura), gastric suction, correction of dehydration and sedatives should be employed. Transfusion is rarely necessary.

Anaphylactoid purpura is commonly benign, the mildest cases requiring only bed rest and treatment of any infection which may be present (most commonly a streptococcal throat infection). Haematuria is a frequent complication, and will in some cases prove intractable, indicating proliferative glomerulonephritis and occasionally

progressing to renal failure. The kidneys in fatal cases have sometimes shown evidence of periarteritis nodosa. Very occasionally, the purpuric skin lesions may become gangrenous.

While the term 'anaphylactoid' has been widely accepted, it must be admitted that this etiology is not definitely proven. The occurrence of purpura in association with urticaria in some cases, however, suggests an allergic factor and antigen–antibody complexes have been demonstrated in the skin and kidneys. Antihistamine drugs are seldom effective. Prednisolone or ACTH relieve the acute symptoms though they do not prevent continuing purpura or haematuria.

ANTIBODY DEFICIENCY SYNDROMES

The lymphoid system, including lymph nodes, tonsils and spleen, is responsible for the production of specific antibodies. Lymphoid tissue has the capacity to react to antigens by proliferation of lymphocytes and plasma cells which, being immunologically competent, can produce specific immunoglobulin in response to antigenic stimulus (p. 24). The thymus appears to be essential for the proper functioning of the lymphoid system, at least in early life.

Deficiency of immunoglobulins may be due to failure of synthesis or, less commonly, to excessive loss, as occurs in the nephrotic syndrome. Though marked hypogammaglobulinaemia is rare, it should be suspected and looked for when an infant or young child suffers from recurrent severe infections especially when they involve different sites in the body.

Thymic alymphoplasia

The most serious form of antibody deficiency is thymic alymphoplasia, which is familial and is characterized by complete immunological incompetence. There is profound lymphopenia and the thymus and lymph nodes are small or rudimentary. The infant fails to thrive and develops cough, diarrhoea and other evidence of infection. Death usually occurs during the first year of life.

Congenital hypogammaglobulinaemia

Congenital hypogammaglobulinaemia or agammaglobulinaemia is the commonest of the antibody deficiency syndromes and is generally inherited as a sex-linked recessive. Severe and frequent infections occur from the age of about a year and there may be effusions into joints. The lymph nodes and tonsils are very poorly developed but the thymus appears normal and there is no deficiency of lymphocytes in the peripheral blood. Treatment consists of replacement of gammaglobulin by periodic injection and the liberal use of antibiotics. A number of other genetically determined immunological deficiency diseases have been described. Deficient production of immunoglobulins may also be an acquired condition, arising either primarily for no apparent reason or secondarily to radiation or immunosuppressive drugs.

These disorders are characterized by general deficiency of immunoglobulins but selective deficiency may also occur. Thus defective synthesis of IgM, with normal or increased levels of IgG, has been found in mongolism and in a few other children with recurrent infections. Selective deficiency of IgG has also been reported occasionally in such children. In these rare *dysgammaglobulinaemias*, the total quantity of plasma immunoglobulin is often within normal limits, so that the disorder may not be recognized unless fractional analysis is undertaken.

CHRONIC GRANULOMATOUS DISEASE

In this disorder of white blood cells, the polymorphs ingest but are unable to kill bacteria which, being protected from antibiotics within the cells, proliferate and cause a granulomatous tissue response. The disease appears to be inherited as an autosomal recessive with a sex modification so that it mainly affects boys. It is characterized by chronic suppurative lesions throughout the body, e.g. lymphadenopathy, skin sepsis, osteomyelitis and pulmonary consolidation, often with abscess formation. Abscesses may occur in other viscera, such as brain or liver. Pericardial and pleural effusions are common.

The infected organs show typical granulomatous changes on biopsy or at necropsy and various pathogenic organisms, principally *Staphylococcus pyogenes* and *Escherichia coli*, are isolated on culture. The defect in the polymorphs can be identified by the nitro-blue tetrazolium test.

Treatment is unsatisfactory, although induction of neutropenia with busulphan and long-term antibiotic therapy have been tried. The condition is usually fatal in early childhood, although a few patients have survived longer.

BIBLIOGRAPHY AND REFERENCES

ALLEN, D. M., DIAMOND, L. K. & HOWELL, D. A. (1960). Anaphylactoid purpura in children. *American Journal of Diseases of Children*, 99, 833.
BARLTROP, D. (1971). Lead poisoning. *Archives of Disease in Childhood*, 46, 233.
BIGGS, R. (1971). *Human Blood Coagulation, Haemostasis and Thrombosis*. Oxford: Blackwell.
BLACKFAN, K. D. & DIAMOND, L. K. (1951). *Atlas of the Blood in Children*. New York: Commonwealth Fund.
BURMAN, D. (1972). Haemoglobin levels in normal infants. *Archives of Disease in Childhood*, 47, 261.
CATHIE, I. A. B. (1950). Erythrogenesis imperfecta. *Archives of Disease in Childhood*, 25, 313.
DAVIS, S. D. and 5 others (1967). The congenital agammoglobulinaemias. *American Journal of Diseases of Children*, 113, 186.
DOXIADIS, S. A. & VALAES, T. (1964). The clinical picture of glucose-6-phosphate dehydrogenase deficiency in early infancy. *Archives of Disease in Childhood*, 39, 545.
FISHBEIN, R. H. (1969). Purpura fulminans. *Journal of Pediatric Surgery*, 4, 320.
FRANGLEN, G. (1970). Immune globulin deficiencies. *British Journal of Hospital Medicine*, 3, 651.
GAIRDNER, D. (1948). The Schönlein-Henoch syndrome (anaphylactoid purpura). *Quarterly Journal of Medicine*, 17, 95.
GAIRDNER, D. (1958). Haematology of infancy. *Recent Advances in Paediatrics*, 2nd series. London: Churchill.
HAWORTH, J. C., HOOGSTRATEN, J. & TAYLOR, H. (1967). Thymic alymphoplasia. *Archives of Disease in Childhood*, 42, 40.
JONXIS, J. H. P. (1957). The occurrence of abnormal haemoglobins. *Scottish Medical Journal*, 2, 1.
KAUDER, E. & MAUER, A. M. (1966). Neutropenias of childhood. *Journal of Pediatrics*, 69, 147.
KOMROWER, G. M. & WATSON, G. H. (1954). Prognosis in idiopathic thrombocytopenic purpura in childhood. *Archives of Disease in Childhood*, 29, 502.
LANCET (1964). Varieties of glucose-6-phosphate dehydrogenase. *Lancet*, ii, 951.
LLOYD, J. K. & BROWN, G. A. (1964). Homozygous thalassaemia in an English child. *Archives of Disease in Childhood*, 39, 625.
OSKI, F. A. & NAIMAN, J. L. (1972). *Haematologic Problems in the Newborn*, 2nd edn. Philadelphia: Saunders.
RICKARDS, A. G. (1955). Megaloblastic anaemia of infancy. *British Medical Journal*, i, 1226.
RIZZA, C. R. & BIGGS, R. (1971). Haemophilia today. *British Journal of Hospital Medicine*, 6, 343.
ROBSON, H. N. & WALKER, C. H. M. (1951). Congenital and neonatal thrombocytopenic purpura. *Archives of Disease in Childhood*, 26, 175.

SMITH, C. H. (1960). *Blood Diseases of Infancy and Childhood*. St Louis: Mosby.
SMITH, R. S. (1965). Iron deficiency and iron overload. *Archives of Disease in Childhood*, **40**, 343.
THOMPSON, E. N. & SOOTHILL, J. F. (1970). Chronic granulomatous disease. *Archives of Disease in Childhood*, **45**, 24.
TIDY, H. (1952). Banti's disease and splenic anaemia. *British Medical Journal*, ii, 1.
ZUELZER, W. W. (1949). Normal and pathologic physiology of the bone marrow. *American Journal of Diseases of Children*, **77**, 482.
ZUELZER, W. W. & OGDEN, F. N. (1946). Megaloblastic anaemia in infancy. *American Journal of Diseases of Children*, **71**, 211.

11 Allergic Disorders

Allergy represents a state of hypersensitivity or 'altered reaction', in which the patient has become sensitized by natural means to a foreign protein, protein-carbohydrate complex, or other substance. Human allergy bears many similarities to anaphylaxis in animals, but in the latter condition hypersensitivity is produced artificially by the injection of a minute quantity of foreign protein, e.g. horse serum, the injection being followed after a latent period by a state in which further injection of the same protein produces profound bronchospasm or shock, the nature of the reaction depending on the species of animal. The exact mechanism by which human allergy is produced is unknown, but in a high proportion of cases it involves: (1) hereditary predisposition; (2) exposure to the sensitizing factor by contact, inhalation, or ingestion by the patient, or by exposure of the mother during pregnancy; and (3) the formation of circulating antibodies (reagins), which have recently been identified with the IgE group of immunoglobulins. The presence of these antibodies on or in the cells alters the cellular reactivity. Subsequent exposure results in union of the sensitizing factor (allergen) with the appropriate antibody and the release of histamine and other pharmacologically active substances, causing an immediate reaction. When the antigen reacts with specifically sensitized cells rather than with circulating antibody, the reaction is delayed, as in tuberculin sensitivity.

All individuals may become allergic, but there is great individual variation in the readiness with which sensitization occurs and the severity of the allergic reaction. The term 'atopy' is used to distinguish the cases of allergy in which the constitutional factor is of paramount importance. It is not clear exactly what the factor is or how it is inherited: it may be a single genetic characteristic or there may be more than one pattern of inheritance. The atopic child is characterized by the ease with which he forms reaginic antibodies and by liability to one or more of the clinical manifestations of atopy, such as infantile eczema, asthma, allergic rhinitis or gastro-intestinal allergy. At least 5 in every 100 children have the atopic constitution, although not all develop symptoms requiring medical attention. In over 60 per cent of cases there is a family history of allergy. It is important to realize that it is the atopic constitution that is inherited and not the particular clinical disorder.

Atopic symptoms may be provoked not only by the specific allergen but also by other agents, such as infection, anxiety, excitement or exercise. The same physiopathological mechanism is probably involved in all cases and it must be assumed that it becomes highly responsive to a variety of stimuli, not all of which involve an antigen-antibody reaction. Allergy is thought to play an essential part in the production of the clinical manifestations of many other diseases such as rheumatism, nephritis, and anaphylactoid purpura, while some cases of migraine may be of allergic origin. But while the importance of allergy in the determination of disease is no doubt much greater than was previously supposed, it is usual to confine the term 'allergic disorders' to those conditions which characterize the atopic child. Since they have certain features in common, these will be considered before the particular syndromes are described.

INVESTIGATION

Every patient in whom an allergic factor is suspected should have a careful family history taken with regard to allergic manifestations in near relatives. These manifestations are not necessarily the same as those observed in the patient; thus in the case of an infant with eczema, one or other parent may give a history of asthma or hay-fever or allergy to a particular food, e.g. eggs or shellfish. In some of these cases there is evidence to suggest that the mother's diet during pregnancy has been responsible for the infant becoming sensitized to ingestants which he has not himself eaten; or allergens may reach him through the mother's milk.

Details of the exact time and circumstances of onset of an attack will often lead to a recognition of the cause. Thus allergic rhinitis occurring consistently in the early summer in Britain will suggest pollen-sensitivity. Asthma, urticaria, or rhinitis occurring only at night should lead to investigation of the bedding, e.g. horsehair mattress or feather pillow, as a possible provoking agent. In some cases the parent will volunteer the information that contact with a particular animal will cause symptoms.

Patients are frequently found to be sensitive to more than one allergen, or to a number of factors including climatic conditions, psychological upsets, mixed dusts, etc. It is not uncommon to find that attacks of asthma are provoked by exposure to a high wind, which may prove to be related either to temperature or to inhalation of dust. House dust raised during cleaning or bed-making is responsible in some cases and it has been shown that the allergenicity of house dust is largely due to a species of mite (Dermatophagoides). Hypersensitivity to insect bites is also common in young children, and very occasionally bee stings are found to provoke an extremely severe reaction similar to anaphylaxis in animals.

Immunization, e.g. to diphtheria or tetanus, should be undertaken with great caution in patients known to be allergic, a trial intradermal test with a minimal amount of the immunizing-agent being made before the full dose is given. Adrenaline should be available in cases in which there is risk of a severe reaction.

Food allergy may be sufficiently obvious to incriminate a particular food on the history alone, e.g. asthma or urticaria occurring rapidly after the food has been eaten. Infants may manifest allergy to a new food by gastrointestinal symptoms, e.g. colic, vomiting or diarrhoea. In some cases it is necessary to carry out skin-testing or to eliminate different foods from the diet one at a time.

The significance to be attached to the psychological history is often difficult to evaluate in the case of allergic patients, particularly asthmatics. Psychological disturbances appear in the case histories with considerable frequency, but when the child is seen for the first time after asthmatic attacks have been occurring for some years, it must be remembered that the state of recurrent invalidism of the child is itself likely to provoke an atmosphere of overanxiety in the household. There is no doubt, however, that domestic tension, whether primary or secondary, reacts adversely on asthmatics particularly, and that a change of environment irrespective of climatic conditions will often produce dramatic relief.

SKIN-TESTING

Skin-testing has been widely used in allergic conditions with the purpose of determining the sensitizing agent, though many allergic children show positive reactions to a large number of different agents without it being possible to incriminate a single one. Nevertheless, a specific reaction when it is obtained is sufficiently valuable to justify the routine use of the investigation in allergic cases.

Tests may be made by intradermal injection or scratch-inoculation, the inner aspect of the forearm being a convenient site. A minute quantity (0·02 ml for intradermal use) of each test reagent is injected or inoculated, and the skin re-examined at short intervals during the next half-hour. A weal at the site of inoculation indicates a positive reaction, the size of the weal, presence of pseudopodia, and associated erythema indicating the strength of the reaction. It is usual to start with 'group testing' for foods, pollens, animal hair, and feathers, using reagents containing a mixture of five or more common allergens, and to proceed to test with individual foods, pollens, etc., when the group to which the patient is sensitive has been determined. Infants are most likely to be found sensitive to foods and older children to inhalants, though skin sensitivity does not necessarily mean that symptoms are produced by the substance concerned.

PRAUSNITZ-KÜSTNER REACTION

It has been found that when the serum of an atopic individual is injected into the skin of one who is not allergic, the area of injected skin will give a positive reaction to the substance to which the allergic donor has become sensitized. This passive transfer of local allergy is occasionally used in the investigation of patients when for any reason, e.g. eczema, it is not practicable to carry out direct skin-testing.

MANAGEMENT

A careful explanation of the nature of allergy must be given to the parents and it should be made clear to them that, although treatment can relieve symptoms, the underlying atopic constitution of the child cannot be changed. Apart from measures appropriate to the particular form of allergy, three lines of general treatment are available. If the specific allergen can be determined, the patient may be kept from contact with it, by changing the environment, eliminating a particular food, or other means; alternatively, hyposensitization may be attempted. Bronchodilator drugs or one of the antihistamines may be used to relieve symptoms or abort an attack. Steroid therapy may be used in selected cases, e.g. status asthmaticus which has failed to respond to adrenaline (see below). In addition, the child and his family must be helped to adjust to his disability; occasionally the emotional disturbance may be severe enough to require expert psychotherapy.

HYPOSENSITIZATION

The aim here is to eliminate or reduce the child's allergic response by injection or ingestion of increasing amounts of the allergen. In the case of inhalants, the amount given at the first injection should be less than that which will produce symptoms, and at each succeeding injection, given at weekly intervals, the amount should be doubled so long as no symptoms are produced. In the case of foods, minimal amounts of the substance to which the patient is sensitive are introduced into the diet and increased daily.

Hyposensitization is not consistently successful, but should be attempted when a specific allergen can be isolated and when it is not possible for the patient to avoid contact with it. In cases of hay-fever, hyposensitization (which will take two to three months by weekly injections) should be completed before the pollen season begins. It may have to be repeated each year for three or more years. The number of injections required is less if an alum-precipitated pyridine extract of the allergen is used.

Allergic (vasomotor) rhinitis

Cases may be divided into those in which the allergen is a pollen ('hay-fever') and those in which other inhalants are responsible. The first group shows a well-marked seasonal incidence of symptoms, whereas in the latter, symptoms may occur whenever the patient comes in contact with the allergen. In both, the symptoms include nasopharyngeal discomfort followed by a profuse mucous nasal discharge, congestion which involves the turbinates and frequently the accessory sinuses also, lachrymation, paroxysmal sneezing, and general malaise similar to that experienced at the onset of a common cold. Cough or deafness occurs in some cases. The temperature may be slightly raised but is typically normal. The onset of symptoms is usually abrupt, and cessation may be equally rapid. Examination of the nose during an attack shows that the mucosa, particularly of the inferior turbinates, is pale, swollen, and oedematous, and is covered with clear mucous exudate which may subsequently become purulent if infection is superadded.

Hay-fever. Sensitization to particular pollens or spores will depend on the type of flora to which the child is exposed, and is most likely to occur when exposure is prolonged and frequent. Hay-fever is uncommon in infancy, but the incidence rises after the age of 5 years and more rapidly in adolescence. Boys and girls are equally affected, and a familial incidence of allergic manifestations is common.

Since the atmosphere in Britain contains the maximum amount of wind-borne pollens during the period from mid-May to the end of August, the great majority of cases of hay-fever occur during this time. In other countries the seasonal incidence will differ. Climatic conditions will also affect the incidence to some extent from year to year. Amongst the commoner pollens causing symptoms are those of the various meadow grasses.

Non-seasonal allergic rhinitis. In these cases the sensitizing agent is usually an inhalant other than pollen; orris root and other cosmetic preparations, house dust, feathers, and horsedander are the most common. Food sensitivity is occasionally manifested by rhinitis, and bacterial allergy is also a possible causative factor.

TREATMENT. If it is impossible to remove the cause or to obtain satisfactory hyposensitization, symptoms may be relieved by local applications of ephedrine or adrenaline. The reduction of oedema resulting from these local applications will relieve obstruction of the sinuses also, since the swollen mucosa is apt to block the ostia. Good results have been obtained in a proportion of cases by the use of antihistamine drugs. Operations on the nose or tonsils are contra-indicated until the allergic condition has been treated.

Asthma

This condition represents a symptom-complex of which the essential features are periodic paroxysms of wheezing dyspnoea with prolonged expiration. The dyspnoea is caused by obstruction of the smaller bronchi and bronchioles by viscid mucus, oedema and spasm of smooth muscle. Long-standing cases commonly show emphysema and some degree of thoracic deformity. Allergic asthma cannot always be distin-

guished on clinical grounds alone from obstructive bronchitis in younger patients, and, indeed, recurrent bronchitis may prove to be the forerunner of more typical asthma in later childhood. In *cardiac* and *uraemic asthma*, due to cardiac and renal failure respectively, the previous history and clinical features will indicate the primary cause.

In the majority of cases of childhood asthma, there is a family history of allergic disorders among close relatives. The condition frequently follows infantile eczema or is associated with allergic skin manifestations. Even when these latter are absent, the skin will often be found to be dry and slightly scaly. Both sexes are affected, but the condition is more than twice as common in boys as it is in girls. Asthma affects 3 to 5 per cent of all schoolchildren in Britain.

AGE OF ONSET. Approximately one-third of all cases of asthma originate in the first decade of life, and the onset of symptoms occurs more frequently in the first than in each subsequent year of the decade.

ALLERGEN. As indicated above, asthma may be initiated by inhalants or ingestants to which the patient is sensitive, inhalants being more commonly responsible in older children and ingestants in infancy. Attacks may be precipitated by psychological upsets, changes in temperature, exercise, excessive laughter, etc. *Infection*, particularly of the upper respiratory tract, has an important role in the genesis of asthma in the atopic child. Secondary infection of the lung commonly occurs when the condition has been operative for some considerable time.

CLINICAL FEATURES. The asthmatic attack is often preceded by malaise, constipation, coryza, headache, and irritability. Usually in the early hours of the morning, the child wakes with severe dyspnoea which makes sleep impossible; the feeling of suffocation which the attack occasions is often extremely frightening to a young child, and increases his distress. It is characteristic of the respiration that the expiratory phase is greatly prolonged and is associated with wheezing. The excursion of the thorax is reduced, the chest being fixed in almost full inspiration despite the fact that the external muscles of respiration are thrown into action. In the severest cases the child becomes cyanosed and prostrated. Cough is usually slight or absent at the beginning of an attack, but later there may be considerable amounts of mucopurulent sputum. Asthmatic attacks commonly last two to seven days. The frequency of their occurrence varies greatly, some patients having only occasional attacks at intervals of several months or more, whilst others show a much shorter periodicity. The more frequent the attacks, the greater is the effect on the general health. In cases of even moderate severity, the amount of invalidism occasioned by the condition is likely to interfere seriously with the child's education, social activities and general health. Attacks which follow respiratory infections are clinically less characteristic, and are more like those of acute obstructive bronchitis, especially in the younger child. The temperature is higher, and there is usually more cough and sputum.

SEQUELAE. The mechanical interference with expiration occasioned by bronchial obstruction leads to functional emphysema. When asthmatic attacks are frequent and occur over a long period, the lung may become secondarily infected, and many patients show some degree of bronchiectasis in later childhood or adolescence. There is almost always some deformity of the thorax when attacks have started in infancy and persisted into later childhood. The antero-posterior diameter of the upper part of the thorax is increased and kyphosis is commonly present,

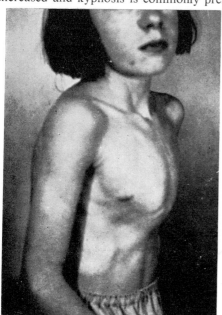

Fig. 11.1   A severe degree of asthmatic deformity, with gross increase in antero-posterior diameter of upper thorax and marked kyphosis.

while the lower ribs are flattened anteriorly, the costal angle increased, and the excursion of the bases diminished. The patients are usually round-shouldered, slender, and poorly nourished.

DIAGNOSIS. In atopic asthma, the family history and occurrence of other allergic manifestations will usually leave little question as to the diagnosis. In young children in whom asthma follows respiratory infection, the distinction between 'asthma' and 'recurrent bronchitis' is less clear-cut, and the diagnosis must rest on the assessment of the clinical features of the attack and other evidence of the atopic constitution. Blood examination will commonly show an eosinophilia in asthmatic cases, and skin-testing may indicate the responsible allergen.

In infants and young children, the sudden onset of continuous wheezing (particularly when this follows a paroxysm of coughing) should always suggest the diagnosis of inhaled foreign body.

TREATMENT. This may be divided into treatment of the acute attack, management between the attacks, and specific prophylaxis.

The acute attack. If this is heralded by premonitory symptoms such as headache and irritability, the child should be given 8 to 30 mg of ephedrine and a sedative, e.g. phenobarbitone, before dyspnoea becomes acute. When dyspnoea is already present, the child should be supported in the sitting position and will often prefer to lean forward on a bed-table. Ephedrine may bring relief or aminophylline (2 to 5 mg per kg body weight) may be given by oral, intramuscular or intravenous route or in a rectal suppository. Sublingual isoprenaline (2·5 to 5 mg) or oral orciprenaline (5 to 10 mg) may be effective in older children. In severe attacks, adrenaline may be administered in small doses by subcutaneous injection (0·1 to 0·5 ml of a 1 in 1000 solution) but care must be taken if the child has already been given a bronchodilator drug and adrenaline is better avoided if possible in very young children, because it may cause undesirable tachycardia by stimulation of β_1 receptors. Sedation with oral promethazine hydrochloride (10 to 25 mg) or dichloralphenazone (225 mg to 1·3 g depending on age), or alternatively an intramuscular injection of trimeprazine tartrate (0·6 mg per kg) will relieve anxiety and allow the child to rest. Corticosteroids will often relieve status asthmaticus when other agents have failed. In such severe cases, a large intravenous dose of hydrocortisone, with administration of moist oxygen and correction of the associated metabolic disturbance, will usually effect a dramatic improvement, though death occasionally occurs in very severe status asthmaticus.

Management of the asthmatic child between attacks. The role of psychological factors in the etiology of asthma makes it highly important that the child should be handled with understanding and that his activities should not be restricted more than necessary, for there is a real danger of invalidism being increased by parental overanxiety or domestic friction. The improvement which often occurs with removal from home surroundings, e.g. to a convalescent home, is sometimes due more to psychological than physical factors. Nevertheless, it is found that in some cases climate and physical environment are so important in precipitating attacks that a change of residence is justifiable. Every case must be carefully investigated before such a change is advised; a full psychological history should be taken as well as an investigation of possible allergens in the home before it is assumed that a change of climate (e.g. from country to town in a pollen-sensitive patient, from mountains to sea or vice versa) will be beneficial. The number of cases in which change of climate is really necessary is quite small.

Except in those cases in which particular ingestants are responsible for asthma, the diet need only be restricted to the extent that heavy meals at night are avoided, and the foods commonly found to cause digestive upsets in childhood are eliminated.

If frequent attacks or continuous, mild symptoms necessitate long-term bronchodilator drug therapy, oral ephedrine, choline theophyllinate or orciprenaline may be used. Patients who obtain relief from the use of an adrenaline or isoprenaline nebulizer may find that its ready availability gives confidence which tends to reduce the number of attacks. Pressurized aerosols should be avoided, however, as there is some evidence that the recent increase in the number of deaths from asthma is attributable to misuse of these preparations.

Disodium cromoglycate is valuable for regular preventive therapy, especially when the bronchoconstriction is labile, and the inhalation of this drug as a fine powder (3 to 6 capsules daily) may reduce the need for other drugs, including corticosteroids.

Breathing and postural exercises are advisable in every case in which attacks are at all frequent, and can be begun from the age of 2 or 3 years. The aim of these is to encourage diaphragmatic respiration and full excursion of the lower ribs and to improve posture.

The use of corticosteroids should generally be restricted to severe asthma which is interfering seriously with the education and social activities of an older child. It may rarely be advisable to give steroids to cut short asthmatic attacks in young children when these are causing progressive deformity of the chest. In general, however, the occasional use of steroids is unwise because the child and his parents may come to rely on them, because they may interfere with growth, and because the side-effects, though uncommon, may have worse consequences than the asthma itself. There may be fewer side-effects with corticotrophin, but there is a risk of severe allergic reaction which may however be avoided by using the synthetic preparation, tetracosactrin. With both of these, the need for parenteral injection is a disadvantage.

PROPHYLAXIS. When skin-testing reveals one or more specific allergens, every effort must be made to remove these from the environment. When the child is found to be sensitive to feathers or horsehair, a non-allergenic rubber mattress and pillows covered with impermeable material should be used. Household pets (cats, dogs, birds, etc.) may have to be sacrificed if they are found responsible, but this is seldom necessary. The child's bedroom should be kept as free from dust as possible by vacuum or damp cleaning and by excluding all dust-harbouring furnishings, stuffed or woolly toys, etc. In cases of food allergy, the particular foods must be eliminated from the diet, and prolonged cooking may reduce the liability to allergic reactions. Hyposensitization should be attempted when this is practicable, though in cases with multiple sensitivity it is not always possible. Upper respiratory infections, either of the tonsils and adenoids, or of the sinuses, should receive appropriate treatment, and the use of antibiotics or vaccines in patients with recurrent or chronic respiratory infection is sometimes helpful. Psychotherapy should be instituted in appropriate cases.

PROGNOSIS. Owing to the varied clinical pattern of asthma, prognosis can only be given in general terms. Patients whose symptoms have onset during the first two years of life are likely to be severely affected and may develop permanent thoracic deformity. Prognosis will, however, be affected by early diagnosis and treatment, and if it is possible for the child to avoid contact with the allergen, or to be hyposensitized to it, the risk of permanent lung damage is correspondingly reduced. There is a general tendency for children to improve at about the time of puberty, which may be marked by complete remission of symptoms. In many cases, however, patients who have been free from asthma throughout adolescence relapse when they are exposed to a sudden change of environment, e.g. army personnel sleeping in barracks or on overseas service.

Infantile (atopic) eczema

Although the terms 'eczema' and 'dermatitis' are used to describe a number of conditions having no common etiology, the majority of cases of eczema occurring in infancy are allergic in origin. In these the skin represents the 'shock organ' as the nasal mucosa does in hay-fever and the lung in asthma. Atopic eczema is seen most commonly in infants between the ages of 2 months and 2 years, but may also occur in older children. A substantial proportion of the infantile cases develop other allergic manifestations later, the commonest sequel being asthma.

ETIOLOGY. The atopic infant's skin is peculiarly sensitive and eczema is the response to a variety of stimulants, especially sensitization to ingestants. There is evidence that sensitization may occur through the placenta or the mother's milk before the allergen has been included in the infant's own diet although eczema is uncommon in wholly breast-fed infants, and often starts after the introduction of cow's milk. In older children, inhalants are more frequently responsible. Contact dermatitis, which is of great importance in adult life (e.g. in industry), is less common in infancy, but it may occur from soaps, toilet preparations, or clothing.

CLINICAL FEATURES. The cheeks and forehead are the sites first affected, and in most cases the condition remains limited to these areas. In some instances the eczema extends to the scalp and limbs, while in the severest cases the whole body is affected, the skin being red, oedematous, and giving rise to intense itching. In some children who have had eczema in infancy, lesions persist in the antecubital fossae or behind the knees and contact dermatitis elsewhere develops readily. Eczema may be *wet* (exudative) or *dry*, and is

commonly associated with erythema; a combination of wet and dry lesions not infrequently occurs. The majority of infantile cases, however, are principally exudative. In the latter the eruption starts with the appearance of erythema and papulo-vesicular lesions, on which crusts form, and which subsequently exude fluid (Plate 16). In the dry form the affected areas are red and scaly, and the lesions are not vesicular.

The condition is extremely irritating, and is rapidly made worse by scratching. Most severe and long-standing cases show innumerable excoriations, lichenification, and frequently secondary infection also. Affected infants are often found to be overweight, the condition tending to improve when weight is lost and to reappear when it is regained. Exposure to sunlight or cold may exacerbate the condition. Owing to the constant irritation, loss of sleep may necessitate prolonged sedation.

Eczematous infants should not be vaccinated, or brought into close contact with a recently vaccinated individual, owing to the danger of their developing generalized vaccinia. Immunization or injection of horse serum should also be avoided. Infection with the virus of herpes simplex may cause a severe reaction (*Kaposi's varicelliform eruption*), a cause of high, unexplained fever in an eczematous infant.

DIAGNOSIS. The condition with which infantile eczema is most likely to be confused is seborrhoeic dermatitis. Here the scalp is more affected than the face, the crusts are greasy rather than scaly, and since the lesions are not irritating, excoriations are not present. Pityriasis of the scalp may simulate the lesions of atopic eczema, the differential diagnosis depending on the site and the demonstration of the pityrosporon. In secondarily infected cases the lesions of atopic eczema may be masked by staphylococcal lesions or impetigo.

Skin-testing is seldom useful in determining the responsible allergen, since positive tests are commonly given to many or all reagents. It is sometimes helpful to remove possible agents one at a time from the diet or environment, and to observe the effect on the condition.

TREATMENT. Except in the mildest cases, this is apt to be tedious and prolonged. Infants should be breast-fed if possible and artificially fed infants usually do better on a half-cream or skimmed dried or evaporated milk formula, the carbohydrate content being kept low. In those rare cases in which cow's milk cannot be tolerated, a soya-bean preparation can be substituted. Soft solids are added to the diet one at a time, particular attention being paid to the tolerance of egg-white and egg-yolk, and to wheat-containing foods. Orange juice and cod-liver oil are also possible allergens.

If it is found that soap is irritating during acute exacerbations, washing in warm saline, or oiling with olive oil, will usually be satisfactory.

Prevention of scratching is an essential part of treatment, though it is extremely difficult to achieve over long periods. The arms should be splinted at the elbow, so that movement is allowed but the hands cannot reach the face. Since these infants frequently learn to rub the face on the pillow if their hands are restrained, it may be found effective to cover the pillow with a smooth material (e.g. Cellophane) on which friction does little damage. Antihistamine drugs relieve itching to some extent, but have no other effect on the lesions. Regular sedation is often necessary.

Local treatment. In the acute exudative stage, crusts may be removed with starch poultices or hydrogen peroxide and calamine lotion applied. When the eczema has dried, $\frac{1}{2}$ to 2 per cent hydrocortisone or prednisolone skin lotions or creams may be applied sparingly in moderate or severe cases. In mild chronic eczema, crude tar or ichthammol paste may be effective and is considerably cheaper.

PROGNOSIS. Infants with atopic eczema are not only liable to develop other allergic manifestations, but are particularly subject to intercurrent and secondary skin infections. In the majority of cases the eczematous condition improves or disappears spontaneously towards the end of the second year. It has been estimated that asthma occurs later in approximately 30 per cent of these cases.

Urticaria ('*Hives*')

The appearance of weals on the skin occurs in normal individuals from the action of various external agents such as stinging nettles or insect bites and stings. In atopic individuals, the reaction to such agents is often excessive and urticaria is also liable to occur from a much greater variety of causes, such as ingestants, inhalants, psychological upsets, heat, cold, sunlight, infections, and drugs. Urticarial weals commonly occur in susceptible individuals after the ingestion of foods such as shellfish, strawberries or eggs. The process producing the weal consists of capillary dilatation, reflex dilatation of the surrounding arterioles causing flushing, and local oedema resulting from increased capillary permeability. The weal appears as a pink or white raised area of irregular shape surrounded by erythema, and is commonly associated with intense itching or stinging.

In infants and children, urticaria is almost always superficial. *Giant urticaria* (angioneurotic oedema) involving the subcutaneous tissues is rare before adolescence, but may occur in cases of drug allergy.

Papular urticaria ('heat spots') is commonly seen in childhood and usually occurs during the warmer months. It may prove an annual irritation for several years but usually ceases before puberty. The weals are seldom large, and occur in crops, mainly over the limbs and trunk. A papule or small vesicle appears in the centre of the weal, and persists after the latter has subsided. The itching is intensified by warmth and is often worst at night; it results in scratching and excoriation, often followed by lichenification. Insect bites are the commonest cause, and if fleas and lice have been excluded, a repellent should be used. Local treatment with calamine lotion containing 0·5 per cent menthol or phenol may relieve irritation.

Papular urticaria is frequently mistaken for varicella (in cases in which the lesions vesiculate or become crusted) or scabies (when the lesions are clustered about the wrists and between the fingers, and when itching at night is particularly pronounced).

Other varieties of urticaria seen in childhood are those associated with purpura (p. 250) or parasitic infestation, and *dermographism*. In the latter condition the skin is abnormally sensitive to tactile stimuli. Gentle scratching or even stroking the skin produces a line of erythema succeeded by a linear weal. In the rare condition of *urticaria pigmentosa*, weals are followed by the appearance of small pigmented patches which may persist for several years, but usually disappear at puberty. The lesions contain large numbers of mast cells. The etiology of urticaria pigmentosa is unknown, but the condition is probably not related to the allergic types of urticaria.

TREATMENT. An acute attack of urticaria or angio-neurotic oedema can be relieved by the injection of adrenaline hydrochloride, and in some cases antihistamine drugs will control the condition over a longer period. Such treatment is only palliative and not curative. The primary cause must be looked for and, if possible, eliminated. If the patient has been taking any drug (particularly aspirin, salicylate, chloral, barbiturate or sulphonamide), the effect of stopping the drug should be observed. The stools should be examined for ova and parasites and any source of local infection dealt with.

Serum sickness

Susceptible individuals are liable to have severe reactions following the administration of serum, either within a few hours or more commonly seven to twelve days later. Symptoms include urticaria, fall in blood pressure, collapse, severe joint pains, nausea, and rigors. While these symptoms are of much less frequent occurrence with the sera now commercially available, it is always advisable to test an allergic patient for sensitivity or to withhold serum treatment unless absolutely necessary.

Immediate reactions due to anaphylaxis in a patient who has previously received serum are similar but more severe, and are more liable to prove fatal. The attack must be treated promptly with adrenaline.

Gastro-intestinal allergy

In addition to the various manifestations described (asthma, urticaria, etc.), allergy may be manifested by digestive disturbances, viz. severe vomiting, colic and diarrhoea. Elimination of the allergen, usually a food, responsible for symptoms is more effective than hyposensitization, and may ultimately lead to loss of hypersensitivity. Allergy to cow's milk protein occasionally causes vomiting and diarrhoea in infants and may necessitate feeding with a synthetic milk, which must be supplemented by vitamins and amino acids to prevent the development of deficiency syndromes.

BIBLIOGRAPHY AND REFERENCES

AAS, K. (1969). Allergic asthma in childhood. *Archives of Disease in Childhood*, **44**, 1.
BRITISH MEDICAL JOURNAL (1971). Mites and house dust allergy. *British Medical Journal*, ii, 601.
CODE, C. F., HURN, M. & MITCHELL, R. G. (1964). Histamine in human disease. *Proceedings of Staff Meetings of the Mayo Clinic*, **39**, 715.
CREAK, M. & STEPHEN, J. M. (1958). The psychological aspects of asthma in children. *Pediatric Clinics of North America*, **5**, 731.
DAWSON, B., HOROBIN, G., ILLSLEY, R. & MITCHELL, R. G. (1969). A survey of childhood asthma in Aberdeen. *Lancet*, i, 827.
DEAMER, W. C. (1960). Allergy in childhood. In *Advances in Pediatrics*, vol. 9. Edited by S. J. Levine. London: Interscience Publishers.
GLASER, J. (1956). *Allergy in Childhood*. Springfield, Ill.: Thomas.
HILL, L. W. (1955). The treatment of eczema in infants and children. *Journal of Pediatrics*, **47**, 141.
HILMAN, B. C. (1967). The allergic child. *Annals of Allergy*, **25**, 620.
JONES, R. S. & BLACKHALL, M. I. (1970). Role of disodium cromoglycate (intal) in treatment of childhood asthma. *Archives of Disease in Childhood*, **45**, 49.
SIEGEL, S. C. (1965). ACTH and corticosteroids in the management of allergic disorders in children. *Journal of Pediatrics*, **66**, 927.
SHERMAN, W. B. & KESSLER, W. R. (1957). *Allergy in Pediatric Practice*. St Louis: Mosby.
SILVER, H. & DOUGLAS, D. M. (1968). Milk intolerance in infancy. *Archives of Disease in Childhood*, **43**, 17.
SMITH, J. M., HARDING, L. K. & CUMMING, G. (1971). The changing prevalence of asthma in schoolchildren. *Clinical Allergy*, **1**, 57.

12 Rheumatic and Collagen Disorders

(See also anaphylactoid purpura, p. 251; acute nephritis, p. 285)

The rheumatic disorders include juvenile rheumatism (rheumatic fever; acute and subacute rheumatism); Sydenham's chorea; and rheumatoid arthritis. The association between juvenile rheumatism and chorea is sufficiently close for chorea in childhood to be regarded as typically a rheumatic disorder, though at least some cases occurring after puberty are thought to be non-rheumatic. Rheumatic carditis is a complication of juvenile rheumatism, whether the latter occurs in acute or subacute form or in association with chorea.

The term 'collagen disorders' has been used to describe a wider group of conditions characterized by damage to mesenchymal tissues, and including not only juvenile rheumatism and rheumatoid arthritis but also lupus erythematosus, dermatomyositis, periarteritis nodosa, and scleroderma. Anaphylactoid purpura and acute nephritis have features linking them with the collagen disorders and are sometimes grouped with them.

JUVENILE RHEUMATISM

Juvenile rheumatism was until recently one of the most important causes of recurrent invalidism and early death; but it is still difficult to provide a satisfactory clinical definition which will embrace all cases and exclude non-rheumatic conditions. When the condition presents with joint swellings and fever (*acute rheumatism, rheumatic fever*), and particularly when rheumatic nodules or cardiac lesions are present, the picture is clear-cut and definitive. But in its subacute form, characterized by recurrent limb and joint pains, fatigue, pallor, loss of weight, etc., rheumatism may be closely simulated by many other diseases and will in some cases only be recognized after the heart has become affected.

Pathologically, the diagnostic lesion is the Aschoff node which is found in the heart muscle, connective tissues, muscles, and other mesodermal tissues. The nodes are situated in the vicinity of blood vessels, and show endothelial proliferation, the presence of giant-cells, round-cell infiltration, and necrosis.

ETIOLOGY

Although a number of etiological factors have been described, their mode of interaction is not clearly established.

HEREDITY

The familial incidence of juvenile rheumatism is well known. Allowing for the fact that both infection and adverse social conditions are likely to affect several members of a family, there is evidence that there exists a hereditary predisposition to rheumatism. There is some evidence, not confirmed by all investigators, that susceptibility may be inherited as a recessive character. Although this is not proven it is generally accepted that the disease will become manifest when susceptible individuals are exposed to the conditions necessary to produce it. There appears to be no clear racial predisposition or immunity.

SEX AND AGE INCIDENCE

While case series of chorea show a definite preponderance of girls over boys, the incidence of juvenile rheumatism without chorea is approximately equal in the two sexes or slightly higher in boys than girls. The age-onset of acute rheumatism is maximum at 7 to 9 years, and it is rare before 3 years of age. The incidence rises sharply after the age of 3 years, but in less than 20 per cent of all childhood cases is the onset before the age of 5.

ENVIRONMENTAL AND SOCIAL CONDITIONS

Juvenile rheumatism is predominantly a disease of the poorer social groups and is probably related to overcrowding, as might be expected in view of the role of streptococcal infection in etiology. The incidence also appears to be affected by damp housing and subsoil. Nevertheless, the occurrence of the disease in widely different climates makes it unlikely that damp is more than a contributory factor.

SEASON AND CLIMATE

In 1678 Thomas Sydenham observed that rheumatism occurred most frequently in the autumn and this is probably still true in Britain, although in New York the highest incidence is in April and the lowest in October. Formerly juvenile rheumatism was a disease of temperate climates but in recent years it has become less common and less severe in Europe and North America, whereas it has greatly increased in incidence in the tropics. This increase may be due, at least in part, to the effects of modern travel in spreading streptococcal infection to susceptible populations.

INFECTION

It has long been recognized that throat infections or scarlet fever caused by group A beta-haemolytic streptococci frequently precede attacks of acute rheumatism. The initial infection, which may be mild or undetected, is likely to be followed by a latent or silent period of from ten to twenty days, during which the patient appears well, before the manifestations of rheumatism appear. This applies both to the primary attack and to relapses. Throat swabs examined for haemolytic streptococci at the time of the rheumatic manifestations, i.e. two to three weeks after the throat infection has subsided, may prove negative. This sequence of events has been explained by a sensitization of susceptible patients to haemolytic streptococci, and the rheumatic lesions have been regarded as allergic phenomena, though the evidence is inconclusive. Experimentally, lesions comparable to those of rheumatic carditis and periarteritis nodosa have been produced by anaphylactic hypersensitivity, not only to streptococci. Studies of the anti-streptolysin titre of the blood in rheumatic patients who have suffered from streptococcal infections show that the titre may rise for some considerable time after the acute infection has subsided, and this finding has been related to the clinical manifestations of rheumatism. Auto-immune mechanisms may be involved in pathogenesis, since streptococcal antigens which exhibit cross-reactions with heart tissue have been demonstrated (Kaplan, 1963). Alternatively, it is possible that rheumatic lesions are due to persisting infection by streptococci in L forms.

CLINICAL FEATURES

Rheumatism must be regarded as a disease affecting the whole patient, with a predilection for certain organs of which the heart is by far the most important. It has been said of rheumatism by Lasêgue that 'it licks the joints, the pleura, and even the meninges, but it bites the heart'.

GENERAL SYMPTOMS

In a severe attack of acute rheumatism, the onset is sudden and frequently occurs two to three weeks after a throat infection. There is high fever, usually up to 39·5°C (103°F). The fever may be associated with swelling, redness, and acute pain of one or more joints, or pain and stiffness of the joints may occur without swelling. Swelling, when present, is mainly periarticular and there is little effusion into the joint. It is characteristic of the joint involvement that the pain or swelling in one joint will subside rapidly to be followed by similar pain or swelling of another. The wrists, knees, and ankles are those most commonly affected. If pain and swelling remain localized to one or more joints without any tendency to move, non-rheumatic arthritis should be suspected. In some acute cases, severe shifting muscle pains take the place of joint pains. The child is pale, sweating is pronounced, and the pulse-rate is raised. A soft apical systolic murmur is commonly heard at this stage, and the first heart sound is muffled in the mitral area. These findings give little indication of the degree of subsequent heart involvement. The urine is scant, of high specific gravity, and often shows a trace of albumin (febrile albuminuria).

The characteristic attack of acute rheumatism described above is now rare and subacute or even subclinical episodes are much more common. In these the onset is more insidious, and it is not very uncommon to find children who have developed a severe cardiac lesion without ever having been kept in bed. There may be a history of repeated throat infections, though this is not

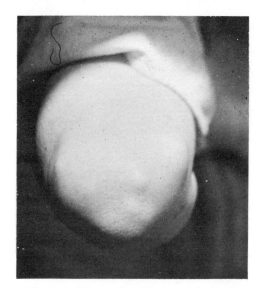

Fig. 12.1   Rheumatic nodules round the elbow.

always obtained. The child has usually become pale and apathetic, and has flagged in both physical activities and school work. Loss of weight, or failure to gain weight, is frequently an early indication of rheumatic disease. Recurrent limb pains are a most important symptom, and since these are often discounted as 'growing pains', the distinction between true rheumatic pains and non-rheumatic pains due to faulty posture or fatigue may be considered in detail (Table 12.1).

The distinction is often difficult to make with absolute certainty, and every aspect of the case must be considered in reaching a diagnosis. It must be remembered that the child who is unhappy and emotionally upset will often complain of somatic disturbances, of which fatigue, loss of appetite, and aching pains are among the most common; while a rheumatic child who is in a state of chronic ill-health is likely to be miserable and apathetic also. The erythrocyte sedimentation rate may be helpful in establishing a diagnosis, as it is likely to be raised in active rheumatism. A raised antistreptolysin titre provides confirmatory evidence of previous streptococcal infection. In any doubtful case both the waking and the sleeping pulse rate should be observed.

RHEUMATIC NODULES

These are small subcutaneous nodules occurring principally over bony points, around the joints, along tendon sheaths and in the occipital

Table 12.1

	Rheumatic pains	Non-rheumatic pains
Character	Sharp and shooting	Aching
Site	Variable; principally limbs and shoulders	Between shoulders, in lumbar region, and backs of knees
Time of onset	Principally on waking	In evening and after prolonged standing
Effect of exercise	Commonly diminished	Increased
Effect of salicylates	Relieved	Usually unaffected
Postural defects	Frequently absent	Commonly present

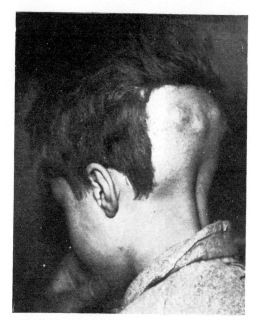

Fig. 12.2   Rheumatic nodules in occipital region.

region. Their structure is similar to that of the Aschoff node. They are almost always multiple, arising in crops, and may appear and disappear with surprising rapidity.

Rheumatic nodules are evidence of rheumatic activity, and almost always indicate cardiac involvement; they occur as a late rather than as an early manifestation of an acute rheumatic episode but are now much less commonly seen than formerly.

PULMONARY LESIONS

Collapse of the base of the left lower lobe occurs mechanically when there is a large pericardial effusion or gross cardiac enlargement. Pulmonary oedema and evidence of back pressure are found in cases with cardiac failure. It is believed by some that a specific type of rheumatic pneumonia occurs, commonly associated with pleurisy over the affected area.

HAEMORRHAGE

Epistaxis is a not uncommon symptom in juvenile rheumatism, and is occasionally so severe as to require transfusion. Haemorrhagic nephritis and purpura are rare complications.

SKIN LESIONS

The most important of these are erythema marginatum and erythema nodosum, though neither is a common manifestation of rheumatism. The former appears as pale rose-coloured rings of erythema on the back, trunk, or thighs; it is unlikely to be seen in the absence of carditis. These lesions fade rapidly but may reappear with exacerbations of the disease. A variety of other erythematous and urticarial lesions are occasionally seen. *Erythema nodosum* of rheumatic origin is clinically similar to the condition occurring as the result of tuberculous infection (Fig. 15.6), and occasionally following the administration of sulphonamides; it is a manifestation of skin hypersensitivity.

ABDOMINAL PAIN

Pain referred to the abdomen is relatively common, and is occasionally so severe as to cause difficulty in diagnosis. In some of these cases it is attributable to a non-specific mesenteric adenitis following the throat infection; in others it is superficial and related to the abdominal muscles.

Rheumatic carditis

The incidence of cardiac involvement in cases of acute rheumatism has been variously assessed owing to the different criteria of involvement adopted by different observers; some hold that in almost every case the heart is affected to some extent, others that a diagnosis of cardiac involvement should be reserved for those patients showing permanent damage. Whichever view is adopted, every child with acute rheumatism should be regarded as being in danger of cardiac damage while the condition is active. The danger appears to be considerably greater in rheumatism than in chorea without other rheumatic manifestations, although long-term studies show that carditis with permanent sequelae occurs more often in 'pure' chorea than was formerly believed. In some cases of rheumatism, the heart will be found functionally normal after convalescence, and may either remain so or show evidence of damage following a subsequent relapse. In others a clearly recognizable cardiac lesion will appear early and persist, or occasionally the onset of carditis is fulminating and rapidly fatal. The danger of cardiac damage occurring insidiously in children with subacute rheumatism who have remained ambulant is a very real one, and is increased by the prescription for them of salicylates, which may remove the danger signal of pain without removing the risk of carditis. If the child is suffering from active rheumatism, he should be at rest; if the pains complained of are non-rheumatic, it is unlikely that salicylates will relieve them.

PATHOLOGY. It was previously believed that when rheumatism attacked the heart, the pericardium, myocardium, and endocardium were all affected to a greater or less extent in every case. While lesions of the myocardium and endocardium are almost always demonstrable at necropsy when there is pericarditis, it is doubtful if the pericardium is necessarily involved in all cases with endocarditis. The characteristic lesions of the myocardium (Aschoff's nodes) are widely disseminated, but are found principally around the coronary arterioles. Rheumatism shows a predilection for particular parts of the endocardium, the mitral valve being affected more frequently than the aortic valve, the tricuspid valve less commonly, while the pulmonary valve is rarely involved. The lesions of the endocardium are primarily inflammatory (valvulitis) and commonly result in the formation of small firm vegetations immediately proximal to the free margin of the valve and on the chordae tendiniae; the inflammatory changes are followed by cicatrization, which results in distortion and immobility of the affected valves. Since the complete picture takes some years to develop, valvular stenosis of the type commonly seen in adult life is comparatively rare in childhood.

In pericarditis, there are roughening and adhesion of the pericardial surfaces due to organizing serofibrinous exudate or to the pouring-out of pericardial effusion. The changes frequently begin posteriorly, where the pericardium is reflected from the great vessels, and subsequently spread to the anterior surface of the heart. Pleuro-pericardial adhesions may form when the parietal pericardium is extensively involved.

CLINICAL FEATURES. The child who is developing rheumatic carditis is pale and tends to be dyspnoeic on slight exertion, or to avoid exertion altogether. Tachycardia is a most important sign and there is softening of the first heart sound with a soft apical systolic murmur. When the child is under observation at rest in bed, it is advisable to chart the sleeping and waking pulse rates separately. If the sleeping pulse rate is within 10 beats a minute of the waking rate, and when it remains persistently above ‚100 per minute, carditis should be suspected. The erythrocyte sedimentation rate is raised, and while this is not a specific test for rheumatism, repeated estimations provide a valuable indication of the progress of the case. The E.S.R. tends to be higher in cases with carditis than in those in which the heart is not involved, and provides an approximate index of severity. (A sudden fall in sedimentation rate, however, is sometimes observed in the terminal stage of cardiac failure.) The blood shows some degree of anaemia, and there is a moderate leucocytosis. The electrocardiogram may show not only an increased PR interval but also inversion of T waves or notching of P waves in acute rheumatism, but is of little help at this stage in determining whether permanent cardiac damage is developing.

As the condition progresses, carditis will be indicated by the pulse rate remaining high despite the subsidence of fever on salicylate therapy. The apical systolic murmur tends to become harsher, is conducted toward the left axilla, and is brought out on exertion. A localized middiastolic murmur may be heard in the mitral area, and this is often associated with reduplication of the second mitral sound. There is gradually increasing cardiac enlargement.

Although more significance should be attached to the appearance of a diastolic murmur than to a systolic murmur, particularly if the latter is not conducted to the axilla, cases are sometimes seen in which a middiastolic murmur disappears entirely and leaves an apparently normal heart. In most cases, however, in which a diastolic murmur appears, the heart is permanently affected. The diastolic-systolic 'bellows murmur' is characteristic of established mitral disease in childhood; the middiastolic murmur may subsequently appear earlier in diastole and gradually become converted into the harsh presystolic murmur accompanied by a thrill more commonly observed in mitral stenosis in adult life.

Although it is not uncommon to find the aortic valve affected at necropsy, clinical evidence of aortic disease is much less frequently detected in childhood than is evidence of mitral disease. Aortic vegetations or cicatrization may give rise to a rough systolic murmur in the aortic area conducted into the neck, and aortic regurgitation to a soft diastolic murmur best heard down the left border of the sternum. When there is well-marked regurgitation, enlargement of the left ventricle and a collapsing pulse will be demonstrable.

The occurrence of pericarditis is marked by increasing pallor and prostration, a rise of pulse rate, and often by the recurrence of pyrexia; nodules may appear concurrently. The child often complains of precordial pain and dyspnoea. On examination, a to-and-fro friction rub (which appears more superficial than the endocardial murmurs) is often transient and disappears when pericardial effusion occurs. The area of cardiac dullness is then greatly enlarged, the sounds muffled, and radiological examination shows a characteristic globular cardiac shadow. The effusion seldom if ever requires aspiration.

Cardiac failure is only likely to occur before the age of 12 in those cases in which the heart has been affected early or extremely severely. The majority of cases which break down before adult life do so at puberty or in early adolescence, so that a review of cases seen in a children's hospital is apt to give a too optimistic impression of the disease. The signs of cardiac failure are increasing dyspnoea, a rising pulse rate, enlargement of the liver, and the appearance of oedema.

DIAGNOSIS. The character of rheumatic pains, migratory joint swellings, cardiac signs, subcutaneous nodules and the response to salicylate therapy, together with the blood count, erythrocyte sedimentation-rate, and antistreptolysin titre, all help to establish the diagnosis. (The presence of an abnormal serum protein, C-reactive protein, has been used as evidence of activity, though like the E.S.R. it is not a specific test for rheumatism.) The conditions most likely to be confused with acute rheumatism are anaphylactoid purpura, osteomyelitis, septic arthritis, and rheumatoid arthritis. The diagnosis of anaphylactoid purpura with joint pains will depend on the presence of the characteristic purpuric lesions. In the other three conditions, the pain and swelling are not migratory as in rheumatism, and are not effectively relieved by salicylate therapy. In acute osteomyelitis the temperature and leucocyte count tend to be higher than in rheumatism; localized tenderness is more likely to be helpful than radiological examination in establishing the presence of a bony lesion. Septic arthritis commonly follows a previous infection and the diagnosis can be made by aspiration of joint fluid. The diagnosis of rheumatoid arthritis is discussed below. Poliomyelitis, in which limb pains and tenderness may be present in the early stages, will be distin-

guished by the association of neck and back stiffness and examination of the cerebrospinal fluid. Leukaemia should be excluded when the presenting symptoms are pallor and limb pains, the diagnosis being confirmed by blood and marrow examination.

TREATMENT. In all cases of acute or subacute rheumatism the essential treatment is rest in bed until signs of activity have disappeared. The position adopted by the child in bed is not important unless there is serious cardiac involvement, when he should be propped up in a semi-sitting position. Subsequent progress will be determined by the response of the pulse, clinical evidence of cardiac involvement, the E.S.R., and possibly by the C-reactive protein reaction. At least four weeks' bed rest is generally necessary, although in mild cases the child need not be completely confined to bed towards the end of this period. The total duration of restricted activity will seldom be less than three months.

In the immediate treatment of acute rheumatism associated with fever and joint or limb pains, sodium salicylate given in adequate dosage (e.g. 120 mg per kg body weight per day in divided doses), or one of the more palatable aspirin preparations, will relieve symptoms and pyrexia rapidly. Indeed, if fever and pain are not relieved within two days, the diagnosis of rheumatism should be questioned. It is doubtful if salicylates have any effect on rheumatic carditis and it is unnecessary to maintain a high blood salicylate level. Salicylate poisoning is evidenced by vomiting, headache, and tinnitus, and these symptoms are an indication for reducing (or temporarily omitting) the dosage. An initial course of penicillin serves to eradicate streptococcal infection, but will not otherwise affect the rheumatic symptoms.

There is some evidence that corticosteroids given in the early stages have a beneficial effect on rheumatic heart disease and patients with signs of carditis should have a course of corticosteroid and aspirin for six weeks or longer. Initial dosage of steroid is determined by the severity of the disease and, after control has been achieved, the dose is progressively diminished, e.g. prednisone 60 mg daily for a week, decreased by 10 mg each week. Aspirin may be continued after termination of steroid therapy in an attempt to avoid recurrence of symptoms on withdrawal of steroids.

The use of digitalis is contraindicated in early carditis, which often shows signs of improvement when corticosteroids are started. The relief obtained by digitalization of children with extreme tachycardia, however, is sometimes sufficient to justify its trial, while in cases with cardiac failure and dyspnoea or oedema it should certainly be used. Dyspnoeic patients should be nursed in oxygen, and if there is much oedema diuretics may be helpful.

The long-term treatment of rheumatic children will include regular supervision, so that relapses can be detected and treatment instituted as early as possible, routine prophylaxis (see below), and regulation of the child's activity so that cardiac function is not overstrained. Children who have sustained no cardiac damage should return to full and unrestricted activity. A persistent apical systolic murmur which is not conducted to the axilla should not be interpreted as evidence of cardiac damage if cardiac function and radiographic examination of the heart are normal.

Where the heart has definitely been affected, it may be necessary to limit activity, but only to the extent that tolerance is not exceeded. This may mean prohibiting competitive games at school and possibly restricting swimming and other energetic sports. Such restrictions should not be maintained longer than necessary, for in many cases the heart becomes remarkably well compensated, and it is just as undesirable to turn these children into chronic invalids by forbidding all normal activities as it is to allow decompensation to occur from neglect. In severely affected cases, prolonged inactivity may be necessary and it is sometimes advisable for the child to attend a special school and to learn a sedentary trade.

PREVENTION. The prompt and adequate treatment with penicillin of streptococcal throat infections reduces the incidence of acute rheumatism, while the prolonged administration of penicillin or sulphonamide is of value in preventing recurrence of rheumatism. Prophylactic treatment, e.g. phenoxymethyl penicillin 125 mg twice daily, should be given for 10 years from the last attack or until the age of 18 years, whichever is the longer period. Sulphadimidine 0·5 g twice daily is also effective and, despite the risks of toxic effects and bacterial resistance, it compares well with penicillin for prolonged use. Benzathine penicillin in doses of 1,200,000 units by intramuscular injection once a month is the prophylactic method of choice if regular oral administration cannot be adequately supervised. More intensive antibiotic cover, using cephalo-ridine or erythromycin if the child is already receiving penicillin, should be given at the time of dental extractions. Tonsillectomy should be advised if the tonsils have become chronically or repeatedly infected, but is not otherwise indicated.

PROGNOSIS. The expectation of life of the individual patient depends very largely on whether the heart is affected, the age at which carditis occurs, and the severity of the lesions. In patients who escape carditis in childhood, the likelihood of relapse and carditis occurring in adolescence or adult life is not high; in those affected in early childhood, the prognosis tends to be worse than when carditis occurs later. In the past 20 years, not only have the incidence and severity of juvenile rheumatism decreased, but the mortality rate and the relapse rate have both shown striking reductions. The complication of bacterial endocarditis can be more effectively controlled, while surgery can relieve established mitral stenosis.

CHOREA

The type of chorea described by Sydenham ('St Vitus's dance') is frequently included as a manifestation of juvenile rheumatism, and cases of rheumatism and chorea are considered together for statistical purposes. In the majority of cases it will be found that rheumatic symptoms have figured in the previous history of choreic patients, though it is rare for acute rheumatism and chorea to occur simultaneously. While there is good reason to regard chorea as essentially rheumatic in origin, uncomplicated cases present certain differences from acute rheumatism which are of prognostic importance. Thus the E.S.R. is raised in only approximately 50 per cent of cases of chorea, the incidence of carditis is significantly lower in uncomplicated cases than in acute rheumatism (see above), and girls are affected two to three times as frequently as boys. The average age of onset is also slightly higher than in the case of acute rheumatism, viz. 10 years to puberty in chorea, as compared with 7 to 9 years in rheumatism.

Chorea has been described as a diffuse meningo-encephalitis, affecting principally the cerebral hemispheres, basal ganglia, and pia-arachnoid; the cerebrospinal fluid is normal with the possible exception of calcium-content which has been found to be reduced. Since it is rare for uncomplicated cases of chorea to die during an acute attack, our knowledge of the pathology is scanty and it is difficult to reconcile the findings which have been described in some fatal cases with the complete remission of symptoms during sleep and with the recovery which normally occurs.

There is no doubt that emotional factors play an important part in precipitating symptoms in many cases. Overpressure of school work, sudden fright, or emotional distress appear frequently in the case histories. It is often claimed that choreic children are 'nervous' or 'highly strung' before the onset of symptoms.

CLINICAL FEATURES

The onset may be sudden or insidious. Most frequently, the child is said to have become clumsy, tripping-up or dropping things, and abnormally tearful on little or no provocation. If the mother is asked whether she allows the child to help with the washing-up, she will very often say she has had to stop it owing to breakages. Complaint is sometimes made of inattentiveness or 'fidgetiness' at school.

Examination will show the presence of frequent, purposeless, jerky movements, which may be unilateral and are commonly associated with facial grimaces or rapid changes of expression. The movements, which are a series of broken and inco-ordinated sequences and which are not repetitive, tend to be increased if the child is asked to carry out any fine movement such as unbuttoning her dress or tying a bow. The handwriting reflects the lack of co-ordination. In the active phase of the disease, the writing is large and irregular, or the child may find herself unable to write more than a number of meaningless scrawls. As recovery takes place, the writing shows a corresponding improvement and may be used as a graphic record of progress. The outstretched hands cannot be maintained steadily in the same position, and often assume the 'dinner fork' position, flexed at the wrist with the fingers extended at the metacarpo-phalangeal joints. This position, however, is often seen in the absence of chorea, and the unsteadiness and writhing movements of the hands are more characteristic of chorea.

In the severest cases, the movements are so violent that the child is in danger of flinging herself out of bed and the sides of the cot must be padded to prevent injury. The movements cease

during sleep. Loss of speech is a symptom which may cause great anxiety to the parents, but if the diagnosis is certain they can be reassured that speech will be recovered.

The tendon reflexes are commonly exaggerated, and the 'sustained knee-jerk' when present is characteristic, the leg flying forward and remaining extended for several seconds before relaxation occurs. The plantar reflex is normal.

Hemichorea is the description given to cases of chorea in which the condition is unilateral, and *chorea mollis* to those cases in which flaccidity, usually of one limb or of both limbs of the same side, takes the place of choreic movement. In the latter condition the tendon reflexes may be reduced or even absent.

DIAGNOSIS

While the fully developed picture of chorea is unmistakable, minor manifestations may be confused with tics (habit spasms), or hemichorea and chorea mollis with hemiplegia or poliomyelitis. The distinguishing feature of tics, e.g. grimaces, shoulder shrugging, etc., is that the performance is consistently repeated in the same manner, and represents a series of co-ordinated movements in which the various muscles involved work in harmony. Often the movement will be repeated on request, but concentration on carrying out a particular performance will tend to abolish the tic rather than to exaggerate it.

In differentiating chorea from choreo-athetoid cerebral palsy, the previous history is particularly valuable. Other manifestations of brain damage will usually be found in choreo-athetosis.

COURSE AND PROGNOSIS

Recovery from an attack of chorea almost invariably occurs although the duration is very variable. There is a considerable likelihood of recurrence, and in each subsequent attack the risk of carditis is increased. The ultimate prognosis in patients developing carditis is the same as that in other types of rheumatism.

TREATMENT

The patient should be kept in bed for at least four weeks, or for longer if movements recur on resumption of activity. A persistently raised E.S.R. or evidence of carditis are indications for further bed rest, as in rheumatism. Sedatives are likely to be required in the more active cases, particularly when insomnia is a symptom. Salicylates are valueless in the absence of other manifestations of rheumatism, since patients are normally afebrile. A variety of 'specific' treatments have been used, but have been largely discarded either owing to toxic reactions or to lack of evidence of their value. It is important that, as far as possible, the child should be guarded against the factors which may have precipitated the attack, e.g. excessive home-work, when full activity is resumed, since a return to previous conditions may cause an immediate relapse.

JUVENILE RHEUMATOID ARTHRITIS (STILL'S DISEASE)

The syndrome described by Still (1897), viz. polyarthritis associated with splenic and lymphatic enlargement, is typically one of early childhood, and is now considered as a particular manifestation of juvenile rheumatoid arthritis.

ETIOLOGY

This is unknown, and although the disease is usually regarded as infective in origin there is little indication of the infecting agent. Examination of the blood, synovial fluid, etc., has in most hands proved negative, though in some instances streptococci have been isolated. Focal sepsis can rarely be incriminated with any confidence. The possibility of an endocrine factor, with suppression of adrenal cortical function, is under investigation. In some respects the disease appears to form a link between juvenile rheumatism and rheumatoid arthritis of adults, since the onset may closely resemble that of acute

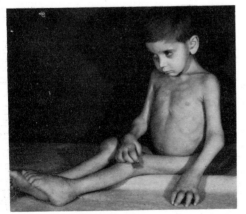

Fig. 12.3 Still's disease, showing swelling of elbows, wrists, interphalangeal joints, knees, and ankles.

rheumatism, transient nodules may appear, and pericarditis is a not uncommon complication.

The condition occurs in both sexes, and although some series have shown a preponderance of girls, the difference in sex incidence is not as great as in adult life. It may start at any age of infancy or childhood but the peak age of onset is between 2 and 5 years.

PATHOLOGY

The joint swelling is mainly due to infiltration of the periarticular tissues. The capsules and synovial membranes are thickened and hyperaemic. Pitting of the articular cartilages and fibrosis of lymph nodes suggesting a chronic inflammatory reaction have been described.

CLINICAL FEATURES

The onset may be *abrupt*, with high fever, irritability and tachycardia, and usually, though not always, with painful swelling of numerous joints (knees, ankles, elbows, wrists, interphalangeal joints, etc.). More often the disease starts *insidiously*, in which case stiffness and fusiform swelling of the joints of fingers, hands, and wrists are commonly the first indications. Swellings of the larger joints, e.g. the knees, which may be symmetrical and associated with low-grade pyrexia, are occasionally the presenting signs. It is not uncommon for a single joint, usually the knee, to be stiff and swollen for some weeks before any other joint is involved. The cervical spine is frequently affected causing the child to move her head slowly and stiffly.

The disease is marked by repeated exacerbations and remissions. As a general rule the child is left more seriously incapacitated following each attack and with more joints involved. The E.S.R. is raised during periods of activity, and a pink, macular rash may appear fleetingly, usually on the trunk. There is a variable leucocytosis, which may be considerably higher than that seen in acute rheumatism. A decrease in plasma albumin with elevation of gamma and sometimes alpha-2 globulins is evidence of rheumatoid activity. The Rheumatoid Factor, as demonstrated by the Rose-Waaler or Latex slide tests, is much less frequently present in the blood in juvenile rheumatoid arthritis than it is in the adult disease.

Wasting is a striking feature and affects not

only the muscles of the limbs but the whole body. Contractures and deformities occur unless they are prevented by splintage, and ankylosis of affected joints is a late sequela. These children may be in continual discomfort, if not severe pain, which is increased by movement of any of the affected joints. They become anxious and miserable and their general condition rapidly deteriorates. Severe anaemia occurs in long-standing cases and iridocyclitis is an occasional late complication.

Lymphadenopathy usually occurs early and during each exacerbation. It is often generalized, though the axillary and inguinal nodes may be enlarged to a greater extent than other groups. The nodes are not acutely tender and do not suppurate. *Splenomegaly*, when it occurs, is of moderate degree. *Hepatomegaly* is present in a minority of cases.

BONE CHANGES

There is a general rarefaction of the skeleton which is most marked around the affected joints, and growth of the limbs is retarded.

CARDITIS

Mild isolated pericarditis manifest by electrocardiographic changes and a friction rub is an occasional complication which usually disappears in a few days or weeks. Rarely, more severe pericarditis or myocarditis occurs early and leads to cardiac failure. Endocarditis is seldom seen.

TREATMENT

No treatment provides certain cure. Corticosteroid therapy gives rapid symptomatic relief but unfortunately relapse frequently occurs when it is stopped or substantially reduced. In mild rheumatoid arthritis, an attempt should be made to treat the disease without recourse to steroids. Stiffness of joints may be relieved by heat in the form of warm baths, hot packs or hot paraffin wax. Salicylates help to relieve pain. The child should exercise daily, putting each affected joint through its full range of movement. Adequate rest and a good diet should be assured. If corticosteroids are required, prednisone may be given initially in a total daily dosage of 60 mg (4 divided doses of 15 mg) for a few days, this being gradually reduced to a maintenance dose of 10 mg daily and continued for at least six months.

Thereafter cautious attempts should be made to reduce the dose to the smallest which will prevent relapse. The total duration of corticosteroid treatment will seldom be less than one or two years. Growth retardation, the masking of infection, peptic ulcer and osteoporosis leading to vertebral collapse are hazards of prolonged therapy and X-rays of the spine should be taken periodically.

As an alternative to prednisone, corticotrophin may be given by injection and is preferable for very long-term therapy since the growth inhibiting effect is less. The use of gold preparations, phenylbutazone and immunosuppressive drugs such as cyclophosphamide should be confined to cases of very severe rheumatoid arthritis in which corticosteroids are ineffective or contraindicated. Other measures include the prevention of contraction deformities, and the treatment of anaemia, if necessary by transfusion. Occupational therapy is most desirable in view of the chronicity of the disease.

COURSE AND PROGNOSIS

The course is very variable and only a small proportion of patients recovers completely at an early stage. In most cases the course is prolonged, though steroid therapy may effect a remission enabling the child to lead a fairly normal life. Apparent arrest of the disease may occur after one or more years and the majority of patients eventually make a complete functional recovery. In some cases of severe rheumatoid arthritis, the disease is progressive, resulting finally in complete invalidism. A few patients die from intercurrent infection or pericarditis; those in whom the condition persists into adult life show the picture of adult rheumatoid arthritis.

OTHER COLLAGEN DISORDERS
Dermatomyositis

The manifestations of this rare inflammatory disorder of unknown etiology appear principally in the muscles, skin, and subcutaneous tissues. The muscles are at first tender and swollen, but subsequently become atrophied and contracted. An erythematous skin rash appears first on the cheeks and eyelids, where it is typically violet in colour; there is associated circumoral pallor (Plate 18). The rash subsequently spreads to the trunk, limbs and knuckles, shows a patchy distribution, and may be both erythematous and urticarial. The subcutaneous tissues become inelastic. An insidious onset is associated with stiffness and muscle weakness, and is followed by low-grade temperature and progressive disability which may include involvement of the muscles of respiration or deglutition. The chronic and frequently fatal course of the disease is only temporarily influenced by steroid therapy, which may nevertheless keep the disease process in check, until spontaneous recovery occurs, though this is unusual.

Lupus erythematosus

The disseminated form of the disease is rare in childhood, and has an even worse prognosis than in later life. The most characteristic lesion is an erythematous 'butterfly' rash over the cheeks and nose, but all the mesenchymal tissues are affected, as evidenced by the occurrence of anaemia, pyrexia, painful swelling of the joints, hepatosplenomegaly, endocarditis, and renal lesions. It is thought that autoimmunization may be responsible for the appearance of atypical antibodies. The L.E. cell phenomenon is a specific diagnostic test, and the changes found on renal biopsy are characteristic. Although steroid therapy may relieve symptoms, it does not appear to affect the outcome.

Periarteritis nodosa

This is a pathological condition of the small and medium arteries, occurring in a number of the collagen disorders, e.g. anaphylactoid purpura, dermatomyositis, and some cases of juvenile rheumatism. The walls of the vessels become thickened and may show aneurysmal dilatation.

Scleroderma

This chronic inflammatory disease of the skin and subcutaneous tissues occurs in a localized and relatively benign form, and also as a more generalized condition involving the muscles, heart, and viscera. Both types are rare in childhood. The affected areas of skin become fibrosed and 'hidebound' to the subcutaneous tissues. Treatment is largely palliative, and owing to the possible occurrence of spontaneous remissions or cure, it is uncertain whether vasoactive drugs or corticosteroid hormones are effective.

BIBLIOGRAPHY AND REFERENCES

BREWER, E. J. (1970). *Juvenile Rheumatoid Arthritis*. Philadelphia: Saunders.
CARDIAC SOCIETY & BRITISH PAEDIATRIC ASSOCIATION (1944). Report on the care of rheumatic children. *British Heart Journal*, **6**, 99.
CLARK, N. S. (1946). Dermatomyositis in childhood. *Archives of Disease in Childhood*, **21**, 160.
CRUICKSHANK, R. & GLYNN, A. A. (1959). *Rheumatic Fever*. Oxford: Blackwell.
FAGER, D. B., BIGLER, J. A. & SIMONDS, J. P. (1951). Polyarteritis nodosa in infancy and childhood. *Journal of Pediatrics*, **39**, 65.
FEINSTEIN, A. R. & LEVITT, M. (1970). The role of tonsils in predisposing to streptococcal infections and recurrences of rheumatic fever. *New England Journal of Medicine*, **282**, 285.
HADFIELD, G. (1938). The rheumatic lung. *Lancet*, ii, 710.
ILLINGWORTH, R. S. (1958). Rheumatic fever. *Recent Advances in Paediatrics*, 2nd series. London: Churchill.
JONES, T. D. (1944). The diagnosis of rheumatic fever. *Journal of the American Medical Association*, **126**, 481.
KAPLAN, M. H. (1963). Immunological relationship of group A streptococcal strains and human heart tissue. *American Heart Journal*, **65**, 426.
LENDRUM, B. L., SIMON, A. J. & MACK, I. (1959). Relation of bed rest in rheumatic fever to heart disease. *Pediatrics*, *Springfield*, **24**, 389.
LINDBJERG, I. F. (1964). Juvenile rheumatoid arthritis. *Archives of Disease in Childhood*, **39**, 576.
MARKOWITZ, M. & KUTTNER, A. G. (1965). *Rheumatic Fever*. Philadelphia: Saunders.
MAYER, F. E., DOYLE, E. F., HERRERA, L. & BROWNELL, K. D. (1963). Declining severity of first attack of rheumatic fever. *American Journal of Diseases of Children*, **105**, 146.
MEDICAL RESEARCH COUNCIL AND AMERICAN HEART ASSOCIATION (1955). Treatment of acute rheumatic fever in children: a co-operative clinical trial of ACTH, cortisone, and aspirin. *British Medical Journal*, i, 555.
MORTIMER, E. A. (1971) The role of the pediatrician in rheumatic fever control. *Pediatrics*, **47**, 1.
NEALE, A. V. (1949). Polyarteritis in childhood. *Archives of Disease in Childhood*, **24**, 224.
SCHLESINGER, B. E., FORSYTH, C. C., WHITE, R. H. R., SMELLIE, J. M. & STROUD, C. E. (1961). Observations on the clinical course and treatment of 100 cases of Still's disease. *Archives of Disease in Childhood*, **36**, 65.
SMYTH, C. J. (ed.) (1959). Rheumatism and arthritis: review of American and English literature of recent years. *Annals of Internal Medicine*, **50**, 366.

STILL, G. F. (1897). On a form of chronic joint disease in children. *Medico-Chirurgical Transactions*, **80**, 47.
SYMPOSIUM ON SCLERODERMA (1971). *Mayo Clinic Proceedings*, **46**, 83.
WALLGREN, A. (1938). Rheumatic erythema nodosum. *American Journal of Diseases of Children*, **55**, 897.
WEDGWOOD, R. J. (ed.) (1963). Symposium on collagen diseases. *Pediatric Clinics of North America*, **10**, 855.
WORLD HEALTH ORGANIZATION (1957). Prevention of rheumatic fever. *Technical Report Series. World Health Organization*, no. 126.
ZUTSHI, D. W., FRIEDMAN, M. & ANSELL, B. M. (1971). Corticotrophin therapy in juvenile chronic polyarthritis (Still's disease) and effect on growth. *Archives of Disease in Childhood*, **46**, 584.

13 Diseases of the Genito-urinary System

The various congenital malformations of the genito-urinary tract considered in Chapter 5 play a considerably more important part in the determination of disease during infancy and childhood than they do in adult life. Acute nephritis also is a disease occurring predominantly in childhood, while nephrotic syndrome occurs twice as frequently in children as in adults, the maximum incidence being between 2 and 4 years. With the exception of nephroblastoma (Wilms' tumour), malignant disease of the genito-urinary tract is rare before puberty. Urinary infection is common at all ages and the importance of pyelonephritis in early life as a cause of adult renal disease has become more evident in recent years. The general techniques of investigation are similar to those adopted in the case of adults, e.g. urinary examination, pyelography and cystourethrography, ultrasonography, cystoscopy, renal biopsy and estimation of renal function, but may have to be adapted to the age and size of the child.

URINARY EXAMINATION

Although the collection of specimens of urine from young children and infants may prove time-consuming, urinary examination is an essential routine procedure, particularly since infection of the urinary tract may present with misleading symptoms, e.g. convulsions or diarrhoea. A mid-stream specimen of urine voided into a sterile container or, in the case of infants, a specimen collected in a sterile plastic bag attached over the cleansed penis or vulva will suffice for most purposes. If required, an uncontaminated specimen may be obtained from the infant's bladder by suprapubic needle aspiration. Catheterization should be undertaken only when essential, with great care to avoid trauma or the introduction of infection. Collection of the complete urinary output during the twenty-four hours can be effected by use of a specially-designed plastic bag from which urine is drawn at short intervals (Baldwin *et al.*, 1962).

The reaction and specific gravity of the urine should be measured and tests carried out for the presence of protein, sugar, acetone, bile and phenylketones. An uncentrifuged specimen should be examined microscopically for red cells, leucocytes, crystals, casts and bacteria. Large numbers of pus cells and bacteria are generally seen in infected urine and the finding of an occasional leucocyte or erythrocyte should not necessarily be interpreted as evidence of pyuria or haematuria. The number of leucocytes can be accurately estimated using a chamber-counting method: more than 20 leucocytes per mm³ in a clean urine specimen is suggestive, though not diagnostic, of infection. A count of the total cellular elements in a 24-hour specimen (Addis count) is sometimes of value, e.g. in assessing recovery following nephritis. Bacteriological culture of the urine is necessary when evidence of infection is sought, for the absence of pus cells cannot be taken as indicating absence of infection. Urine must be examined immediately after voiding or refrigerated if there is likely to be more than one hour's delay. Bacterial counts may help to distinguish true urinary tract infection from contamination: repeated counts of over 100,000 organisms per ml in fresh specimens collected under proper conditions usually indicate that infection is present. The presence of bacteria on microscopy of the stained sediment from fresh centrifuged urine is also an indication of infection.

Proteinuria

If qualitative tests show the presence of protein, the percentage present should be estimated by the Esbach method (traces of protein shown by the Albustix strip method, which is very sensitive, can generally be ignored). The significance to be attached to proteinuria may be obvious from the other constituents of the urine, e.g. erythrocytes or casts, or from the evidence of disease elsewhere, e.g. nephrotic oedema, cardiac failure. A transient proteinuria may occur in healthy newborn infants.

Febrile proteinuria occurs readily in infancy and childhood in the presence of pyrexia, and while it indicates a toxic effect on the kidneys, it usually disappears with the subsidence of fever and implies no permanent damage.

Orthostatic proteinuria occurs in approximately 10 per cent of normal children over 10 years of age, and may be produced by violent exercise or prolonged standing in a greater number. In most cases, it is of no clinical significance, but the diagnosis should only be made when renal disease has been excluded. Protein is absent from the first morning specimen passed immediately on rising.

Selectivity of proteinuria is a useful index of probable response to steroids in the nephrotic syndrome. The clearance of proteins by the glomeruli is selective, being inversely proportional to molecular weight. High selectivity is correlated with minimal changes in the kidneys and a good response to steroid therapy, while selectivity is impaired or lost in severe membranoproliferative disease.

Haematuria

Red blood cells may be present in the urine in such small numbers that they can only be recognized microscopically, or haematuria may be such that the urine has the appearance of almost pure blood; if the urine is 'smoky', blood will be present in considerable amount. The urine may be red in haemoglobinuria, porphyrinuria and after eating beetroot or red sweets, and such discolouration should not be mistaken for haematuria. Pink staining of an infant's napkin with urates may also be a source of error. The possible causes of haematuria are very numerous, and haemorrhage may occur at any site from the renal glomerulus to the prepuce. The following are the more important causes:

Blood diseases. These include anaphylactoid and thrombocytopenic purpura, leukaemia, scurvy, sickle cell anaemia and haemorrhagic disease of the newborn. Haemophilia seldom gives rise to spontaneous haematuria in the absence of trauma.

Trauma. A common form of trauma in childhood is due to insertion of foreign bodies into the urethra. Lesions of the prepuce or meatus will usually be obvious on external examination. Occasionally the male urethra may be ruptured by a fall astride a hard object. Penetrating wounds or crush injuries involving the kidneys will almost invariably result in profuse renal haemorrhage. Calculi may also cause traumatic haematuria.

Inflammatory and infective conditions. The commonest cause of haematuria in childhood is acute nephritis. Pyelonephritis and cystitis may be complicated by haematuria. Generalized infections may cause renal haemorrhage from embolism or infarction, and thrombosis of renal vessels occasionally occurs in marasmic infants. Tuberculosis is an uncommon cause of haematuria in childhood.

The meatal ulcer or blister which sometimes occurs in male infants following circumcision causes bleeding at the beginning of micturition when the scab is detached by the stream of urine.

Congenital abnormalities. Of the many congenital abnormalities of the genito-urinary tract, polycystic kidneys and haemangioma of any part of the tract are the only ones likely to cause haematuria in the absence of secondary infection.

Neoplasms. In infancy and childhood the only primary neoplasm of the genito-urinary tract which is at all common is nephroblastoma (Wilms' tumour), and haematuria is not usually the presenting symptom. Bladder tumours (sarcoma, papilloma, etc.) are very rare in this age group.

Recurrent haematuria. Recurrent attacks of haematuria in childhood may occur spontaneously or after exercise or minor respiratory infection. There are usually no symptoms but the child may complain of malaise or loin pain. The causes of haematuria listed above must be excluded by investigation, but renal biopsy is not indicated unless there are other indications of glomerulonephritis, e.g. persistent proteinuria or impaired renal function. Recurrent haematuria is commoner in boys than in girls and the outlook is generally good in those cases with no demonstrable cause. Occasionally the condition is familial when the prognosis must be more guarded, since the haematuria may be due to familial progressive glomerulonephritis.

Pyuria

As in the case of blood in the urine, pus may originate at any level of the genito-urinary tract. The genitalia should be examined to exclude contamination by vaginal discharge in girls or from balanitis in boys. Urethritis rarely occurs in boys before puberty, but in girls the urethra is likely to be infected in vulvovaginitis.

When pus originates above the urethra, it is important to establish whether there is bacterial infection of the urine, which is likely in childhood to be due to stagnation of urine secondary to congenital malformation (Fig. 5.32). In the differential diagnosis of acute abdominal pain associated with pyuria, it should be remembered that an inflamed appendix lying against the ureter may be responsible for pus appearing in the urine.

Aminoaciduria

It has been estimated that normal children excrete approximately 2·5 mg α-amino acids per kg body weight daily. In massive aminoaciduria the excretion may be 10 to 50 times this amount. This latter may be due either to defects of intermediary amino acid metabolism in various organs, or to failure of tubular reabsorption or both. In the first group are included a number of inborn errors of metabolism associated in some instances with disorders of the central nervous system. Of these, phenylketonuria (p. 188) is recognized by testing the urine with ferric chloride or the test can be made with Phenistix on a recently wetted napkin. Other inborn errors of amino acid metabolism (Chapter 7) have been recognized by chromatography. Cystine crystals are seen in the urine in cystinuria.

INVESTIGATIONS

In all cases of urinary infection, the organism and its sensitivity to antibiotics should be identified by culture and the urinary tract should be visualized: if infection is chronic or recurrent, renal function tests should also be carried out. When culture is consistently negative for pyogenic organisms and the tuberculin test is positive, a 24-hour specimen of urine should be examined for tubercle bacilli.

In patients showing haematuria or proteinuria the investigations will depend on the suspected diagnosis. In acute nephritis, estimations of blood urea, urinary output, and blood pressure will provide the information required during the acute phase.

CYSTOURETHROGRAM. This is a simple procedure which can be carried out even in the youngest infants and will sometimes provide useful information. A straight X-ray of the abdomen is taken, and the infant is then catheterized, using the largest soft rubber catheter that can be passed without trauma. Contrast medium is then injected into the bladder through the catheter, and when the bladder is distended, the catheter is clipped and an X-ray taken. Reflux into the ureters should be regarded as probably pathological. It is sometimes possible in this way to demonstrate gross abnormalities of the bladder, ureters, or renal pelves. Fluoroscopy and serial films taken during micturition may demonstrate posterior urethral obstruction due to valves and vesico-ureteral reflux not evident previously. The contrast medium should be washed out with physiological saline when the procedure is completed.

INTRAVENOUS AND INTRAMUSCULAR PYELO-GRAPHY. The intravenous or intramuscular injection of a substance which is radio-opaque when excreted by the kidney provides a useful method of visualizing the renal tract by radiography. The results are often less satisfactory in children than in adults, partly owing to the difficulty of avoiding gas shadows in the intestine; even when serial X-rays are taken at five-minute intervals after injection, it is not always possible to obtain complete views of even a normal urinary tract. However, the method will often provide conclusive evidence of localized pathology e.g. hydronephrosis (Fig. 13.1), and the risk of misinterpreting the results lies principally in attaching too much importance to negative findings.

Owing to the risks of excessive irradiation, a careful check should be kept on the number of exposures to which the child is subjected.

CYSTOSCOPY AND RETROGRADE PYELO-GRAPHY. In many cases these provide the only reliable method of determining whether the urinary tract is abnormal on one or both sides. In the case of congenital abnormalities it is particularly important to ensure that both kidneys are present before operative procedures are carried out, since a unilateral hydronephrosis or hydro-ureter may be associated with absence of the other kidney. Specimens of urine from both ureters can be obtained for examination at the same time.

Although a specially designed cystoscope is necessary for use in infants and young children, the procedure is usually practicable even during the first year of life.

RENAL FUNCTION TESTS. Most of the tests of renal function devised for adults can be adapted for use in older children (Behrendt, 1962), but in

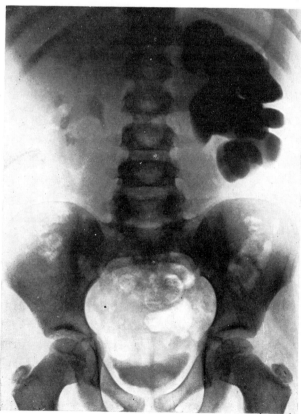

Fig. 13.1   Intravenous pyelogram, showing large left hydronephrosis, with contrast medium also present in normal right renal pelvis and lower part of bladder.

infancy there are obvious difficulties in obtaining timed or complete specimens of urine and objections to limiting fluid intake. Of the tests in general use, the capacity for concentrating and acidifying the urine and the urea clearance test are probably the most valuable. The interpretation of the results of the latter test involves correction for surface area. In the case of older children, accurately timed specimens of urine are obtained one and two hours after administration of urea (1 g per year) and specimens of blood at half and one and a half hours, the urea content of the blood and urine being estimated. The calculation is based on the amount of blood cleared of urea per minute. For infants under 2 years of age, a similar test using the total amount of urine passed in 24 hours has been devised.

INFECTION

Pyelonephritis

The term pyelitis implies infection limited to the renal pelvis but in most if not all cases so described the infection extends to the kidney (pyelonephritis) and sometimes to the bladder also. The term urinary tract infection is often used in preference to pyelonephritis, since it is not usually possible to define the anatomical location of the infection on clinical grounds, and it may be limited to the bladder.

Urinary infection is common in infancy and early childhood, and slightly less so during the later school years, increasing again in frequency at adolescence in girls. In earliest infancy boys are more often affected than girls, but later girls are affected three to five times as frequently as boys. Infection may be acute or chronic, the latter often following repeated acute attacks.

ETIOLOGY. Pyelonephritis may be primary, or secondary either to infection elsewhere or to obstruction. In chronic or recurrent infections, congenital malformation should always be suspected as the primary cause, and obstruction will frequently be found responsible for acute attacks in male infants. The various sites at which congenital obstruction may occur are shown in Figure 5.32. In most instances the infection appears to be an ascending one, the short female urethra contributing to the ease with which this occurs and accounting for the higher incidence in girls. The fact that *Escherichia coli* is found to be the infecting organism in a high proportion of cases suggests faecal contamination as a common cause. Other organisms, including staphylococci, streptococci, *Pseudomonas pyocyanea*, and the typhoid-dysentery group, are found in 10 to 20 per cent of cases. Reflux of urine from the bladder up the ureters is important in the genesis of pyelonephritis. It is probable that the infection may be blood-borne in some cases, though in these also urinary stasis is likely to be a determining factor.

Upper respiratory infection precedes the onset of pyelonephritis in a significant number of cases, though the etiological relationship is not clear. *Diarrhoea* is more commonly a sequel of pyelonephritis in infancy than a predisposing cause, but may precede the occurrence of pyuria. *Debilitating conditions* of all kinds increase the liability to urinary infection and variations in protective immunological mechanisms affect the susceptibility of the renal tract to infection. In a very high proportion of infants with myelomeningocele, the urinary tract becomes infected early.

PATHOLOGY. This varies from local inflammatory changes in the pelves and calyces to extensive destruction of kidney tissue with involvement of the ureters and bladder. Small abscesses may be scattered throughout the renal tissue, or the kidney substance may be reduced to a shell surrounding a bag of pus (*pyonephrosis*). When there is obstruction of the urinary tract at a lower level, one or both ureters are likely to be dilated and also filled with pus. Fibrosis and scarring of the remaining renal parenchyma are liable to occur in the most chronic cases. In the more acute, haemorrhage into the renal substance or ureters is an occasional finding.

Involvement of the bladder (*cystitis*) varies from a mild inflammatory reaction to a severe haemorrhagic or bullous cystitis. In those cases in which there has been long-standing obstruction at or below the neck of the bladder, the bladder-wall is likely to be hypertrophied. A congenital diverticulum of the bladder is occasionally responsible for infection occurring in this region.

CLINICAL FEATURES. In view of the varied pathology, it will be understood that the clinical picture will vary from a single acute attack, often benign and of short duration, to that of chronic and progressive renal failure. The symptom-complex will also differ in infancy and later childhood, since in young infants frequency and dysuria may be unsuspected, and the picture be overshadowed by secondary symptoms such as diarrhoea and vomiting or anaemia.

The *acute attack* may either arise without warning or be preceded by an upper respiratory infection. A high rise of temperature, shivering, or (in infants) a convulsion is often the first symptom. Older children will commonly complain of frequency, dysuria, or pain in the loins, or a small child who has previously been dry may suddenly become enuretic. Younger infants will often be found to scream and draw up the legs during or after micturition, and refusal of feeds, vomiting, or diarrhoea may rapidly lead to dehydration. As a general rule the infant with acute pyelonephritis appears severely ill, but urinary infection may merely cause failure to gain weight and microscopy of urine is therefore an essential part of the investigation of any infant who is not thriving. Unless the condition responds rapidly to treatment, anaemia is likely to develop in younger infants.

Repeated examination of the urine is sometimes necessary to establish the diagnosis, since in some cases pus will be absent from the first specimens examined, and subsequently appear in large amounts. Occasionally bacilluria precedes frank pyuria, or haematuria may obscure the true diagnosis unless the urine is examined microscopically and cultured, with bacterial colony count (see above) in cases of doubt. Cystitis is commonly associated with appearance of a considerable quantity of mucus in the urine.

Chronic or recurrent pyelonephritis is often insidious in onset, and patients come under observation for a variety of symptoms, including enuresis, recurrent pyrexia, lassitude, headache, anaemia and interference with growth, in addition to the more obvious ones of frequency and dysuria. The last is likely to be most marked when there is associated cystitis. Persistent vesico-ureteric reflux in recurrent urinary infection is likely to cause progressive renal damage. In chronic cases extensive damage may already have occurred, and investigation shows a corresponding impairment of renal function. Since there is a high likelihood of congenital malformation being present, full investigation and visualization of the urinary tract are essential. It is particularly important to determine whether the condition is unilateral or bilateral, and whether both kidneys are present. In chronic atrophic pyelonephritis there is often clubbing of calyces and loss of renal substance radiologically: renal biopsy may help to establish the severity of the disease.

COURSE AND PROGNOSIS. The duration of the acute attack depends to a large extent on early diagnosis and treatment. The temperature is often irregularly raised for five to ten days, but in cases which fail to respond to treatment the duration is considerably longer. In infancy, in which period the majority of cases occur, the complications of diarrhoea and vomiting, anaemia, and disturbances of acid-base balance render the prognosis more serious than in later childhood, and patients may succumb after the urinary infection has apparently become controlled. Although in many cases of acute urinary infection, recovery is complete, it is most important to ensure adequate follow-up to avoid overlooking acute recurrences or chronic pyuria. Absence of symptoms is not necessarily an indication that the infection has been eradicated and, if follow-up is inadequate, pyelonephritis may continue unrecognized for years, eventually causing irregular contraction and scarring of the kidneys with renal insufficiency in later life.

Whenever obstruction is responsible for urinary stasis, infection is almost certain to recur unless the obstruction can be relieved. In chronic cases in which the kidney is already severely damaged, the prognosis depends principally on whether the lesion is unilateral or bilateral. If one kidney is able to function normally, removal or drainage of the affected kidney is usually curative. When both kidneys are partially destroyed, however, there is a much greater danger of progressive renal failure even when the active infection can be controlled.

TREATMENT. The aim of therapy is in the first instance to render the urine sterile, and subsequently to correct any cause of obstruction which may be present. Chemotherapy has proved of the greatest value in treatment provided that it is adequately prolonged (for at least six weeks). Although in most cases the infecting organism is *E. coli*, it is essential to culture the organism and determine its sensitivities. In *E. coli* infections, a sulphonamide, e.g. sulphadimidine, is the drug of choice. Infections with proteus should be treated with streptomycin or ampicillin, or, if resistant, chloramphenicol, provided that care is taken to avoid overdosage and blood dyscrasia. Polymyxin or colomycin is indicated if the infection is due to *P. pyocyanea*, unless the organism is sensitive to tetracycline. Other therapeutic agents which may be used in selected cases of resistant urinary tract infection include nitrofurantoin, nalidixic acid, neomycin, kanamycin and erythromycin. Therapy may have to be given over a long period or changed if resistance develops.

Adequate fluid intake should be ensured and particular care is necessary in the case of infants who develop diarrhoea or vomiting, since they are especially liable to develop dehydration. Severe anaemia may necessitate transfusion of blood.

After the acute illness has subsided, investigation of the urinary tract should be undertaken to identify any congenital malformation. Careful technique including cystourethrography will reveal such anomalies in about half of all children with urinary infection. If evidence of an organic lesion causing obstruction is found, surgical correction should be undertaken when the patient is in a fit state to stand operation. Surgery should also be considered when gross vesico-ureteric reflux is present in infancy or early childhood, though lesser degrees may respond to chemotherapy and regular emptying of the bladder by the technique of triple micturition.

Carbuncle of the kidney and perinephric abscess

These conditions are both considerably rarer in childhood than in adult life. The former represents a localized abscess within the kidney and results from bacterial metastasis. Perinephric abscess arises from infection of the perirenal tissue which may extend from an abscess of the kidney, or arise from infection elsewhere, e.g. appendix abscess. The symptoms in both cases simulate acute pyelonephritis, but are more persistent and associated with a greater degree of toxaemia and leucocytosis; pain and localized tenderness in the loin are usually evident, and a mass may be palpable. The thigh on the affected side is usually flexed and extension is painful. The child should be carefully examined for evidence of suppuration elsewhere. Surgical drainage of the abscess will be necessary; when the kidney is extensively involved, nephrectomy is usually indicated.

Cystitis

Inflammation of the urinary bladder should always be regarded as secondary to some primary cause which must be found and remedied. Excretion of drugs in the urine may cause chemical irritation and foreign bodies inserted into the bladder will cause traumatic inflammation, often followed by infection. The presence of a congenital diverticulum or fistula or a vesical calculus is also liable to lead to secondary infection. The association of cystitis with pyelonephritis has been referred to above. Cases in which no primary cause is found within the bladder itself, and in which there is no evidence of a primary urethritis or vulvovaginitis, should be investigated for obstruction below the trigone. In boys a posterior urethral valve is probably the commonest cause, but a defect of the neuromuscular mechanism of the outlet of the bladder is sometimes held to be responsible. Infection of the bladder may also occur as a complication of spinal cord lesions. The infecting organisms in cases of childhood cystitis are commonly *E. coli*, staphylococci, or streptococci, but other organisms are occasionally responsible.

CLINICAL FEATURES. Acute cystitis is characterized by pyrexia, shivering, urgency, frequency, and scalding pain on micturition, which may be referred to the tip of the penis or to the perineum. There is commonly suprapubic discomfort and tenderness. The urine contains pus and mucus, and blood may also be present. *Chronic cystitis* gives rise to similar though less severe symptoms.

TREATMENT. General treatment and antibiotic therapy are as described for pyelonephritis. The primary cause of the cystitis should be identified and dealt with appropriately. It is inadvisable to undertake cystoscopy during an acute attack of cystitis, and when possible the urine should be rendered sterile before this is carried out. It may, however, be necessary to remove a foreign body as a matter of urgency.

Urethritis

Gonococcal infection of the male urethra is rare before puberty, although it may be contracted at any age. Non-gonococcal infection may be caused by the insertion of foreign bodies, particularly when these have lodged in the urethra and caused partial obstruction. If the wall of the urethra is perforated, a *periurethral abscess* may result and require surgical drainage. Urethritis also occasionally complicates balanitis and erythema multiforme (Stevens-Johnson syndrome). In these cases the urethritis usually subsides within one or two weeks with attention to general hygiene and local cleanliness.

In girls urethritis is liable to complicate vulvovaginitis.

Vulvovaginitis

This condition is seen in female children of any age, but especially in the first five years of life, for at this time the vagina is easily infected by organisms of low virulence. Bacteriological examination of the vaginal discharge shows a great variety of organisms, including *E. coli*, staphylococci, streptococci, and diphtheroids, although in many cases there appears to be no infecting organism. Occasionally *Candida albicans*, *Trichomonas vaginalis* or the *Herpes simplex* virus is present. Gonococcal infection is now rare but it is important to recognize it as early as possible owing to its high infectivity.

Gonococcal vulvovaginitis is characterized by redness and swelling of the external genitalia and a profuse greenish-yellow purulent vaginal discharge. The urethra is frequently involved, when the lips of the meatus are reddened and swollen. The infection is liable to extend to the rectum. Other complications are relatively rare.

When a case of gonococcal vulvovaginitis in childhood comes under observation, careful investigation of the source of infection must be made. Infection may be acquired by sexual exposure but more frequently is due to accidental contamination.

TREATMENT. Regular bathing and the administration of penicillin will effect cure in the majority of cases. A small proportion will relapse after the initial course, which must then be repeated. Every patient should be kept under observation for at least some months after vaginal, rectal, and urethral swabs have been found negative, and the parents warned that any signs of a relapse should call for prompt investigation.

Non-gonococcal vulvovaginitis is seen in debilitated children when personal hygiene has been neglected, but may occur in any child. An important though unusual cause is the presence of a foreign body in the vagina, and any such matter must be removed as a preliminary to treatment. Occasionally threadworms invade the vagina from the bowel and cause local irritation. Masturbation, which is often blamed, is more likely to occur as the result of irritation than to cause it, but the habit may be responsible for persistence of symptoms. The vaginal discharge is usually scanty but may have a faint odour and stain the clothing yellow or brown. When a foreign body is present the discharge is often blood-stained and offensive.

TREATMENT. Apart from removal of local causes, treatment consists essentially of attention to the general health and hygiene of the child; the under garments should be changed frequently. Daily baths and scrupulous cleanliness will usually be the only local treatment required; douching is contraindicated. In those cases due to thrush, nystatin suspension should be applied. Antibiotic or sulphonamide therapy will be indicated in appropriate cases. The duration of the condition varies considerably, depending on the general health; although there is a tendency to relapse, the general prognosis is good.

Balanitis and posthitis

Inflammation of the glans (balanitis) and of the prepuce (posthitis) is commonly the result of phimosis, or of adhesions between the glans and prepuce, with retention of smegma. The prepuce becomes swollen and oedematous, there is a foul-smelling sero-purulent discharge from the orifice and micturition is painful.

TREATMENT. Smegma should be removed, the glans and prepuce washed, and penicillin cream applied. When retraction of the prepuce is impossible, the sac should be irrigated with saline and penicillin solution instilled until the acute infection has subsided. In cases with extreme phimosis and much oedema it is occasionally necessary to incise the prepuce dorsally, but whenever possible it is advisable to wait until the acute infection has subsided and then to carry out circumcision.

Orchitis and epididymitis

Infection of the testicle and epididymis before puberty is rare; mumps, the commonest cause of orchitis in adolescence, very seldom affects the infantile testicle.

Pain and swelling of the testicle due to trauma should be distinguished from *torsion* of the spermatic cord. The latter is almost invariably associated with congenital malformation or maldescent of the testicle, and since the blood supply of the organ is cut off, leads to gangrene or atrophy unless the condition is relieved surgically. Torsion should be suspected when there is sudden onset of severe pain and swelling of an abnormally mobile or maldescended testicle, associated with shock and vomiting, without a previous history of trauma.

TREATMENT. If torsion has been excluded, the treatment of orchitis and epididymitis consists of bed rest and elevation of the scrotum, with systemic treatment of infection when this exists. Orchitis due to trauma usually subsides spontaneously without permanent injury.

URINARY CALCULI

The presence of stones in the urinary tract gives rise to symptoms which vary with the site and the size, contour, and composition of the stones. The incidence appears to depend to some extent on race, diet, and climate, urinary calculi being commoner in hot climates amongst the malnourished, and in regions where the water either contains much alkaline deposit or is abnormally hard. The incidence of vesical calculi in childhood has decreased greatly in countries where the standard of living has improved.

Calculi are described as *primary* when they form in sterile urine without a central nucleus, and *secondary* when crystalline deposit occurs around a foreign body, blood-clot, or cellular debris. Stagnation of urine is a predisposing cause.

Stones of different composition vary in their radio-opacity, the least opaque being those composed of uric acid or urates, and the most opaque those containing calcium, e.g. calcium oxalate, phosphate, or carbonate, and the cystine stones which may occur with cystinuria. Frequently stones are of mixed composition.

Renal calculi may either occur within a single calyx, or fill the pelvis of the kidney. They are single or multiple and faceted. Symptoms are often minimal until obstruction and infection have caused extensive destruction of the kidney.

A stone which passes into the ureter is likely to cause attacks of intense pain, often accompanied by haematuria, vomiting, and dysuria. Typically the pain radiates from the loin to the inguinal or subinguinal region or testis, but in young children it is often less clearly localized.

Stones which have successfully negotiated the ureter will usually be passed spontaneously from the bladder, though they are sometimes held up in the urethra. When there is obstruction at the bladder outlet, however, a small stone may form the nucleus of a vesical calculus. The symptoms of vesical calculus are frequency, dysuria, and suprapubic pain, sometimes associated with difficulty in starting micturition or with sudden obstruction to the stream.

DIAGNOSIS. Symptoms suggesting the possibility of urinary calculi call for a full urological investigation. Intravenous pyelography will help to distinguish between a stone and a calcified mesenteric lymph node adjacent to the ureter or bladder. Cystoscopy and retrograde pyelography will localize the position of the calculus more accurately, and will demonstrate lesions such as stenosis of the ureteric orifice which may prevent a ureteric stone passing into the bladder. Radio-opaque foreign bodies will also be recognized by radiography.

TREATMENT. A considerable proportion of small stones are passed spontaneously. Large renal calculi will require removal through the renal pelvis, or nephrectomy may be indicated if pyonephrosis has developed. Vesical calculi should be removed by suprapubic cystotomy. D-Penicillamine may be effective in reducing calculus formation in cystinuria.

ENURESIS DUE TO ORGANIC DISEASE

Enuresis may be the presenting symptom in a variety of diseases both within and without the genito-urinary system. Although no organic disease is present in the great majority of patients with enuresis, this possibility should always be excluded before it is considered to be a functional disorder (see p. 392).

In taking the history, it should be established whether the child has previously been dry and has regressed to a state of enuresis or whether control has never been established, and whether enuresis occurs every night or is intermittent. Enquiry should be made with regard to other symptoms possibly related to genito-urinary disease, e.g. frequency, urgency, dysuria, recurrent pyrexia, etc. The act of micturition may demonstrate difficulty in starting, an obstructed flow or dribbling incontinence following urination. Occasionally the history indicates that an excessive urinary output is responsible for enuresis. The urine must be carefully examined for evidence of infection and other abnormalities and full urological investigation is generally indicated. Occasionally enuresis is the presenting symptom in children with polyuria due to chronic nephritis, diabetes insipidus or diabetes mellitus.

Enuresis may be associated with mental subnormality, since subnormal children commonly fail to establish effective bladder control or acquire it late. Nocturnal epilepsy is also a possible cause of bed-wetting which can usually be ruled out by a carefully taken history. It is not uncommon for enuresis to occur in young children as the result of acute or chronic illness of any kind and to disappear when the general health is restored.

Enuresis must be distinguished from incontinence of urine, i.e. urinary dribbling through an inadequate urethral sphincter. Congenital malformation of the bladder neck or posterior urethra may result in dribbling or overflow incontinence and in such cases a greatly enlarged bladder may be palpable through the abdominal wall. Sudden wetting on rising from bed or a chair should suggest the possibility of an ectopic ureter.

Lesions of the spinal cord are responsible for incontinence in only a very small proportion of all children complaining of wetting and minor abnormalities of the lumbo-sacral spine demonstrable radiologically are never likely to account for enuresis. Every patient should, however, be examined to exclude incontinence from organic nervous disease, with particular reference to spina bifida.

BRIGHT'S DISEASE (Nephritis, nephrosis, and nephrosclerosis)

The term Bright's disease has been used to describe a heterogeneous group of conditions characterized by inflammatory, degenerative, or sclerotic changes in the kidneys. Numerous classifications have been suggested in which attempts have been made to wed the clinical and pathological findings. The two, however, often make uneasy bedfellows. It appears simplest to exclude infections of the kidney and to describe the pathological features separately from the clinical syndromes observed in childhood, recognizing that in some instances the etiology is not understood and that one type of disturbance may be complicated or overlap another.

Glomerulonephritis

The term glomerulonephritis includes those conditions in which the structure and function of the glomeruli are primarily affected. Tubular changes, consisting of dilatation, focal necrosis and atrophy, are sometimes seen as secondary phenomena.

PATHOLOGY. Understanding of the pathology of glomerulonephritis and its use as a guide to therapy has been greatly enhanced by the introduction of percutaneous renal biopsy.

In kidneys described as showing *minimal changes*, some of the glomeruli are normal, while in others there are slight increases in the mesangial matrix with focal hypercellularity. Occasional small, obsolete glomeruli may be observed.

Proliferative glomerulonephritis describes a group of lesions characterized by the proliferation, in varying degrees and combinations, of mesangial cells (in the glomerular stalk), endothelial cells (lining capillaries) and epithelial cells (of Bowman's capsule). In the diffuse proliferative and exudative nephritis which follows streptococcal infection, there is diffuse glomerular enlargement with proliferation of both mesangial and endothelial cells and infiltration of capillaries with polymorphs. There may be occasional crescents of epithelial cells which eventually undergo fibrosis causing scarring and glomerular obliteration. Crescents are more prominent in the nephritis of anaphylactoid purpura (p. 252), which may also show focal mesangial proliferation affecting some glomeruli segmentally. Membranoproliferative nephritis is characterized by mesangial proliferation and thickening of capillary walls due to infiltration by mesangial fibrils and cells.

In *focal glomerulosclerosis*, glomeruli show all degrees of abnormality from minimal changes to complete sclerosis. Many show segmental involvement which differentiates the lesion from minimal change, in which partly sclerosed glomeruli are not seen.

Epimembranous nephropathy is a non-inflammatory condition in which there is dense subepithelial thickening in the basement membrane without cellular proliferation. It is rare in this country.

In far-advanced glomerulonephritis of any type, the structure of the kidney may be so altered that specific glomerular changes cannot be recognized and the only possible pathological diagnosis is *chronic glomerulonephritis*.

Acute nephritis (Acute glomerulonephritis)

In this condition damage to the capillaries of the glomerular tufts gives rise to haematuria; the present evidence suggests that this is only one manifestation of extensive capillary involvement throughout the body. In its typical form, acute nephritis follows an acute streptococcal infection, usually of the upper respiratory tract, after a latent period of ten days to three weeks. During this latent period, which is comparable to that observed preceding the manifestations of acute rheumatism or anaphylactoid purpura, antibody to the bacteria is formed. There is good evidence that glomerular damage is caused by an immune reaction to the deposition of antigen—antibody complexes on the basement membranes.

INFECTION. Group A beta haemolytic streptococci are the organisms most commonly responsible for the primary infection. Only certain strains are nephritogenic, type 12 being especially common. Less frequently, pneumococcal infections or staphylococcal skin infections are responsible. The liability to nephritis does not necessarily depend on the clinical severity of the previous infection, which is often found to have been overlooked or untreated. Cold and exposure are probably important as predisposing causes in so far as they relate to infection.

AGE AND SEX INCIDENCE. Both sexes are affected, though boys more frequently than girls. No age is immune. The disease may appear in the first year of life, but the peak incidence is in the fifth year, when upper respiratory infections also have an increasingly high incidence.

CLINICAL FEATURES. Owing to the variable severity and distribution of the renal lesions, the clinical picture may be marked by little disturbance of general health, or be ushered in with violent headache, convulsions, vomiting, anuria, and gross hypertension. Most commonly, how-

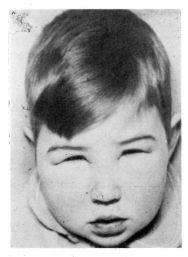

Fig. 13.2   Facies at onset of acute nephritis, showing oedema of eyelids.

ever, haematuria or oedema of the eyelids (Fig. 13.2) is the first complaint, though it may be found on enquiry that this has been preceded by general malaise. The child has often appeared well during the latent period following the initial infection and preceding the nephritic manifestations. Headache, shivering, pain in the loins or abdomen, frequency and dysuria are commonly associated with the haematuria; the temperature may be raised at onset but sometimes there is no fever. The child appears pale, and there is a variable degree of oedema of the face, legs, genitalia, and sacral region; even when no swelling has been noticed, it is usually possible to demonstrate pitting oedema over the tibiae. The blood pressure is raised to some extent, except in the mildest cases, but usually returns to normal within a few days of onset. Severe hypertension with headache, retinal changes and convulsions is exceptional. The urine is scanty and appears smoky or resembles pure blood; numerous blood and granular casts are present, and the protein content is greater than is accounted for solely by the haematuria. Anuria lasting more than 24 hours indicates severe renal damage. The blood urea is likely to be raised at onset, and falls to normal as the acute phase of the disease subsides. The blood cholesterol and plasma-protein values are usually within normal limits. The E.S.R. is raised. Culture from a throat swab may be positive for beta haemolytic streptococci but, even if this is negative, evidence of recent infection is usually obtainable by estimating the serum antistreptolysin-O titre, which is raised in 90 per cent of cases. The serum level of β_{1C}-globulin is low but rises as recovery takes place.

COURSE AND PROGNOSIS. The general prognosis is considerably better in childhood cases than in those occurring in adult life. Of the childhood cases showing frank haematuria, over 95 per cent may be expected to make a complete recovery. As a general rule, those children who show much haematuria and little oedema at onset are likely to do better than those in whom oedema is more marked than haematuria. Death during the acute phase is rare, but may occur as the result of encephalopathy, anuria, or cardiac failure. In the most favourable cases, a sudden increase in urinary output with a corresponding fall in weight often occurs after a few days. The signs and symptoms subside within three to six weeks of onset, red cells disappear more gradually from the urine, and though slight proteinuria or raised erythrocyte sedimentation rate may persist for a longer period, the kidney function is left unimpaired. Recovery is possible even when urine examination shows abnormalities for a year or more, but the prognosis becomes worse the longer that haematuria persists. Persistent heavy proteinuria and low levels of serum β_{1C}-globulin, serious impairment of renal function or other atypical features should suggest the possibility of membranoproliferative nephritis and indicate the need for renal biopsy.

DIAGNOSIS. Typical cases with macroscopic haematuria are likely to cause little difficulty in diagnosis if oedema and hypertension are present at onset, and the condition follows a streptococcal infection. Renal biopsy is not necessary for diagnosis, but if it is carried out in the acute stage, the typical changes of diffuse proliferative and exudative glomerulonephritis are seen. Biopsy after some months usually shows only residual mesangial proliferation.

Other causes of haematuria such as scurvy, urinary calculi, or nephroblastoma can be excluded by the absence of other signs of the disease, and haematuria complicating pyelonephritis will be recognized by the presence of pus and organisms in the urine. Attacks of subclinical glomerulonephritis are only likely to be diagnosed by routine examination of the urine, which will be found to contain protein and possibly casts and a few red cells following an acute infection. Since febrile proteinuria only occurs during the course of an infection and is unassociated with haematuria, it is unlikely to cause confusion in diagnosis. Nephritis associated with anaphylactoid purpura represents a more serious condition than simple poststreptococcal nephritis, since some of these cases have severe proliferative glomerulonephritis with extensive crescent formation and die ultimately with renal failure. A serious and often fatal form of nephritis may also occur in epidemic form in association with haemolytic anaemia and thrombocytopenia (haemolytic-uraemic syndrome).

TREATMENT. The child should be kept in bed until the acute symptoms have subsided, gross haematuria and proteinuria have ceased and the E.S.R. is falling. Rest in bed need not be enforced after this stage and the child may get up if he wishes to. If there is a return of symptoms or haematuria, however, it is wise to return him to bed, even although there is little evidence that early ambulation affects the outcome adversely. Patients who have made a clinical recovery should be kept under observation with repeated urine examination for at least a year. Upper respiratory infections should be treated with antibiotics and in the acute phase it is a wise precaution to give all patients penicillin. If the tonsils are chronically infected they should be removed under a penicillin screen *after the acute phase is passed*, but the operation should never be undertaken unless it is really necessary. Chronic sinus infection should also receive attention.

Diet. At the onset, both food and fluid should be restricted, and glucose drinks are all that are required by mouth. When there is much vomiting, ice should be sucked to relieve thirst. As the acute symptoms diminish or, in milder cases, as soon as the urinary output is known to be satisfactory the diet can be rapidly increased by the addition first of carbohydrate and subsequently of fat and protein. Prolonged restriction of protein is unnecessary. It is advisable to maintain a low salt diet as long as there is any evidence of oedema or restricted urinary output. Persistent anuria associated with severe vomiting will necessitate feeding by gastric tube (or by the intravenous route), using a preparation designed to reduce the catabolism of body protein and to replace vomited electrolytes.

Hypertension. Rising blood pressure can be countered by rest and phenobarbitone, with hypotensive agents if necessary. Reserpine (0·07 mg per kg) or reserpine combined with hydralazine hydrochloride (0·1 mg per kg) may be given intramuscularly and repeated 12 hours later if required. Convulsions due to hypertensive encephalopathy require immediate treatment, and intramuscular injection of 50 per cent magnesium sulphate (0·2 ml per kg body weight) is of proved value. Lumbar puncture may also help to relieve cerebral symptoms.

Cardiac failure, which may also occur with severe hypertension, will necessitate sedatives and digitalization.

Prolonged anuria has been successfully treated in selected cases by peritoneal dialysis or by use of the artificial kidney.

The nephrotic syndrome

This is characterized by generalized oedema, gross proteinuria, reduction of the total plasma proteins with alteration of the albumin:globulin ratio, and a raised blood cholesterol. It does not represent a single disease entity, and the variable pathology indicates that a similar clinical picture is produced in various ways. In the majority of cases the cause is unknown but in some the condition may be a manifestation of glomerulonephritis, quartan malaria or lupus erythematosus while in others it may be a reaction to a drug, e.g. troxidone. Renal biopsy helps to distinguish the underlying cause and gives information of use in prognosis. The kidney may show minimal or no changes but in about 10 per cent of cases there is focal glomerulosclerosis or proliferative glomerulonephritis, and these children are more likely to have hypertension, haematuria and loss of selective proteinuria. The term nephrosis, if used at all, should be reserved for those cases in which there are no glomerular changes. In general, patients with pure nephrosis or with minimal changes respond to steroid therapy and have a better prognosis than those with more advanced proliferative and membranous changes, which are likely to be irreversible.

CLINICAL PICTURE. In the great majority of cases, the first complaint is the insidious or relatively rapid appearance of oedema. A previous history of haematuria is rare, and although there may be evidence of preceding infection, e.g. streptococcal or pneumococcal infection of the upper respiratory tract, or mixed skin infection, many cases give no indication of previous ill health. The oedema is usually first noticed as swelling of the eyelids, face, or ankles, the first often being most marked on waking and sometimes causing difficulty in opening the eyes. The oedema tends at first to fluctuate and disappear temporarily, but subsequently becomes generalized, involving the sacrum, genitalia, abdominal wall, and serous cavities. Ascites usually becomes gross (Fig. 13.3).

The blood pressure is typically not raised, though hypertension may occur in the terminal stages. The child becomes listless and anorexic and there may be vomiting and diarrhoea.

URINE EXAMINATION. During the periods in which oedema is accumulating, the urinary output is reduced and the specific gravity is raised. Protein is present, often in very great amount. Casts are also present and are of various types, mainly granular. The occurrence of red cells in the urine is very variable; in some cases they are consistently absent, in others a few cells are present from time to time, and in others again they are more consistently present and in larger numbers. Loss of oedema is accompanied by diuresis, with reduction of the specific gravity of the urine; proteinuria, however, usually persists.

BLOOD EXAMINATION. The blood urea is not significantly raised unless there is terminal renal failure. The blood cholesterol is raised, often to 400 mg per 100 ml or more. While the total plasma protein content is lowered, the albumin is reduced to a much greater extent than the globulin, and the ratio of the two is correspondingly altered. Elevation of the alpha and beta globulins may result in the total globulin level being normal, despite reduction in the gamma fraction. It has been found that the threshold point for the appearance of oedema is reached when the albumin falls below 1·2 g per 100 ml, a lower point than that observed in adults.

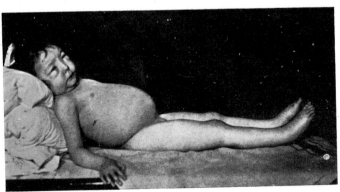

Fig. 13.3   Nephrotic syndrome. Girl aged 5 years, showing ascites and gross oedema of face and legs.

PROGNOSIS. In cases of childhood nephrotic syndrome, a recovery rate of approximately 30 per cent was claimed before antibiotics or steroid therapy were available. Death from intercurrent infection, e.g. pneumococcal peritonitis, is now exceptional, and though it is too early to assess accurately the long-term recovery rate following steroid therapy, recent surveys suggest that it may approach 70 per cent at 10 years. The ultimate prognosis in those cases of the nephrotic syndrome with membranoproliferative glomerulonephritis or focal glomerulosclerosis is poor. Apparent clinical recovery with loss of oedema but persistent proteinuria is only too often followed by subsequent relapse and ultimately by death from renal failure.

TREATMENT. Management of a condition which may have a duration of months or years should aim at encouraging the child to lead as normal a life as practicable within the limits of the disability and at maintaining the morale of the parents. Gross oedema at onset or during periods of relapse will necessitate bed-rest and support of the scrotum if affected; paracentesis is occasionally required to relieve extreme abdominal distension due to ascites. Restriction of salt to less than 2 g sodium daily is also indicated during exacerbations of oedema and during steroid therapy but otherwise the diet must be made as attractive as possible to maintain nutrition. Normal activity should be encouraged during remissions as far as consistent with avoidance of cold and exposure. Any infection should receive prompt treatment with the appropriate antibiotic.

Steroid therapy appears to have improved the prognosis in nephrosis, and has certainly reduced the disability resulting from oedema. Prednisolone or prednisone has been found superior to both cortisone and ACTH. (In some clinics, however, it is the practice to start treatment initially with ACTH and follow with prednisolone.) The dosage of prednisolone recommended, irrespective of age or weight, is 60 mg daily in divided doses for 10 days, followed by 40 mg daily for a further 10 days, followed by 20 mg daily. This last dosage is gradually reduced to a maintenance dose of 10 or 15 mg. Since some children respond to a six weeks course of steroid and do not relapse thereafter, such a short course may be tried initially and only followed by long-term low-dosage maintenance therapy if a relapse occurs (Arneil & Lam, 1966). An intermittent high-dosage regimen is an alternative form of treatment, which can maintain the child in good health for long periods and is remarkably free from side-effects. Prednisolone is given in a dose of 60 to 80 mg daily for three consecutive days in each week, no steroid being given on the other four days. This regimen can be continued for many months or years if necessary. Owing to the particular risks of infection during steroid therapy, some authorities advocate routine antibiotic prophylaxis. If the child is under careful supervision, however, immediate treatment of infection when it occurs is probably equally satisfactory.

Renal biopsy is not necessary in all cases of nephrotic syndrome but if clinical evidence suggests membranoproliferative disease, biopsy should precede steroid therapy, since in some cases the hormone may aggravate the disease.

In a small proportion of cases, not necessarily confined to those with severe renal lesions, there is no response to steroid therapy. In others, frequent relapses will necessitate prolonged therapy with undesirably high doses of steroids. In such steroid-dependent children, who usually show minimal changes on renal biopsy, the use of cyclophosphamide may allow the reduction or withdrawal of steroid therapy.

In cases in which steroid therapy has failed to produce diuresis and relief of oedema, frusemide (0·5 mg per kg daily) or chlorothiazide (500 mg b.d. increasing to 2 g b.d. if necessary) will sometimes prove successful. Potassium chloride (2 to 4 g daily) should be given during chlorothiazide therapy.

Nephrosclerosis

Generalized nephrosclerosis is usually the end-result of chronic glomerulonephritis or pyelonephritis. Nephrosclerosis secondary to primary hypertension also occurs in childhood but is extremely rare.

The features of advanced nephrosclerosis are polyuria, the urine being of low specific gravity and containing only a trace of protein and occasional casts; retardation of growth; nitrogen retention and increasing impairment of renal function; and a variable degree of hypertension, the last being in general less marked in childhood than in adult life. The condition progresses to terminal uraemia and renal failure, characterized by convulsions, diarrhoea, vomiting, dyspnoea, and death.

OTHER RENAL DISORDERS

Congenital hypoplasia of the kidneys

Small malformed kidneys which have limited function may suffice to allow growth and development for a time but eventually give rise to infantilism and renal rickets. They frequently become infected and are often associated with other congenital malformations of the urinary tract. It is noteworthy that the presenting symptoms, viz. thirst, polyuria, and failure to thrive, may be present for long periods and associated with a severe degree of nitrogen retention before the blood pressure is raised to a corresponding extent. The condition is, however, ultimately fatal, and treatment can only be directed to relief of symptoms.

Renal acidosis

Primary renal acidosis (*Lightwood syndrome*) is a rare disease of infancy characterized by defective reabsorption of bicarbonate and excretion of hydrogen ion by the renal tubules, and resulting in chronic acidosis in the presence of an alkaline urine. Clinically the infants fail to thrive. Vomiting is associated with constipation. With alkaline and diuretic therapy a proportion of the patients recover.

Renal acidosis is also a feature of the oculo-cerebrorenal syndrome of Lowe (see p. 190).

BIBLIOGRAPHY AND REFERENCES

ARNEIL, G. C. & LAM, C. N. (1966). Long-term assessment of steroid therapy in childhood nephrosis. *Lancet*, ii, 819.
BALDWIN, E. M., CLAYTON, B. M., JENKINS, P., MITCHELL, J. & RENWICK, A. G. C. (1962). Collection of urine and faeces in children. *Archives of Disease in Childhood*, 37, 488.
BARNETT, H. L. (1966). Pediatric nephrology. *Archives of Disease in Childhood*, 41, 223.
BEHRENDT, H. (1962). *Diagnosic Tests for Infants and Children*, 2nd edn. London: Kimpton.
CAMPBELL, M. F. (1951). *Clinical Pediatric Urology*. London: Saunders.
CHISHOLM, J. J. (1959). Clinical significance of aminoaciduria. *Journal of Pediatrics*, 53, 303.
EDELMANN, C. M. (ed.) (1971). Pediatric nephrology. *Pediatric Clinics of North America*, 18, 347.
FANCONI, G. (1954). Tubular insufficiency and renal dwarfism. *Archives of Disease in Childhood*, 29, 1.
HELLER, R. H., JOSEPH, J. M. & DAVIS, H. J. (1969). Vulvovaginitis in the premenarcheal child. *Journal of Pediatrics*, 74, 370.
HENDRICKSE, R. G., GLASGOW, E. F., ADENIYI, A., WHITE, R. H. R., EDINGTON, G. M. & HOUBA, V. (1972). Quartan malarial nephrotic syndrome. *Lancet*, i, 1143.
ILLINGWORTH, R. S., PHILPOTT, M. G. & RENDLE-SHORT, J. (1954). A controlled investigation of the effect of diet on acute nephritis. *Archives of Disease in Childhood*, 29, 488.
LIGHTWOOD, R. C., PAYNE, W. W. & BLACK, J. A. (1953). Infantile renal acidosis. *Pediatrics, Springfield*, 12, 628.
LYONS, E. A., MURPHY, A. V. & ARNEIL, G. C. (1972). Sonar and its use in kidney disease in children. *Archives of Disease in Childhood*, 47, 777.
MACGREGOR, M. (1970). Pyelonephritis lenta. *Archives of Disease in Childhood*, 45, 159.
MEADOW, S. R., GLASGOW, E. F., WHITE, R. H. R., MONCRIEFF, M. W., CAMERON, J. S. & OGG, C. S. (1972). Schönlein-Henoch nephritis. *Quarterly Journal of Medicine*, 41, 241.
PARSONS, L. (1927). The bone changes occurring in renal and coeliac rickets. *Archives of Disease in Childhood*, 2, 1.
PRYLES, C. V. (1965). Percutaneous bladder aspiration and other methods of urine collection for bacteriologic study. *Pediatrics, Springfield*, 36, 128.
RILEY, H. D. (1968). Pyelonephritis. *Advances in Pediatrics*, vol. 15. Chicago: Year Book Medical Publishers.
SMELLIE, J. M. (1970). Acute urinary tract infection in children. *British Medical Journal*, iv, 97.
WHITE, R. H. R. (1970). Glomerulonephritis in children. *British Journal of Hospital Medicine*, 3, 746.

14 Disorders of the Respiratory Tract

(See also allergic rhinitis, p. 257; asthma, p. 258; atelectasis, p. 41; congenital malformations, p. 102; diphtheria, p. 340; mycotic infections, p. 362; neonatal pneumonia, p. 55; neoplasms, p. 232; pertussis, p. 345; respiratory distress syndrome, p. 49; tuberculosis, p. 326; and virus infections, p. 351.)

UPPER RESPIRATORY TRACT

While treatment of disease of the upper respiratory tract forms a somewhat specialized field, infection of the nose, pharynx, ears, and paranasal sinuses plays such an important role in childhood disease that familiarity with the presenting signs and symptoms is essential in assessing the general health of a child and the clinical picture of such various conditions as nephritis, rheumatism, bronchiectasis, and gastroenteritis. This applies also to the indications for tonsillectomy, the operation often being recommended without adequate reason, or without considering both the child as a whole and the environment in which he lives.

In the young infant, the short Eustachian tube and the danger of food being regurgitated into the nasopharynx render him particularly liable to infection of the middle ear, and provide an important reason for the infant being fed sitting up rather than lying supine. Infection of the lymphatic tissue of the nasopharynx becomes more common after the age of 3 years than in infancy, though this is at least partly related to the increased likelihood of exposure to infection. Rapid growth of lymphoid tissue is, however, physiological in middle and later childhood. The infant or young child is most likely to acquire his infections in the home, whereas the school child has enlarged his circle of contacts, and the classroom, buses, and the cinema provide additional sources of infection, although the home, and particularly the sleeping quarters, still remains of outstanding importance. Children develop no absolute immunity to upper respiratory tract infection, although an acute infection is usually followed by a period of temporary immunity, and there does appear to be some individual variation in susceptibility.

Nasal obstruction

It is often assumed that a child who keeps his mouth open has nasal obstruction. This is not necessarily the case, and the nasal airway should first be tested by observing the breath patterns on a mirror or the movement of a wisp of cotton-wool held before each nostril while the child is breathing normally. If there is evidence of obstruction the nose should be inspected, using a nasal speculum and head mirror; if necessary, swollen turbinates must be contracted by local application of a constricting agent.

Deflection of the nasal septum, occurring either as a congenital malformation or as the result of trauma, may be found responsible for unilateral obstruction. Radical operation for its correction should not be undertaken in childhood, though removal of a spur or manipulative correction is sometimes indicated.

Chronic rhinitis and infection. Chronic nasal catarrh resulting in nasal obstruction is in the great majority of cases the result of infection. (Allergic rhinitis is more liable to occur in recurrent acute attacks, though an allergic basis should be considered in chronic cases also.) The commonest type of chronic rhinitis is that in which there is hypertrophy of the nasal mucosa. Much more rarely in childhood the mucosa is atrophic, in which case the nose is filled with hard crusts and the breath becomes offensive.

Chronic nasal obstruction causes *habitual mouth-breathing*, which may produce deformity of the face, nasopharynx, and chest. Young children should therefore be taught to blow the nose effectively with the nostrils patent, and to breathe through the nose rather than the mouth. Frequent clearing of the nostrils by blowing the nose will be effective in most infections and antibiotics are seldom necessary. If required, the appropriate one, usually penicillin or ampicillin, should be given for at least two weeks. Oily solutions should never be instilled into the nose of an infant owing to the danger of inhalation pneumonia. In all cases of chronic rhinitis, infection of the paranasal sinuses should be excluded.

Polypi, occurring in the anterior or less commonly in the posterior nares, occasionally complicate chronic rhinitis and add to the degree of nasal obstruction. They are readily removed, but are liable to recur if chronic infection remains untreated or if there is underlying cystic fibrosis.

Foreign bodies, such as beads or peas, are often inserted into the nose by young children. If they become fixed in position, they produce a foul purulent nasal discharge which may be blood-stained. Removal of the foreign body and cleansing of the nose will result in rapid cessation of symptoms.

The common cold (*Acute rhinitis, coryza*)

This acute infectious disease, which has an incubation period of from one to six days, is not only one of the commonest disorders of childhood, but is responsible for complications in the younger age groups which far outweigh the severity of the initial symptoms. A virus, most commonly a rhinovirus, can be isolated in a minority of cases.

The incidence of colds in the population as a whole shows peak periods in the early autumn, in January and February, and often a third in the early summer. Infants are comparatively seldom affected during the first two months of life if proper precautions are taken by attendants, but in later infancy and early childhood infections become more frequent. Very few children show more than a transient immunity following an acute infection, though there is probably some individual variation in susceptibility which is not accounted for by exposure and environment.

CLINICAL FEATURES. The manifestations of the disease differ considerably in infancy and later childhood, general symptoms being more severe and the likelihood of complications greater in infants than in older children. These general symptoms include pyrexia, lassitude, anorexia, and, in infants, diarrhoea or vomiting and difficulty in sucking. In older children the disease picture resembles more closely that occurring in adults, viz. a period of itching and discomfort in the nasopharynx, followed by sneezing and a seromucoid nasal discharge which rapidly becomes mucopurulent owing to the presence of secondary invading organisms. The nasal mucosa becomes swollen and hyperaemic and subsequently denuded. Since the mucosa of the paranasal sinuses is continuous with that of the nose, the infection involves the sinuses to a greater or less extent, and may also extend to the larynx and trachea.

COMPLICATIONS. Gastroenteritis, laryngotracheobronchitis, pneumonia, and otitis media are all serious complications in infancy, but are less likely to occur in childhood. Chronic sinusitis is liable to follow repeated acute infections at any age. Cervical lymph node enlargement is due to secondary infection.

DIAGNOSIS. While there is little difficulty in diagnosing the typical case, it is often impossible clinically to draw a sharp distinction between a cold and influenza when the former is associated with severe general symptoms. The catarrhal symptoms occurring at the onset of measles or pertussis may be misdiagnosed as a common cold if a history of contact is not obtained; in the case of measles there is associated lachrymation and conjunctivitis, with the early appearance of Koplik spots, while in pertussis the catarrh is more generalized and accompanied by cough even before the paroxysms become characteristic. Allergic rhinitis should be suspected when there is a history of allergy, a typical seasonal incidence, or when the discharge remains mucoid and symptoms respond to adrenaline or antihistamine drugs.

COURSE AND PROGNOSIS. In the absence of complications, the primary disease usually runs a short course of a few days to a week or more, and is essentially benign. Persistence of symptoms should suggest a complication, e.g. sinusitis.

. TREATMENT AND PROPHYLAXIS. There is no specific treatment, although many have been advocated. General symptoms, particularly pyrexia, are an indication for bed rest for two or more days, during which time the child should be isolated and provided with ample fluids. Aspirin is generally helpful at this stage but is better avoided in infancy. Antibiotic therapy has no effect on the primary infection, but may be of value in the treatment of complications. In the case of infants, the blocked nostrils should be cleansed with cotton-wool. Older children obtain relief of local symptoms from the use of vaso-constrictive drops or benzedrine inhalation, but this should not be long continued.

Epistaxis

Bleeding from the nose, occurring as the result of trauma, mucosal congestion, or the presence of a local lesion, is a common symptom in childhood, and is usually controlled spontaneously or by inserting cotton-wool soaked in adrenaline and applying pressure. When bleeding is recurrent or prolonged, the nasal mucosa should be examined. The commonest findings are a dilated vessel or a scab lying on the nasal septum immediately within the anterior chamber,

bleeding occurring whenever the affected area is scratched. Cauterization or application of a fused chromic acid bead to the vessel will effect cure. When bleeding is persistent it will be necessary to pack the nose.

Uncontrollable epistaxis is most likely to occur in childhood as a symptom of a haemorrhagic or blood disease, viz. purpura, haemophilia, or leukaemia, and in these blood transfusion may be necessary. Hypertension is rarely the responsible factor. Epistaxis may also occur as a symptom of generalized infections or of acute rheumatism.

Sinusitis

The paranasal sinuses consist of the maxillary antra, the frontal sinuses, the anterior and posterior ethmoidal cells, and the sphenoidal sinus. Of these the frontal sinuses are not significantly developed until the fourth to sixth year, and are seldom infected before later childhood. The sphenoidal sinus is confined to cartilage in early childhood, and does not exist as an air-containing space within the sphenoid bone until the age of 9 years or later. The maxillary antra, though present as air-containing cells at birth, enlarge downwards throughout childhood, so that in infancy their anatomical relationship to the nose differs from that in adult life. The ethmoidal cells are also present at birth, enlarging gradually during childhood.

Infection of the maxillary antra and ethmoidal cells is common even in early childhood, and some involvement of the lining mucosa is likely to occur in the course of every upper respiratory infection. The factors on which the transience or chronicity of the infection will depend are the drainage of the sinuses, i.e. patency or blockage of the ostia and effectiveness of ciliary action, and the frequency and severity of upper respiratory infections.

Acute sinusitis, occurring during a cold, will be evidenced by discomfort, local tenderness and headache, and is associated with acute nasal obstruction. The condition normally subsides as the ostia become patent. In more severe infections there may be localized pain or even oedema over the antrum, and X-ray shows a fluid level or complete opacity. Examination of the nose is likely to show the presence of pus in the middle meatus, though this may be absent with complete blockage of the ostia. Immediate treatment should aim at shrinkage of the nasal mucosa to promote drainage. Vasoconstrictive drops and oral decongestants are often effective. Appropriate antibiotic therapy is indicated.

Complications of acute sinusitis include otitis media, osteomyelitis of the maxilla, meningitis, cavernous sinus thrombosis, and orbital cellulitis.

Chronic sinusitis. Though possibly overdiagnosed, chronic infection of the paranasal sinuses is recognized as an important cause of chronic ill-health in childhood and as a contributory factor in the etiology of rheumatism, nephritis, and bronchiectasis. The local signs and symptoms may be minimal, or include recurrent cold, headache, and localized tenderness. A chronic nasal or postnasal discharge is very commonly present, resulting in mouth-breathing or recurrent cough. Careful search should be made for associated causes of nasal obstruction, e.g. infected adenoids, deflected nasal septum, or polypi. The possibility of nasal allergy should always be considered.

Radiological examination will usually demonstrate infection of the maxillary antra, but is sometimes misleading. Proof puncture is required to establish the diagnosis, the contents of the antra being aspirated and examined bacteriologically. Chronic rhinitis must be treated as already indicated, and any cause of chronic nasal obstruction removed. In cases of chronic sinusitis in which there is associated infection of the adenoids, adenoidectomy will be required; tonsillectomy, however, should only be undertaken if it is necessary on other grounds.

Operation on the antra, other than antral puncture and washouts, should never be undertaken during childhood until full trial of conservative treatment and antibiotic therapy has been made.

Tonsils and adenoids

These represent part of the lymphatic system of the fauces and nasopharynx, and normally grow rapidly during middle and later childhood. The size of the tonsil alone gives little indication of its health, for many children have large, smooth tonsils projecting well beyond the anterior pillars with no evidence whatever that the organs are infected or are causing symptoms.

The normal function of the tonsil in early life is generally regarded as being one of catchment and phagocytosis, infection being dealt with locally in the first instance, with the production of some degree of immunity. It is only when repeated infections have rendered the tonsils useless for this purpose, and have reduced them to a nidus of chronic infection that tonsillectomy is indicated. In such cases the adenoids should be removed with the tonsils, but it is not equally true that when the adenoids require removal, e.g. as a cause of nasal obstruction, the tonsils should necessarily be removed at the same time. This applies particularly to adenoidectomy which may be necessary in very young children. It must be realized that removal of the tonsils cannot itself prevent fresh infections of the fauces occurring; but a healthy upper respiratory tract will be less likely to be affected than one in which chronic infection is constantly present, e.g. in the crypts of chronically infected tonsils.

Acute tonsillitis

The most important infecting organism is the haemolytic streptococcus, though mixed bacterial infections and viral infections (adenovirus, enterovirus) frequently occur. The tonsils are swollen, bright red, and may be covered with small white patches which represent pus exuding from the crypts. In bacterial cases the purulent exudate sometimes coalesces to form a yellowish-white pseudo-membrane which is limited to the tonsillar area; in this respect, and in its colour, the pseudo-membrane differs from the gelatinous membrane of diphtheria which often extends on to the fauces or soft palate. In *Vincent's angina* the tonsil is likely to be ulcerated with slough formation, and other lesions in the mouth are often present. Acute tonsillitis may occur at any age, but is less common in infancy than in early childhood.

SYMPTOMS. The temperature often rises to 39·5°C (103°F) and the child appears flushed and distressed. The pulse is rapid, and the respiration-rate may be raised (particularly in infants), though to a less extent than when there is pulmonary involvement. Occasionally in infancy the infection will be ushered in by a convulsion. Young children seldom refer the symptoms to the throat, though there may be difficulty in swallowing. Thirst, lassitude, and anorexia are usual symptoms, and may be associated with vomiting or diarrhoea in infants. Complaint of abdominal pain is common. Earache frequently occurs in young children, and the ear-drums should be examined throughout the attack.

DIAGNOSIS. This is only likely to be overlooked through failure to examine the throat, as may occur when no complaint of sore throat has been made. In all cases a throat swab should be examined. This will also serve to establish the diagnosis of Vincent's angina, in which condition there is commonly associated stomatitis and foetor oris.

COMPLICATIONS. The commonest complication in infants is *otitis media*, and in older children *cervical adenitis*. In the latter condition the lymph nodes in the anterior cervical triangle become enlarged and tender; if they progress to suppuration, the pus must be evacuated. With antibiotic therapy, however, the cervical nodes subside in the majority of cases without abscess formation.

Peritonsillar abscess (*quinsy*) should be suspected if there is increasing pain, dysphagia, difficulty in speech, and salivation. Inspection of the throat will show a fluctuant swelling above one or other tonsil, and displacement of the uvula towards the unaffected side. An abscess will require drainage by incision, either through the superior crypt of the tonsil or through the soft palate. *Oedema of the larynx* is a rare but serious complication which may necessitate tracheotomy.

TREATMENT. During the acute stage, the child should rest in bed and an adequate fluid intake should be assured. Appropriate antibiotic therapy should be started as soon as the bacterial diagnosis has been made, and continued for at least ten days. Where the infection is due to a group A haemolytic streptococcus, penicillin is indicated. Gargles are of little value, but spraying the throat with normal saline or a suspension of aspirin will often give symptomatic relief.

Vincent's angina usually responds rapidly to penicillin and to local application of hydrogen peroxide to the ulcerated areas.

Streptococcal tonsillar infections call for particularly careful supervision, owing to the danger of nephritis or rheumatism developing two to three weeks after the initial attack. In all cases the urine should be examined for the presence of red cells and protein until the risk of nephritis is past.

Chronic tonsillitis

There is no sharp dividing line between recurrent attacks of acute tonsillitis and chronic tonsillitis. In the latter condition the tonsils are sometimes considerably enlarged but more frequently

are small, sclerosed, and 'craggy'; pus or cheesy material can be expressed from the crypts. The tonsillar lymph node at the angle of the jaw is usually chronically enlarged.

Adenoids

Simple hypertrophy of the lymphoid tissue of the nasopharynx results in nasal obstruction, snoring, and mouth-breathing, particularly when the nasopharynx is poorly developed. This hypertrophy may occur at any age, and in some instances is due to allergic rhinitis.

Infection of the adenoids commonly occurs in association with chronic rhinitis, sinusitis, or otitis media, and also results in hypertrophy. Although in these cases the adenoids are only one of the tissues sharing in the more general infection, the presence of chronically infected lymphoid tissue in the nasopharynx tends to perpetuate the infection of the ears or sinuses.

Infection of the adenoids also occasionally leads to infection of the retropharyngeal lymphoid tissue and abscess formation. *Retropharyngeal abscess* due to pyogenic infection must be distinguished from the more deeply situated type of abscess secondary to tuberculous disease of the cervical spine (p. 337). The infecting organism is usually a haemolytic streptococcus. The abscess gives rise to dysphagia and head retraction, and there is often associated dyspnoea, pyrexia, and shock. On digital examination of the pharynx a fluctuant swelling can be palpated. The abscess should be opened and the pus aspirated, care being taken to avoid the latter being inhaled.

Tonsillectomy

The decision as to whether the tonsils are to be removed should never be made lightly, and should be based on the history, the condition of the tonsils, the general health of the child, and a consideration of the child's environment. Indications are a history of repeated acute infections or of peritonsillar abscess: and tonsils which are so grossly enlarged as to cause obstruction or are small, irregular, and sclerosed with chronic enlargement of the cervical nodes. Tuberculous adenitis is also an indication for tonsillectomy, provided that there is not an active primary focus elsewhere which makes an immediate operation an unjustifiable risk. In considering the general health of the child, symptoms such as anorexia, lassitude, or loss of weight should never be attributed to the tonsils unless there is confirmatory evidence that these are infected. There is also little to justify tonsillectomy as a routine in cases of juvenile rheumatism or nephritis, and the operation should only be undertaken if it is indicated on other grounds. Much importance attaches to the child's environment, since little benefit can be expected from tonsillectomy if recurrent attacks of tonsillitis are due to continuous contact with infection in the home which is allowed to continue. In such cases tonsillectomy may be found unnecessary if the child can be removed from infection, and if the operation is undertaken it is additionally important that the child's environment should be improved.

Sinusitis and otitis media are more likely to be indications for adenoidectomy than for tonsillectomy, and there is some evidence to suggest that these infections, and also recurrent respiratory infections, are more rather than less frequent in tonsillectomized children than others.

The age of the child should be taken into consideration. It is generally undesirable to perform tonsillectomy before the age of 3 to 5 years, save in exceptional circumstances. Usually it will be found that the indications in the younger age groups are for adenoidectomy rather than tonsillectomy.

The operation should not as a rule be undertaken within six weeks of an acute infection, during an epidemic of poliomyelitis, or during the periods when upper respiratory infections are most prevalent. Every care should be taken to avoid exposure to infection after operation.

COMPLICATIONS. Unskilled operative technique and anaesthesia are still responsible for some avoidable complications such as pulmonary collapse or lung abscess due to inhalation of infected material. Haemorrhage is usually controllable by pressure or suture. A transient bacillaemia may follow the removal of tonsils in which active infection is present, and in patients where there are particular risks, e.g. those with congenital heart disease, the operation should be performed under antibiotic cover. Earache is a very common post-operative complaint; this is usually of short duration.

Any residual tonsillar tags are extremely liable to hypertrophy or to become reinfected and to require subsequent removal.

Adenoidectomy

This is undertaken in all cases in which tonsillectomy is performed, but may be required inde-
pendently. Chronic sinusitis, otitis media, and nasal obstruction, when associated with adenoid hypertrophy or infection, are indications for operation. Adenoidectomy should not be postponed on account of age if it is otherwise indicated, since delay may result in chronic deafness or other avoidable disability. Cor pulmonale with cardiac failure may rarely occur in predisposed children, due to hypoventilation resulting from chronic nasopharyngeal obstruction. If the syndrome is recognized early enough, removal of tonsils and adenoids effects a cure.

THE EAR AND MASTOID

EXTERNAL AUDITORY CANAL

The presence of wax in the canal usually gives rise to no symptoms unless it becomes impacted or swollen, when deafness occurs. Similarly foreign bodies inserted into the ear are often symptomless until they result in local infection or deafness. Removal should only be undertaken by an expert, as there is a real risk of causing further damage. Syringing must not be employed when a foreign body consists of vegetable matter, e.g. a pea, owing to the danger of swelling and impaction.

Infection of the canal (*otitis externa*) is uncommon in childhood, but may arise from a purulent otorrhoea and persist after the discharge from the drum has ceased. *Furunculosis* of the canal gives rise to great pain and local swelling, only relieved when the furuncle has been incised or burst. Treatment of otitis externa aims at keeping the canal clean and dry, and the lumen patent, while the topical application of a suitable antibiotic is indicated in chronic cases.

Acute otitis media

Acute infection of the middle ear is one of the more common and important diseases in paediatric practice. While any severe respiratory infection is liable to involve the Eustachian tube and middle ear in both infants and children, infants are especially susceptible. In some cases the regurgitation of milk is thought to be responsible for infection occurring, and the shortness and direction of the tube in infancy are undoubtedly contributory factors. Blockage of the orifice of the tube by adenoid tissue also interferes with drainage and results in the stagnation of secretions.

The mastoid antrum, which consists of a single cell at birth and around which groups of air-containing cells subsequently develop during early childhood, is in such close connection with the middle ear that infections of the latter are likely to involve the mucosa of the mastoid antrum to a greater or less extent.

CLINICAL FEATURES. In acute catarrhal otitis media, which is a frequent accompaniment of the common cold, there may be little pain or pyrexia, older children complaining of transient deafness or noises in the ears. The tympanic membrane is at first retracted, with some loss of lustre. Subsequently there may be pain and bulging of the drum and rupture of the drum may occur. Many cases, however, subside spontaneously.

In purulent otitis media, pain (particularly at night) is often severe, being indicated in young infants by screaming, head rolling, pulling at the ears, and restlessness. The temperature may rise abruptly to 39·5°C (103°F) or higher, and is occasionally associated with convulsions or meningism. There is often transient tenderness over the mastoid process. The drumhead shows reddening of the margin and subsequently generalized infection and loss of light reflex; bulging of the posterior area of the drum indicates that pus is under pressure and requires release by myringotomy. In some cases clear or haemorrhagic bullae appear over the tympanic membrane (*myringitis bullosa*).

COMPLICATIONS. If the acute infection fails to subside, the condition passes into one of *chronic otitis media*, associated with perforation of the drum and chronic or intermittent otorrhoea, which may be mucopurulent or thick and offensive. If there is a marginal perforation situated superiorly, with cholesteatoma formation, there is a risk of intracranial spread of infection and surgical treatment is usually necessary.

Untreated chronic otitis media is frequently associated with deafness and may prove extremely resistant to treatment. It is important that the external auditory canal should be kept dry and clean; alcohol drops and an appropriate antibiotic should be used. Infected adenoids should be removed. Mastoidectomy is only rarely necessary. A long-standing perforation may be closed by myringoplasty if it has been dry for six months.

Serous otitis media. Affecting mainly children of 3 to 7 years, serous otitis media may develop insidiously or after inadequate antibiotic treat-ment for purulent otitis media. A sticky mucoid material accumulates in the middle ear, causing conductive hearing loss ('glue ear'). The condition may persist for months and treatment by drainage is not always effective.

Mastoiditis. Infection of the mastoid cells and antrum may be acute or chronic, and result either from an attack of acute otitis media or from an exacerbation of a more chronic condition. When mastoid infection persists after adequate drainage of the middle ear has been obtained, the aural discharge may become more profuse or cease altogether. Continued pyrexia, local tenderness, and oedema over the mastoid are important findings, and if these are associated with signs of meningeal irritation, swinging temperature, or rising pulse rate, the condition should be regarded as an emergency. The prompt and adequate treatment of otitis media with antibiotics has rendered mastoidectomy now comparatively seldom necessary.

Sinus thrombosis (p. 378). Thrombosis of the lateral sinus is a serious complication which is liable to be overlooked until infection has passed beyond this site or thrombosis has extended to other cerebral sinuses. The condition should be suspected if a high rise of temperature associated with a convulsion occurs after the original infection.

Meningitis. Extension of the infection to the meninges is evidenced by increased pyrexia,

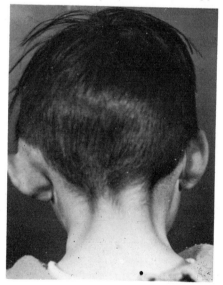

Fig. 14.1   Mastoiditis with abscess formation and displacement of left ear.

convulsions, and signs of meningeal irritation. Lumbar puncture will show the presence of purulent fluid and organisms, though a sterile meningeal reaction sometimes precedes the appearance of frank meningitis. Intensive antibiotic therapy, depending on the infecting organisms, must be instituted immediately.

Cerebral abscess. This serious complication of otitis media often develops insidiously, though the history may give evidence of transient meningeal irritation following the acute infection of the ear. A history of an aural discharge which has ceased one or more weeks before the occurrence of headache, vomiting, pyrexia, and bradycardia is very suggestive. The abscess is commonly situated in the temporal lobe and less frequently in the cerebellum. Localizing signs are often minimal, though in cerebellar cases there may be evidence of ataxia or nystagmus. The patient is usually lethargic or semi-comatose. Papilloedema is a most important diagnostic sign, though it may also occur with sinus thrombosis.

Lumbar puncture is contraindicated in the presence of raised intracranial pressure. The treatment consists of surgical drainage and antibiotic therapy.

Infantile gastroenteritis. While there is evidence that otitis media *may* precipitate diarrhoea and vomiting in infancy, and that in particular epidemics a considerable proportion of infants have such infections, the relationship is not constant and otitis may be secondary to the vomiting. Nevertheless it is important to consider upper respiratory infection as a possible etiological factor in any case of gastroenteritis.

TREATMENT. Antibiotic therapy has had a major effect on the treatment of infections of the ear. Most acute infections subside rapidly under this form of treatment, which does not however invalidate the general principle that pus in a confined space requires drainage. This may be effected in some cases by clearing the nose, nasopharynx, and Eustachian tubes, but when pus is causing bulging of the tympanic membrane, myringotomy is likely to be required. This has the advantage over spontaneous rupture that drainage is better through a free incision reaching the base of the cavity than through a small perforation situated high up. There is immediate relief of pain and the temperature falls as drainage is established. In uncomplicated cases, healing of the drum is subsequently complete without impairment of hearing. Otitis media cannot be considered cured, however, unless hearing has been restored to normal.

Deafness

The incidence of deafness amongst schoolchildren in Britain has been estimated as from 52 to 83 per thousand. Local authorities are obliged to provide special training for deaf children over the age of 2, although in only about 12 per thousand schoolchildren will special educational arrangements be necessary. In more than half the cases attending special schools, deafness is of prenatal origin, due in most instances to malformation of the cochlea and associated structures. In the majority of these cases the etiology is unknown; in others the defect is the result of maternal rubella occurring during the period of organogenesis, or is genetically determined. Deafness may be caused by birth injury or anoxia or may result from postnatal meningitis (most commonly meningococcal), in which case either the middle ear or eighth nerve may be affected; from haemolytic disease; or from mumps. In a proportion of acquired cases deafness is the sequel of otitis media. Deafness in early infancy will interfere with the acquisition of speech and the use of words as vehicles for thought, with all that this implies. In the case of children who become deaf after speech has been acquired, and language is already the currency of thought, training is in many ways easier: but even children of 6 or 7 years may regress in speech to a very great extent unless training is methodically undertaken and long continued.

A rough classification of deafness can be made according to the degree of hearing loss. Children who are *hard of hearing* are those who can hear the human voice, and in whom speech will be acquired spontaneously, though often imperfectly. The *partially hearing* are those who can appreciate amplified sound, and for whom acoustic aids will make acquisition of speech possible. The *profoundly deaf* are those in whom appreciation of sound is absent or so limited that speech cannot be acquired spontaneously when the condition dates from infancy (*deafmutism*); education in these cases has to be effected through lip-reading, tactile sensation, and other methods.

It is important to determine as soon as possible whether an infant's backwardness in vocalizing and other behaviour patterns dependent on normal hearing is the result of deafness or mental defect or both. A skilled observer may be able to suspect deafness during the first three months of life, and an intelligent mother will often notice that an infant will pay no attention to the human voice or to other sounds such as clinking of the milk bottle unless these are made within his range of vision. The infant often makes cacophonous noises bearing little similarity to the normal 'baby talk' of a healthy infant which is influenced by hearing speech long before recognizable words are formulated. Screening for deafness should be undertaken in all children as soon as possible after 6 months of age. If deafness is not detected at that time, the most frequent presenting symptom is failure to speak, and deafness should always be considered when a child is brought with this complaint or on account of speech defect which may be the result of partial deafness.

More detailed testing of hearing requires specialized techniques, since it is desirable to know not only the degree of deafness but the range of pitch over which deafness extends. For infants and young children specially designed play material and standardized tests with the human voice and other sounds are used. Older children are assessed more accurately by audiometry, which should be undertaken routinely at school entry.

In ascertaining educational needs, children with defective hearing are graded according to the special provisions required, the decision depending on total assessment of the child and not on hearing loss alone. Many children with slight hearing loss require no special arrangements. In other cases, it may be possible to undertake education in normal schools if the necessary facilities can be provided, e.g. the child who is hard of hearing sitting in the middle of the front row, or the partially hearing being provided with acoustic aid. Yet other children require education in special schools. For the pre-school child, skilled training in a special day or residential nursery is desirable. The profoundly deaf will always require special training, and the best results are usually obtained in residential schools.

THE LARYNX AND TRACHEA
Stridor

Harsh, noisy respiration is a symptom requiring the most careful investigation, since although it may be of little clinical importance it is often an indication of disease of extreme severity. It may be caused by obstruction at the level of the larynx or immediately above or below this site. In cases dating from birth without other evidence of disease, *congenital laryngeal stridor* (p. 103) is often a benign and transient condition requiring no treatment, though secondary infection may result in a severe degree of obstruction. It is essential to visualize the larynx to exclude conditions requiring surgical intervention. Other causes of stridor in infancy considered elsewhere are *laryngismus stridulus* (p. 155), which will be associated with other evidence of tetany; *retropharyngeal abscess* (p. 295); diphtheria (p. 340); and pressure of enlarged lymph nodes on the trachea. Similar pressure symptoms may arise from an enlarged heart or thyroid gland or from a constricting vascular ring.

Acute laryngitis (laryngitis stridulosa). Acute infection of the larynx varies in severity from a comparatively mild condition (*croup*) seen in older infants and children as an extension of an upper respiratory infection to one of extreme severity, carrying a very high mortality in young infants.

Viral croup is commonly due to respiratory syncytial virus or adenovirus, though other viruses such as para-influenza or measles virus may be responsible. It usually affects children under 3 years of age and is preceded by coryzal symptoms. The child often wakes from sleep with dyspnoea and crowing respiration, which alarm both him and his parents, but fever is seldom high and the systemic disturbance is mild unless the infection extends to the lower respiratory tract.

Acute epiglottitis is a potentially dangerous condition which causes rapid respiratory obstruction and is often accompanied by septicaemia. The inflamed epiglottis appears as a bright red swelling behind the tongue. Antibiotics including chloramphenicol should be given pending the results of bacterial examination, since many of these cases are due to *Haemophilus influenzae* type b. In those in which a virus is responsible, antibiotic therapy may control secondary infection.

Laryngotracheobronchitis. This represents the most severe type of laryngitis in which the infection extends to the trachea and bronchi. Although in some cases the infection results in little exudate and settles rapidly, it is impossible to predict at onset whether the condition will progress into one with acute respiratory obstruction. There is rapid onset of dyspnoea and cyanosis. The larynx is acutely inflamed and oedematous, and becomes occluded by tenacious secretion which also blocks the bronchi and may cause pulmonary collapse.

In all cases of croup the atmosphere should be humidified and oxygen administered for respiratory distress. It must be remembered that the 'mild' case may pass rapidly into a state of suffocative dyspnoea, and aspiration of muco-purulent secretions or tracheostomy may be necessary at short notice. Diminution of cyanosis on giving oxygen does not necessarily indicate improvement. When epiglottitis is suspected, laryngeal examination should not be undertaken without facilities for immediate relief of respiratory obstruction, e.g. tracheostomy, since there is a danger of precipitating complete obstruction from laryngospasm.

Oedema of the larynx occasionally complicates acute infections of the neck or results from inhalation of steam from a boiling kettle. The larynx may also be affected in the nephrotic syndrome or in angioneurotic oedema. Oedema of the larynx is characterized by severe dyspnoea and cyanosis, and may necessitate intubation or tracheostomy.

Foreign body. Lodgement of a foreign body in the immediate vicinity of the larynx, usually in the pyriform fossa, will give rise to a varying degree of obstruction, depending on the size and shape of the object. Stridor and indrawing of the lower thorax will usually be preceded by a paroxysm of coughing. Since in young children there is often no clear history of a foreign body having been inhaled, sudden onset of stridor in the absence of infection should always suggest this possibility. Radiological examination will only serve to localize a radio-opaque object, and laryngoscopy will be required in any case of doubt and when removal of the foreign body is attempted.

Papilloma of the larynx is a rare cause of laryngeal obstruction in childhood; obstruction is likely to be preceded by a history of hoarseness. Diagnosis must be made by laryngoscopy, and treatment may involve repeated removal owing to the tendency of these tumours to recur.

THE BRONCHI, LUNGS, AND PLEURA

In considering disease of the lower respiratory tract in infancy and childhood, certain physio-logical differences related to age must be borne in mind. The muscle of the bronchiolar walls in infancy is not adapted to the calibre of the bronchioles, and there is consequently greater liability to collapse. Displacement of the mobile mediastinum occurs readily in childhood. Mechanical and obstructive factors are of particular importance in respiratory disease in early life, and respiratory embarrassment is an even greater risk to the infant than to the older child. Interpretation of X-rays must also be related to age, e.g. crying (and consequent venous engorgement) will result in great increase in the width of the upper mediastinal shadow in infancy which may be misinterpreted as a pathological finding.

While many different infective agents may be responsible for lower respiratory tract infections in early life, the respiratory viruses are of first importance. Surveys have shown that respiratory syncytial virus, adenoviruses, para-influenza viruses or picornaviruses are present in a high proportion of cases. Since viruses are generally uninfluenced by antibiotic therapy, there is thus little justification for the indiscriminate use of antibiotics in childhood respiratory infections. While hard and fast rules cannot be laid down, there are good grounds for suggesting that antibiotic therapy should be reserved for seriously ill children, those from whom pathogenic bacteria have been cultured or who are believed on other grounds to have a bacterial infection, and selected children in whom the development of secondary bacterial infection would be especially undesirable.

Bronchitis and bronchiolitis

Acute bronchitis commonly represents an extension of an acute upper respiratory infection, or occurs as a complication of measles or pertussis; chronic bronchitis may follow repeated acute attacks, but is more closely related to persistent upper respiratory tract infection, e.g. chronic sinusitis. Bronchitis is in general considerably commoner in the younger age groups, though it occurs at all ages. Overcrowding and infection in the home are important etiological factors, and though no social class is exempt, chronic bronchitis is frequent amongst the poorer sections of the community. Malnutrition predisposes to respiratory infections, which are also more common in obese infants and young children. Infections are commonly of mixed type, including pneumococci, *H. influenzae*, streptococci, and staphylococci, but the bacteria found may be secondary invaders following a virus infection.

CLINICAL FEATURES. The most severe and lethal type of respiratory infection occurring in infants is laryngotracheobronchitis which has been considered above, but the trachea is involved to some extent in all cases.

Obstructive bronchiolitis (capillary bronchitis) starts with coryza and rapidly progresses to restlessness, cough, dyspnoea and wheezing simulating asthma. This type occurs most frequently in epidemic form in infancy and respiratory syncytial virus (R.S.V.) is commonly isolated. Fine crepitations are heard throughout the lungs and there may be diffuse mottling radiologically, with patchy areas of emphysema and collapse.

Acute bronchitis is manifested by cough and pyrexia, which may follow or coincide with an upper respiratory infection or the onset of measles, or precede the more characteristic paroxysms of pertussis. The temperature is often 38°C (100° or 101°F), and is seldom over 39°C (102°F) unless the condition is complicated by bronchopneumonia. The degree of dyspnoea varies greatly, being most marked in infants and sometimes very slight in older children. Typically, the respiration rate is little raised, except in early infancy. Some evidence of bronchial obstruction, however, is usually present. As a general rule, the cough is at first dry, irritating, and non-productive, and subsequently becomes 'loose' though sputum is usually swallowed by younger children. Violent coughing may result in vomiting, and older children will often complain that the cough is painful. Substernal discomfort due to tracheitis is also a common complaint.

On examination of the chest, rhonchi and scattered rales, their nature depending on the stage of the disease and character of the secretions, are heard throughout both lungs; fine rales and sibilant rhonchi are heard when the bronchioles are involved, and harsh rhonchi when there is much secretion in the large bronchi. The percussion note is not impaired in uncomplicated cases.

Chronic bronchitis is characterized by persistent or intermittent cough, usually worst at night and on waking in the morning. There is little or no pyrexia. The child's general condition and nutrition are usually poor, and thoracic deformity is sometimes present when the condition is

of long duration. The presence of unremitting cough, finger clubbing, or localized rales which are consistently present in one area should suggest that bronchiectasis has already developed. Examination of the nasopharynx may show a trickle of muco-pus, indicating chronic sinus infection. The sinuses should be investigated in all cases.

DIAGNOSIS. The constitutional symptoms in acute bronchitis are in general less severe than those in bronchopneumonia, and there will be no clinical or radiological evidence of consolidation. In children in whom there is abrupt onset of cough and dyspnoea without pyrexia, the possibility of inhaled foreign body being responsible should be considered.

Asthma can usually be distinguished in older children on the history and nature of the attack, but it may be difficult to draw a sharp distinction between allergic and infective bronchiolitis in young infants.

COURSE AND PROGNOSIS. In the great majority of cases an attack of acute bronchitis lasts from one to two weeks, the patient only being febrile during the first few days. Obstructive bronchiolitis of early infancy is a serious and sometimes fatal condition but recovery is rapid once the acute stage is past. However, there is always some risk of bronchial occlusion occurring, and in marasmic patients the likelihood of bronchopneumonia complicating the initial infection is greater. A high proportion of infants who die from respiratory tract infections have major congenital abnormalities.

In chronic bronchitis the prognosis depends to a great extent on the successful elimination of chronic sinus infection when this is present and on the improvement of environmental conditions. The longer the condition persists, the greater is the likelihood of bronchiectasis developing.

TREATMENT. Bed rest during the period of pyrexia and confinement to a warm room until symptoms are relieved are indicated during the acute attack. While a humid atmosphere may be of value during the dry or viscid stage of bronchitis, it can be a danger when the child is already drowning in his own secretions. A humidifier should not be used when bronchopneumonia has developed.

Infants who are restless, cyanosed or dyspnoeic should be nursed in oxygen, though this is seldom necessary for older children with uncomplicated bronchitis. Since most cases are viral in origin, antibiotics are unlikely to be beneficial but treatment with a broad-spectrum antibiotic is indicated in severe cases to lessen the risk of complications and in cases of known bacterial infection. Attention must be paid to fluid and electrolyte balance and digoxin may be required for cardiac failure. Occasionally bronchoscopy and aspiration are necessary when the secretions are fibrinous or so profuse that they are causing bronchial occlusion. Naso-tracheal intubation and mechanical ventilation may be life-saving when respiratory failure is imminent.

In chronic bronchitis the first aims of treatment should be to eliminate upper respiratory infection, to improve the general nutrition and environment of the child, and to institute postural drainage and breathing exercises. Drug therapy when it is employed should as far as possible be adjusted to the stage of the disease. A non-productive irritating cough which is interfering with sleep is an indication for a sedative, e.g. chloral or amylobarbitone, or for a cough suppressant, e.g. codeine or pholcodine, but if the cough is due primarily to muco-pus in the naso-pharynx (which is apt to be most irritating at night), treatment must be directed to the upper respiratory tract. Drugs should never be used to suppress a cough which is serving to raise sputum, nor should drugs such as belladonna be given with the purpose of 'drying up' the secretion, i.e. rendering it more viscid.

The use of expectorants to liquefy viscid secretion, on the other hand, appears rational though it is dubiously effective. Amongst those commonly used are ammonium chloride, ipecacuanha, and potassium iodide. Ephedrine or orciprenaline may prove effective in relieving bronchial spasm. In some cases prolonged antibiotic therapy, e.g. a small daily dose of ampicillin, may be justified to prevent frequent exacerbations.

Inhaled foreign body

A foreign body which will pass the larynx is unlikely to obstruct the trachea, but may lodge in any part of the bronchial tree, most commonly the right main bronchus or right lower lobe bronchi. Among the foreign bodies which are apt to be inhaled are pins, tin-tacks, beads, and vegetable matter. Peanuts are particularly irritating and cause an intense inflammatory reaction. A tooth, fragment of tonsil, or blood-clot may act

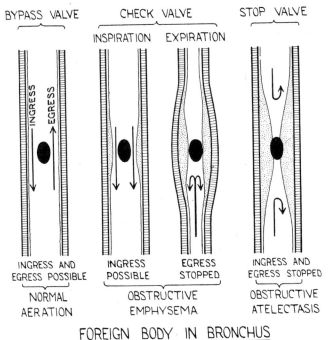

FOREIGN BODY IN BRONCHUS
(REDRAWN AFTER JACKSON)

Fig. 14.2 Foreign body in bronchus, showing mechanism of production of obstructive emphysema and collapse. (*After* Jackson.)

as a foreign body, and care is necessary in operations on the mouth or nasopharynx to avoid inhalation of material during anaesthesia. Foreign bodies lodged in the trachea may produce tracheal 'flutter', wheezing, dyspnoea, cough, and cyanosis. In the bronchial tree the signs and symptoms will depend to some extent on whether obstruction of the lumen is partial or complete, though in all cases there is likely to be cough and production of offensive sputum which may be blood-stained. Three types of obstruction may occur (Fig. 14.2): (1) partial obstruction, when both ingress and egress of air past the foreign body is possible; (2) a check-valve action, in which ingress is possible, but egress impossible owing to the smaller lumen of the bronchus during expiration; in this case obstructive emphysema beyond the foreign body will result; and (3) complete obstruction, in which both ingress and egress of air are blocked, and collapse of the lung beyond the obstruction occurs.

The longer the obstruction persists, the greater is the likelihood of a *lung abscess* or *bronchiectasis* developing beyond the obstruction.

DIAGNOSIS. Although there is often no clear history of inhalation given, the condition should be suspected whenever there is sudden and unexplained onset of cough and wheezing, especially when the sputum is blood-stained. Clinical evidence of emphysema or pulmonary collapse will be confirmed by radiological examination, which will serve to demonstrate a radio-opaque foreign body and may also be of considerable help in localizing a non-opaque object, such as a peanut.

TREATMENT. Removal of the foreign body by bronchoscopy is the first essential, though this may present great difficulty in the case of small objects which have reached the peripheral bronchi or foreign bodies of vegetable origin which fragment readily. Subsequent treatment will depend on the degree of peripheral lung damage which has occurred, though even in the case of a lung abscess it will sometimes be found that once free drainage has been obtained the cavity heals spontaneously. Antibiotic therapy should always be given when there is evidence of secondary infection.

Bronchiectasis

Dilatation of the bronchi, usually associated with stagnation of secretion and secondary infec-

tion, occurs readily in childhood, though much less commonly since broad-spectrum antibiotics came into general use. Congenital cysts of the lungs communicating with bronchi may simulate saccular bronchiectasis, and should be distinguished from the acquired variety which arises from degeneration of the bronchial wall and secondary dilatation. This is most commonly *cylindrical* in the larger descending bronchi, while the smaller bronchi may show *saccular* or *fusiform* dilatation. A localized type of *collapse bronchiectasis* arises when there is collapse of a lobe or of a whole lung, following obstruction of the lumen of a bronchus by a foreign body, tuberculous material, or a plug of sputum. In these cases the bronchi within the collapsed area are crowded together, lose their elasticity and become dilated.

Chronic upper respiratory infection is an important etiological factor in those cases which are not due to mechanical obstruction. The condition is likely to be progressive if there is constant inhalation of organisms from a nidus of infection in the sinuses, and muco-pus continually reaches the descending bronchi from this source.

CLINICAL FEATURES. In non-obstructive cases the history frequently dates from an attack of pneumonia or pertussis. The clinical findings may be very similar to those of chronic bronchitis, but the cough tends to be more constantly present throughout the year and localized rales are consistently present, most commonly below the scapulae. Any part of the lung may be involved, however, though the lower lobes are much more frequently affected than the upper.

In obstructive cases there is likely to be evidence of collapse (localized dullness and impaired air entry), but since a collapsed lower lobe may lie within the paravertebral fossa and is often reduced to small size, it is sometimes difficult to demonstrate except on radiological examination.

The *sputum* is variable in amount and appearance. In the advanced case with heavy anaerobic infection, the sputum is abundant, purulent and offensive. Haemoptysis occasionally occurs. In milder cases the sputum is less diagnostic, and is sometimes minimal especially when antibiotics have been used. Violent coughing on waking usually raises a quantity of sputum which has accumulated during the night, and postural drainage at intervals throughout the day will generally result in further sputum being raised.

Clubbing of the fingers is a valuable diagnostic sign and is evidenced by curvature of the nails in their long axis, violet discoloration of the nail-beds, and slight swelling of the soft tissues.

The child may appear well-nourished if anorexia and toxaemia have been controlled by antibiotic therapy but often there is poor nutrition with retardation of growth. In advanced cases wasting, cyanosis of the lips, and deformity of the chest are evident.

RADIOLOGICAL DIAGNOSIS. It is often possible to suspect bronchiectasis from the straight X-ray, which may show a mottled area of infiltration, most commonly in the cardiophrenic angles; in these cases there is a general increase of lung markings running down from the hilum. The appearance of collapsed lobes is described on p. 331.

The only satisfactory method of determining the nature and extent of the bronchiectatic lesions, however, is by radiological examination after injection of radiographic oil (bronchography). As a preliminary, the child should be given a course of postural drainage in order to empty the cavities.

TREATMENT. Environmental conditions and the general health and nutrition of the patient should be fully investigated and any upper respiratory infection cleared up. Cystic fibrosis should always be excluded. Every case must be carefully assessed as to the extent and localization of the lesions and whether these are reversible. In general, patients with unilateral lesions, especially when confined to a single lobe, are likely to benefit most from surgical treatment. Except in selected cases of collapse bronchiectasis, it is usually advisable for the child to have a period of postural drainage after any existing upper respiratory infection has been dealt with before surgical removal of the affected area (segmental resection, lobectomy, or pneumonectomy) is carried out. A more conservative attitude may be adopted in very mild and early cases, when postural drainage, physiotherapy, and attention to the general health, may result in considerable improvement if not cure. When the lesions are diffuse and bilateral, incomplete removal of the diseased areas will almost certainly be followed by subsequent extension, and the relative merits of surgical and conservative treatment must be considered in terms of temporary improvement rather than permanent cure. The use of the mucolytic drug, n-acetyl cysteine, as an aerosol has been advocated. Antibiotic therapy is principally of value in reducing the risk of operative procedures and in preventing complications. In inoperable cases, and particularly those associated with cystic fibrosis, the organisms are liable to develop resistance to successive antibiotics.

COURSE AND PROGNOSIS. The disease is essentially a chronic one, and except in the earliest cases seen before the lesions are irreversible, the bronchial damage is likely to be slowly progressive. Complete surgical removal of affected areas gives a reasonable prospect of subsequent good health if the child can be protected from further infection. Intensive and prolonged medical treatment may at least arrest or delay the progress of the disease, though complete recovery can only be hoped for in a small proportion of all cases.

THE PNEUMONIAS

The time-honoured classification of pneumonia on an anatomical basis, viz. *lobar pneumonia*, *bronchopneumonia*, etc., is difficult to sustain when applied to infantile and childhood cases, since the distribution of the lesions is so frequently atypical. Against a purely etiological classification such as bacterial infection, virus infection, fungus infection, aspiration pneumonia, etc. must be placed the difficulty of obtaining sputum for examination at the onset of pneumonia in infancy and the facts that in many cases a mixed bacterial, or bacterial and virus, infection is present, and that the same organism may be responsible for different clinical types. For the present purpose, it appears best to describe pneumococcal pneumonia as a separate entity, to include under 'bronchopneumonia' the various pneumonias characterized by extensive involvement of the bronchial walls and to consider the atypical pneumonias as a separate group. For practical purposes, the important distinction is now between pneumonias which respond to antibiotic therapy and those which do not, though with the development of resistant strains there is increasing necessity for the early recognition and testing of the infecting agent.

Pneumococcal pneumonia (*Primary*, 'lobar' *pneumonia*)

The disease may follow a cold or arise suddenly without previous evidence of infection.

Cold and exposure are regarded as predisposing causes, but the condition is only slightly more frequent amongst malnourished and debilitated infants and children than in those who have previously been in good health. The incidence is highest in the winter and spring, and in cold, wet climates. The disease occurs throughout childhood, and although the incidence is maximum in the second year of life, pneumococcal pneumonia is considerably commoner than bronchopneumonia after the age of infancy.

The infection enters by way of the respiratory passages, and causes inflammation of the alveoli which become filled with exudate (stage of congestion). The stage of red hepatization which follows is characterized by consolidation of the affected area, which is not necessarily demarcated by the boundaries of a lobe, and the outpouring of red and white cells, fibrin, and organisms into the alveoli and bronchioles. This is followed by grey hepatization, in which leucocytes predominate in the alveoli, and finally by resolution, during which stage the alveolar and bronchiolar exudate liquefies and is expectorated. An important finding is that the bronchial and bronchiolar walls are little involved and that after complete resolution the lung tissue is left functionally normal, without the interstitial fibrosis which commonly follows a bronchopneumonia. The pleura shares in the congestion of the underlying lung and may become covered with sero-fibrinous exudate. Unless the pneumonia is complicated by empyema, the pleural exudate absorbs.

CLINICAL FEATURES. The onset is abrupt and the sudden rise of temperature to 39·5°C (103°F) or more can often be accurately timed. In infants and younger children the initial pyrexia is sometimes associated with signs of meningeal irritation (*meningism*), or with a convulsion. The respiratory rate is raised to a relatively greater degree than the pulse rate, the respiration : pulse ratio changing from the normal 1:4 or $3\frac{1}{2}$ to 1:2. The alae nasi can be seen in movement. The patient is usually flushed and obviously dyspnoeic, with a short, painful cough. Cyanosis when present is likely to be only slight; infants may appear pale and prostrated, particularly when there is much vomiting or diarrhoea at onset. Pain referred to the abdomen most often occurs when the pneumonic process affects the lower lobes; right-sided abdominal pain associated with vomiting may simulate appendicitis,

but it will be found on inspection that the abdomen moves freely on respiration, and the raised respiratory rate will serve to distinguish the two conditions.

Examination of the chest frequently shows no definite evidence of consolidation at first, though the breath-sounds may be reduced over the affected area during this time and pleural friction may be heard. Subsequently, localized dullness, transient moist sounds, and ultimately bronchial breathing are detected over the pneumonic area. With antibiotic therapy, signs of consolidation are likely to persist for a variable number of days after the temperature and respiration have fallen to normal.

COMPLICATIONS. The commonest of these are *empyema*, occurring two to three weeks after the onset of symptoms, and *acute otitis media*, which may appear more rapidly. Lung abscess, pneumococcal meningitis, peritonitis, arthritis, and pericarditis are all rare complications.

DIAGNOSIS. The established clinical picture in childhood is usually sufficiently clear-cut to present little difficulty in diagnosis, though radiological examination is desirable. In collapse of lung and pleural effusion there is likely to be less temperature reaction, and the white blood count (which shows a high leucocytosis in pneumonia) will be little raised. The presence of herpes, though suggestive of pneumonia, is not diagnostic. Before signs of consolidation have appeared, marked meningism or convulsions may suggest the presence of meningitis; if radiological examination is not definitive, it is better to undertake lumbar puncture than to risk delay in treatment of a meningitis. In meningism the cerebrospinal fluid is clear, sterile, and under increased pressure, with little or no increase in cellular and protein content and no reduction of sugar.

In infants the diagnosis is often more difficult, owing to atypical temperature reactions and distribution of the pulmonary lesions, while complications such as abdominal distension or diarrhoea and vomiting may mask the primary symptoms. In such cases X-ray of the chest is essential. In general the raised respiratory rate is the most important single diagnostic sign, but even this is considerably less reliable in infancy than in childhood.

COURSE AND PROGNOSIS. Even before chemotherapy became available it was not uncommon to see abortive cases, particularly in infants, in which the temperature and respiration fell to normal before the fourth day. In the majority of all cases, however, the temperature and respiratory rate remained elevated for four to eight days, usually falling by crisis and less frequently by lysis. An atypical course was more common in infancy than in later childhood, when the disease tended to follow the adult pattern more closely. Except in early infancy, the prognosis was good, and although resolution was in some cases delayed it was usually complete.

Antibiotic therapy has now made it rare for a case to follow the 'natural' course, adequate treatment usually effecting a fall in temperature, respiration- and pulse-rate within forty-eight hours, with a corresponding relief of symptoms. The mortality has been greatly reduced in infants, and in childhood (in which age period it was always low) the mortality is now minimal in uncomplicated cases. The incidence of complications has also been reduced.

TREATMENT. Penicillin therapy alone will prove promptly effective in the great majority of cases of pneumococcal pneumonia, but in severe infections it may be advisable to combine two antibiotics. Since in young infants the clinical picture is less clear-cut, and there is a greater likelihood of pneumonia being due to a penicillin-resistant staphylococcus, it is advisable to start treatment with a broad-spectrum antibiotic.

Infants should be nursed in oxygen in a semi-upright position as long as dyspnoea or cyanosis persists. For older children, the room should be well ventilated, and if the child can be kept warm, nursing in fresh air or by an open window will sometimes be found to give more relief than too warm an atmosphere. Although skilled nursing is still desirable for the comfort of the patient, the duration of toxaemia and fever is now so much reduced that many patients can safely be treated in the home.

Bronchopneumonia

This category includes a much more heterogeneous group of cases than that described above. A variety of infecting organisms is found, including staphylococci, streptococci, H. influenzae type b, and (rarely) Friedländer bacilli, alone or in combination, while in some cases there is evidence of a virus infection followed by secondary invasion by bacteria. Pneumococcal infection may also produce the clinical and pathological picture of bronchopneumonia rather than that of the typical pneumococcal pneumonia.

In bronchopneumonia the walls of the bronchioles and bronchi are involved, and the consequent interstitial inflammation is likely to result in incomplete resolution and subsequent fibrosis. The lesions also tend to be diffuse, multi-focal, and bilateral, but confluent areas of bronchopneumonia may simulate lobar pneumonia on clinical and radiological examination.

The disease is frequently secondary to a previous illness, e.g. measles, pertussis, influenza, bronchitis, and is more likely to occur in ill-nourished and debilitated infants. The incidence is highest in the first year of life, and staphylococcal pneumonia is largely confined to this age period except in cystic fibrosis. Aspiration pneumonia, due to the inhalation of food, vomitus, or infected material, and lipoid pneumonia from inhalation of oily nasal drops, are also most likely to occur in the youngest age group.

CLINICAL FEATURES. Since the disease is often secondary to previous infection, it will usually be found that an abrupt or more insidious rise of temperature is superimposed on an existing low-grade fever. The pyrexia is more irregular, and in untreated cases more persistent than in typical pneumococcal pneumonia. Similar evidence of respiratory embarrassment occurs, but there is a greater tendency to cyanosis and cough is generally a more prominent sign.

In young infants, the distinction between obstructive bronchiolitis and bronchopneumonia cannot readily be made on clinical grounds, but in the latter cyanosis and prostration are generally greater, wheezing is less and there is radiological evidence of consolidation. Occasionally, severe bronchopneumonia may present in early infancy with circulatory failure and collapse.

The lung lesions frequently show a patchy distribution and a tendency to migrate. If they are diffuse, signs of consolidation may be indefinite and are often obscured by those of generalized bronchitis.

COMPLICATIONS. Staphylococcal pneumonia frequently leads to the formation of minute abscess cavities, and if one or more of these rupture through the pleura, a localized pneumothorax or a pyopneumothorax is produced. Infections with H. influenzae sometimes cause surgical emphysema, rupture of an alveolus leading first to localized emphysema of the mediastinum, and this in turn spreading to the superficial tissues of the neck or extending over the trunk. Cardiac failure is responsible for death in a proportion of fatal cases. Of late complications, pulmonary fibrosis, delayed resolution, and chronic bronchitis or bronchiectasis are the most common.

COURSE AND PROGNOSIS. Since the disease occurs predominantly in early infancy, the general prognosis, even with antibiotic therapy, is not uniformly favourable. The mortality has, however, been greatly reduced in recent years. Patients who recover are more likely to be left with some residual damage to the lung or bronchi than is the case in pneumococcal pneumonia, and there is a greater likelihood of subsequent attacks.

TREATMENT. General treatment is essentially the same as for bronchitis or bronchiolitis. A broad-spectrum antibiotic such as ampicillin should be used at least until the sensitivity of the organism has been determined. Recovery should be followed by a period of convalescence with final radiological examination to make sure that resolution is complete.

Primary atypical pneumonia

This is a mixed group rather than a separate disease entity, since atypical pneumonia may develop in the course of a number of known viral infections, while in many clinically similar cases no virus has yet been identified. Epidemics have been described, affecting principally adults but also children. In some of these, *Mycoplasma pneumoniae* (Eaton agent) has been the organism responsible. The signs and symptoms are less clear-cut than in the pneumonias described above, and the diagnosis is often made only on radiological examination, or from the failure to respond to antibiotic therapy, though improved facilities for virus culture are making accurate diagnosis more practicable. The onset is insidious, with malaise, anorexia, headache and persistent cough which may be paroxysmal; the temperature is variably raised but the respiratory rate may be normal. Radiological examination shows enlargement of the hilar shadow with patchy, soft infiltration of the lung. In some cases, cold agglutinins appear in the blood.

Although fatal cases have occurred in young infants, the disease usually runs a benign though protracted course with recovery. Treatment is largely symptomatic, and antibiotic therapy is typically ineffective. Atypical pneumonia due to

M. pneumoniae is generally more severe than when due to a virus but may respond to tetracycline.

Lung abscess

Solitary abscess of the lung is rare as a sequel of pneumonia, though multiple small abscesses are not uncommon in staphylococcal pneumonia. Most examples of solitary abscess occur as the result of inhalation of a foreign body, or following operations on the mouth or nasopharynx.

A localized abscess is most likely to form in the periphery of the lung, and consists of an area of necrosis and liquefaction involving both the bronchi and parenchyma of the lung, and surrounded by a variable degree of inflammatory infiltration. The breath becomes foul, pyrexia and evidence of toxaemia usually occur, and localized dullness may be manifest on clinical examination. Although cough is always present, the nature of the sputum will depend on whether the abscess is draining through a bronchus. When there is bronchial obstruction, sputum is minimal; the sudden clearing of a bronchus will result in the expectoration of large amounts of extremely foul sputum. The diagnosis can often be suspected from the history, e.g. onset of symptoms some few days after an operation or inhalation of a foreign body, and will be confirmed by radiological examination. A fluid level seen within the abscess cavity is diagnostic but may be obscured by surrounding infiltration.

Whenever an inhaled foreign body is responsible, or the abscess is not draining naturally, bronchoscopy and removal of the obstruction should be undertaken. If drainage can be established by way of the bronchi, some patients will recover spontaneously and completely; but when the condition is of long standing, surgical drainage to the exterior may be necessary. There is always considerable danger of aspiration of infected sputum producing a suppurative bronchopneumonia, and antibiotic therapy should be given.

Idiopathic pulmonary haemosiderosis

Recurrent haemorrhage into the lung is occasionally responsible for patchy consolidation and deposition of haemosiderin ('brown induration of the lungs') associated with blood-stained sputum, and resulting in secondary anaemia, hepatosplenomegaly, and cardiac failure. Diagnosis depends on the finding of haemosiderin in the phagocytes of the sputum, or on lung puncture. If primary cardiac disease, lupus erythematosus, and polyarteritis are excluded as possible causes of haemosiderosis of the lungs, there remain cases where the etiology is obscure. An abnormal immunological response to the ingestion of cow's milk has been suggested as a possible factor, and the effect of removing milk from the diet should be tried. Transfusion may be required to combat anaemia. The prognosis is poor.

Gangrene of the lung

This is rare in childhood, and though extensive necrosis may occasionally follow pneumonia, the etiology in many cases is obscure. The rapid disintegration of large areas of lung tissue results in foetor of the breath and sputum (which often contains Vincent's organisms and spirochaetes), toxaemia, pyrexia, and wasting. While early cases may respond to antibiotic therapy, pneumonectomy is likely to be required. The mortality is high.

Pulmonary collapse

Collapse of lung with secondary air absorption is most likely to occur from bronchial occlusion or from the presence of air or fluid in the pleural cavity. Extreme abdominal distension, paralysis of the diaphragm or respiratory muscles, and chest wounds are also possible causes. Bronchial occlusion may be due to blockage of the lumen of the bronchus by a foreign body, caseous material, a plug of mucus or sputum, or infiltration of the bronchial wall; pressure from without, e.g. from tuberculous or malignant lymph nodes, is most likely to produce occlusion when the bronchial wall is also infiltrated.

The radiological appearances of collapse of

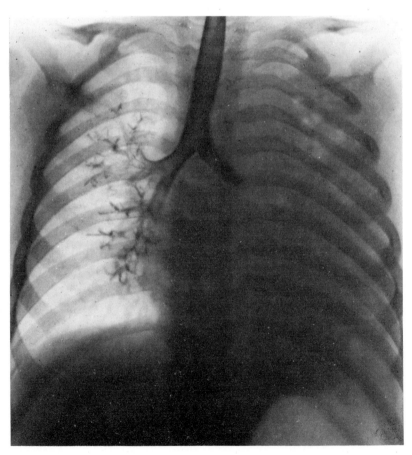

Fig. 14.3   Obstruction of left main bronchus by foreign body (bronchogram).

the various lobes are described on p. 331. Massive collapse of the whole of one lung is most likely to arise from blockage of a main bronchus (Figs. 14.3 and 14.4) by a foreign body or by secretion following operation; contralateral trauma to the chest-wall is rarely responsible in childhood cases. At necropsy, a collapsed lung, lobe, or lobule is seen to be reduced in size and airless; there will be compensatory emphysema of the remaining lung tissue if the collapsed area is at all extensive.

The symptoms vary with the cause. They may be similar to those of pneumonia in post-operative cases, while in lobar collapse due to tuberculosis, slight dyspnoea or wheezing may be the only indication that collapse has occurred. In massive collapse of the lung there is diminished movement of the affected side, impaired percussion note, and diminished or absent breath-sounds. The heart and mediastinum are displaced towards the affected side. Smaller areas of collapse (Fig. 14.8) will give rise to similar but more localized signs.

COURSE, PROGNOSIS, AND TREATMENT. Although in many cases the collapsed area will re-expand spontaneously, bronchoscopy should not be delayed if it is thought that bronchial obstruction is responsible. If collapse is allowed to persist, there is a considerable likelihood of the affected area becoming fibrosed or the site of collapse bronchiectasis. Inhalation of CO_2 in oxygen and breathing exercises are often valuable. When collapse is due to pressure from without, e.g. pleural effusion, treatment is that of the primary condition.

Emphysema

Overdistension of the alveoli with air and loss of elasticity of the area of lung involved occur as the result of collapse of neighbouring lung tissue

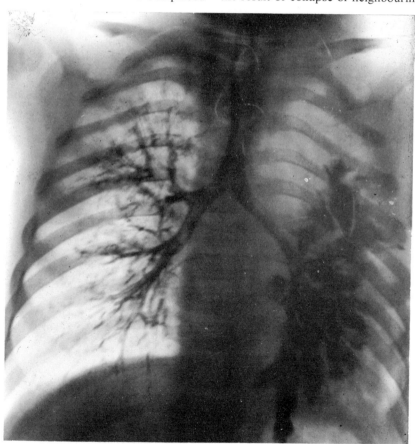

Fig. 14.4   The same case as Fig. 14.3, showing extensive bronchiectasis in left lung beyond site of obstruction.

(*compensatory emphysema*) or of obstruction to the egress of air from the bronchi (*obstructive emphysema*). The latter may be due to the presence of a foreign body in a bronchus but is more commonly the result of bronchospasm in chronic asthma. The chest tends to become barrel-shaped, movement is diminished, and the affected area is hyperresonant. There is expiratory dyspnoea or wheezing and exercise tolerance is impaired. Radiological examination will show diminished excursion of the chest and diaphragm and increased translucency of the affected area. Treatment is that of the primary cause. Rupture of an emphysematous bulla is occasionally responsible for pneumothorax.

Congenital lobar emphysema may cause acute and rapidly increasing respiratory distress in early infancy. A valvular type of bronchial obstruction is present; lobectomy is usually indicated.

Pulmonary embolism

Pulmonary embolism is rare in infancy and childhood. When an embolus lodges in the pulmonary artery, there is sudden onset of pain, dyspnoea, collapse, and blood-stained sputum. The condition is most likely to occur following operations in malnourished children; fat embolism occasionally results from fracture of a long bone. If the condition is not immediately fatal, the child must be sedated and kept at complete rest in an oxygen tent. Heparin is probably of value. Any existing infection must be treated.

Cystic fibrosis (*Fibrocystic disease of the pancreas, mucoviscidosis*)

Cystic fibrosis is a generalized disorder of the exocrine glands characterized by progressive pulmonary disease, pancreatic insufficiency and abnormally high sweat electrolytes. It is considered here because the brunt of the disease generally falls on the lungs and the degree of lung involvement determines the fate of the patient. Cystic fibrosis is inherited as an autosomal recessive, the gene being present in approximately 1 in 22 of the British population, and the disease occurs about once every 2000 births. A high proportion of affected children die early, but more are now surviving into adult life as the result of improvements in treatment.

PATHOGENESIS. Mucous glands throughout the body secrete abnormal mucus, which accumulates in the ducts and causes dilatation of the glands. The tenacious viscid secretions obstruct major organ passages, leading to changes in the organs themselves. In the lungs, failure to remove bronchial secretions results in widespread bronchiolar obstruction with areas of collapse and emphysema. Infection follows and the mucopurulent material blocks the bronchi, while invasion of the bronchial walls leads to fibrosis and ultimately to bronchiectasis. These changes are generalized in both lungs, the upper lobes being involved to a greater extent than the lower.

Staphylococcus aureus is the principal pathogenic organism, though *Pseudomonas aeruginosa* is also frequently present. Chronic hypoxia and increasing pulmonary hypertension lead to right ventricular hypertrophy and eventually to cor pulmonale with right heart failure.

In the pancreas, dilatation of acini secondary to obstruction of the ducts gives the cystic appearance seen histologically, while blockage of the bile canaliculi causes progressive cirrhosis of the liver.

CLINICAL FEATURES. The manifestations of cystic fibrosis are protean and include neonatal intestinal obstruction, failure to thrive, malabsorption and recurrent respiratory infection. In *meconium ileus*, which affects about one-tenth of

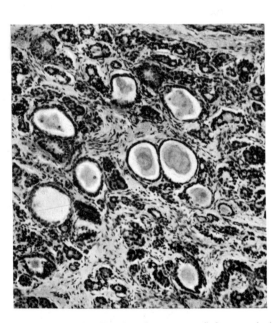

Fig. 14.5 Cystic fibrosis of pancreas (infant aged 4 months). Pancreas shows dilated acini and ducts containing inspissated secretion. Other acini are atrophied. Inter- and intralobular stroma is increased. H. and E. × 160.

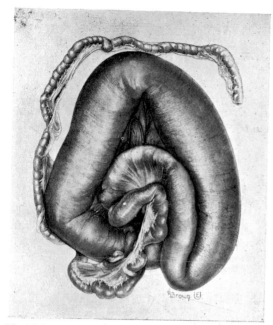

Fig. 14.6   Meconium ileus in a newborn infant, showing greatly dilated loop of ileum surrounded by small, empty colon.

Most infants with cystic fibrosis fail to thrive from the early weeks, although some progress reasonably well for months or even years and then cease to do so as infection and malabsorption begin to interfere with growth and nutrition. Typically the appetite is good and often it is voracious, but chronic pyogenic infection may cause anorexia. Although the lungs are usually normal at birth, the characteristic pulmonary changes can occur at any time, even in the newborn period. Early respiratory manifestations may be attributed at first to bronchitis or pneumonia, and sometimes to pertussis if the cough is spasmodic. Gradually the cough becomes more continual, the chest assumes a barrel shape and persistent moist sounds may be heard on auscultation of the lungs. Increasing airways resistance is indicated by rising residual lung volume and decreasing vital capacity. Radiologically, opacities appear and increase throughout the lung fields, being most prominent in the hilar regions. Chronic sinusitis and nasal polypi may be troublesome.

Further progression of the chronic lung disease, punctuated by acute exacerbations, leads to a more or less permanent state of dyspnoea with productive cough and cyanosis; eventually cardiac failure is precipitated. The degree of abnormality of the stools depends on the extent

infants with cystic fibrosis, the meconium is abnormally tenacious, obstructing the lower intestine and causing great dilatation of the proximal ileum, while the terminal ileum and colon are usually small and contracted. In fetal life, the intestinal wall may perforate to cause sterile meconium peritonitis, while failure to evacuate the bowel after birth results in intestinal obstruction, manifest as abdominal distension and bilious vomiting. Masses of viscid meconium may be palpable through the abdominal wall. Radiologically there are dilated loops of bowel without fluid levels and there may be a granular appearance due to bubbles of air in the meconium.

At laparotomy, it may be necessary to resect part of the bowel and ileostomy is generally performed. Thereafter attempts are made to wash the abnormal meconium from the intestine with saline, to which liquefying agents may be added. The mortality from meconium ileus is high and most of the survivors will subsequently develop other manifestations of cystic fibrosis. It should be noted, however, that neonatal obstruction with meconium is not always due to cystic fibrosis, since sticky meconium may be found occasionally in otherwise normal infants, while a meconium plug may be an indication of Hirschprung's disease.

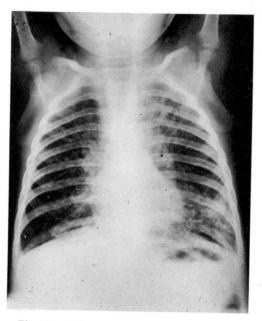

Fig. 14.7   Pulmonary changes in cystic fibrosis.

of involvement of the pancreas. Typically they are bulky, pale and greasy, indicating steatorrhoea, and have a characteristically offensive odour due to their content of partly digested protein. While the majority of children with cystic fibrosis show both respiratory and intestinal symptoms, some have pulmonary disease with no steatorrhoea while a few escape respiratory changes, perhaps for years, and show the distended abdomen and abnormal stools of malabsorption.

In severe cystic fibrosis, the combination of respiratory and pancreatic disease leads to gross failure to thrive. Cirrhosis of the liver and prolapse of the rectum may occur as complications. Such children are likely to die in infancy or early childhood. In other cases, however, symptoms may be quite mild for long periods or may be controlled so well by treatment that adolescence or adult life is reached before disability becomes serious.

DIAGNOSIS. Any newborn infant with intestinal obstruction and any infant or child who fails to thrive or has recurrent respiratory infections or abnormal stools should be suspected of having cystic fibrosis. Suspicion should also be aroused if siblings are reported to have died from any of these disorders, or from gastroenteritis or congenital heart disease.

The diagnosis is confirmed by demonstrating raised levels of chloride and sodium (over 60 mEq/l) in sweat obtained from a small area of skin by iontophoresis of pilocarpine and collected on weighed filter paper for analysis. The fat excretion test (see p. 163) is usually abnormal but the xylose excretion test is normal, since the intestinal mucosa is not affected. In nearly all cases, trypsin is absent from pancreatic juice collected by duodenal intubation.

TREATMENT. As in all chronic handicapping diseases, the child with cystic fibrosis must be helped to live as normal a life as his condition permits. Nutrition should be maintained by ensuring a full diet with ample protein and added vitamins. Pancreatin is given before each meal to replace absent enzymes and a liberal intake of salt should be encouraged, especially in hot weather when sweating may cause excessive loss of electrolyte. The respiratory passages must be kept as clear as possible by regular breathing exercises and postural drainage. Antibiotics are given freely in acute respiratory infections, while intermittent or continuous antibiotic prophylaxis

will be required as the disease becomes established. Bacteriological control of therapy is essential because the staphylococcus so quickly becomes resistant to antibiotics. As symptoms increase, inhalation of nebulized water vapour or mists containing bronchodilator drugs, liquefying agents or other substances, may give relief. In advanced pulmonary disease oxygen and digitalis will be necessary.

THE PLEURA

The pleura will be involved to some extent in any inflammatory, tuberculous, or neoplastic disease of the underlying lung. Thickening of the pleura adjacent to one or more of the interlobar septa will often render these visible radiologically; since such pleural thickening may persist for many years, the appearance does not necessarily indicate active disease. In the great majority of cases of pneumonia there will be some plastic exudate over the surface of the visceral pleura during the early stages of the disease, giving rise to pain; a purulent exudate (empyema) is more likely to occur some little time after the onset of pneumonia. Occasionally there is a sterile pleural effusion in cases of pneumonia which have received inadequate treatment, or in the course of acute rheumatism.

Most non-purulent pleural effusions seen in childhood, however, are of tuberculous origin, and this etiology should be assumed until tuberculosis has been excluded. Neoplastic disease involving the lung or pleura is a rare cause of effusion in childhood, and such effusions are likely to be blood-stained and may contain malignant cells.

While most empyemata and effusions arise in the pleural cavity, localized collections of pus or fluid may be situated between the interlobar septa or over the diaphragm. Lateral views of the chest are essential in these cases for accurate diagnosis.

Blood in the pleural cavity (*haemothorax*) is only likely to appear as the result of trauma; malignant disease and tuberculosis are very rare causes in childhood. *Chylothorax* (the presence of chylous fluid in the pleural cavity) is extremely rare in childhood, and occurs from rupture of the thoracic duct into the pleural cavity.

Pleural *transudates* occur in children with generalized oedema due to renal or cardiac disease. Aspiration to relieve respiratory embar-

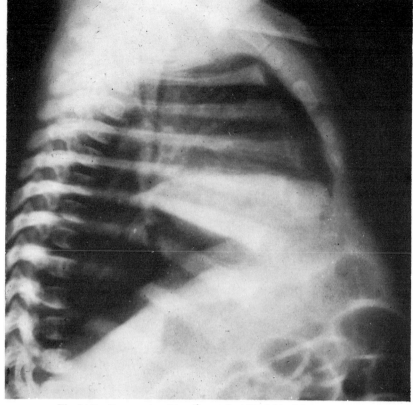

Fig. 14.8   Pneumonia with collapse of middle lobe of right lung.

rassment is only of transitory value, treatment being that of the primary disease.

Pneumothorax

Air may be introduced into the pleural cavity accidentally during thoracocentesis, or as the result of penetrating wounds of the chest wall. Spontaneous pneumothorax is of much less common occurrence in childhood than in adult life, and tuberculosis is rarely responsible. Rupture of a cyst or emphysematous bulla is a possible cause and may occur during a paroxysm of pertussis or asthma. The majority of cases are the result of staphylococcal pneumonia or lung abscess, the rupture of an abscess through the pleura introducing air or more commonly air and pus into the pleural cavity (*pyopneumothorax*). Influenzal pneumonia is also sometimes complicated by the rupture of alveoli resulting in tracking of air into the mediastinum (mediastinal emphysema) followed by more extensive surgical emphysema or pneumothorax. *Pressure pneumo-*

thorax occurs when a valve-like opening into the pleural cavity results in the progressive filling of the cavity with air during respiration.

Spontaneous pneumothorax (Fig. 14.9) causing collapse of the whole lung is characterized by sudden onset of dyspnoea and cyanosis. On examination, the affected side is immobile and hyperresonant, with absence of breath sounds. The heart and mediastinum are displaced to the opposite side. Small localized pneumothoraces may only be discovered on radiological examination. If the symptoms are progressive, as in a pressure pneumothorax, a measured volume of air should be slowly removed to relieve pressure and closed drainage instituted. Unless there is severe respiratory embarrassment, however, pneumothorax should in general be treated conservatively. The treatment of pyopneumothorax is that of empyema.

Empyema

Pus in the pleural cavity, or less commonly

between interlobar septa, is usually secondary to pneumonia. The incidence and mortality of pneumococcal empyema have been greatly reduced since the introduction of antibiotic therapy, and the mortality from staphylococcal empyema in young infants, which was previously extremely high, has shown an impressive reduction, although it must still be considered a condition of grave prognosis. Streptococcal empyema is also more frequently seen in infants than in older children, and though the prognosis is less good than in pneumococcal empyema it has been greatly improved by appropriate therapy.

CLINICAL FEATURES. Pneumococcal empyema should be suspected whenever there is a recrudescence of fever with dyspnoea or chest pain following a pneumonia which has incompletely resolved. The signs of pleural exudate are often preceded by a pleural rub which disappears when the pleural surfaces are separated by the purulent effusion. There are then typically diminished movement, dullness, and diminished breath sounds over the site of the empyema, though these signs may be altered by the thin chest wall in infancy.

In staphylococcal empyema the clinical features are similar, but there is a greater likelihood of associated pneumothorax.

DIAGNOSIS. Aspiration of the pleural cavity should be carried out as soon as an empyema is suspected, and in the case of encysted effusions may occasionally have to be done under fluoroscopy. As a general rule, the needle should be inserted over the lower portion of the area of maximum dullness. Failure to obtain pus is often due to aspirating at some arbitrary point rather than over the major accumulation of pus, or to using too small a needle. In early cases the effusion will be sero-purulent, but whereas

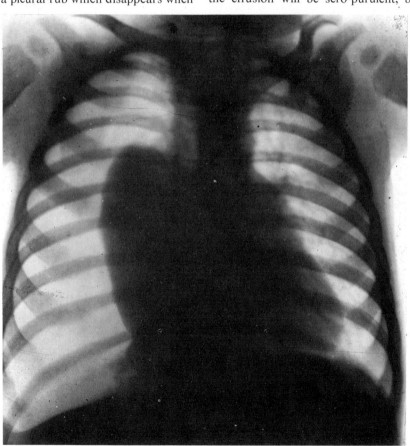

Fig. 14.9   Spontaneous pneumothorax with complete collapse of right lung. Note absence of lung markings in right side of thorax.

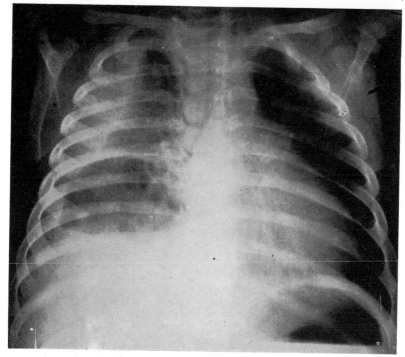

Fig. 14.10   Empyema on right, secondary to staphylococcal pneumonia.

pneumococcal effusions tend to become thicker and walled off, staphylococcal and streptococcal effusions often remain thin and watery. It is most important that the infecting organism should be determined as soon as possible and its sensitivity to therapeutic agents tested.

TREATMENT. The appropriate antibiotic should be given systemically, and good results have been obtained by the injection of penicillin or other antibiotic into the pleural cavity, with or without proteolytic enzymes. Repeated aspirations and antibiotic therapy may make surgical drainage unnecessary, but it is generally advisable to institute continuous closed drainage of the pleura as early as possible, the aim being to re-expand the lung as drainage of pus is effected. In all cases, expansion of the lung should be aided by physiotherapy and breathing exercises during convalescence.

Epidemic pleurodynia (*Epidemic myalgia; Bornholm disease*)

Epidemics of severe pain referred to the chest or upper abdomen have been described amongst school children, in whom the onset is usually characterized by associated pyrexia and vomiting. The pain is lancinating and most severe on respiration. When referred to the abdomen, the pain is superficial, suggesting muscular involvement. A small proportion of cases develop aseptic meningitis. A pleural rub may be heard in some cases, but there is no effusion. The disease runs a short benign course with complete recovery. Various strains of group B Coxsackie viruses have been isolated in different epidemics, and virological confirmation of the diagnosis should be made if possible. Treatment is symptomatic, and consists of rest, strapping of the chest, and administration of analgesics.

BIBLIOGRAPHY AND REFERENCES

ANDREWES, C. H. (1966). Rhinoviruses and common colds. *Annual Review of Medicine*, **17**, 361.

APLEY, J. (1953). The infant with stridor. *Archives of Disease in Childhood*, **28**, 423.

BEALE, A. J., MCLEOD, A. J., STACKIW, W. & RHODES, A. J. (1958). Isolation of cytopathogenic agents from the respiratory tract in acute laryngotracheobronchitis. *British Medical Journal*, i, 302.

BIRRELL, J. F. (1952). Chronic maxillary sinusitis in children. *Archives of Disease in Childhood*, **27**, 1.

CLARK, N. S. (1964). Mechanism and management of childhood bronchiectasis. *Biochemical Clinics*, **4**, 113.

CLYDE, W. A. & DENNY, F. W. (1967). Mycoplasma infections in childhood. *Pediatrics, Springfield*, **40**, 669.

CROOKS, J. (1954). Non-inflammatory laryngeal stridor in infants. *Archives of Disease in Childhood*, **29**, 12.

COURT, S. D. M. (1968). Epidemiology and natural history of respiratory infections in children. *Journal of Clinical Pathology*, **21**, suppl. 2, 30.

DAVIS, C. M. (1966). Inhaled foreign bodies in children. *Archives of Disease in Childhood*, **41**, 402.

DI SANT'AGNESE, P. A. & TALAMO, R. C. (1967). Pathogenesis and physiopathology of cystic fibrosis of the pancreas. *New England Journal of Medicine*, **277**, 1287, 1344, 1399.

EMERY, J. L. (1953). Pulmonary thrombosis. *Archives of Disease in Childhood*, **28**, 187.

EWING, I. R. & EWING, A. W. G. (1944). The ascertainment of deafness in infancy and early childhood. *Journal of Laryngology and Otology*, **59**.

FIELD, C. E. (1949). Bronchiectasis in childhood. *Pediatrics, Springfield*, **4**, 21, 231, 355.

GARDNER, P. S. (1968). Virus infections and respiratory disease of childhood. *Archives of Disease in Childhood*, **43**, 629.

GARDNER, P. S., ELDERKIN, F. M. & WALL, A. H. (1964). Serological study of respiratory syncytial virus infections in infancy and childhood. *British Medical Journal*, ii, 1570.

GLOVER, J. A. (1948). The paediatric approach to tonsillectomy. *Archives of Disease in Childhood*, **23**, 1.

GRIFFITHS, M. I. (1953). Pulmonary atelectasis in young children. *Archives of Disease in Childhood*, **28**, 170.

HEINER, D. C., SEARS, J. W. & KNIKER, W. T. (1962). Multiple precipitins to cow's milk in chronic respiratory disease. *American Journal of Diseases of Children*, **103**, 634.

HOLZEL, A. *et al.* (1965). Virus isolations from throats of children admitted to hospital with respiratory and other diseases. *British Medical Journal*, i, 614.

JONES, R. S. (1972). The management of acute croup. *Archives of Disease in Childhood*, **47**, 661.

JONES, R. S., OWEN-THOMAS, J. B. & BOUTON, M. J. (1968). Severe bronchopneumonia in the young child. *Archives of Disease in Childhood*, **43**, 415.

LAWSON, D. (1972). Cystic fibrosis—assessing the effects of treatment. *Archives of Disease in Childhood*, **47**, 1.

MACARTNEY, F. J., PANDAY, J. & SCOTT, O. (1969). Cor pulmonale as a result of chronic nasopharyngeal obstruction. *Archives of Disease in Childhood*, **44**, 585.

PEACH, A. M. & ZAIMAN, E. (1959). Acute laryngo-tracheo-bronchitis. *British Medical Journal*, i, 416.

PRYLES, C. V. (1958). Staphylococcal pneumonia in infancy and childhood. *Pediatrics, Springfield*, **21**, 609.

REPETTO, G. *et al.* (1967). Idiopathic pulmonary haemosiderosis. *Pediatrics, Springfield*, **40**, 24.

RUSSELL, G. (1971). Childhood croup. *Practitioner*, **206**, 781.

SIMPSON, H. & FLENLEY, D. C. (1967). Arterial blood gas tensions and pH in acute lower respiratory tract infection in infancy and childhood. *Lancet*, i, 7.

WARIN, J. F., DAVIES, J. B. M., SANDERS, F. K. & VIZOSO, A. D. (1953). Oxford epidemic of Bornholm disease. *British Medical Journal*, i, 1345.

WHETNALL, E. & FRY, D. B. (1964). *The Deaf Child*. London: Heinemann.

15 Communicable Diseases and Other Infections

(See also common cold, p. 292; congenital syphilis, p. 35; epidemic pleurodynia, p. 315; infantile diarrhoea, p. 169; infectious hepatitis, p. 167; pneumonia, p. 304; neonatal conjunctivitis, p. 56; thrush, p. 55; vulvovaginitis, p. 283)

'Communicable' or 'infectious' diseases are those which are due to living organisms and are transmissible from man to man or from animal to man. The distinction from other infections is somewhat arbitrary, since the same organisms may give rise to different manifestations of disease, the infection being readily transmissible in one instance and not in another. The age group at risk will also influence infectivity, e.g. *Staphylococcus aureus* being particularly liable to spread among infants in a newborn nursery.

NOTIFICATION

In order to control the spread of infectious diseases in the community, there is a statutory obligation in England and Wales to notify the Health Authority when any one of the following conditions is diagnosed:

Anterior poliomyelitis and polioencephalitis (acute)
Anthrax
Cerebrospinal fever
Cholera
Diphtheria and 'membranous croup'
Dysentery (amoebic or bacillary)
Encephalitis
Enteric (typhoid or paratyphoid) fevers
Erysipelas
Malaria
Measles
Ophthalmia neonatorum
Pertussis
Plague
Pneumonia (acute influenzal and acute primary)
Puerperal pyrexia
Relapsing fever
Scarlet fever
Smallpox
Tuberculosis (all forms)
Typhus fever.

In some localities rubella and epidemic jaundice are also notifiable; in Scotland, 'continued fever' is notifiable, but measles is not. Chicken-pox is made notifiable in the presence of an outbreak of smallpox. Many Local Authorities make it obligatory for head teachers to notify the Health Authority of all cases of infectious disease occurring among schoolchildren.

TRANSMISSION

Infection may occur by *inhalation* through the respiratory tract, by *ingestion* into the alimentary tract, or, in the case of certain diseases, through the skin or mucous membrane by *inoculation*. In most of the communicable diseases, infection enters predominantly or exclusively by one route, e.g. typhoid and the enteroviruses by the alimentary tract; malaria by inoculation; pertussis, influenza, measles, etc., by inhalation. As in the case of tuberculosis, however, certain infections may enter by any one of the three routes. The principal means by which infection occurs are as follows:

Direct contact with a patient suffering from the disease, either in classical or minor form. This may involve droplet inhalation or contact with excretions or skin lesions.

By the medium of a carrier, i.e. an individual who harbours and can transmit the infection without himself suffering from the disease, or when convalescent from the disease. Carriers are a particular danger in the spread of typhoid fever, dysentery, poliomyelitis, diphtheria, and meningococcal infection.

By fomites, i.e. contaminated bedding, clothing, toys, etc.

Inhalation of contaminated dust particles.

Ingestion of contaminated food or water.

By insect vectors, the infection either being inoculated by the bite of an infected insect, e.g. typhus, malaria, or being conveyed to food on the legs of flies.

By auto-infection or inoculation, e.g. threadworm ova conveyed from the anal region to the mouth by the patient's hands.

CONTROL OF INFECTION

The decision as to whether a particular patient suffering from an infectious disease should be removed to a place of isolation for the safety of the community rests ultimately with the Health Authority and will usually depend on the danger and virulence of the infection, the facilities for isolation in the home, the risk of younger children being infected, the severity of the case, and the isolation accommodation available during an epidemic. Attendance at school, travelling by public conveyance, and visiting public places are prohibited during the isolation period of a notifiable disease.

Disinfection and disinfestation of fomites, and disinfection of rooms in which patients have been nursed, should be carried out according to the requirements of the Health Authority.

'INEVITABLE INFECTIONS'

Certain of the communicable diseases are so widespread, or assume epidemic proportions with such regularity, that comparatively few children escape them. These are sometimes known as the 'inevitable infections' and include measles (in an unvaccinated community), chickenpox, rubella and, until recently, pertussis. Mumps, though having a high incidence in middle childhood, is often delayed until adolescence or early adult life. Scarlet fever, while predominantly a disease of childhood, affects a considerably smaller proportion of the childhood population, and should be regarded as only one possible manifestation of haemolytic streptococcal infection.

All these infections give a more or less permanent immunity in the great majority of cases, and while second attacks can and do occur, they are exceptional. Since such congenital immunity as may be possessed by the newborn infant is transitory, the high incidence of these infections in childhood is explicable on the basis of exposure of a non-immune community, contact being particularly liable to occur when the child reaches school age.

ACTIVE IMMUNIZATION

Active immunization should normally be undertaken in Britain against diphtheria, tetanus, pertussis, poliomyelitis and measles (B.C.G. inoculation for protection against tuberculosis in newborn infants or tuberculin-negative schoolchildren is considered on p. 324). Vaccination against the enteric fevers (typhoid and paratyphoid) is highly desirable for those visiting southern Europe, while immunization against yellow fever, plague, cholera, typhus, etc., is only indicated in the case of children passing through or residing in tropical areas where these diseases are endemic. Immunization against rubella is recommended for older girls. Although immunization against both scarlet fever and mumps is possible, it is not in either case recommended as a routine. Immunization against the influenza virus also has not been widely practised in children, owing to the temporary character of the immunity conferred and the number of strains of virus involved. It may, however, be desirable in a closed community if an epidemic is anticipated. Vaccination against smallpox has been abandoned as a routine measure, although repeated vaccination throughout early life should still be the policy for those living in endemic areas of the world.

All the routine immunization procedures should if possible be carried out in infancy, in order to protect the individual during the most vulnerable period of life. In the case of diphtheria and tetanus immunization, the antigen employed is a modified toxin or toxoid, and in the case of pertussis, measles and poliomyelitis a vaccine. In each instance the antigen is designed to stimulate the maximum production of antibodies compatible with the antigen being innocuous.

Both *antidiphtheritic* and *antitetanus immunization* can be regarded as combining a very high degree of efficient protection with a minimum of risk. Apart from occasional tenderness at the site of injection and very rare general reactions (headache, vomiting, and malaise) which are transient, the only serious hazard has been that of 'provocation poliomyelitis' developing in the limb into which diphtheria antigen or pertussis vaccine, alone or in combination, had been injected. This risk has been minimized by the general use of poliomyelitis vaccination. Virtual elimination of diphtheria in the community is obtained when over 60 per cent of the pre-school and school population is effectively immunized. Antidiphtheritic immunization of older patients should be preceded by a *Schick test* to determine whether natural immunity has already developed.

Antipertussis immunization, using a vaccine of killed organisms, gives a reasonable measure of protection, and in immunized patients who develop whooping cough an attack is likely to be modified. Cerebral degeneration following pertussis immunization very occasionally occurs, and immunization should not be performed in an infant who has had convulsions, or continued when a convulsion is provoked by the first injection. In view of the high mortality and morbidity for which whooping cough was previously responsible, however, immunization is fully justified.

Poliomyelitis vaccination, after a somewhat disastrous début, when the vaccine produced by one laboratory was found to contain living virus capable of inducing the disease, has proved safe and many millions of injections have been given. The Salk vaccine, which was at first most widely used in Britain, consists of inactivated virus given by injection. Recently, however, increasing use has been made of trivalent oral vaccines prepared from Sabin's living attenuated strains of virus. In very young infants the presence of maternal antibodies will have an inhibitory effect on antibody response, but from 3 months of age Sabin poliovaccine gives effective immunity against all three types of virus. It is given by mouth in three doses at 4 to 8 week intervals, and a further dose should be given during the second year or at school entry.

Measles vaccination is now recommended for all children who have not been protected by a previous attack of the disease. Live attenuated measles virus vaccine is used, one injection being given at the beginning of the second year. A mild febrile reaction may occur and children who have had convulsions, are receiving corticosteroids or are allergic to egg should not be vaccinated.

Rubella vaccination should be offered to all girls between 11 and 14 years of age, the object being to establish immunity before they reach child-bearing age rather than to eradicate the disease from the community. A single injection of live attenuated virus vaccine is given.

Vaccinia and vaccination

Jenner in 1798 showed that infective material from the lesions of vaccinia or cowpox, a disease of cattle, could be utilized for the protection of humans against smallpox. This protective inoculation proved so successful in reducing the incidence and mortality of smallpox that infantile *vaccination* with suitably prepared calf lymph was made obligatory, though allowance was made for conscientious objection. Compulsory vaccination of infants was abandoned in 1948, since less than 37 per cent of infants had in fact been vaccinated in the decade 1936–46. Although the proportion increased subsequently in some areas of the country, it fell as low as 10 per cent in others, and recent smallpox epidemics have emphasized that the general population is very inadequately protected. However, in view of the diminishing incidence of smallpox throughout the world, this is no longer considered to be a

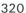

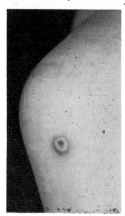

Fig. 15.1   Primary vaccination on eighth day; multiple-pressure method.

matter for concern, and in 1971 routine vaccination was abandoned in Britain as a national policy.

If it is to be carried out, primary vaccination should be effected between 1 and 5 years, preferably during the second year. The skin in the lower deltoid area is cleansed and dried, after which the lymph is expressed on to it (the thigh, which is sometimes selected as the site of inoculation in female infants, is less satisfactory, owing to the risk of faecal contamination). Scarification through the lymph is made as a single linear scratch 3 to 6 mm in length, care being taken not to draw blood. The alternative multiple-pressure method consists of pressure with the point of a needle held tangentially, made 10 to 20 times over an area 2 mm in diameter, after which the lymph is allowed to dry.

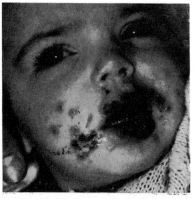

Fig. 15.2   Vaccinia occurring seven days after primary vaccination in an infant aged 11 months; umbilicated lesions on cheeks, lips, tongue, and palate.

Successful primary vaccination is indicated by the formation of a papule at the site of inoculation, appearing on the third or fourth day, becoming vesicular on the fifth, and pustular on the eighth to tenth day. There is often considerable local reaction during the stage of vesiculation, sometimes accompanied by general malaise and enlargement of the axillary lymph nodes. The local reaction subsides gradually, and the pustules form crusts which separate, leaving an area of scarring which is permanently recognizable. Contraindications to vaccination are infantile eczema, skin sepsis, corticosteroid therapy and hypogammaglobulinaemia. Vaccination must not be carried out during pregnancy, since the fetus may die of vaccinia.

Since the immunity afforded by vaccination gradually diminishes, revaccination is advisable every seven years or more frequently if smallpox is prevalent in the community. The response to revaccination is often accelerated and represents a modified reaction with little constitutional disturbance. Vesiculation should, however, occur for the reaction to be regarded as a satisfactory 'take'.

COMPLICATIONS. If primary vaccination is properly carried out during the second year, the risk of complications is small.

Generalized vaccinia may result from auto-inoculation by scratching, or as the result of implantation from the blood. The primary vaccination papule may show some delay in appearance, but the course of the primary lesion is otherwise normal. Secondary papules followed by vesiculation, pustulation, and scarring appear over the body while the primary lesion is still active. The prognosis is generally good, though deaths have occurred in young infants.

Localized auto-inoculation from a vaccination lesion may produce a secondary lesion at any site. The reaction is accelerated, and healing follows the normal course.

Post-vaccinal encephalomyelitis. The clinical manifestations are closely similar to those of encephalomyelitis following specific fevers (p. 361). The condition is rare at all ages, but the risk is greatest when primary vaccination is carried out at school age, as may be necessary during a smallpox epidemic when infantile vaccination has not been practised.

The immediate mortality may be as high as 30 to 40 per cent, milder cases usually making complete recovery,

Immunization regimen

The object of the regimen selected is to obtain the maximum immunity compatible with a limited number of injections and medical visits. For this purpose diphtheria, tetanus, and pertussis antigens are combined in a 'triple vaccine' and the recent tendency has been to give oral poliomyelitis (attenuated) vaccine at the same time.

Officially recommended schedules have been modified in the light of experience and practice varies from area to area. One regimen which represents a reasonable compromise between what is desirable and what is acceptable is as follows:

Age	Vaccine
4 to 6 months	Diphtheria/tetanus/pertussis+oral polio-vaccine given at the same time on each of three visits at not less than four weeks interval
12 months	Measles vaccination (live attenuated vaccine)
15 to 18 months	Smallpox vaccination (if desired)
School entry	Diphtheria/tetanus+oral polio vaccine
8 to 12 years	Smallpox revaccination Possibly measles revaccination (uncertain)
Over 12 years	B.C.G. (for tuberculin-negative children) Rubella vaccination (girls)

PASSIVE IMMUNITY

The value of providing passive, transient immunity against infections to which children have been exposed depends largely on the risks involved if the disease is contracted. There is little purpose in attempting to protect children against chickenpox, rubella, and mumps, since complications are unlikely to occur. In the case of measles it may be advisable to protect younger infants and severely ill children, e.g. when a case occurs in hospital. The most effective method is by the use of gamma-globulin, in a dosage of 2 ml intramuscularly. Gamma-globulin has almost entirely replaced the use of convalescent serum, owing to the risk of post-inoculation hepatitis when the latter is employed.

Antitoxic sera are used mainly in prevention or treatment of diphtheria and tetanus. Adrenaline should be at hand and a test dose of serum given first in case of reaction (p. 263).

Tetanus antitoxin in dosages of 1500 to 20,000 units should be given in all cases where there is risk of infection of a wound unless the patient has already been immunized, in which case an injection of 0·5 ml toxoid should be made.

Exposure to smallpox should call for immediate vaccination, which is likely to prevent the disease if effected within seven days and modify the attack if carried out between the seventh and tenth day following exposure. Since active immunity is so rapidly developed, passive immunization is not indicated.

TUBERCULOSIS

Tuberculosis is still 'the most important specific communicable disease in the world' (W.H.O., 1964), and the progress that has been made toward its eradication in particular countries must be seen in perspective against this global background. It is liable to be exacerbated at any time by war, economic depression or other factors lowering the general standard of living. While the last two decades have witnessed a striking reduction in tuberculous mortality and morbidity in Britain (to which improved social conditions, antituberculosis measures, including provision of safe milk, and specific chemotherapy have all contributed), it should be remembered that there has been a general downward trend in the tuberculosis death rate in Britain since 1870, which began before Koch's discovery of the tubercle bacillus and preceded any organized attempts to combat the disease. The war of 1939–45 caused a sharp rise in the death rate, but this fell rapidly in the post-war years to reach the expected point on the downward trend.

Before chemotherapy became available, the death rates of the youngest age groups were much higher than the general death rate for 'non-respiratory' forms of the disease, including abdominal tuberculosis, tuberculous meningitis, and miliary tuberculosis. The remarkable fall in the total deaths from all forms of tuberculosis in infancy and childhood which has occurred during the past 20 years in England and Wales is shown in Table 15.1. The great reduction in mortality, however, should not obscure the facts that the risk of dissemination is greatest in the youngest age groups, that the disease has not been eradicated in the indigenous population, and that fresh sources of infection are liable to be introduced by immigration.

INCIDENCE

For purposes of comparison between different years, neither the death rate nor the number of notifications provides a wholly satisfactory indication of incidence. Thus the introduction of mass radiography in schools will bring to light a number of unsuspected infections which will be notified without a corresponding rise in the death rate or any true increase in incidence. On the other hand, the introduction of new forms of therapy has radically altered the prognosis in previously fatal types of the disease and has lowered the death rate disproportionately.

Table 15.1   Deaths from tuberculosis (all forms) in infancy and childhood. England and Wales 1949–69

| Year | Age (years) | | |
	0 to 1	1 to 4	5 to 14
1949	163	602	383
1959	15	36	21
1969	3	9	3

Tuberculosis varies from a fulminating disease to a symptomless infection, and the number of children in the community who have successfully overcome their infection is substantially greater than the number who show evidence of active disease. In some children, however, tuberculous infection is responsible for a variable period of general ill-health and failure to thrive, with the risk of breakdown and dissemination before the primary lesion is fully healed. Many of these are treated for minor symptoms without the underlying cause ever being recognized, while a few develop the more serious clinical manifestations described below. The prevalence of tuberculous infection, whether active or healed, in childhood communities can be determined by tuberculin testing, except where widespread B.C.G. inoculation in infancy has been adopted.

TUBERCULIN TESTING

Infection with mycobacteria, including *M. tuberculosis*, produces a state of altered skin reactivity, which usually develops within six weeks of infection and persists permanently, though differing in degree in different individuals and in different stages of the disease. This is utilized as the basis of skin testing with old tuberculin (O.T.) or purified protein derivative (P.P.D.), a positive reaction demonstrating that the child has at some previous time been infected and has developed a specific sensitivity.

Mantoux test. This consists of the injection of 0·1 ml of a known dilution of old tuberculin

intradermally, usually using 1 in 1000 dilution, or 1 in 10,000 if a strong reaction is expected. Alternatively, P.P.D., 5 tuberculin units (T.U.) in 0·1 ml may be employed. The injection must be carried out with a fine intradermal needle, using a special syringe from which 0·1 ml can be accurately delivered. The test is read at the end of 48 hours, by which time 'false positive' reactions will have faded. A positive reaction (Fig. 15.3) is shown by erythema surrounding the site of injection, and an area of induration 5 mm or more in diameter. The double Mantoux test, consisting of simultaneous skin testing with tuberculin and with antigen to one of the atypical mycobacteria, is a reliable means of differentiating tuberculosis from other mycobacterial infection, especially when coupled with the history relating to duration of signs and possibility of contact.

Heaf test. This is a multiple-puncture test, using an automatic punch releasing six needles which puncture the skin evenly to a depth of 1 or 2 mm as desired. The test is read in three to seven days; positive reactions vary from a ring of indurated puncture scars to a large area of induration with blister formation and are graded I to IV. The test is less painful and time-consuming than the Mantoux test, and is particularly suitable for screening large numbers of children. It is not sufficiently precise, however, for accurate discrimination between those who have been infected with tuberculosis and those who have not, since a grade I or II reaction may signify infection with mycobacteria other than mammalian tubercle bacilli. Though the proportion of non-specific grade II reactions is relatively low in Britain, it is high in some other countries, e.g. Nigeria.

INTERPRETATION. A positive tuberculin test usually means that the child has at some time had a tuberculous lesion, however small, and has developed skin sensitivity. Since a positive reaction will normally be given by a patient who has received B.C.G. vaccination (see below), it is essential to know whether this procedure has been carried out. If the Mantoux reaction is positive but the reaction to 5 T.U. of P.P.D. is less than 12 mm of induration, the possibility of avian or other atypical mycobacterial infection should be considered and differential Mantoux testing carried out (Keay & Edmond, 1966). A negative reaction usually means either that the child has never had a tuberculous lesion, or that the latter is of such recent origin that skin sensitivity has not yet developed. Occasionally sensitivity may be lost in the terminal stages of disseminated tuberculosis or in the acute stage of infections such as measles.

The importance to be attached to a positive reaction in an unvaccinated child depends largely on his age and on the prevalence of the disease where he lives. In low-prevalence areas it is advisable to assume that a positive reaction at any age indicates active disease until this has been disproved. After the age of 5, increasing numbers of children in successive age groups show positive reactions without active disease being present. From the age of 5 onward, therefore, a negative reaction is of value in contra-indicating a diagnosis of tuberculosis but a positive reaction is of decreasing value in diagnosing active disease. Recent figures for England and Wales indicate that less than 10 per cent of children have become tuberculin-positive by about 13 years of age, though there is considerable regional variation.

SOURCE OF INFECTION

The great majority of cases of childhood tuberculosis are acquired by contact with an infected adult, and in the case of infants and pre-school children the nidus of infection is likely to be found in the home or immediate family circle. Intimacy of contact and frequency of exposure are of even more importance than over-crowding, the greatest risk being to an infant who is being cared for by an infected mother with positive sputum. Visits to a tuberculous relative, e.g. a grandmother, may prove lethal if the infant is handled, kissed, and coughed over, or allowed to play in a room containing particles of sputum.

Whereas overcrowding *per se* will not introduce tuberculosis into a tubercle-free family, once it is introduced, overcrowding, a low standard of living, and a number of children exposed will increase the likelihood of spread. Older children, whose social circle is expanding, are more likely to acquire infection outside the family, but the home still remains an important source of infection. It is frequently found that when the remainder of the family is investigated following the diagnosis of tuberculosis in a child, an unsuspected infection in a parent or older sibling will be discovered. Owing to the particular vulnerability of the younger age groups, it is most important that nurses, nursery helps, schoolteachers, and others having the care of young children should themselves be free from active disease.

Infection with bovine tuberculosis by the ingestion of infected milk has been almost eradicated by the production of tuberculin-tested milk, pasteurization, and the use of dried milk for infant feeding. It is now very rare to see clinical tuberculosis of bovine origin except occasionally in children receiving fresh milk direct from the farm. While effective pasteurization will kill tubercle bacilli in milk, it is a wise precaution to boil liquid milk not obtained from an attested herd or reputable dairy. There is still a slight risk of acquiring bovine tuberculosis from an adult whose lesion acquired many years previously has broken down.

PROPHYLAXIS

Since tuberculosis is still widespread in most underdeveloped areas of the world, and is constantly being reintroduced from these into low-

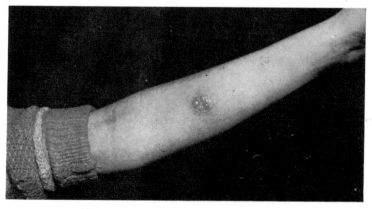

Fig. 15.3   Mantoux reaction: strongly positive.

prevalence areas, there is comparatively little likelihood of an individual avoiding all contact for the whole of his life span. Indeed, there is no doubt that many individuals develop some degree of immunity by repeated minimal exposure, but that this immune reaction may break down if the exposure becomes too heavy or if nutritional and environmental conditions are sufficiently adverse. In dealing with infants and young children, it must be remembered that their capacity for developing immunity is lower and they are liable to succumb to a degree of exposure which might prove innocuous to the adult.

The effect of the standard of living of the community on the tuberculous mortality has already been emphasized, but it must be realized that raised nutritional standards, improved working conditions, and better housing will not themselves prevent the spread of tuberculosis unless at the same time the sources of infection are identified and removed. Most cases of tuberculosis are found in ordinary clinical practice but other methods of case-finding are necessary, including examination of contacts, tuberculin testing of children and examination of immigrants. Mass radiography is still useful where prevalence is high, but in low-prevalence areas is being superseded by selective radiography of high-risk groups.

ARTIFICIAL IMMUNITY

This may be produced by vaccination with the bacillus of Calmette-Guérin, a strain of bovine tuberculosis which has become non-virulent on prolonged cultivation outside the body. Intradermal injection of 0·1 ml of the vaccine will give 80 per cent protection of tuberculin-negative schoolchildren. The method has been widely adopted in Britain where the great majority of tuberculin-negative children are vaccinated before leaving school. B.C.G. vaccination should also be given to tuberculin-negative contacts of new cases, and newborn infants should be vaccinated if there is a family history of tuberculosis. In the case of infants of tuberculous mothers, the infant must be separated from the parent if possible at the time of birth. Successful vaccination is indicated by the appearance of a nodule at the site of injection, usually ten days to four weeks after vaccination, and by the tuberculin test becoming positive shortly afterwards. It is most important that the infant or child should not be incubating tuberculosis at the time of vaccination, and also that he should be removed from any exposure until the tuberculin reaction has become positive. Formation of a pustule at the site of injection is not uncommon but abscesses of the axillary lymph nodes are very rare when freeze-dried vaccine is used.

SPECIFIC THERAPY

The principal antibiotic and chemotherapeutic agents available are the streptomycins, para-aminosalicylic acid (PAS) and isonicotinic acid hydrazide (isoniazid). Subsidiary antituberculous agents include pyrazinamide, prothionamide, rifampicin and ethambutol but their use is rarely necessary in children. Of the streptomycins, streptomycin sulphate and chloride are less toxic than dihydrostreptomycin, and are generally preferred. Isoniazid has the great advantage over other agents that it passes readily into the cerebrospinal fluid and is also active intracellularly.

The use of steroids in combination with adequate specific therapy has been advocated in tuberculous meningitis, lymphadenitis, and pleurisy but their value is unproven. In very severe illness, they may maintain life long enough for chemotherapy to be effective. The steroid most frequently used is prednisone in a dosage of 1 mg per kg daily for four to six weeks.

Resistance. The emergence of strains of tubercle bacilli resistant to specific therapy is not only a disaster for the patient but also a menace to those whom he is liable to infect. Resistance can largely be avoided by adequate therapy and suitable combination of agents. Streptomycin should never be used alone in the treatment of tuberculosis, but should be combined with PAS or isoniazid or both. Similarly, resistance to PAS alone develops readily. (If initial treatment includes all three drugs, the risk of an organism resistant to one of them escaping is reduced.) Resistance to isoniazid has proved a less serious risk than was previously expected, but combined therapy, e.g. with PAS, is generally advocated when oral therapy over a long period is necessary. The duration of adequate treatment, viz. a minimum of 18 months and of two years in all cases of pulmonary tuberculosis and tuberculous meningitis, makes it essential that the regular taking of oral drugs should be properly supervised. When supervision is difficult, as in developing countries, intensive treatment with streptomycin, isoniazid and pyrazinamide for six months is a possible alternative.

Toxicity. A small proportion of patients undergoing prolonged streptomycin treatment develop vestibular disturbances or eighth nerve deafness, particularly when the antibiotic is used intrathecally. Occasionally the drug causes vomiting, pyrexia or skin eruptions. PAS, though often well tolerated, may produce nausea, vomiting, or anorexia in younger children. Isoniazid appears to be the least toxic of the specific agents, but occasionally produces allergic symptoms, constipation, or peripheral neuropathy. Pyridoxine deficiency, a risk in older patients, is unlikely to occur in childhood.

Dosage. Streptomycin, when given by intramuscular injection, is used in a dosage of 40 mg per kg body weight daily up to a maximum of 1 g daily. (The dosage for intrathecal use, which is still controversial, is up to 100 mg daily for older children and 25 mg for infants.) PAS, which is given orally in four divided doses, has a wide safety margin, and a daily dosage of 200 mg per kg is probably optimal. Isoniazid is also given orally in two or four divided doses, the daily dosage being 10 to 20 mg per kg.

Indications. Chemotherapy has little effect on the lymph node enlargement of the *primary complex*, but it is indicated in all active primary infections in childhood on the grounds that the risk of haematogenous spread (see below) and therefore the incidence of post-primary infection is lessened. In the case of infants under two years of age, when the risk of dissemination is greatest, it is advisable to use streptomycin and isoniazid initially, followed by PAS and isoniazid for a minimum of 2 years. A similar course of intensive treatment may be adopted with older children who are acutely ill at the onset of the primary infection or in whom there is extensive lung involvement. In less severe but active primary infections, 18 to 24 months treatment with PAS and isoniazid (without streptomycin) is indicated. Unvaccinated older children who are found to have a positive tuberculin-test on routine examination, but who show no clinical or radiological evidence of active disease, should be kept under regular observation and treated promptly if there is subsequently any evidence of activity.

Miliary tuberculosis should also be treated initially with intramuscular streptomycin and isoniazid, in order to obtain the maximum bactericidal effect immediately. When the acute stage of the disease has passed, treatment should be continued with PAS and isoniazid for at least 2 years. Since the response to treatment will depend to a considerable extent on early diagnosis, the duration of streptomycin and isoniazid treatment must depend on the progress of the individual case.

Tuberculous meningitis still provides a somewhat controversial therapeutic problem. Excellent results are obtained by prolonged intrathecal streptomycin therapy, combined with intramuscular streptomycin and oral PAS and isoniazid, although this involves daily lumbar puncture for several weeks. Oral therapy with PAS and isoniazid is continued for at least one year, and preferably two. Many authorities have been reluctant to abandon a regimen of proved efficacy, but there is some evidence that equally good results can be obtained without intrathecal administration of streptomycin. A suitable course consists of intramuscular streptomycin 1 g daily for one month, or until the C.S.F. pressure is normal, followed by twice-weekly injections for six months; and oral isoniazid 20 mg per kg daily until the patient is clinically well, followed by 10 mg per kg daily for at least two years together with PAS daily. In the case of patients who are critically ill, some authorities use intrathecal isoniazid (10 mg in 3 ml normal saline) in addition for the first two weeks. Steroid therapy is referred to above (p. 324).

Bone and joint tuberculosis. Treatment with intramuscular streptomycin and PAS is now regarded as useful supportive therapy though it does not replace the classical orthopaedic methods, and the effects are seen mainly in the patient's general condition rather than in the speed of radiological healing.

CLASSIFICATION

The broad distinction into *respiratory* and *non-respiratory* forms of tuberculosis is often used for compiling health statistics and may be elaborated into one based on the tissues principally involved, e.g. osseous, meningeal, peritoneal, lymphatic, etc. Ranke's classification of tuberculosis into *primary*, *secondary*, and *tertiary* stages, depending on the degree of hypersensitivity and resistance, is attractive but not wholly acceptable. It is probably simplest to distinguish primary tuberculosis and its complications on the one hand from post-primary tuberculosis on the other, the latter term encompassing lesions caused by reactivation of quiescent primary tuberculosis and by fresh exogenous infection in sensitized individuals. For the present purpose, the clinical manifestations of tuberculosis will be considered in relation to the principal site of disease.

PORTAL OF ENTRY

With rare exceptions, tubercle bacilli enter the body through mucous membrane, the commonest portal being the respiratory tract. Much less frequently, the site of entry is the alimentary tract, the tonsil, the nasal mucosa, the middle ear, the vagina, or the skin. Placental transmission is occasionally responsible for congenital tuberculosis. In this instance, tubercle bacilli from a placental metastasis reach the fetal liver by way of the umbilical veins.

In addition to these natural routes, inoculation of tubercle bacilli is a real danger if therapeutic injections are made using faulty techniques and tuberculous abscesses have been observed at the site of penicillin injection.

INTRATHORACIC TUBERCULOSIS

Primary infection of the lung

This is of the greatest importance in infancy and childhood since the large majority of cases of tuberculosis, whether classified as respiratory or non-respiratory forms, do in fact originate from pulmonary infection. The primary stage covers the period of formation of the *primary complex*, consisting of the primary focus in the lung parenchyma, lymphatic transmission of infection from this focus to the mediastinal lymph nodes draining the affected area, and enlargement of these nodes. There is probably always a transient bacteraemia in the early stages. During a period

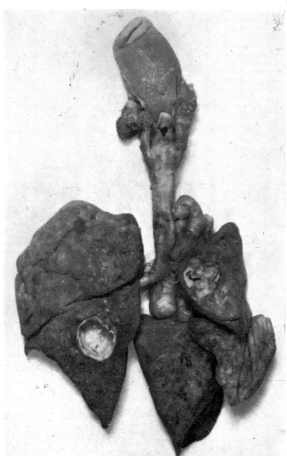

Fig. 15.4   Primary tuberculous foci showing cavitation, associated with caseating tracheobronchial lymph nodes, in a young infant.

of approximately six weeks following the primary infection, the child develops hypersensitivity, which is demonstrable clinically by the tuberculin reaction of the skin (see above).

The primary focus may be found in any part of the lung, but is generally subpleural and in the right upper lobe. The lesion develops from the inhalation of a particle of sputum or dried dust containing living tubercle bacilli which passes through the bronchi and bronchioles to lodge in an alveolus. This leads to the formation of a small area of tuberculous pneumonia surrounded by an area of infiltration. In cases of fatal tuberculosis the primary focus appears at necropsy as a central area of caseation approximately the size of a pea, surrounded by tuberculous granulation and a variable degree of fibrosis depending on the extent of healing which has occurred. In some cases satellite tubercles also surround the primary focus. In young infants the primary focus may liquefy, producing a ragged irregular cavity (Fig. 15.4). In patients who have successfully overcome the infection, the primary focus becomes densely calcified and encapsulated with fibrous tissue.

Tuberculous enlargement of mediastinal lymph nodes is almost invariably secondary to a primary lung infection, and careful search will seldom fail to reveal a primary focus within the appropriate area. In some cases a line of tubercles will mark the peribronchial and perivascular lymphatic channels by which the infection has been conveyed, and, in healed cases, calcification of the whole complex (primary focus, lymphatic channels, and mediastinal nodes) may be demonstrable radiologically.

Considerable enlargement of the affected lymph nodes occurs, and there is likely to be extensive caseation and giant-cell formation within the nodes directly draining the primary focus. Healing is characterized by calcification and fibrosis, but even when clinical recovery from the primary infection occurs, living tubercle bacilli may remain within the affected nodes for long periods, and the disease be reactivated by intercurrent infection.

The primary focus is commonly surrounded by an area of *infiltration* which may be partly allergic and exudative in nature, or may represent true tuberculous involvement. These lesions should be distinguished radiologically from localized pleurisy and areas of pulmonary collapse.

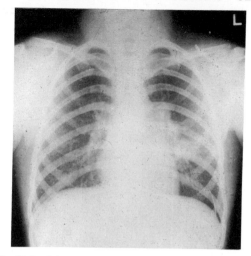

Fig. 15.5   Primary tuberculous complex showing enlarged hilar lymph nodes.

CLINICAL PICTURE. This varies from such slight disturbance of general health that the condition passes unrecognized, to one characterized by fever, abdominal pain, lassitude, cough, anorexia, loss of weight, and pallor, though it is rather exceptional for symptoms to point clearly to the lungs as the site of the disease, and cough is often minimal in infants. The incubation period of 4 to 8 weeks following the primary infection is silent, the febrile reaction when it occurs appearing at the time that hypersensitivity is established and the tuberculin reaction has become positive.

Physical examination frequently fails to reveal evidence of pulmonary disease at this stage; indeed, if there is unequivocal evidence of localized dullness or impaired air entry, it is probable that this is due to a complication, e.g. pulmonary collapse, or that the condition is not tuberculous. It must be recognized that physical examination of the chest alone is a quite unreliable basis for early diagnosis, and that such signs as may occur with heavy primary infiltration are not pathognomonic; this being so, primary tuberculosis should be suspected in cases presenting with the rather vague symptoms of fatigue and general ill-health when no adequate cause for them is found.

Erythema nodosum. Although this is neither diagnostic of tuberculosis nor confined to the primary stage, it is a sufficiently frequent manifestation of the allergic state developing with the

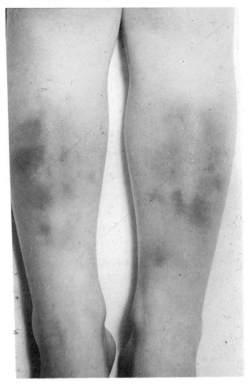

Fig. 15.6   Erythema nodosum.

formation of the primary complex to be considered in the clinical picture of the disease. The lesions appear rapidly over the shins (Fig. 15.6), being much less frequently seen on the thighs or arms. They consist of raised indurated areas from 1 to 3 cm in diameter, at first erythematous and subsequently fading until they have the appearance of old bruises. There may be localized pain and tenderness, and a transient febrile reaction. They tend to disappear over a period of a week or more, but may recur.

Every child with erythema nodosum should be suspected of suffering from tuberculosis until the diagnosis has been disproved. In high-prevalence countries, up to 80 per cent of cases of erythema nodosum are in fact tuberculous although the proportion is now much lower in Britain. An exactly similar lesion may result from sensitivity to streptococcal infection or to drugs, especially sulphonamides.

DIAGNOSIS. When a history of exposure, the clinical picture described above or the occurrence of erythema nodosum suggests the presence of a primary infection of the lung, it is essential to carry out further investigations.

Tuberculin testing and X-ray of the chest should be employed as a routine, and other investigations include estimation of the erythrocyte sedimentation rate, which will be raised in the presence of active disease, and examination of the sputum or stomach washings for tubercle bacilli (see below).

It is most unlikely that an uncalcified primary focus will be clearly recognizable on X-ray, though a heavy primary infiltration may appear as a diffuse shadow around it. More commonly, the enlarged hilar lymph nodes produce an X-ray shadow which is suggestive of tuberculosis, although it must be remembered that some degree of hilar node enlargement occurs in other conditions, e.g. pneumonia or leukaemia. The appearance of the hilum must be interpreted in relation to the child's age. Thus in infants the 'normal' hilum is barely visible, whereas in older children the hilar shadow becomes larger and denser with increasing age (Fig. 15.5).

Examination of sputum and stomach washings. It is exceptional for children to produce sputum voluntarily, and the most satisfactory method is to obtain such sputum as has been swallowed during the night by gastric lavage. The stomach is washed out with sterile water in the early morning before food has been taken, and the washings are centrifuged. The deposit is examined directly for tubercle bacilli and also inoculated into a guinea-pig or cultured: the nature of acid-fast bacilli found on direct examination should always be confirmed. It may be necessary to repeat gastric lavage three or more times.

The demonstration of tubercle bacilli will clinch the diagnosis, but the absence of tubercle bacilli will not contra-indicate it. Many children apparently pass through the stage of primary infection without producing tubercle bacilli in the sputum, but the percentage in which organisms are found depends to some extent on the number of examinations made in each case.

COURSE. In the great majority of children acquiring their infection after the age of 5 years, the primary complex heals by calcification and fibrosis. This process of healing may occur rapidly or be delayed over a period of many months, during which time the child can never be considered out of danger of an exacerbation or dissemination of the disease. In cases where the progress of the disease is not arrested at the primary stage, the primary focus may undergo progressive caseation, with a likelihood of haematogenous spread or aspiration pneumonia in untreated cases. Similarly, progressive caseation of the mediastinal nodes may result in one of the following sequelae:

1. Transmission of tubercle bacilli to the bloodstream by way of the thoracic duct, with dissemination.
2. Erosion of a blood vessel, and direct passage of tubercle bacilli into the blood-stream, with dissemination.
3. Generalized mediastinal involvement (tuberculous mediastinitis). This is likely to cause brassy cough, stridor, or wheezing dyspnoea, particularly in infancy.
4. Erosion of a bronchus, with aspiration of caseous material throughout the lungs (tuberculous bronchopneumonia of aspiration type).
5. Localized extension from the hilum of the lung of a caseous pneumonic process.
6. Pressure on bronchial walls, or infiltration and erosion of a bronchus, causing blockage of the lumen and collapse of lung.

TREATMENT of the primary infection will aim at arresting the progress of the disease at the earliest possible stage, and its success will largely depend on early diagnosis. The child must be removed from the risk of further infection at least until healing is established. Bed rest is indicated initially until the E.S.R. has returned to normal, the child is gaining weight satisfactorily, and radiological examination shows that the lesion is not progressing. As the febrile reaction is seldom of long duration, the temperature is a less valuable index of progress than are the weight-gain and E.S.R. A liberal diet with vitamin D supplements is required.

For all children with primary tuberculosis, whether symptomatic or not, a period of 18 to 24 months treatment and supervision will be indicated. The role of chemotherapy is considered above. Bed rest is not necessary in the case of older children who show no evidence of activity or parenchymal involvement. Every case must be considered individually in deciding the routine to be followed, and if there is any doubt as to healing of the primary complex it is advisable to err on the side of caution.

Pleurisy

The type of pleurisy most commonly observed in childhood is the *exudative* or *pleural effusion*, which is usually related more or less closely to the primary stage of tuberculosis. (Caseous pleurisy, i.e. tuberculous empyema, either of haematogenous origin or due to rupture of a caseous focus through the pleura, is rare.) Exudative pleurisy occurs when the primary focus, or less commonly a secondary focus, lies in the immediate vicinity of the pleura. The condition occurs most commonly in later childhood and adolescence.

CLINICAL FEATURES. The onset is often sudden, and accompanied by high fever, acute pain in the chest, and dyspnoea. Careful enquiry, however, will usually reveal that the acute symptoms have been preceded by a period of general ill-health. Although it is not always possible to determine accurately the time interval between the primary infection and the occurrence of pleurisy, symptoms of the primary stage may have been noted three months to a year before the manifestations of pleural effusion.

The physical signs will depend on the size and localization of the effusion. A pleural rub, which disappears with the appearance of the effusion, may be heard at onset. When a massive effusion fills one pleural cavity, there will be displacement of the heart and mediastinum toward the opposite side, since the mediastinum is more mobile in childhood than in later life. There is diminished movement and air-entry on the affected side, and stony dullness over the site of effusion. (Owing to thinness of the chest-wall and the smaller amount of fluid in the thorax, however, an effusion is sometimes mistaken for pneumonic consolidation in young children.)

When the effusion is *interlobar* in position, the physical signs are less clear-cut, and a lateral X-ray will be required for accurate localization (Fig. 15.7b).

DIAGNOSIS. Although an X-ray should be taken to determine accurately the extent of the effusion, and the appearance of as much of the lung fields as are visible, the physical signs will usually be sufficient to indicate the need for a diagnostic aspiration. The needle should be inserted over the area of maximum dullness, and 5 to 10 ml of fluid withdrawn for examination.

The fluid is typically straw-coloured and has a clear or slightly ground-glass appearance, being readily distinguishable from a purulent fluid. On microscopic examination it is found to contain polymorphs at the onset of the effusion, and subsequently lymphocytes. Tubercle bacilli are rarely seen on direct examination, but may be demonstrable in about a third of cases on culture.

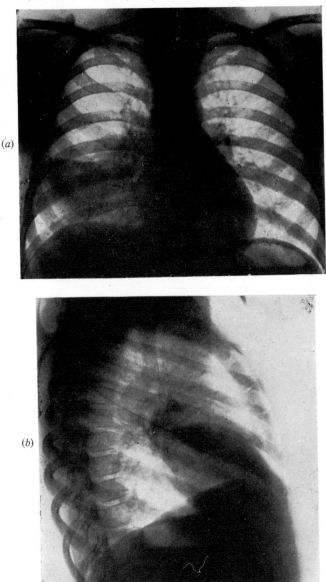

(a)

(b)

Fig. 15.7   Interlobar pleural effusion lying between right upper and right middle lobes, with partial collapse right middle lobe. (a) In this A.P. view the opacity is sharply demarcated above and the costophrenic angle clear. (b) In this lateral view the opacity extends to the sternum. (Compare with Fig. 15.8.)

A diagnosis of tuberculous pleural effusion may be made if the tuberculin reaction is positive and may be confirmed if necessary by pleural biopsy.

TREATMENT. This is on the lines indicated for primary infection, but it is most important that it should be sufficiently prolonged and a minimum of 18 months chemotherapy and supervision is required. In the great majority of cases, further removal of fluid after the first diagnostic aspiration is unnecessary, although some authorities have recommended drainage and injection of streptomycin into the pleural cavity. The use of systemic streptomycin and of oral PAS and isoniazid will be determined by the degree of parenchymal lung involvement and by the progress of the case.

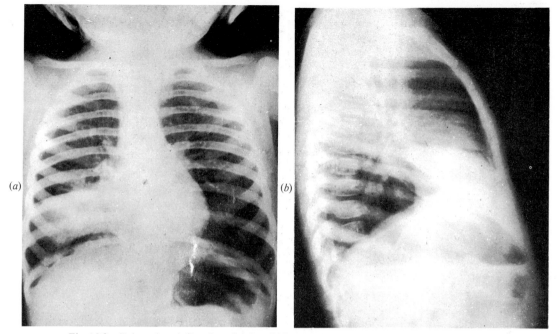

Fig. 15.8   Tuberculous infiltration of right middle lobe. The A.P. view (*a*) is similar to that of interlobar pleural effusion, but the lateral view (*b*) shows that the opacity involves the whole of the right middle lobe and is based on both sternum and diaphragm.

COURSE AND PROGNOSIS. The course varies considerably, and it is not uncommon for pyrexia to persist for three or more weeks; the E.S.R. usually remains elevated for a considerably longer period. Favourable signs are weight gain, which is often remarkably rapid after pyrexia has subsided, and a falling E.S.R. Progress must be checked by regular radiological examination.

The size of the effusion bears little relationship to the extent of pulmonary involvement, and in many cases it will be found that when a massive effusion absorbs, the lung is only slightly affected. In cases with more extensive pulmonary involvement the prognosis is that of the primary disease but, as a general rule, the ultimate prognosis is good.

Collapse of lung

This is a common complication of primary tuberculosis in childhood. Pressure on a bronchus from without, or blockage of the lumen by granulation tissue, an eroding lymph node, or caseous material within, will cause absorption collapse of the area of lung supplied by the bronchus. (More rarely, partial bronchial obstruction will result in obstructive emphysema peripherally.)

Depending on the site of the obstruction, the collapsed area will represent the whole of a lung, the whole of a lobe, or part of a lobe. The commonest site for a segmental lesion is the middle lobe of the right lung. The radiological appearances of collapse of two lobes are shown

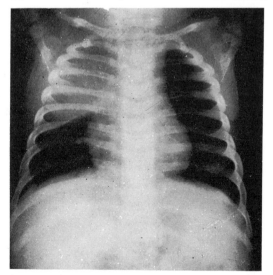

Fig. 15.9   Collapsed right upper lobe. Male infant aged 4 months.

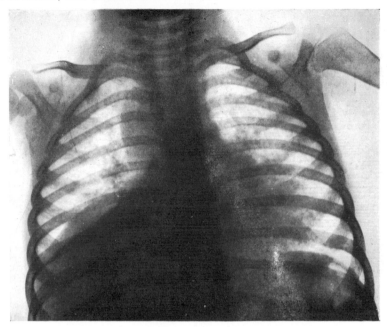

Fig. 15.10   Collapsed right lower lobe, secondary to gross enlargement of hilar nodes. Triangular shadow obscures right cardiophrenic angle.

in Figures 15.9 and 15.10. Thus collapse of the right or left upper lobe gives a sharply demarcated shadow at the apex, with a concave lower margin, and collapse of the right or left lower lobe a triangular shadow across the cardiophrenic angle, with a concave upper margin. The shadow of a collapsed left lower lobe is often obscured by the heart shadow, and may be better seen in a semioblique view. Collapse of the right middle lobe gives a shadow in the A.P. view having a sharply demarcated upper margin corresponding with the interlobar septum between the upper and middle lobe, and a more diffuse lower margin which does not obscure the costophrenic angle. The distinction from an interlobar effusion is made on the lateral view (Fig. 15.7b). Since the portion of the lung which is not collapsed will tend to expand to take the place of the collapsed lobe, it usually appears more translucent than the opposite lung field. Physical examination will show impairment of percussion note and diminished air entry over the collapsed area.

TREATMENT. Although collapsed areas will sometimes re-expand either spontaneously or following breathing exercises and inhalation of CO_2, it is generally advisable to undertake bronchoscopy as soon as the diagnosis has been made. In some cases it will be found possible to remove an obstruction of the lumen, though in others, due to pressure from without, this will not be feasible. General treatment is that of primary tuberculosis.

COURSE AND PROGNOSIS. While removal of an obstruction within the lumen of the bronchus will facilitate re-expansion, it is seldom the only factor involved, and collapse frequently recurs. In most cases, re-expansion will depend ultimately on the degree of involvement of the bronchial wall and the decrease in size of the adjacent lymph nodes. Although complete re-expansion is possible after a period of many months, it becomes less likely the longer that collapse continues, and in about half of all segmental lesions there are permanent abnormalities such as fibrosis and bronchiectasis, though these are often symptomless.

Tuberculous bronchopneumonia

This arises from inhalation of caseous material into the bronchial tree. It may originate by ulceration of a caseating lymph node through the wall of the bronchus, by extension of a caseating primary focus to involve a bronchus, or by haematogenous spread. Both lungs are likely to be involved though often to an unequal extent.

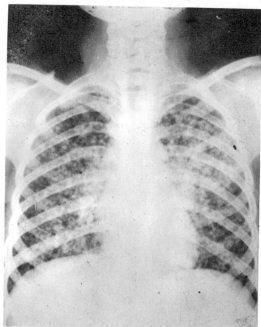

Fig. 15.11   Tuberculous bronchopneumonia. The mottling is coarser than in miliary tuberculosis (compare Fig. 15.12).

CLINICAL PICTURE. After a period of general ill-health, weight loss, and pallor, the temperature gradually rises or less frequently there is high pyrexia of sudden onset; cough and dyspnoea almost invariably appear. As the disease progresses, there is wasting, often accompanied by diarrhoea and vomiting. The physical signs are those of a generalized bronchopneumonia. The tuberculin reaction is strongly positive except in the terminal stages, and tubercle bacilli are commonly present in the sputum.

The radiological picture (Fig. 15.11) shows generalized lesions throughout both lung fields simulating confluent miliary tuberculosis, though the shadows are considerably larger.

COURSE AND PROGNOSIS. Before the advent of specific therapy, the condition carried a high mortality at all ages. Now, however, good results follow the use of streptomycin, PAS and isoniazid.

Post-primary infection

This may be haematogenous, bronchogenic, or due to fresh exogenous infection after the primary focus has healed. An infraclavicular focus, unassociated with enlargement of the corresponding lymph nodes, is seen less commonly in childhood than in adolescence or adult life, but may occur at any age. An apical focus is seldom recognizable radiologically until calcification has occurred. The progress of post-primary infections in children is in general more rapid, and marked by a greater tendency to caseation with less formation of fibrous tissue than in adults, but nevertheless chronic forms of the disease with extensive cavitation do occur.

Tuberculous pericarditis

This is a rare complication of caseating pulmonary lesions, direct extension to the pleural pericardium resulting in an exudative or caseous effusion. Cardiac embarrassment will necessitate aspiration of the pericardial sac. The prognosis is poor, though recovery is possible with intensive chemotherapy.

DISSEMINATED TUBERCULOSIS

While the primary complex in the lung is the commonest site from which tubercle bacilli enter the blood-stream (either directly into a blood vessel from the primary focus or mediastinal nodes, or indirectly via the thoracic duct), primary foci elsewhere may also act as the source of blood-stream infection. A transient bacillaemia probably almost always occurs early in a primary infection and the fact that healed tubercles may be found in patients dying from other causes suggests that disseminated foci of infection commonly occur, but quickly heal. Bone and joint tuberculosis represent types of blood-borne dissemination in which the infection has become localized to particular organs. The term 'disseminated tuberculosis' is generally applied, however, to more generalized dissemination, viz. miliary tuberculosis and tuberculous meningitis, both of which occur more readily in the first two years of life than in the older age groups.

Miliary tuberculosis

This may be acute or chronic, the most fulminating type of infection being seen in infants during the first twelve months of life, and usually occurring shortly after the primary infection. The pulmonary lesions are often detectable radiologically before the diagnosis can be made with certainty by other means. The most characteristic picture is a generalized 'snow storm' appearance, with minute pin-head shadows scattered uniformly throughout both lung fields (Fig.

15.12). A similar radiological appearance is sometimes seen in the lipidoses or in xanthomatosis, or during resolution of a post-measles bronchopneumonia.

The symptoms and physical signs are often very indefinite until the disease is far advanced. Loss of weight and energy or failure to thrive may be the first complaint. The temperature is usually irregularly raised, or a gradually mounting temperature, associated with abdominal symptoms and splenomegaly, may at first suggest a diagnosis of typhoid fever. Pulmonary symptoms are seldom diagnostic, but cough, dyspnoea, and cyanosis indicate heavy pulmonary involvement. Examination of the lungs may then show scattered rales or crepitations, though the disease is often remarkably silent. Tubercle bacilli will usually be found in the gastric washings. The fundi should be examined for choroid tubercles and the chest X-rayed, though both may be negative in the early stages. It will also be found that the Mantoux test is unreliable in the presence of an overwhelming infection.

Once almost invariably fatal, acute miliary tuberculosis can now usually be cured if effective chemotherapy is instituted early. There is still a significant mortality in cases diagnosed late or complicated by malnutrition or other disease. At

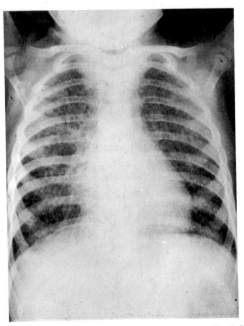

Fig. 15.12   Miliary tuberculosis showing generalized fine mottling giving 'snowstorm' appearance.

necropsy, greyish-white tubercles are found scattered throughout the lungs and other viscera, the spleen usually being heavily involved.

In the chronic form of the disease, in which bacillaemia is intermittent or of short duration and the infection less heavy than in the acute type, the progress of the disease is much more prolonged and there may be healing of individual tubercles while the disease is still active.

TREATMENT is considered on p. 325.

Tuberculous meningitis

Involvement of the meninges frequently occurs in the course of generalized miliary tuberculosis, and the majority of cases of tuberculous meningitis coming to necropsy show some evidence of miliary spread. The two conditions, however, are not necessarily associated, and tuberculous meningitis is often not explicable as a local manifestation of acute miliary tuberculosis. Thus a high proportion of cases of tuberculous meningitis show a focus of infection within the central nervous system which is of earlier origin than the meningitis. Such foci are often multiple and represent small tuberculomata seeded from a primary focus elsewhere, one or more of which has reached the surface of the brain and from which tubercle bacilli have been shed into the subarachnoid space. An intense exudative reaction is set up, and the infection disseminated throughout the meninges by way of the cerebrospinal fluid. The great majority of childhood cases of tuberculous meningitis occur within three months of the primary infection.

The symptoms appear insidiously in a previously healthy child and are at first vague and difficult to interpret. A slight character change may be noted by the mother, the child appearing irritable, anorexic, and disinclined to play. Transient headache is a frequent complaint, and this tends to become more severe and persistent as the disease progresses. Loss of weight sometimes precedes definite evidence of meningeal irritability, but often the child is well nourished when he first comes under observation. This *period of invasion* lasts a week or more, the length of history depending to some extent on the care with which the child has been observed. Alertness for the possibility of tuberculous meningitis should lead to diagnosis at this stage.

The second stage of the disease is that in which meningeal irritation becomes manifest. The child is fretful, resents examination, and tends to lie facing away from the light. There is stiffness of the neck, and Kernig's sign is usually positive. Other neurological signs are very variable, and may change within a matter of hours. In untreated patients, this *stage of irritability* also lasts approximately a week.

From irritability, the child passes into the terminal *stage of coma*. The eyes are staring, the abdomen carinated, and there is often marked wasting (Fig. 15.13). The signs of meningeal irritation become more obvious and convulsions or hyperpyrexia often occur shortly before death.

DIAGNOSIS. A tuberculin test and lumbar puncture should be carried out immediately the

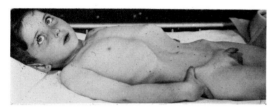

Fig. 15.13   Advanced tuberculous meningitis, showing staring facies and carinated abdomen.

condition is suspected. The tuberculin reaction is likely to be strongly positive in the early stages of the disease, though reactivity may subsequently be lost. Choroidal tubercles are visible in about half of all cases. X-ray of the chest may reveal hilar lymph node enlargement or miliary tuberculosis.

Examination of the cerebrospinal fluid should be carried out as soon as possible after lumbar puncture, since estimation of cells and sugar content will be unreliable after prolonged standing. The fluid is at first clear, though under increased pressure, later becoming ground-glass or cloudy. The cellular content varies from 20 to several hundred cells per mm^3, the cells being predominantly lymphocytes. The sugar content, which is normally approximately 80 per cent of that of the blood, is reduced; this finding is particularly valuable in the differential diagnosis from poliomyelitis, in which condition the sugar content is unaltered. The protein is increased; in the late stages the chlorides may be reduced. If the fluid is allowed to stand, a 'spider-web' clot forms in the test tube; this clot should be examined for the presence of tubercle bacilli, which can be found in a high proportion of cases.

TREATMENT is considered on p. 325. The prospects of recovery in early cases are now good. Whichever programme of treatment is used, the results are likely to be greatly influenced by the stage at which the patient comes under intensive treatment. Early diagnosis is of outstanding importance in prognosis, since those late cases which survive are most likely to show residual sequelae.

ABDOMINAL TUBERCULOSIS

The types of infection to be considered are (1) tuberculous enteritis, (2) tuberculous mesenteric adenitis, and (3) tuberculous peritonitis. All are now rare in Britain but may very occasionally occur when an infant ingests organisms from infected sputum or in untreated milk.

Tuberculous enteritis

When primary infection occurs through the alimentary tract there are usually no symptoms, the primary complex consisting of a small ulcer in one of the Peyer's patches (usually near the lower end of the ileum), and enlargement and caseation of the corresponding mesenteric lymph nodes.

Rarely, the bowel wall is heavily infected and caseous, when perforation is liable to occur, with secondary infection of the peritoneal cavity or the formation of faecal fistulae. In these cases there is diarrhoea and wasting, the stools containing mucus, pus, and tubercle bacilli.

Tuberculous mesenteric adenitis

Infection of the mesenteric lymph nodes occurs from entry of tubercle bacilli through the intestinal mucosa or from the blood-stream, in which case the primary focus will usually be found in the lung. Investigation should therefore include not only a tuberculin test but an X-ray of the chest and examination of stomach washings. In the great majority of cases, there is little disturbance of general health, and calcified abdominal nodes are sometimes found accidentally after spontaneous healing has occurred. In young infants, however, there is a greater danger of caseation and spread to other groups of nodes, leading to tuberculous peritonitis or generalized dissemination.

Such symptoms as occur are often indefinite, and include anorexia, loss of weight, pallor, and lassitude. Vague abdominal pain and tenderness are not uncommon in older children, and there may be diarrhoea. The tuberculin test is positive and the E.S.R. is raised.

Tuberculous peritonitis

The peritoneum is not infrequently involved in miliary tuberculosis. Tuberculous peritonitis may also arise from isolated foci of haemic origin, or from rupture of the ulcerated bowel wall or a caseous mesenteric node.

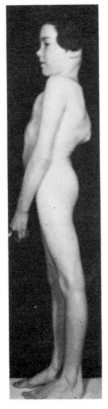
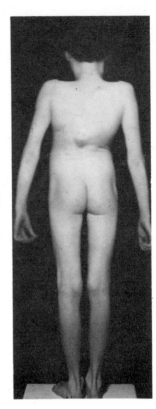

Fig. 15.15   Tuberculosis of spine, showing kyphosis and postural deformity.

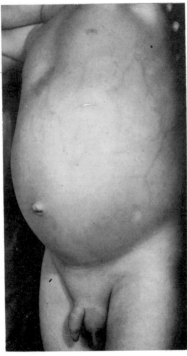

Fig. 15.14   Tuberculous peritonitis with ascites and left orchidoepididymitis; distension of abdomen, eversion of umbilicus, and venous dilatation. Infant aged 20 months.

The type of onset will vary with the origin of the infection; when this is alimentary, the picture will at first be that of mesenteric adenitis, followed by abdominal distension and wasting. Ascites resulting from an isolated haemic focus is more likely to be of rapid onset, with great enlargement of the abdomen. In patients in whom caseation and adhesions are the predominating lesions, the abdomen has a doughy feel.

With specific therapy the prognosis has been considerably improved but there is a risk of dissemination until complete healing has occurred. Subsequently adhesions may give rise to obstruction.

TUBERCULOSIS OF BONES AND JOINTS

Tuberculous infection occurring in the bones and joints is often the first manifestation of the disease recognized, but is always secondary to a primary infection elsewhere. Over 80 per cent of cases in Britain are secondary to a focus in the lung and are due to a human strain. The infection of the bone is blood-borne, the tubercle bacillus being particularly liable to settle in an area of cancellous bone immediately adjacent to a joint and subsequently to infect the joint. The sites most commonly involved are the spine and hip, which together comprise two-thirds of the infections seen in childhood; the third most common site is the knee.

Although it is often difficult to evaluate the

importance of minor trauma occurring weeks or months before there is clinical evidence of tuberculous infection, it is thought that this frequently serves to produce a site of lowered resistance.

Tuberculous spondylitis

From a focus in the body of a vertebra, the infection extends to cause progressive destruction and caseation, with subsequent collapse of the vertebral body. This in turn produces gradually progressive kyphosis, while the extrusion of caseous material into the spinal canal may result in pressure on the spinal cord. One or more of the vertebral bodies may be affected, the lesion appearing most commonly in the lower dorsal region.

Pain and limitation of movement are the most common early symptoms, though the former is by no means constantly present and may be referred to the abdomen. Occasionally it will be found that paralysis, e.g. paraplegia, has already developed by the time the child comes under observation. The presence of a 'cold' lumbar or psoas abscess should always indicate investigation of the spine as the most probable source of infection. Cervical infection may present as a deeply situated retropharyngeal abscess causing respiratory embarrassment.

Radiological examination of the spine will readily distinguish deformities due to tuberculosis from congenital malformations. Osteomyelitis of the spine is usually a more acute process with high leucocytosis. The tuberculin test in cases of tuberculous spondylitis will be positive.

Treatment consists essentially of immobilization of the affected area, prolonged chemotherapy and attention to the general nutrition and health. Surgical procedures such as spinal cord decompression, removal of tuberculous debris and spinal fusion may be required.

The prognosis in childhood is better than in adult life, and there is a prospect of good functional recovery if treatment is undertaken early and is sufficiently prolonged.

Tuberculosis of the hip

Lesions in the region of the hip may be either intra-articular or extra-articular, the former including acetabular and synovial infection, and the latter lesions of the head and neck of the femur and of the ilium.

The child comes under observation on account of *pain*, which is often referred to the knee, is intermittent, and may wake the child from sleep ('starting pain', due to relaxation of muscular spasm), and *limping*. Examination will usually show wasting of the thigh and buttock on the affected side, and possibly shortening of the leg if the lesion has been present long enough. Limitation of movement at the hip joint can usually be demonstrated.

The association of pain, limp, wasting, and limitation of movement should indicate the diagnosis, the only other conditions likely to present a similar picture being Perthes' disease and traumatic lesions. The 'irritable hip' syndrome of young children simulates tuberculous hip disease but subsides rapidly on rest with traction; the cause is often uncertain but may be trauma in some cases.

The diagnosis of tuberculosis can be confirmed radiologically, though in the earliest lesions rarefaction around the joint is often the only demonstrable finding. The tuberculin test will be positive, and a primary focus may be found elsewhere.

The general principles of treatment are again chemotherapy, immobilization with some form of traction, attention to the general health, and slow return to activity under careful supervision. In selected cases, surgical removal of diseased bone will hasten recovery.

Tuberculosis of other joints

Infections of the knee, ankle, elbow, wrist, shoulder, etc. are characterized by pain and swelling of the affected joint and by wasting and muscle spasm. Tenderness is less marked than in the case of septic or rheumatoid arthritis, there is no leucocytosis and the tuberculin test is positive. A direct biopsy from the affected area will establish the diagnosis in cases of doubt. Treatment consists essentially of chemotherapy with immobilization in the optimum position, since fibrous ankylosis may occasionally follow healing.

Tuberculous dactylitis

This is seen rarely in disseminated infections in infants. The phalanges of the fingers are affected and there may be associated tuberculosis of the metacarpals. The painless, spindle-shaped swellings of the fingers are not unlike those of syphilitic dactylitis (Fig. 4.8), from which they are distinguished by the positive tuberculin test and negative Wassermann reaction.

The osseous lesion of sarcoidosis also resembles tuberculous dactylitis: in this rare condition, the tuberculin test is generally negative but the intradermal Kveim test is sometimes of diagnostic value, though its specificity is doubtful. The bone lesions may be associated with sarcoid lesions of the skin, lymph nodes and eyes. Biopsy may be required to establish the diagnosis.

TUBERCULOSIS OF OTHER ORGANS

Tuberculous cervical adenitis

The usual portal of entry is the tonsil, or less commonly the mouth or adenoids, the cervical lymph nodes then forming a part of the primary complex. The condition, which was formerly common but is now very rare in Britain, was predominantly due to bovine infection. It is also possible, however, for cervical node enlargement to occur as a result of haematogenous spread secondary to a primary lung infection. A human strain is then likely to be responsible.

In an increasing number of cases, cervical lymphadenitis is due to acid-fast bacilli which are neither human nor bovine tubercle bacilli. These atypical mycobacteria, which include *M. avium*, may be resistant to anti-tuberculous drugs but respond to erythromycin.

CLINICAL PICTURE. Gradual and painless enlargement of the lymph nodes occurs on one or both sides of the neck. The nodes at first remain discrete and have a rubbery consistency but later they are liable to undergo caseation, and to become adherent to the skin (Fig. 15.16). Rupture of a caseating node through the skin will produce a chronic sinus; the surrounding skin then becomes chronically indurated (*scrofulo-*

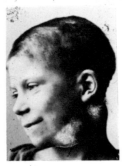

Fig. 15.16   Caseating tuberculous lymph nodes of neck.

derma) and may ulcerate. Nodes which have not ruptured commonly heal with fibrosis and calcification.

DIAGNOSIS. The tuberculin test is helpful in distinguishing tuberculous adenitis from other types of cervical adenitis, especially in young children. If the reaction is weakly positive atypical mycobacteria should be excluded (see p. 322). Cervical adenitis due to pyogenic infection tends to be more acute and painful: when partially treated with penicillin, the nodes may remain large and then resemble tuberculous nodes. In Britain, inadequately treated pyogenic infection is a far more common cause of indolent cervical adenitis than is tuberculosis. The diagnosis of lymphosarcoma, leukaemia, and Hodgkin's disease is considered in Chapter 9, and that of glandular fever on p. 355. In all cases the lungs should be X-rayed in order to determine whether a primary lung infection or mediastinal adenopathy is present.

TREATMENT. This should be conservative in the early stages of the disease, with chemotherapy and attention to the general health and nutrition of the child. The tonsils should be removed when the nodes have subsided, unless a primary infection of the lung is present. Operative removal of the nodes is the treatment of choice in atypical mycobacterial infection and should be undertaken if tuberculous nodes enlarge further or begin to soften, or when caseation has already occurred.

Genito-urinary tuberculosis

Apart from involvement in miliary tuberculosis, the *kidney* is much less commonly the site of chronic tuberculosis in children than in adults. When infection occurs it is always secondary to tuberculosis elsewhere. The renal lesion is usually discovered at necropsy or on routine examination of the urine of children with pulmonary tuberculosis. Frequency or haematuria are occasionally presenting symptoms, but more commonly protein and pus are found in an acid urine in the absence of pyogenic organisms. The centrifuged deposit of a 24 hour specimen of urine will show tubercle bacilli on direct examination or on culture.

Since it is necessary to determine whether the condition is unilateral or bilateral, intravenous pyelography should be carried out, and a specimen of urine from each ureter obtained by ureteric catheterization for bacteriological examination.

Haematogenous infection of the *epididymis* and secondary involvement of the body of the *testis* are both rare, but occur occasionally in infants and young children who have a primary focus of infection elsewhere. Chemotherapy has greatly improved the prognosis in genito-urinary tuberculosis and surgical treatment is rarely necessary.

Tuberculosis of the skin

With the exception of erythema nodosum and scrofuloderma, the only skin lesions of tuberculous origin which are likely to be seen in childhood are tuberculides. Primary infection of the skin is rare, and lupus vulgaris, though it may start in childhood, is seldom seen in advanced form at this age.

Tuberculides. These are papulonecrotic or nodular lesions varying in size from a pin's head to several millimetres in diameter and having a purplish-red colour. They appear following a primary infection, usually of the lung, or during generalized miliary tuberculosis. Treatment is that of the primary infection.

Tuberculosis of the eye

Three types of lesion occur, viz. primary infection, which is very rare, haematogenous infection, and allergic reaction. Haematogenous lesions include *tubercles of the choroid*, which are seen in tuberculous meningitis, and *tuberculous iridocyclitis*.

Phlyctenular conjunctivitis is an allergic manifestation for which tuberculous infection elsewhere in the body is responsible and most cases occur six months to a year after the primary infection.

The lesions consist of 'phlyctenules' or nodules on the conjunctiva or cornea, which are composed of an aggregation of polymorphs surrounded by mononuclear and occasional giant cells.

Photophobia, lachrymation and blepharospasm are often so severe as to make examination difficult without an anaesthetic. In some cases secondary staphylococcal infection results in a purulent discharge. If neglected, the condition may progress to extensive ulceration and scarring of the cornea. Although the first attack usually subsides within a few days recurrences are common.

During the acute phase, the eye should be irrigated with normal saline and hydrocortisone eye drops should be instilled; the child should be nursed in a darkened room as long as photophobia is present.

OTHER BACTERIAL INFECTIONS

Septicaemia and bacteraemia

The presence of living bacteria in the bloodstream may be a transient phenomenon, e.g. following the removal of septic tonsils or secondary to a septic focus elsewhere, giving rise to few general symptoms other than a sudden rise in temperature; to this the term *bacteraemia* is applied. When organisms are present in the blood for sufficiently long and in sufficient number to cause severe general symptoms, the condition is one of *septicaemia*. Neither can be regarded as a specific disease, since a number of infections with organisms of high invasive power may either begin or terminate with septicaemia, while transient bacteraemia is even more frequent. Thus meningococcal and typhoid infections normally pass through a septicaemic phase, while bacteraemia is a feature of a considerable proportion of cases of lobar pneumonia. Other organisms which have a high virulence but low invasive power, such as *Corynebacterium diphtheriae* and *Clostridium tetani*, are unlikely to produce septicaemia, their remote effects being due to the elaboration of toxins.

CLINICAL FEATURES. Septicaemia should be suspected when there are high, swinging temperature and severe toxaemia which are out of proportion to the local infection. The spleen readily becomes enlarged, and haemorrhagic manifestations may occur. When there is disseminated abscess formation, the condition is described as *pyaemia*.

DIAGNOSIS. The bacteriological diagnosis depends on the demonstration of organisms by blood culture, which should be repeated several times if necessary. Although there is perhaps a greater likelihood of obtaining a positive culture if blood is taken when the temperature is rising, this is not necessarily the case, and in early infancy the temperature reaction may be no indication of the severity of the infection.

TREATMENT. This will depend on the causative organism, and on its sensitivity to antibiotic therapy. When an effective antibiotic is available, response to treatment may be rapid and complete. In order to avoid delay, it is generally advisable to start treatment immediately with a broad spectrum antibiotic pending the results of sensitivity testing of the causative organism.

Diphtheria

Infection with *Corynebacterium diphtheriae* is characterized by (1) the formation of exudate or pseudomembrane at the site of infection, (2) constitutional symptoms, and (3) remote degenerative changes caused by the exotoxin. The varying severity of the disease depends on a number of factors, including host resistance, the virulence of the infecting organism, the site of infection, and the length of time elapsing before specific treatment is instituted. Three types of organism, the gravis, intermediate, and mitis, can be identified, which are usually related to the clinical severity of the disease, though exceptions to this occur.

The pseudomembrane is generally greyish-white in colour and consists of organisms, necrotic epithelial cells, leucocytes, and fibrin. Above the glottis the membrane is adherent, and bleeding occurs from the raw surface when it is removed. Below the larynx, the membrane is often less adherent.

The toxin, which is elaborated at the site of the membrane, is disseminated by the blood-stream and also to some extent by the perineural lymphatics of the nerves supplying the infected area. Although it affects almost all tissues, it has a particular affinity for cardiac muscle, renal tissues, and the nervous system. Cardiac muscle undergoes extensive toxic myocarditis, and the conducting mechanism is also involved. Toxic degenerative changes occur in the parenchyma of the kidneys and liver. The peripheral nerves show histological evidence of a toxic peripheral neuritis.

Diphtheria rarely occurs under 6 months of age, but carries its highest mortality in older infants and pre-school children.

CLINICAL TYPES. Cases are sometimes classified as follows:

Anterior-nasal, in which only the anterior nasal mucosa is involved, and toxaemia is absent or slight. These cases are marked by a high degree of host immunity, but are infectious to others. The only symptom may be blood-stained nasal discharge, usually bilateral.

Laryngeal (*membranous croup*), in which membrane involves the larynx, with or without extensions downwards to the trachea and bronchi. Mechanical obstruction and swelling of the larynx give rise to stridor on inspiration, cyanosis, and respiratory embarrassment, which may be fatal unless promptly relieved.

Faucial, involving the tonsils and/or pillars of the fauces. The membrane is readily visible, but since the onset of the disease is often insidious and no complaint is made of sore throat by young patients, the infection may be well advanced before diagnosis is made unless the throat is examined as a routine.

Nasopharyngeal. Here the membrane not only involves the tonsils and pillars but extends to the palate, uvula, pharynx, or post-nasal mucosa. Extensive necrosis and haemorrhage may cause a distinctive foetor, and toxaemia is severe. The cervical lymph nodes are enlarged and swelling and oedema of the neck may give rise to a so-called 'bull-neck' appearance which is of bad prognosis.

Non-respiratory infections include skin lesions, indolent ulcers, umbilical, vulval, and aural infections. The degree of toxaemia is very variable, but paralysis occasionally follows comparatively small lesions.

CONSTITUTIONAL SYMPTOMS. Except in the very mildest cases, the child with diphtheria appears pale and toxic, and prostration is often quite out of proportion to the degree of pyrexia; the temperature seldom rises above 39·5°C (103°F) and is usually little raised, e.g. 38°C (100·4°F). When the nasopharynx and larynx are affected, there may be cyanosis and dyspnoea. The pulse is rapid and feeble or irregular; in some cases bradycardia due to heart-block occurs. Early cardiac failure and sudden death are liable to occur during the initial toxaemia, and cardiac failure may also occur later, e.g. two to three weeks from onset. Electrocardiographic changes and elevated serum transaminase levels will confirm the presence of myocarditis. If this phase is safely passed, there is very rarely any residual evidence of cardiac damage. Proteinuria is commonly present in the early stages of the disease, and may persist for weeks but no permanent renal damage results.

Paralysis. Palatal paralysis commonly appears during the third week, and causes nasal speech and regurgitation of fluids through the nose. When the paralysis extends to the pharynx, it is accompanied by dysphagia and cough. Ocular paralyses occur later than palatal paralysis, and include strabismus and paralysis of accommodation.

Of the various manifestations of peripheral neuritis, diaphragmatic paralysis is the most serious and is revealed by lack of movement of the upper abdomen. The commonest manifestations are ataxia and absence of the deep tendon reflexes. Peripheral neuritis may occur late, e.g. two months or more after the primary infection.

TREATMENT. The first essential of treatment is prompt diagnosis and immediate administration of antitoxin. The doses recommended are: for mild cases, 10,000 units intramuscularly; for moderate cases, 15,000 to 30,000 units intramuscularly or intravenously; and for severe cases, 50,000 to 100,000 units intravenously. If more than 20,000 units are required, the intravenous route should be used. The risk of anaphylaxis should be remembered and a preliminary test for sensitivity made by subcutaneous injection of 0·05 ml antitoxin. While the diagnosis of diphtheria should be confirmed bacteriologically, antitoxin administration should never be delayed if clinical examination indicates it. Penicillin or erythromycin should be administered until swabs are negative, in order to reduce the carrier-state.

Local treatment. In any patient with stridor, laryngoscopy and aspiration of membrane should be promptly undertaken, followed by intubation or tracheotomy. Intubation, though often effective, has the disadvantage that the tube may be coughed out or become blocked by membrane within the trachea. Preparation for tracheotomy should always be made. The use of humidified air and of sedatives is usually indicated.

General treatment. In no disease is absolute rest more essential, owing to the risk of sudden cardiac failure, and in all except the mildest cases a minimum of six weeks bed rest will be required. A fluid diet is usually best during the early stages, though palatal paralysis will necessitate the thickening of feeds or nasal feeding. Glucose should be given intravenously in severely toxic cases. Peripheral neuritis or cardiac complications will be indications for prolonged rest, and oxygen should be given when there is respiratory embarrassment; patients with diaphragmatic or intercostal paralysis may benefit from nursing in a respirator.

PROGNOSIS. Unless death occurs from cardiac or respiratory failure during the first four weeks, the ultimate prognosis is good. Even patients who have had severe myocardial damage may expect a perfect functional recovery.

Scarlet fever

It is now generally accepted that scarlet fever is only one manifestation of haemolytic streptococcal infection, and that no sharp distinction can be drawn between cases showing an exanthem and others in which the manifestations are only those of a streptococcal sore throat. Occasionally a scarlet fever rash follows haemolytic streptococcal infection of wounds or burns. The results of infection are (1) local and pyogenic, and (2) constitutional, due to circulation of diffusible exotoxin. Throat swabs during the acute phase at onset are likely to show a profuse growth of group A haemolytic streptococci, but several different types are sometimes isolated in the same epidemic.

CLINICAL FEATURES. The incubation period is commonly two to five days and the onset is sudden. A rise of temperature to 39·5°C (103°F) or more is accompanied by headache, vomiting, and sore throat. The child appears flushed, with circumoral pallor, and examination of the throat shows inflammation of the tonsils and fauces, and flushing or stippling of the soft palate. The tongue is at first furred with projection of the papillae ('white strawberry tongue'), subsequently becoming clean and generally reddened ('red strawberry tongue').

The *rash* or *exanthem* appears one to two days after the initial rise of temperature, and is typically a fine punctate erythema. Although it often appears first on the neck and extends to the trunk and face, the distribution and appearance are variable. Fine, branny desquamation of the skin, including that of the palms and soles, occurs during the third and fourth weeks.

COMPLICATIONS. The cervical lymph nodes are commonly enlarged. Infection of the nose, sinuses, or middle ear are important complications, since the discharges are infectious.

Proteinuria frequently occurs during the pyrexial phase of scarlet fever, but is usually transient; nephritis, however, is liable to occur during the third week, irrespective of the severity of the initial infection.

Acute rheumatism is uncommon but may be initiated by scarlet fever in the same way as by other throat infections. Rheumatic arthritis must be distinguished from 'serum sickness' and also from the much rarer streptococcal arthritis which occasionally occurs: the latter is marked by high pyrexia and leucocytosis, and fails to respond to salicylate therapy. Haemorrhage or sudden death from myocarditis may occur in severe scarlet fever.

TREATMENT. Penicillin is the antibiotic of choice and should be given in large doses. Isolation is advisable until cultures have shown that the patient is free from streptococcal infection.

Erysipelas

This also is one of the manifestations of group A haemolytic streptococcal infection, the portal of entry in this case being the skin or mucous membrane. Infection may follow wounds, burns, or operations, or occur at the junction of skin and mucosa. The disease is contagious but not highly so and the infection is commonly acquired by contact with other clinical types of streptococcal infection.

The disease is first manifested by a rise of temperature, vomiting, or convulsions associated with the appearance of a red, indurated area at the site of infection. The skin lesion has a raised irregular margin and tends to advance to adjacent areas. Vesiculation, desquamation, or abscess formation frequently occur behind the advancing edge. There is commonly a high leucocytosis.

Before the era of chemotherapy, the disease in infancy carried a very high mortality but the great majority of cases now respond rapidly to penicillin.

Osteomyelitis

Although not regarded as a communicable disease, pyogenic infection of bone may appropriately be considered in association with other streptococcal and staphylococcal infections. In infancy more than 50 per cent of cases are streptococcal infections, whereas in older children the great majority are staphylococcal, although osteomyelitis due to Gram-negative bacilli is becoming more common. Other organisms are rarely responsible. Skin sepsis or upper respiratory or pulmonary infection may provide the portal of entry for haematogenous spread, but in many cases the site of primary infection is obscure. Osteomyelitis is of much commoner occurrence in childhood than in adult life, and boys are affected twice as frequently as girls.

Acute osteomyelitis. Although any bone may be infected, the commonest site is the juxta-epiphyseal region of the metaphysis of a long bone. Localized pain, tenderness, and swelling with oedema are associated with pyrexia and high leucocytosis. In some fulminating cases there is rapid formation of a subperiosteal abscess; blood culture may show the presence of the infecting organism. Since the lesion commonly lies in the vicinity of a joint, a mistaken and sometimes disastrous diagnosis of rheumatism may be made. It must be remembered that the swellings in acute rheumatism tend to move from joint to joint, the tenderness is not localized to bone, the pyrexia responds to salicylates, and the white blood count is not raised to the same extent as in acute osteomyelitis. The differential diagnosis of scurvy has been considered (p. 157). Radiological examination is unlikely to demonstrate rarefaction in acute osteomyelitis for several days after the onset of symptoms, after which time local destruction of bone may be clearly recognizable.

Chronic osteomyelitis. Failure to localize and overcome the infection will result in sequestrum formation, spread of infection to the shaft of the bone, and often secondary lesions elsewhere. Constitutional symptoms and pyrexia are less marked than in acute cases, but there is usually progressive anaemia and wasting.

TREATMENT. Acute osteomyelitis should be treated with large doses of penicillin, e.g. 1 to 2 million units daily in three-hourly doses. When the infection is due to a penicillin-resistant staphylococcus, cloxacillin should be used. If treatment is begun sufficiently early, surgical intervention will be unnecessary in many cases, though subperiosteal abscess formation will require aspiration or drainage and whenever pus is under pressure it must be released. The prognosis is good.

In more chronic cases, surgical removal of sequestra is likely to be necessary. Antibiotic therapy has not only reduced the risks of operation, but has made more conservative surgery possible.

Bacterial infections of the central nervous system

On the slightest suspicion of meningitis, and before any treatment is started, lumbar puncture should be carried out and blood taken for culture. If there is evidence of bacterial infection in the cerebrospinal fluid, therapy should be instituted without delay.

Bacterial meningitis progresses so rapidly, especially in infancy, and so quickly causes irreparable damage to the central nervous system, that the use of combinations of anti-

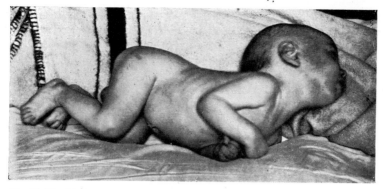

Fig. 15.17   Meningococcal meningitis with head retraction; infant aged 4 months.

bacterial agents in much larger doses than are commonly employed is justified. Although newer antibiotics such as ampicillin are tending to replace chloramphenicol, the latter antibiotic is of such proven efficacy that it can still be recommended for severe meningitis, despite its known toxicity.

The following combinations of therapeutic agents are recommended in order to prevent the emergence of resistant strains, and to obtain maximal concentration at the site of infection with a minimum of delay. Where a sulphonamide is indicated, either sulphadiazine or sulphadimidine may be used.

Meningococcus—sulphonamide plus
   penicillin
Pneumococcus or streptococcus—penicillin
   plus sulphonamide plus chloramphenicol
Haemophilus influenzae—ampicillin or
   chloramphenicol plus sulphonamide
Colon bacilli—streptomycin plus
   chloramphenicol plus sulphonamide
Salmonellae—chloramphenicol plus
   streptomycin
Pyocyaneus—polymyxin plus streptomycin or
   carbenicillin.

Meningococcal meningitis and septicaemia
(*Cerebrospinal fever*)

The meningococci form a group of organisms varying in virulence and antigenic properties. Infection commonly occurs by way of the nasopharynx, and results first in a blood-stream infection (*meningococcaemia*) followed by infection of the meninges and cerebrospinal fluid. A purulent exudate then occurs throughout the subarachnoid space, being most evident over the base of the brain. Carriers are common, and are the principal source of transmission. The disease assumes epidemic proportions in the winter or spring. Although the disease is most liable to affect infants and pre-school children, older children and young adults often form a higher proportion of those affected during epidemics, particularly when they are living in overcrowded conditions.

CLINICAL FEATURES. The incubation period is normally two to four days, and rarely as long as ten days. The onset is in most cases abrupt with high fever. Convulsions and vomiting are common presenting symptoms in infants, while older patients are likely to complain of intense headache and photophobia. Stiffness of the neck is almost always present when there is meningeal involvement, but in young infants there may be only a little fullness or bulging of the fontanelle without neck stiffness. Head retraction may be an early sign in infants and papilloedema may occur. Kernig's sign is positive in older children but only in a small proportion of infants. Restlessness, drowsiness, or coma are frequent findings. The appearance of a rash within twenty-four hours of onset is a helpful diagnostic sign, but is by no means constant, particularly in

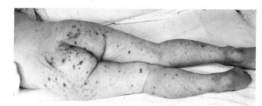

Fig. 15.18   Meningococcal septicaemia, showing haemorrhagic rash.

sporadic cases; the rash consists of scattered purplish spots or more extensive haemorrhagic areas which may become necrotic in fulminating cases. Herpes often appears later.

While the majority of cases in early life are of sudden onset, it is possible for the disease to appear more insidiously, with little pyrexia and few localizing signs. These subacute and chronic cases are the ones in which there is most likelihood of the basilar cisternae being involved (*posterior basic meningitis*), with subsequent development of hydrocephalus.

COMPLICATIONS. Cases in which treatment is given late or is inadequate are liable to develop a block in the circulation of the cerebrospinal fluid with progressive *hydrocephalus*. Before chemotherapy was available, this was a common complication but is now rare. *Subdural collections of fluid* may occasionally persist or accumulate after the acute phase, even in patients who have received full treatment. These require aspiration. Terminal *bronchopneumonia* may be found in fatal cases.

Deafness, due to involvement of the eighth nerve with ultimate destruction of the labyrinth, is of increasing importance, since it is liable to occur in infants who have been otherwise successfully treated. The disability is likely to be permanent.

Optic atrophy is occasionally due to direct involvement of the optic nerve and results in partial or complete blindness. Ocular palsies are uncommon.

Mental defect may be a late complication of the disease, but is unlikely to occur with early and adequate treatment.

Arthritis, *ophthalmia*, and *otitis media* are complications which usually respond rapidly to adequate treatment.

Adrenal haemorrhage with collapse and prostration (*Waterhouse-Friderichsen syndrome*) is a most serious complication of the septicaemic and fulminating types of the disease, but prompt treatment with hydrocortisone hemisuccinate (50 to 100 mg) and noradrenaline will be life-saving in some cases. Supportive therapy includes intravenous glucose-saline infusion and oxygen.

TREATMENT. Sulphadiazine or sulphadimidine is a most effective drug if the patient is given an adequate initial dose, e.g. 150 to 200 mg per kg body weight, followed by a total of 150 to 200 mg per kg body weight daily in divided doses four-hourly for seven or more days depending on progress. The drug is given orally as soon as practicable, but vomiting or coma may make it necessary to give the initial doses by intramuscular injection or intravenously into a glucose-saline infusion. Penicillin in full doses should be given in addition for the first few days. A dramatic response is usually observed within 24 to 48 hours. When treatment is started early, the prognosis is good, even in infants. Daily lumbar puncture is unnecessary if the patient is progressing satisfactorily, and, indeed, a diagnostic lumbar puncture at onset and one or more cerebrospinal fluid examinations after the temperature has settled, will be all that are required.

DIAGNOSIS. Although the diagnosis can be suspected from the history and clinical signs in cases presenting with meningitic signs, lumbar puncture and blood culture are required to determine the causative organism. The cerebrospinal fluid in these cases will be under increased pressure, cloudy or frankly purulent, containing large numbers of polymorphonuclear cells and forming a clot on standing. The protein content is raised and the sugar content reduced. Gram-negative diplococci which are typically intracellular but may also be extracellular are usually readily demonstrable in acute cases. In chronic cases, and occasionally in very early cases, organisms may be scanty, and a higher proportion of lymphocytes is sometimes found. The organisms should be further identified by culture. Septicaemic cases without meningeal involvement will be diagnosed on blood culture, and the organisms may also be identified in the skin lesions. The white blood count shows a high polymorphonuclear leucocytosis in acute cases.

Differential diagnosis from other types of purulent meningitis will be made on the history and demonstration of the causative organism; from tuberculous meningitis by the more insidious onset of the latter and the cerebrospinal fluid findings; and from benign lymphocytic meningitis by the character of the fluid and the absence of organisms in that disease. Difficulty is only likely to arise in those rare cases of meningococcal meningitis in which the cell count of the cerebrospinal fluid is relatively low, when lymphocytes predominate, and when organisms are scanty; or when inadequate antibiotic treatment has been given empirically before carrying out lumbar puncture.

Other purulent meningitides

In all acute cases the signs are similar to those described above, but the purpuric rash is rarely seen. The cerebrospinal fluid is purulent, the sugar content reduced, and diagnosis depends on isolation of the causative organism. If no bacteria are cultured, a viral infection may be suspected but sometimes meningococci are difficult to grow. Once cerebrospinal fluid has been obtained, severely ill children should be given chloramphenicol, penicillin, and sulphonamide or kanamycin pending final bacteriological diagnosis. Some authorities prefer to use ampicillin alone in this situation but therapeutic failures have been reported on this regimen. Intravenous fluids and hydrocortisone may be lifesaving in very severe meningitis. The two more important types of purulent meningitis are *influenzal meningitis* and *pneumococcal meningitis*. *Streptococcal meningitis* has been referred to as a possible complication of aural infections; *staphylococcal meningitis* is rare but occurs as a complication of osteomyelitis, sinus thrombosis, skin sepsis, etc. Other pyogenic organisms are rarely responsible for meningeal infection but in the newborn infant, *Escherichia coli* and, less commonly, *Listeria monocytogenes* may cause meningitis.

Influenzal meningitis

This is due to infection with *Haemophilus influenzae*, and bears no direct relationship to virus influenza. It appears to be less common in Britain than in the U.S.A., but sporadic cases are seen amongst infants in the latter part of the first year and during the second year of life, and more rarely in older children. In most cases meningitis follows an upper respiratory infection.

Chloramphenicol should be given, 10 to 20 mg per kg initially followed by 50 to 100 mg per kg daily in four divided doses (half these doses in the newborn infant). Alternatively, ampicillin 200 mg per kg may be given daily by injection. Antibiotic should be combined with full doses of a sulphonamide and treatment should be prolonged. The mortality, which was previously extremely high, has been substantially reduced by the use of specific therapeutic agents, but the prognosis is still considerably less good than that of meningococcal meningitis and sequelae are frequent. Subdural effusion should be suspected if fever persists despite adequate therapy, and subdural taps should be performed.

Pneumococcal meningitis

This occurs most frequently in infants as a complication of upper respiratory infection or pneumonia. The importance in etiology of birth injury and trauma, causing lesions of the dura, is recognized; when such lesions are suspected, surgical exploration and repair of the dura should be undertaken after the infection has been controlled. The purulent exudate is situated principally over the vertex, the base of the brain and spinal meninges being less involved. Treatment consists of 2 to 10 mega units daily of crystalline penicillin in divided doses, combined with sulphonamide and chloramphenicol. (Since the cerebrospinal fluid may be thickly purulent on first lumbar puncture, it is the practice in some clinics to give an initial intrathecal injection of 10,000 units benzyl penicillin at this time.) There is still a significant mortality and a proportion of infants who survive are left with permanent defect or paralysis.

Pertussis (*Whooping cough*)

Pertussis is a specific infectious disease characterized by paroxysmal cough, and caused by *Bordetella pertussis*, which can be cultured on 'cough plates', using a blood-containing medium. The organism grows on the epithelium of the trachea and bronchi, and produces an endotoxin which is thought to sensitize nerve endings in the respiratory tract, and also possibly to have toxic effects on the central nervous system. A closely similar organism, *Bord. parapertussis*, and a number of viruses, including adenoviruses and the respiratory syncytial virus, can cause a clinically indistinguishable condition.

The incidence and severity of the disease have both declined in recent years but mortality is still appreciable in infants under 12 months of age, particularly if deaths from secondary bronchopneumonia are added to those directly due to pertussis itself. The disease occurs throughout the year and epidemics are likely to occur in alternate years. One attack usually provides lasting immunity, but second attacks may occur, usually in later life when immunity has waned.

CLINICAL FEATURES. The incubation period is from seven to 14 days. The onset is characterized by a catarrhal stage lasting seven to 14 days, during which the child has coryza, cough, and slight pyrexia, and is highly infectious.

The cough gradually becomes more severe and

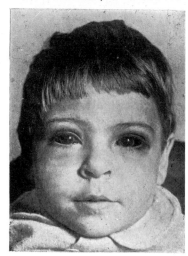

Fig. 15.19   Bilateral conjunctival haemorrhage due to pertussis.

assumes a paroxysmal character. A prolonged series of violent expirations, during which the child's face becomes suffused or cyanotic, is followed by a sudden indrawing of breath which produces the typical 'whoop'. Very frequently a paroxysm of coughing ends in vomiting, and this adds to the difficulty of feeding young ·infants. The paroxysms are usually worst at night but are readily initiated during the day by a variety of stimuli. After two to three weeks they become less frequent and severe, but it is not uncommon for a transient recrudescence of cough and vomiting to occur in the sixth or seventh week of the illness. The length of time during which paroxysms persist varies greatly in different cases, and the total duration of cough depends also on whether secondary respiratory infection occurs. Although the paroxysm is usually characteristic, the whoop is not a constant occurrence and is often absent in the immunized child, who is likely to have a mild attack of the disease.

COMPLICATIONS. *Haemorrhage* from the nose or into the conjunctiva frequently occurs during a paroxysm, and petechial haemorrhages of the brain are seen in fatal cases.

Convulsions are probably due in most instances to cerebral anoxia or more rarely to haemorrhage, but may indicate an effect of the endotoxin on the brain.

Ulceration of the frenum of the tongue is not uncommon in infants whose lower incisors have erupted.

Respiratory complications. Laryngitis and

otitis media occur frequently, and bronchitis invariably, during the catarrhal stage of the disease; bronchopneumonia may develop either early or late, and is the most serious of the common complications.

Emphysema of some degree is an almost inevitable result of a severe attack of pertussis. Pulmonary collapse is common, though the collapsed areas usually re-expand spontaneously.

DIAGNOSIS. The diagnosis may be suspected during the catarrhal stage of the disease in the presence of an epidemic or following contact, but usually paroxysmal cough is the first symptom to suggest it. Confirmation is obtained from the white blood count, which shows a high lymphocytosis during the paroxysmal stage and a leucopenia during the catarrhal and convalescent stages, and by culture of *Bord. pertussis* on a cough plate or on a post-nasal swab taken during or just after a paroxysm. The possibility of an inhaled foreign body, which may cause sudden onset of paroxysmal cough, must be remembered in the differential diagnosis.

TREATMENT. While antibiotics have little or no effect on the course of the illness, both erythromycin and chloramphenicol rapidly eliminate the organisms and render the patient non-infectious. The former is preferred for this purpose because of its lower toxicity. The subsequent object of treatment is to prevent secondary infection of the respiratory tract, and penicillin is generally used. Antispasmodics and sedatives, such as scopolamine and phenobarbitone, have little effect in controlling paroxysms.

Since feeding often provokes a paroxysm of coughing followed by vomiting in infants, it may be necessary to feed a second time after vomiting has occurred, the second feed being more readily retained. Oxygen therapy and intensive care techniques may be necessary in seriously ill infants.

Brucellosis (*Undulant fever; abortus and Malta fevers*)

The milk of cattle infected with *Brucella abortus* and of goats infected with *Br. melitensis* is liable to cause long-continued fever in man, the two types of infection being known as abortus and Malta fever respectively. The incidence of *Br. abortus* infection in children in Britain is not certainly known, but is probably considerably higher than the relatively small number of reported cases would suggest, particularly in country districts. With effective pasteurization of milk, however, the risk of infection can be reduced or eliminated.

CLINICAL FEATURES. The clinical picture is variable but the onset tends to be more abrupt in children than in adults. The temperature varies from 38° to 40°C (100·4° to 104°F), and may continue with remissions for six months or more. The child often appears less ill than the continued pyrexia would suggest. Sweating, fatigue, headaches, abdominal discomfort, and joint pains may occur. Splenomegaly and lymphadenopathy are sometimes present. The blood may show anaemia and lymphocytosis, but these are not constant findings.

DIAGNOSIS. The disease may be suspected in cases with unexplained fever of long duration, particularly if the child has consumed unpasteurized milk. Agglutination tests are usually positive in high dilution (1 in 500 or more) as the disease progresses, and a rising titre indicates the diagnosis; tests which only remain positive in lower dilution, e.g. 1 in 80, are suggestive but less diagnostic, as they may be due to previous subclinical infection. Blood culture and urine culture may demonstrate the organism in the early stages of the disease. Skin testing with brucellin may give a positive reaction but is not diagnostic.

TREATMENT. The organisms are sensitive to the tetracyclines and to chloramphenicol; the former should be used in proven cases and may be combined with streptomycin. Treatment is otherwise largely symptomatic, and directed to maintaining the hygiene of the skin and mouth and general nutrition.

Tetanus (*Lockjaw*)

The disease is caused by *Clostridium tetani*, an organism producing highly resistant spores which require anaerobic conditions to germinate. Infection in older children most commonly occurs as the result of penetrating wounds by foreign bodies which have been contaminated by tetanus-containing faeces of domestic animals, particularly horses and sheep; tetanus neonatorum (p. 59) is more likely to arise from umbilical infection. The organism produces a virulent exotoxin which passes by way of the motor nerves to the central nervous system.

CLINICAL FEATURES childhood cases the incubation period varies from two to 16 days,

but occasionally the infection remains latent for much longer periods. The presenting signs are muscular rigidity followed by reflex spasm. Trismus of the jaw and risus sardonicus are characteristic, while in the more generalized forms rigidity of the back, slight opisthotonos, and convulsions occur.

DIAGNOSIS. Trismus due to local infections of the mouth, jaw, or fauces (e.g. quinsy) must be distinguished by local examination and the absence of neck rigidity. Bell's palsy (seventh nerve paralysis) will be unassociated with evidence of muscular rigidity. A lumbar puncture may be necessary to distinguish tetanus from poliomyelitis or meningitis, though trismus is not present in these conditions. The diagnosis of infantile tetany is considered in Chapter 6. The history of a penetrating wound will help to confirm the diagnosis of tetanus, though the disease may follow an injury so slight that it has been overlooked.

TREATMENT. Administration of 100,000 international units (i.u.) of tetanus antitoxin, half intravenously and half intramuscularly, should be undertaken as soon as the diagnosis has been made, and surgical treatment of the wound carried out after infiltration with antitoxin. Penicillin should be given in full dosage but is no substitute for antitoxin. Spasms should be controlled by barbiturates and chlorpromazine. The management of a child with severe tetanus requires the combined skills of paediatrician and anaesthetist, for ventilation and other intensive care techniques may be necessary.

PROPHYLAXIS. Following wounds when there is a risk of infection having occurred, e.g. by contamination with cultivated soil or road dust, children already immunized should be given a 'booster dose' of 0·5 ml toxoid. For unimmunized children, intramuscular injection of 2500 i.u. of antitoxin, preceded by a subcutaneous test dose, may be used but active immunization should follow at once.

PROGNOSIS. The longer reflex spasm is delayed after the original infection, the better the prognosis. As a general rule, deep, extensive, and secondarily infected wounds are more likely to be followed by severe tetanus than superficial ones. In severe generalized tetanus in which antitoxin is given late, the mortality is high, and tetanus neonatorum is very frequently fatal. In cases of local and delayed tetanus complete recovery is the rule.

Bacillary dysentery

The role of dysentery organisms in the causation of infantile diarrhoea has been referred to (p. 169). In Britain the great majority of such infections in both infants and older children are due to *Shigella sonnei; Shig. flexneri* is less common and *Shig. dysenteriae* infection is rare. Dysentery occurs most frequently under conditions of overcrowding and faulty sanitation, when it is transmitted by direct contamination of food or water or by the medium of flies. Epidemics and household infections are not uncommon. The pathological lesion is typically an ileo-colitis with a varying degree of invasion and ulceration of the mucosa of the bowel.

CLINICAL FEATURES. Severe infections in infants may be ushered in by a sudden rise of temperature and a convulsion before the appearance of diarrhoea. Sonne dysentery is in general a milder infection than other types, though severe attacks do occasionally occur in children under 5 years of age. The onset of symptoms is rapidly followed by the occurrence of diarrhoea. While blood intimately mixed with the semifluid stool is very commonly present in the first diarrhoeal motions passed, the amount may be small and be overlooked. Mucus, however, is more consistently present and persists longer than macroscopic blood. There is commonly tenesmus and abdominal discomfort. In older children the only symptoms may be persistent or recurrent diarrhoea. Complications such as arthritis rarely occur in Sonne infections.

DIAGNOSIS. Rectal swabs should be taken to identify the organism, and if the examination is positive, the investigation should be extended to other members of the household. While in Britain blood and mucus in the stools are most commonly due to dysentery, elsewhere Salmonella infections are a more important cause. In acute food poisoning due to staphylococcal contamination, symptoms occur within a few hours of ingesting the infected food, and when food poisoning is due to Salmonella organisms, usually within 12 to 48 hours; in both cases vomiting and prostration are likely to be associated with the diarrhoea. Intussusception, in which condition blood and mucus may be passed in the stools, can be distinguished from dysentery by the characteristic recurrent spasms of pain and by palpation of an intra-abdominal mass.

TREATMENT. Children should be treated in bed and given a low-residue diet during the acute phase, while infants require the general treatment described for gastroenteritis. Oral streptomycin (1 g daily in divided doses for five days) is effective in treatment, and preferable to tetracycline or sulphadiazine alone, owing to the emergence of resistant strains.

Enteric fevers (*Typhoid and paratyphoid fevers*)

Infections with *Salmonella typhi* and with *Sal. paratyphi* B represent similar though distinct diseases, paratyphoid fever being in general less severe than typhoid fever. Both may occur at all ages, though typhoid fever is rare in early infancy.

Infection occurs by ingestion of water, milk, or food contaminated by sewage or by a carrier, and in dealing with an outbreak it is most important to determine the source. After an incubation period of eight to 21 days, the bloodstream is invaded and there is lymphatic involvement of the small intestine, mesenteric nodes, and spleen. The blood usually shows a marked diminution in the number of neutrophils and eosinophils during the second and third weeks, which may be followed by a lymphocytosis.

CLINICAL FEATURES. Such wide variations occur in childhood cases that the clinical picture may be dominated by meningeal, respiratory, or circulatory disturbances and the 'enteric' symptoms thought to be secondary. As a general rule there is malaise and anorexia and the temperature rises gradually over a period of days, but a more abrupt onset associated with headache, convulsions, or meningism may occur in younger patients. During the second week, rose spots may appear on the abdomen or flanks, but these are scanty and may be absent. Slight splenic enlargement occurs during the first week, and hepatomegaly is not uncommon. Diarrhoea is sometimes a presenting symptom in infants, but this is less true of children in whom constipation often occurs during the first week; abdominal pain and distension are commonly present. Perforation and haemorrhage are rare complications, but inflammation of the ileocaecal region may closely simulate appendicitis. When the respiratory system is affected, signs of bronchitis or bronchopneumonia are liable to obscure the diagnosis. Myocarditis may occur in the severest cases. In comparing childhood with adult cases it is generally found that the disease is less severe in children, the pyrexia less prolonged, the incidence of serious complications lower, and there is a greater tendency to relapse.

DIAGNOSIS. This is established by blood culture during the first week, or during the second and third weeks when there is persistent pyrexia. After the tenth day the Widal reaction is likely to be positive, and should be repeated in doubtful cases. Stool and urine cultures may be positive in the second week or earlier.

TREATMENT. The general principles of nursing and isolation are the same as in the case of adults, and symptomatic treatment and hygiene are of major importance. Correction of dehydration is necessary in infants with severe diarrhoea. Chloramphenicol 50 mg per kg should be given daily in divided doses for two weeks or more.

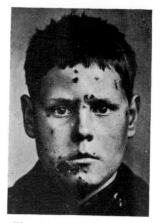

Fig. 15.20   Impetigo of face.

SKIN INFECTIONS

Bacterial infections of the skin are in most instances due to staphylococci or streptococci, the manifestations varying with age and immunity of the patient and the virulence of the infection, while other factors such as lack of cleanliness, hormonal secretions, and allergy may influence the picture in individual cases. Certain families may harbour these infections for long periods, many members of the family being affected at different times. Secondary staphylococcal infection frequently complicates scabies and pediculosis capitis, and is likely to persist if the primary condition remains untreated. Skin infections of the newborn (p. 57) and erysipelas (p. 342) have already been considered.

Impetigo contagiosa

The infection may be either streptoccccal or staphylococcal, and is highly contagious. It is spread by towels, washing utensils, and direct contact. The lesions first appear as vesicles, usually on the face, ears, nostrils, or scalp; the vesicles then become purulent, rupture, and exude a seropurulent discharge which forms loosely adherent crusts (Fig. 15.20). Occasionally the vesicles coalesce to form large bullae. More deeply seated infections are described as *ecthyma*.

Treatment consists of removal of the crusts with cetrimide soap and water followed by application of neomycin/bacitracin or tetracycline ointment. Systemic antibiotic therapy may be required if local treatment is not rapidly effective. An infected child should be excluded from school and must keep strictly to individual toilet articles, which should be sterilized after use.

Furunculosis

Multiple boils, due to infection of sebaceous glands or hair follicles, may occur in debilitated infants or children of school age. When furunculosis is recurrent, the possibility of underlying disease such as diabetes or hypogammaglobulinaemia should be considered. In infants the lesions occur principally on the scalp and in children on the back or buttocks. General cleanliness and application of hexachlorophene to the skin will help to prevent spread. Hot compresses afford relief in the early stages; incision may be needed when pus forms. Antibiotic treatment must be guided by the sensitivity of the organism. Autogenous vaccines in chronic cases are of value, while improvement of the child's general health and nutrition is essential.

Acne vulgaris

This is a disorder of the sebaceous glands of the face, neck, and trunk which frequently occurs in boys at puberty and rather less commonly in girls at the same age; it is rare in childhood. The gland becomes blocked with sebaceous material and acne bacilli, forming a comedo which is black at the orifice of the gland. Secondary infection leads to the formation of pustules.

Comedones ('blackheads') should be removed with an extractor after thorough cleansing of the area with cetrimide soap and hot water, and a lotion containing precipitated sulphur, zinc sulphate, and potassium sulphate applied. Attention should be paid to the general health and diet: excessive consumption of animal fat should be avoided. Antibiotic therapy is possibly of value if combined with local treatment. Reassurance that

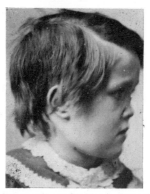

Fig. 15.21   Depressed nasal bridge in congenital syphilis.

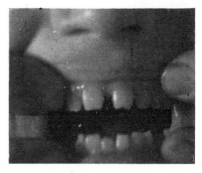

Fig. 15.22   Hutchinson's teeth. Boy aged 10 years.

acne is a common disorder at puberty and will tend to improve spontaneously later is important, though it must not take the place of treatment.

SYPHILIS

Syphilis is a generalized infection caused by a spirochaete, *Treponema pallidum*. The clinical features of the disease at birth and in early infancy are considered on p. 35. In childhood, it is generally the late result of congenital infection and is very seldom acquired postnatally. Juvenile congenital syphilis has become much less common in recent years and is now rarely seen in Britain. Manifestations appearing for the first time during childhood suggest that active infection is still present and that the early lesions have passed unrecognized or have been inadequately treated.

CLINICAL FEATURES. It will usually be found that the untreated patient has been below average height and weight for age for as long as measurements are available. Chronic hepatic and renal dysfunction probably contribute to the retardation of development.

The skin is often dry, wrinkled, and inelastic, and shows irregular pigmentation. Linear scars (rhagades) at the angle of the mouth are characteristic. While the face often appears somewhat abnormal, there is no diagnostic feature except the depressed nasal bridge resulting from ulceration and destruction of the nasal cartilage.

Teeth. The milk teeth are frequently small, irregular, and poorly calcified, but there are no changes in the first dentition which can be attributed exclusively to syphilis, with the possible exception of cup-shaped erosion of the deciduous molars. The second dentition, however, often shows changes which are diagnostic.

The permanent incisors, which are normally wider peripherally than at the gum margin, are likely to be peg-shaped in congenital syphilis, i.e. the sides of the tooth slope inward to the biting edge, due to defective development of the central cusp. The upper central incisors are most commonly affected (Hutchinson's teeth). The biting edge is often notched also, but this is not diagnostic of syphilis, and notched incisors are frequently seen in otherwise normal individuals.

The first permanent molars may show the same type of deformity as the incisors. The crown of the tooth, instead of showing the cusps standing out boldly, is incurved, and the cusps undeveloped, forming small rounded excrescences (Moon's or 'mulberry' molars).

Bones. The destructive bone lesions seen in infancy do not persist into childhood. The commonest type of bone lesion is a diffuse inflammatory thickening of the diaphysis. This gives rise to anterior curving of the tibia, the bone most commonly affected (*sabre tibia*).

Painless symmetrical effusion into joints (Clutton's joints) may occur without evidence of

 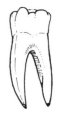

Syphilitic   **Normal**

FIRST MANDIBULAR MOLAR

Fig. 15.23   Syphilitic molar removed from a boy of 14 years, compared with normal.

neighbouring bony involvement. The knees are most commonly affected, but the lesions may be multiple. They must be distinguished from effusions due to rheumatoid arthritis, trauma, and other causes. Destructive lesions of the joints (Charcot's joints) are very rare in childhood.

Viscera. Both liver and spleen may be enlarged, firm, smooth, and non-tender, but hepatosplenomegaly is much less common in childhood than in infancy. Evidence of renal involvement may be shown by proteinuria. The lungs in some cases show extensive fibrosis, radiating fanwise from the hilum.

Eyes. The most common lesion of the eye, *interstitial keratitis*, is generally bilateral and may interfere seriously with vision. It usually develops between 5 and 15 years of age. The first complaint is photophobia or disturbance of vision in one eye, but examination will often show that both eyes are in fact affected, and that there is some degree of associated iridocyclitis. The cornea has a ground-glass appearance, and there is conjunctivitis. Local treatment includes atropinization during the acute phase, and protection of the eyes from strong light. Good results have been obtained from the instillation of $\frac{1}{2}$ to 1 per cent hydrocortisone eye drops, particularly when the lesion is an early one.

Various types of choroido-retinal degeneration occur as the result of congenital syphilis, the most striking appearance being produced by a punctate distribution of pigment, the 'pepper and salt' fundus. In other cases, extensive degeneration and scarring will cause impairment of vision.

Ears. Deafness is a relatively common symptom, and is usually due to involvement of the middle ear or temporal bone rather than to neurosyphilis. The prognosis depends to some extent on early recognition and treatment, but some cases fail entirely to improve once deafness is established.

Nervous system. Meningo-vascular inflammation begins at the time of the general dissemination in intrauterine life but may remain clinically latent for years. The ultimate manifestations are very variable, and include progressive mental retardation, convulsions, paralyses varying from hemiplegia to single cranial nerve palsies, optic atrophy, and hydrocephalus. There may be clinical evidence of syphilitic meningitis, though meningitis is much more commonly present than it is manifest.

The classical adult pictures of tabes dorsalis and of general paralysis of the insane are rarely seen before puberty.

TREATMENT. The treatment of juvenile syphilis is less satisfactory than that of early syphilis, since the disease has been established for a much longer period, and many of the pathological changes are irreversible. Intensive penicillin therapy should be given over a period of 14 days, a course of 7 to 14 million units being administered in divided doses. This initial course should be followed by two courses each of 10 bi-weekly injections of 900,000 units of procaine penicillin in oil, with aluminium monostearate (P.A.M.). Such a regimen will arrest the disease in a substantial proportion of cases, but patients should be kept under long-term observation and re-treated if there is evidence of relapse.

The blood Wassermann reaction is always positive in untreated cases. In congenital neurosyphilis, the reaction is also positive in the cerebrospinal fluid. Tests of cure should provide for three-monthly Wassermann reactions on the blood and, if necessary, the cerebrospinal fluid, at least until the reaction has been negative for two years.

VIRUS INFECTIONS

Recent advances in virus research have included the culture and identification of an increasing number of viruses from the alimentary and respiratory tracts, cerebrospinal fluid, etc., of which the pathogenicity and clinical manifestations are not yet fully clarified. Classification is in many instances still tentative, though it is convenient to speak of the enteroviruses (including the polioviruses, Coxsackie B, and ECHO, or 'enteric cytopathogenic human orphan', viruses); adenoviruses; pox viruses (including smallpox, vaccinia, and molluscum contagiosum); herpes viruses (varicella and herpes); the respiratory viruses, and the myxoviruses (including influenza subtypes A to D and mumps). It is clear that some of the 'new' viruses may give rise to radically different clinical manifestations in different cases, and also that the same clinical picture, e.g. aseptic meningitis, encephalitis, may be associated with a wide variety of viral infections. Thus group B Coxsackie viruses have been identified in cases of epidemic pleurodynia (p. 315), aseptic meningitis, myocarditis of the newborn, infantile paralysis, and encephalitis. ECHO viruses were originally isolated from the faeces of healthy children, but various types have since been found to be responsible for aseptic meningitis, fever with or without exanthem, encephalitis, and summer diarrhoea. Adenoviruses have been identified in association with non-streptococcal tonsillitis, pharyngeal conjunctival fever, primary atypical pneumonia without cold agglutinins, and so on.

At the present time, the progress that has been made in immunization has not been paralleled by similar advances in treatment. With the exception of the mantle viruses, e.g. of psittacosis and trachoma, viruses have in general proved resistant to chemotherapeutic agents, and though the encouraging results with idoxuridine in herpes simplex infection and methisazone in smallpox prophylaxis suggest that effective antiviral therapy comparable to the antibiotics in bacterial infections may ultimately be found, no specific therapy is yet of established clinical value.

Measles (*Rubeola; Morbilli*)

The disease rarely attacks infants under 4 months of age, since the great majority are born with a congenital immunity to the infection which is gradually lost. Between 6 months and 5 years, most unimmunized children are infected and acquire an immunity which is usually permanent. The disease becomes epidemic at short intervals (usually alternate years), epidemics reaching their peak in the late winter and spring. The disease is readily communicable by droplet infection during the catarrhal stage, and becomes less so after the rash has appeared.

CLINICAL FEATURES. The incubation period is 10 to 12 days to the onset of symptoms. The first stage or *enanthem* is characterized by coryza, cough, conjunctivitis, photophobia, and a rise of temperature to about 38·5°C (101·3°F). The throat is injected and the cervical nodes may be slightly enlarged. *Koplik* spots appear during this stage, and are most valuable for establishing early diagnosis. They consist of pinhead erythematous lesions with a paler centre, situated on the buccal mucosa. They fade before or with the appearance of the rash. The facies is often characteristic, the eyelids appearing slightly puffy and the conjunctivae injected. A prodromal erythematous rash, which is not specific, is sometimes seen at this stage. After one or two days the temperature falls, and then rises again abruptly to a higher level, e.g. 39·5°C (103°F) on the fifth or sixth day.

This second rise of temperature ushers in the *exanthem*, a blotchy maculo-papular rash appearing first on the forehead and behind the ears and spreading rapidly over the face, trunk, and limbs. The lesions are often coalescent and very occasionally haemorrhagic. After three or four days, the colour of the rash changes and gradually fades, to be followed by fine, branny desquamation.

During the appearance of the rash the child is often severely ill and delirious, with persistent cough and signs of generalized bronchitis. In uncomplicated cases the temperature falls within two to three days of the exanthem, and there is rapid remission of general symptoms. Although infectivity is much less after the rash has appeared than during the catarrhal stage, it is generally advisable to isolate patients for a further week after the rash has occurred.

COMPLICATIONS. The distinction between the primary disease picture, which includes bronchitis and coryza, and respiratory complications, is somewhat arbitrary. *Laryngitis* is sometimes sufficiently severe to cause obstruction, and *otitis media* occurs in a significant proportion of cases.

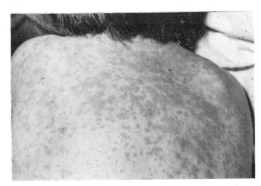

Fig. 15.24   The rash of measles.

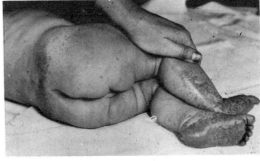

Fig. 15.25   Morbilliform rash caused by a drug (phenytoin).

Bronchopneumonia may occur either during the prodromal stage or later, and is evidenced by persistent pyrexia, dyspnoea, and exacerbation of cough, with scattered rales and signs of patchy consolidation in the lungs.

Encephalomyelitis. This rare sequela of measles occasionally occurs a week or more after the appearance of the rash (p. 361). The insidious development of subacute sclerosing panencephalitis some years later may also be a sequel of measles. In this condition early personality changes and falling off in school performance are followed by myoclonic spasms and convulsions. A characteristic EEG pattern of paroxysmal slow high-voltage waves appears and thereafter progressive intellectual and neurological deterioration ends in death a few weeks to a few years after onset.

PREVENTION. Active immunization against measles is considered on page 319. Its widespread adoption is likely to lead to a rapid decline in the incidence of the disease in childhood.

TREATMENT. Gammaglobulin given before the manifestations of the disease have appeared may suppress or modify the attack. There is no specific treatment for the attack itself. The use of penicillin in severely affected cases is probably of some value in reducing the incidence of complications, particularly otitis media, and antibiotics used in the treatment of bronchopneumonia have certainly lowered the mortality from secondary infection.

Skilled nursing and attention to the hygiene of the skin, mouth and eyes are of great importance.

PROGNOSIS. The great majority of children who contract measles make a successful recovery. Death from measles is now a rare occurrence in this country, though still frequent in some parts of the world, but it should not be forgotten that the annual morbidity directly attributable to the disease is still substantial.

Rubella (*German measles*)

The virus is thought to be harboured in the upper respiratory tract, and transmitted by droplet infection during the prodromal stage. It is less highly infectious than measles, but usually occurs in epidemics every three years or more at the same season. Children are more likely to be affected than infants; one attack gives permanent immunity. In view of the mild character of the disease, there is little advantage in attempting to guard against exposure in childhood; this applies particularly to girls, who will be protected by an attack in childhood against the risk of infection during pregnancy.

CLINICAL FEATURES. The incubation period is 14 to 21 days. Prodromal symptoms are often very slight; they include mild catarrh, sore throat, and enlargement of the posterior cervical and occipital lymph nodes; other nodes including the pre- and post-auricular, axillary and epitrochlear nodes may also be affected. The rash occurs on the second to fourth day and the temperature rises suddenly when the rash has appeared. Pyrexia is of short duration, usually lasting only one to three days, after which symptoms are minimal.

The rash is bright pink in colour, unlike the dusky-red rash of measles. It appears progressively on the face, neck, trunk, and limbs, and fades in the same order, leaving little staining. The lesions are typically discrete pin-head macules, but these may coalesce in various areas.

It is very rare for complications to occur, though occasional examples of purpura or post-infective encephalomyelitis have been described. The possible effects of maternal rubella on the fetus have been considered (p. 34).

DIAGNOSIS. The condition is distinguished from measles by the much less severe catarrhal symptoms, the pink colour of the rash, and the absence of Koplik spots. It should be noted, however, that many children with rubella do not develop a rash. Enlargement of the posterior cervical and occipital nodes is a valuable diagnostic feature. Blood examination may show leucopenia and the presence of Türk and plasma cells in the peripheral blood. Where accurate diagnosis is important, estimation of neutralizing antibodies and culture of the virus from throat washings may be undertaken.

TREATMENT. There is no specific treatment, and in view of the rarity of complications and the short duration of pyrexia, bed rest for three or four days is all that is required.

Roseola infantum (*Exanthem subitum*)

This is primarily a disease of infants aged between 6 months and 2 years and a virus etiology (possibly of the adenovirus group) is generally assumed. The incubation period is five to 15 days, and the onset sudden. The temperature rises to 39·5° or 40°C (103° or 104°F) and persists for three or four days. A macular, rose-red rash appears on the trunk, spreading to the face and limbs, as the temperature falls. The rash usually fades within 48 hours. Lymphadenopathy and relative lymphocytosis may occur. With the exception of convulsions, which are occasionally precipitated by the sudden rise of temperature, there are no complications, and the constitutional disturbance is usually slight. Mild cases are clinically indistinguishable from the minor illnesses with fever and rash caused by enteroviruses.

Pityriasis rosea

This disease has features suggesting a virus infection, but no causative organism has been identified and there is little likelihood of transmission to contacts. A rose-pink or yellowish-pink macular eruption appears approximately a week after an initial 'herald patch' and involves the trunk and upper thighs. There may be a slight rise of temperature, malaise, and local irritation at onset. The eruption lasts for some weeks and disappears spontaneously.

The condition must be differentiated from the exanthemata, ringworm or psoriasis. The mode of onset, the presence of a herald patch, and if necessary scrapings of the lesions (which will show no evidence of fungus infection), should clarify the diagnosis. No treatment is required.

Erythema exudativum multiforme (*Stevens-Johnson syndrome*)

This uncommon syndrome which occurs mainly in children is believed to be a hypersensitivity reaction, though it has some features suggesting a virus infection. In many cases an upper respiratory infection occurs one or two weeks before the typical manifestations, which include pyrexia, stomatitis, conjunctivitis, balanitis, and a rash. The last affects the cheeks, back of the chest and neck, and extends to the trunk, buttocks and limbs. The skin lesions consist of large purplish-red macules which may show a necrotic centre. A urethral discharge may accompany the balanitis. In some cases a pulmonary infection suggesting a virus pneumonia occurs.

Although the condition causes photophobia, dysphagia, and considerable malaise, and is occasionally fatal in the acute stage, it is usually self-limited with complete recovery. There is no specific treatment, though antibiotics may prevent secondary infection and corticosteroids are indicated in severe cases. Particular attention

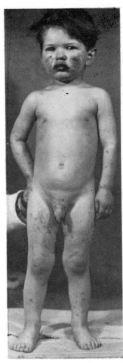

Fig. 15.26   Erythema exudativum multiforme, showing rash on cheeks and extremities, and stomatitis; patient also showed conjunctivitis and balanitis.

should be given to the care of the mouth, conjunctivae, and skin.

Mumps (*Epidemic parotitis*)

The disease is endemic in urban areas and occurs in epidemics during the late winter and early spring. It is spread by direct contact and droplet infection from saliva and the upper respiratory tract, but is not as highly infectious as measles and chickenpox. The virus has been isolated and a vaccine prepared. Children over 5 years of age and adolescents are most commonly affected. One attack usually confers permanent immunity.

CLINICAL FEATURES. The incubation period is 14 to 21 days, or rarely 12 to 28 days. Prodromal symptoms are often absent, but may include pyrexia up to 38·5°C (101·3°F), malaise, and sore throat. The first noticeable symptoms, however, are usually associated with parotid swelling, commonly unilateral, which is painful and causes discomfort on opening the mouth. The other salivary glands are often affected also, though seldom to the same extent as the parotids. The duration of the swelling is very variable; it may

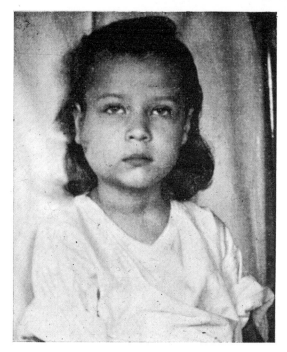

Fig. 15.27   Mumps, affecting principally the right parotid gland. (*Courtesy of* Parke, Davis and Co. Ltd.)

subside within two or three days of onset, or persist for two or more weeks. The temperature is seldom greatly raised and pyrexia usually lasts for only a few days.

COMPLICATIONS. Mumps is a generalized disease and the following complications, which are rare before puberty, are really manifestations of the disease itself. During adolescence, *orchitis* may occur seven to 10 days after the onset of parotid swelling, affecting 10 to 20 per cent of adolescent boys. *Oöphoritis* in girls is indicated by lower abdominal pain; *mastitis* may occur after puberty. *Pancreatitis* giving rise to recognizable symptoms is rare at all ages, but routine examination of the urine may show a temporary increase in urinary diastase. *Meningitis* and *encephalitis*, occurring eight to 10 days after the onset of symptoms, are rare but serious complications, though recovery is the rule. Deafness may result from damage to the inner ear.

TREATMENT. The patient should be isolated and kept at rest until pyrexia and malaise diminish. A fluid diet is usually indicated and the hygiene of the mouth requires attention to prevent secondary infection. There is little evidence that bed rest prevents complications, though when orchitis occurs, bed rest and support of the testicles will be required until the swelling has subsided.

Infectious mononucleosis (*Glandular fever*)

This disease is generally regarded as a virus infection. It is not very uncommon in children, but is liable to pass unrecognized unless an epidemic occurs in an institution and blood examinations are carried out.

CLINICAL FEATURES. The incubation period is probably 10 to 12 days. The onset may be insidious or characterized by sudden rise of temperature associated with sore throat and generalized lymph node enlargement. Splenomegaly occurs during the first week in approximately half the cases. Hepatic enlargement is less frequently present. Skin rashes, which are usually maculo-papular and situated principally on the trunk, frequently occur during the course of the illness, and slight jaundice is common. There may be evidence of meningeal irritation, with an increase of mononuclear cells and protein in the cerebrospinal fluid without alteration in sugar or chloride content.

DIAGNOSIS. The disease should be suspected when sore throat is followed by persistent pyrexia and lymphadenopathy, with or without splenomegaly, a transient rash or jaundice. The peripheral blood shows a white cell count of 10,000 to 20,000 per mm^3 with a high proportion (up to 75 per cent) of mononuclear cells. These cells are thought to be lymphocytic and typically have irregular vacuolated nuclei which are basophilic. The marrow appears normal. The presence of heterophile antibodies is demonstrated by the Paul-Bunnell test, which usually becomes positive during the second week. The blood-and-marrow picture and Paul-Bunnell test serve to distinguish the disease from leukaemia, and also from *acute infectious lymphocytosis*. In the latter condition the bone-marrow and peripheral blood show an increased number of small lymphocytes, and lymph node enlargement is absent.

TREATMENT. There is no specific treatment, with the possible exception of convalescent serum. Antibiotics are useful for the treatment of secondary infection.

Smallpox (*Variola*)

The disease is of world-wide distribution, but the incidence is falling due mainly to programmes of eradication sponsored by W.H.O.

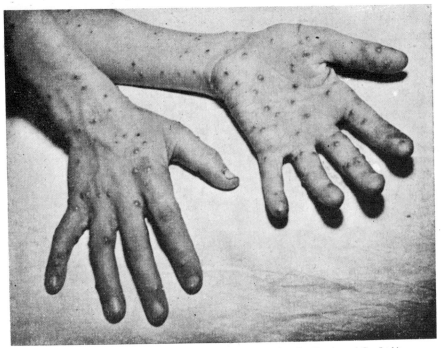

Fig. 15.28   Smallpox pustules on hands. (*Courtesy of* Parke, Davis and Co. Ltd.)

From time to time it is introduced into Britain by travellers from countries where it is still endemic. Such local outbreaks are controlled by isolation of the patients and vaccination and surveillance of contacts and their infrequency has warranted the abandonment of routine vaccination of all infants in this country. Smallpox is highly infectious and may be transmitted by direct contact and droplet infection, by the content of lesions or by crusts and by fomites. Infectivity of the patient persists from shortly before the prodromal symptoms appear until the skin lesions are completely healed. The disease affects all age groups and both sexes; one attack gives lasting immunity.

CLINICAL FEATURES. In its classical form, the disease is of great severity but it has become so much modified in countries where vaccination is widely practised, that it is usual to recognize two clinical types, *variola major* and *variola minor* (alastrim).

Variola major. The incubation period is approximately 10 days, with a range of seven to 18 days. The onset is sudden, with a rise of temperature which may reach 40·5°C (105°F). There is associated headache, vomiting, and pain in the back, and the patient appears severely ill.

After two to four days a transient erythematous rash appears, sometimes associated with petechial lesions in the flexures. This is followed by the typical eruption, which is at first macular and then papular. The papules become vesicular and the vesicles become pustular on the fifth or sixth day, finally forming crusts, which separate after two or three weeks to cause permanent pocking. The eruption may be haemorrhagic in severe cases and, in the most severe, extensive purpura appears at the macular stage.

The distribution and character of the eruption distinguishes the classical form from chickenpox. Thus the lesions are most profuse on the face and extremities and affect the palms and soles. The vesicles tend to be umbilicated and to become confluent. The lesions do not show the same tendency to appear in successive crops as do those of chickenpox, and are therefore mostly at the same stage of maturity at any given time.

With the appearance of the eruption, the temperature falls and remains low until pustulation occurs, when it is likely to show a secondary rise. Subsequent fall to normal occurs on the tenth day in uncomplicated cases.

Variola minor. This is caused by an attenuated strain of virus and represents a mild form of the disease. It is much more likely to be mistaken for chickenpox than is variola major. *Varioloid* is the description sometimes applied to modified smallpox occurring in patients who have been previously vaccinated but in whom immunity has waned.

DIAGNOSIS. In the differential diagnosis from chickenpox, the shorter incubation period, the simultaneous appearance of the lesions, and their distribution and character are the more important distinguishing points, while the occurrence of known cases of smallpox in the community will aid the diagnosis. Laboratory procedures include detection of the virus by direct examination of smears from lesions or by culture; demonstration of a specific antigen in lesions; and demonstration of a rising titre of antibody in the blood.

COMPLICATIONS AND PROGNOSIS. While the mortality from classical smallpox is likely to be over 30 per cent in early childhood, in variola minor it may be less than 1 per cent. The more important complications are skin sepsis and bronchopneumonia, both of which reduce the prospect of recovery. Corneal ulceration, myocarditis, encephalitis, otitis media, and nephritis are occasional complications.

TREATMENT. Vaccination will modify the attack if carried out during the incubation period, but is ineffective later. Antibiotics are probably of some value during the pustular stage of the eruption and in the prevention of secondary infection. The treatment, however, is largely symptomatic, special attention being paid to the eyes, skin and mouth.

Chickenpox (*Varicella*)

This is regarded as one of the inevitable diseases of childhood, and occurs in small epidemics during the winter and early spring. Children of school age are commonly affected and there appears to be a congenital immunity lasting up to six months in the infants of mothers who have had the disease. One attack usually, but not invariably, gives permanent immunity. The virus is primarily dermotropic, and is probably identical with that of herpes zoster. It is conveyed by contact and droplet transmission. Infectivity is thought to last not more than a week from the appearance of the eruption.

CLINICAL FEATURES. The incubation period is 14 to 21 days; the prodromal symptoms, which are transient, include pyrexia, headache, malaise and rash. The typical eruption is characterized

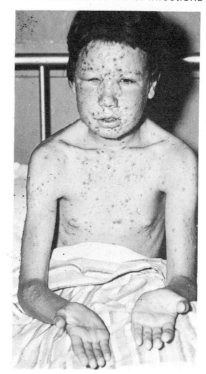

Fig. 15.29   Chickenpox, showing polymorphic eruption.

by crops of pink macules which rapidly become vesicular. The vesicles are superficial, thin-walled and oval, and soon form crusts, the progress from macule to crust lasting only two to four days. Lesions of different stages of maturity are commonly seen at the same time. Separation of the crust leaves a pink scar which subsequently becomes white or invisible, and pocking only occurs if the lesions have been scratched. The distribution of the eruption is centripetal, in distinction to that of smallpox, and though the extremities are likely to be affected to some extent, the trunk is the area principally involved. The lesions may also be profuse on the face and scalp. Constitutional symptoms are likely to be mild and complications other than skin sepsis are infrequent. Encephalopathy with fatty degeneration of the viscera occurs rarely in infants and chickenpox pneumonia very occasionally supervenes. Rare cases of disseminated chickenpox infection have been attributed to corticosteroid therapy.

DIAGNOSIS. Apart from smallpox (see above), the conditions to be considered in differential diagnosis are *herpes*, which may co-exist with chickenpox, *papular urticaria*, *impetigo*, and

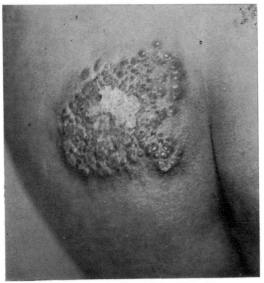

Fig. 15.30   Herpes of buttock.

pemphigus. In the case of papular urticaria, a history of similar lesions occurring in previous years will often be given.

TREATMENT. There is no specific treatment, and as the disease is almost always mild, the principal concern will be the prevention of secondary skin infection and scratching. There is often considerable discomfort and irritation, which will be relieved by daily bathing. When a child on corticosteroid therapy develops chickenpox, the dose of steroid should usually be maintained unchanged.

Herpes

At least two distinct types of herpes virus occur, causing *herpes simplex* and *herpes zoster* respectively. Both infections are characterized by the formation of crops of vesicles and give rise to localized burning or itching.

Herpes simplex, which occurs most commonly on the red margin of the lip and may extend to the face, is a frequent accompaniment of the common cold, pneumonia, and a variety of other acute infections and tends to recur. The virus may also cause stomatitis (p. 160) and necrotizing encephalitis. Herpes simplex infection of eczematous skin may give rise to acute illness with high sustained fever (Kaposi's varicelliform eruption).

Herpes zoster (*shingles*) is due to virus infection of a spinal root ganglion, and is manifested by the appearance of vesicles in the distribution of the corresponding nerve. Common sites are the chest and buttock. Facial herpes sometimes occurs in association with chickenpox, though this is less common in children than in adults. Vesiculation is often preceded by severe itching, and less commonly by transient pyrexia and pain. The condition is in general less severe in children than in adult patients, and vesiculation is normally followed by crusting and recovery.

A zinc-and-starch dusting powder should be used during the stage of vesiculation, and analgesics may be necessary when there is uncontrollable irritation or neuralgic pain. There is no specific treatment.

A herpes virus infection sometimes causes neuritis of the seventh cranial nerve, giving rise to unilateral facial paralysis (*Bell's palsy*). In most instances, however, the cause of the neuritis is obscure. Paralysis is often preceded by upper respiratory infection; it rarely affects children under two years of age. Although the condition is distressing, causing disfigurement and difficulty in speaking and eating, complete recovery is usual after some weeks or months. Treatment includes protection of the cornea and prevention of stretching of the paralysed muscles. Corticosteroids may hasten recovery.

Warts (*Verrucae*)

These are epithelial growths, which may be flat, filiform or pedunculated, occurring in any area, but commonly on the hands, neck, or soles. The virus infection is transmitted by contact, and in the case of plantar warts most commonly by walking barefoot over contaminated surfaces, e.g. in swimming baths. Plantar warts are apt to be depressed to the level of the sole and are painful.

Many treatments have been used, including suggestion, which is sometimes successful, surgical curettage and cauterization under local or general anaesthesia. Local application of trichloracetic acid, salicylic acid, or podophyllin paint may be given a trial particularly when the warts are multiple.

A somewhat similar condition, *molluscum contagiosum*, also due to a virus infection which is autoinoculable, occurs principally on the face, trunk, and buttocks. The lesions consist of raised papules which are of pink or pearly colour with a central dimple from which cheesy material can be squeezed. The lesions should be evacuated or incised and cauterized with silver nitrate or phenol.

Poliomyelitis (*Infantile paralysis*)

The incidence and severity of poliomyelitis did not decrease significantly during the first half of the century but in recent years there has been a dramatic decline in areas where mass vaccination has been practised. The causative organism is a small filtrable virus, of which there are three types, which can be cultured and transmitted to monkeys. The virus is excreted in the faeces, not only by infected patients for weeks after the onset of illness, but also by a high proportion of home contacts. The virus has also been obtained from flies in contact with infected excreta. Since it is exceptional, even in an epidemic, to obtain clear evidence of case to case infection by direct contact, it is assumed that carriers, non-paralytic cases, and possibly insect vectors, are largely responsible for spread. It has been suggested that both contaminated water and milk may be vehicles of transmission.

The portal of entry is usually the nasopharynx or the intestine, the virus reaching the central nervous system by way of motor or sensory nerves or the autonomic nervous system. The infection is likely to be severe in recently tonsillectomized children developing the disease, and tonsillectomy should not be performed during an epidemic. Intramuscular injections, e.g. for immunization, may occasionally be followed by provocation poliomyelitis in the injected limb.

At necropsy in fatal cases, acute oedema of the spinal cord and some degree of encephalitis are seen. The anterior horn cells of the cord and cranial motor nerve nuclei show degenerative changes, the lumbar and cervical areas of the cord being those most affected. In patients who survive, the oedema will subside and permanent damage is likely to be less than suggested by the degree of initial paralysis.

EPIDEMIOLOGY. Sporadic cases occur throughout the year in temperate climates, but most commonly in the late summer or early autumn. Before the introduction of poliomyelitis immunization, epidemics occurred at irregular intervals, usually following a hot dry season; but even in the severest epidemics, only a small proportion of the total population developed clinical evidence of the disease. In most countries the infection fell most heavily on children aged 2 to 5 years, but American figures showed that the age incidence there was gradually changing and that older children and young adults represented a higher proportion of the total cases than in earlier epidemics. In areas where incidence has declined due to vaccination, there is a risk of poliomyelitis occurring in unvaccinated contacts of children receiving oral vaccine.

A syndrome indistinguishable from that of poliomyelitis may be caused by ECHO or Coxsackie viruses.

CLINICAL FEATURES. The incubation period is not accurately known, but is thought to be seven to 14 days. Several clinical types of the disease occur, which are variously classified, e.g. *abortive type*, in which only prodromal symptoms occur; *non-paralytic type*, with clinical evidence of meningeal involvement, but without paralysis (see aseptic meningitis, p. 361); *paralytic type*, which may be further subdivided into those with paralysis of spinal origin, those with brain-stem involvement, etc.; *cerebral type* (polioencephalitis); and *cerebellar type*, characterized by ataxia either without or associated with paralysis. Abortive and non-paralytic cases are most likely to be recognized in the course of an epidemic.

PRODROMAL SYMPTOMS. These do not always occur or may be overlooked, but a high proportion of patients have gastrointestinal or respiratory symptoms, associated with headache and low-grade pyrexia lasting two or more days and occurring approximately five days before the pre-paralytic stage. The temperature falls to normal and rises again as the pre-paralytic stage is reached, giving a double-humped or 'dromedary' temperature chart.

PRE-PARALYTIC STAGE. The temperature rises to 38° or 39°C (101° or 102°F) and there is associated headache and pain in the back. Drowsiness or irritability often occur, but the patient may be mentally alert. On examination the child shows rigidity of neck and back, the latter being an important diagnostic point. If the child is asked to kiss his knees, he is unable to reach them. When he is asked to sit up, he will do so with back held rigidly and support himself with his hands placed on the bed behind him. Kernig's sign is positive. The tendon reflexes may be increased at this stage. A considerable proportion of patients recover without developing paralysis; exercise or fatigue at this stage favours severe muscular involvement.

PARALYTIC STAGE. Paralyses usually appear within three days of onset of the pre-paralytic stage, and before the temperature has fallen to normal. The affected muscles are tender and may be in spasm at first. In the majority of cases paralysis is maximum within a few hours of onset, and tends to diminish as the inflammatory changes in the nervous system subside: but in some instances paralysis progresses for several days. The temperature usually remains raised for four or five days and falls gradually to normal.

Any muscles or muscle groups may be affected, though symmetrical paralysis is exceptional. Paralysis of the paravertebral muscles is apt to be overlooked, the patient subsequently developing a severe scoliosis. The most severe types are those in which there is bulbar paralysis, or in which the respiratory muscles and diaphragm are paralysed.

Polioencephalitis is characterized by increasing drowsiness occurring early and passing into stupor. There are frequently associated cranial nerve and other palsies. Some patients die without regaining consciousness, and those that survive may be left with mental disturbance or severe paralysis.

CONVALESCENCE. The initial paralysis usually diminishes to some extent after a period of two or more weeks, and improvement may continue for several months. The affected muscles become flaccid with loss of tendon reflexes and atrophy, while contraction of opposing muscles will tend to produce severe deformities. When the chronic stage is reached, six months to a year after the initial infection, no further spontaneous improvement can be expected.

DIAGNOSIS. Accurate diagnosis during the prodromal stage is virtually impossible on clinical grounds alone, since the symptoms and signs are in no way specific. With the onset of the pre-paralytic stage, the rigidity of the back, pyrexia, etc., call for a lumbar puncture. The fluid is clear, under slightly increased pressure, and shows 50 to 200 cells per mm³. The cells may be polymorphonuclear at onset, but are typically lymphocytic. The globulin is increased and the sugar and chloride normal; no organisms are found and the fluid forms no clot on standing. These features will distinguish poliomyelitis from tuberculous and other bacterial types of meningitis. The differential diagnosis of aseptic meningitis due to other viruses requires special laboratory techniques. In meningism the cell count will not be significantly raised and there will be evidence of infection elsewhere, e.g. pneumonia. In infective polyneuritis the protein content of the fluid is very high, but the cell count is unlikely to be raised. Once paralysis has occurred, the clinical diagnosis is usually clear, though lumbar puncture may give confirmation if performed within a few days of onset.

Polioencephalitis requires virological studies to distinguish it from other types of encephalitis. Bulbar paralysis is indicated by cranial nerve palsies, nasal voice, regurgitation of fluids through the nose, respiratory distress, inability to cough, accumulation of secretions in the pharynx, and tachycardia. When there is intercostal or diaphragmatic paralysis, the accessory muscles of respiration will be called into play. It is important to assess the extent and nature of the paralysis as promptly as possible, so that progress and treatment can be properly regulated.

TREATMENT. Patients should be kept at rest and isolated during the acute illness. It is advisable to nurse the child lying flat, with bed-boards under the mattress, and a foot-board to prevent foot-drop. Patients with bulbar paralysis should have the foot of the bed raised to assist drainage of secretions, and an aspirator should be used to remove pharyngeal secretions. Positive pressure ventilation through a naso-tracheal or tracheostomy tube may be required. During the acute phase, these children should be given intravenous fluids owing to the danger of inhalation of fluids given by mouth or stomach-tube. Patients with paralysis of the intercostal muscles or diaphragm may require prolonged treatment with a ventilator.

Paralysed muscles must be kept in the position which will prevent deformities from the contracture of opposing muscles. Hot packs or ice bags should be applied to relieve muscle pain and spasm. After all tenderness has disappeared, passive and then active movement should be instituted. There is no specific treatment, convalescent serum having proved valueless. The late treatment, when spontaneous improvement can no longer be expected, is orthopaedic.

Acute viral encephalitis

This is most commonly due to mumps virus, the enteroviruses or herpes viruses, although many other viruses may occasionally be responsible. Within three to four weeks of infection, the child becomes restless, complains of headache and may vomit, and then rapidly lapses into delirium or coma. The temperature may be slightly raised or as high as 41°C (105·8°F). Occasionally, early behavioural changes suggest an emotional disturbance while in other cases convulsions are the presenting feature.

Physical signs are variable and include neck stiffness, cranial nerve palsies and papilloedema. The cerebrospinal fluid is clear, contains 0 to 200 lymphocytes per mm^3 and is bacteriologically sterile. Protein and glucose are normal or slightly increased.

Serum should be sent for antibody studies on admission and 14 days later, a significant rise in specific antibody to a virus indicating the diagnosis. Attempts should be made to isolate virus from faeces, cerebrospinal fluid and throat swabs.

There is no effective specific treatment but good nursing is essential and intensive therapy, including mechanical ventilation, may be required. Recovery usually occurs eventually but is often incomplete, with residual mental retardation, personality changes or paralyses.

Aseptic meningitis syndrome

This term includes a wide range of viral infections or post-infective reactions characterized by meningeal irritation in the absence of clinical evidence of encephalitis. In all there are likely to be neck rigidity, positive Kernig's sign and headache associated with cerebrospinal fluid changes similar to those in viral encephalitis. Viral infections directly responsible for the syndrome include enterovirus infections, mumps, herpes, primary atypical pneumonia, infective hepatitis, lymphocytic choriomeningitis, infectious mononucleosis, and infectious lymphocytosis; the post-infective states following measles, rubella, chickenpox, smallpox, and vaccinia may also give rise to a meningeal reaction but are considered under post-infective encephalomyelitis (see below).

Lymphocytic choriomeningitis (*benign lymphocytic meningitis*) is due to a virus (L.C.M.) transmitted by mice, which can be isolated from the blood and cerebrospinal fluid. The clinical picture is similar to that of other types of aseptic meningitis with associated influenza-like symptoms; the cell count in the cerebrospinal fluid ranges from 150 to over 20,000 lymphocytes per mm^3. The disease normally runs a short course of approximately two weeks, followed by complete recovery, but occasionally fatal cases with encephalitis or myelitis occur.

Post-infective encephalomyelitis

This occasionally follows vaccination, measles, and chickenpox, and still more rarely rubella and smallpox. It is thought that the condition is due to an antigen–antibody reaction, perhaps combined with a direct action of the virus. The clinical picture is somewhat similar in each type, though the mortality is apt to be greater after vaccination and complications commoner following measles. Symptoms appear in the first or second week after the original illness and include somnolence deepening to coma, convulsions, paralyses, incontinence, and papilloedema, associated with pyrexia. Less commonly, there is paraplegia (myelitic type). The cerebrospinal fluid shows a raised lymphocyte count and increased globulin, but no alteration in sugar or chloride content. In fatal cases there is extensive demyelinization and perivascular infiltration of the brain.

The immediate mortality is as high as 30 to 40 per cent in post-vaccinal encephalomyelitis, and lower in other types. In patients who survive, the duration of the acute illness is usually a matter of days. Residual paralyses or mental changes occur in a proportion of cases. Treatment is symptomatic.

Infective polyneuritis (*Guillain-Barré syndrome*)

This rare condition, of which the virus etiology is not established, is characterized by an ascending and symmetrical paralysis, which may follow an acute infection. In the severest forms, respiratory or bulbar paralysis occurs, often associated with facial paralysis. The cerebrospinal fluid shows a very high protein content, e.g. 200 to 800 mg per cent, with little or no cellular increase or alteration of sugar or chloride content.

The majority of childhood cases run a chronic but favourable course, with very gradual return of function. The deep tendon reflexes are absent and are likely to remain so long after recovery is otherwise complete. There is no specific treatment; patients with respiratory or bulbar paralysis will require the same treatment as in poliomyelitis. In view of the chronicity of the disease and the prospect of ultimate recovery, skilled nursing, prevention of respiratory infection, and occupational therapy are particularly important.

Influenza

Studies of influenza epidemics have shown that many different strains of the three main types of influenza virus (A, B and C) may be responsible for the clinical disease and that the findings are not uniform even in the same epidemic. Secondary invading bacteria, including *Haemophilus influenzae*, *Staphylococcus aureus*, and pneumococci, are of varying importance in different epidemics in causing complications. The disease is spread to the respiratory tract by droplets and commonly becomes epidemic in the winter and spring.

CLINICAL FEATURES. Clinical influenza cannot be regarded as a specific disease, and the symptoms in different outbreaks show considerable variation. Pyrexia and constitutional symptoms (malaise, headache, shivering, muscular pains, and prostration) are the most constant; respiratory symptoms, varying from cough and catarrh to bronchopneumonia, occur in a considerable proportion of cases, though they are often mild in relation to the constitutional disturbance. Gastrointestinal symptoms (vomiting, diarrhoea, and abdominal discomfort) are a marked feature of certain epidemics. Nervous symptoms are less common, and must be distinguished from those due to encephalitis.

Children tend to be less severely affected than adults. The primary disease may be difficult to distinguish clinically from the common cold, and the diagnosis usually rests on the presence of an epidemic or known contact. Blood examination may show a leucopenia, but this is not a constant finding.

COMPLICATIONS. Apart from the complications common to most infections involving the upper respiratory tract, viz. otitis media and bronchitis, influenza is in some epidemics followed by a peculiarly virulent and fatal form of bronchopneumonia, characterized by blood-stained sputum, severe toxaemia, and dyspnoea. Patients who recover are apt to be left with pulmonary fibrosis which may subsequently lead to bronchiectasis.

TREATMENT. There is no specific treatment for the primary infection, but antibiotic therapy is of great value in preventing complications and should be used in severe cases or in epidemics in which complications are frequent.

MYCOTIC INFECTIONS

Actinomycosis

Infection with *Actinomyces israeli* is rare in childhood, but is of some importance in the differential diagnosis of chronic suppuration of the face, jaws, neck, or lungs, or following appendicitis. The organism consists of branching filaments, growing anaerobically, but difficult to culture; actinomycotic pus contains yellow 'sulphur' granules, best seen after shaking the pus with saline. The organism exists as a harmless saprophyte in the gastrointestinal tract, becoming pathogenic when it gains entrance to the deeper tissues through a local lesion of the mucosa.

CLINICAL FEATURES. The disease is characterized by its chronicity, the profuse production of granulation tissue, and the tendency of the lesions to break down and suppurate. Owing to the common occurrence of dental caries and the liability of the gums to trauma, the mouth, cheek, and neck form the commonest site of lesions. A hard swelling forms around the root of a carious tooth, or on the face or neck, and later softens and suppurates. The caecum or appendix may be involved after an attack of acute appendicitis. The patient is likely to show evidence of intra-abdominal suppuration, and in chronic cases a large indurated mass may be felt in the right iliac fossa.

Pulmonary infection may be primary or arise by extension from infection of the pharynx or abdomen. A preceding history of inhaled foreign body is sometimes obtained. The clinical picture

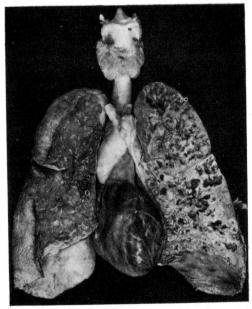

Fig. 15.31 Actinomycosis of left lung, showing multiple abscess cavities.

often simulates a pneumonia with delayed resolution and persistent cough. The diagnosis is likely to be made when a superficial swelling containing thick pus and granules appears over the lower ribs. The affected portion of the lung may be found riddled with abscess cavities (Fig. 15.31), while the opposite lung remains unaffected.

TREATMENT AND PROGNOSIS. The organism is sensitive to sulphadiazine and penicillin, and combined and intensive therapy should be given as soon as the diagnosis is established. Tetracycline is effective also. Unfortunately delay in diagnosis is often responsible for wide extension of the disease. In localized infections, e.g. of the alveolus, surgical removal may be possible.

Aspergillosis

The mould *Aspergillus fumigatus* may occasionally invade the lungs in childhood, forming granulomatous masses visible radiologically as a patchy infiltration. The Aspergillus is resistant to antibiotics and indeed the infection may be favoured by long-term antibiotic therapy. Sulphonamides and nystatin may be effective but the results of treatment are disappointing and the condition may be rapidly fatal.

Dermatomycoses

Fungus infections of the skin and scalp are relatively common in temperate climates and of very frequent occurrence in tropical areas. Children of school age are more commonly affected than infants, particularly when they are using common baths, toilet utensils, etc. The school health service, however, has done much to reduce the incidence of ringworm of the scalp and skin which was previously one of the commonest infections of schoolchildren. The great majority of these infections are caused by Trichophyton (hair, skin, and nails), Microsporon (hair and skin), and Epidermophyton (skin and nails), but since dermal or vaginal infections with Candida may occur, it is essential that the organism should be identified by laboratory means. Griseofulvin (a fungistatic antibiotic) is effective against Trichophyton, Microsporon, and Epidermophyton, but not against Candida. It is given orally, 250 mg two to four times daily, up to a total of 10 mg per kg. Candida infections should be treated with local applications of nystatin.

Ringworm of the hands and feet (*Athlete's foot*)

This common infection usually remains limited to the feet, especially the skin between the toes, which becomes white and macerated. There is considerable irritation and denuded areas bleed when rubbed or scratched. The infection is apt to be very chronic, though showing remissions and exacerbations; reinfection from shoes frequently occurs.

PREVENTION. Since infection is often acquired in swimming baths, these should be provided with foot-baths containing disinfectant, through which all users are required to pass, and floors and bath-mats should be regularly disinfected.

TREATMENT. · Mild infections will usually respond to the use of Whitfield's ointment or other antifungal preparations. The socks should be changed daily and disinfected and a dusting powder used.

Tinea capitis (*Ringworm of scalp*)

This infection may be due to Microsporon or Trichophyton and is liable to become epidemic in schools. The mycelium invades the scalp and subsequently the follicle and shaft of the hair. Small red papules form, the hairs break off, and the affected area becomes largely denuded; in some cases a pustular eruption (*kerion*) occurs. Diagnosis is made by microscopic examination of scrapings of scalp and of infected hairs, or inspection of the hairs under Wood's light. Treatment with griseofulvin is highly effective.

Favus

Infection of the scalp with *Trichophyton schoenleini* is characterized by the formation of pustules followed by crusting and alopecia. Treatment is similar to that of tinea capitis.

Tinea cruris and tinea circinata

The former consists of pinkish-brown scaly marginated lesions, occurring in the groins, scrotum, or perianal region. The lesions of tinea circinata (or corporis) are similar, but occur on any part of the trunk, limbs, or face. Tinea cruris is usually due to an Epidermophyton and is acquired from infected towels or clothing. Tinea circinata is due to a Microsporon or Trichophyton and may be of animal origin. Treatment with oral griseofulvin and topical application of antifungal ointment or paint usually results in rapid cure.

PARASITIC INFESTATIONS

Climate and *standard of living* are of first importance in governing the incidence of parasitic infestation. In many tropical areas malaria represents a major cause of infant mortality and morbidity, and hookworm and ascaris infestations are so common in the childhood population that they are likely to form the background of almost any disease picture. The occurrence of malaria and filariasis will depend primarily on conditions suitable for life of a particular insect vector; infestation by bilharzia and guinea-worm on the presence of the appropriate snail or cyclops respectively in contaminated water; and trichiniasis on the eating of inadequately cooked pork. Only those infestations of clinical importance in temperate climates will be considered here, although it must be remembered that tropical diseases not hitherto seen to any extent in this country are being encountered with increasing frequency, owing to the ease and speed of modern travel.

PROTOZOAN PARASITES

Malaria

Although the Anopheles mosquito is found in certain areas in Britain, and malaria was previously endemic in the fen country, primary infection with malaria in Britain is now practically unknown. It may be encountered occasionally in schoolchildren returning from visits to parents in tropical countries during school holidays.

Unprotected children in malarious countries are liable to retardation of growth and development by repeated attacks of malaria, especially the malignant tertian form, which may cause death in the first few years. Children who survive develop anaemia and hepatosplenomegaly, but a degree of acquired immunity modifies the severity of subsequent attacks. Headache, drowsiness and fever are common symptoms and may occur in Britain in children who have recently arrived from abroad. The parasite may be found in the blood, although examination of several films may be necessary. Chloroquine is the drug of choice for therapy. Children going to malarious areas should be protected by a regular dose of proguanil or pyrimethamine.

Giardia lamblia

Parasites, which appear as trophozoites with eight flagella and also as ovoid cysts, have been found in the stools of pre-school children in residential nurseries. Their pathogenicity is somewhat dubious, and probably depends on the degree of infestation and factors such as gastro-intestinal infections due to other causes. It has been suggested that infestation can cause vague ill-health, abdominal discomfort, failure of fat absorption with the passage of pale bulky stools, and anaemia. Treatment with mepacrine, 25 to 50 mg twice daily for five days, or metronidazole, 50 to 100 mg daily for 10 days, will clear the stools of parasites.

Toxoplasmosis

Infection with *Toxoplasma gondii* may be acquired during infancy or childhood, and although the congenital form of the disease (p. 33) is likely to result in severer disabilities, it is probable that the acquired type is commoner than is generally recognized. Infection should be suspected in cases of unexplained lymphadenopathy with or without fever, maculopapular rash and muscle tenderness. Uveitis frequently occurs. Rare complications include encephalomyelitis, chorioretinitis, pneumonia, and myocarditis. The organism has been identified in the tissues and after transmission to mice, but the diagnosis is usually made by the demonstration of antibodies. Sulphadiazine has been used in treatment, but its effectiveness alone or in combination with pyrimethamine is not yet clearly established.

NEMATODES

The nematode parasites are elongated 'round worms', possessing in their adult state an alimentary canal and unsegmented cuticle, and showing differentiation of the sexes. In the case of threadworms, the ova are embryonated when they are passed in the faeces and are rapidly infective, being conveyed directly from the anal region to the mouth on the child's fingers. Whipworm infection is also of direct type. A modified direct type of infection occurs in the case of *Ascaris lumbricoides*. The ova are not embryonated when passed and become infective outside the body, e.g. in contaminated soil. They also reach the human intestine without an intermediate host, the eggs hatching in the intestine. The larvae then penetrate the intestinal wall, reaching the lungs via the blood-stream, whence they ascend to the trachea, are swallowed, and mature in the intestine. Indirect infection, in which the ova hatch outside the human host into larvae which penetrate the skin and so reach the blood-stream, lungs, trachea, and intestine, is illustrated by the hookworm.

Threadworms (*Pinworms: Oxyuris or Enterobius vermicularis*)

These are the commonest intestinal parasites in temperate climates. Children of all social classes are affected, though the incidence is highest amongst those living in overcrowded conditions. The worms infest the large intestine and particularly the caecum and appendix, the females being approximately 1 cm in length and the males 2 to 5 mm. Maturity is reached in about two weeks from ingestion of the ova. The mature adult female passes from the anus and lays her eggs on the perianal skin; a single female may lay over 10,000 eggs. The perianal irritation caused by the worms results in scratching and infection of the child's hands and nails; auto-reinfection by the mouth then occurs. Other members of the household may also be infected by contamination of food or house dust.

CLINICAL FEATURES. With the exception of anal and perineal pruritus, which may cause insomnia, symptoms are often minimal. Children may, however, become extremely distressed by a condition which their parents regard with obvious disgust, and a variety of nervous symptoms may be provoked by an unsympathetic or too obsessional attitude to the child's condition.

DIAGNOSIS. Adult worms may be recognized in the faeces, though they should be carefully examined to distinguish them from fragments of vegetable matter. The most satisfactory method of routine examination, which should be carried out on other members of the household when a case has been diagnosed, is by swabbing the anal region with a glass rod wrapped in a square of cellophane, followed by microscopic examination of the cellophane mounted in water for the presence of ova.

TREATMENT. Reinfection must be prevented by keeping the child's nails cut short and clean, and by scrupulous cleanliness in food-handling. Scratching should be prevented, e.g. by the wearing of close-fitting pants at night, and the perianal region should be regularly washed and dried.

The treatment of choice is a single dose of viprynium embonate (5 mg per kg), repeated one week later. Alternatively, piperazine elixir, containing the equivalent of 500 mg of the hydrate to 3·5 ml (1 fl dr), may be given daily for one week, the course being repeated if necessary after a week's interval. Infants of normal weight aged 9 months to 2 years require 3·5 ml daily; those between 2 and 4 years 5 ml daily; and children from 4 to 13 years 7 to 10 ml daily. Good results may also be obtained by a single dose of piperazine (100 mg per kg) combined with senna. A repeat dose is advisable two weeks later. Cure should be checked by re-examination of anal swabs. It must be emphasized that success in treatment depends largely on prevention of auto- and familial reinfection.

Ascaris lumbricoides (*Large roundworm*)

Although the distribution of the parasite is world-wide, infestation is uncommon in Britain. The adult worms measure 15 to 35 cm in length, the female being larger than the male; they inhabit the small intestine, whence they may be passed in the faeces, or reach the stomach and be vomited, or crawl from the nose. A mature female lays 25 million or more eggs, which are passed in the faeces, and, when they contaminate the soil, are liable to return to a human host.

CLINICAL FEATURES. The ingestion of large numbers of ova may be followed within five days by pyrexia and respiratory symptoms. When the adult worms reach the small intestine, they seldom give rise to symptoms and their presence is only recognized when a worm is passed in the faeces or vomited. Occasionally large masses of worms cause intestinal obstruction.

DIAGNOSIS. The naked-eye appearance of the adult worm is unmistakable. Examination of faeces may show ova in various stages of development. Eosinophilia (up to 10 per cent) frequently occurs, and may be associated with urticaria.

TREATMENT. Piperazine (as used in the treatment of threadworms) is the drug of choice. Bephenium hydroxynaphthoate in a single dose of 2·5 to 5 g is also effective.

Ancylostoma duodenale (*Hookworm*)

Ancylostomiasis is rare in Britain, but local outbreaks occasionally occur. The larvae penetrate the skin when the child walks over infected ground, causing local inflammation at the portal of entry. They are carried by the blood-stream to the lungs, and pass by way of the trachea to the oesophagus and small intestine. The adult worms are 1 to 1·5 cm in length and possess two pairs of teeth with which they attach themselves to the mucosa of the small intestine.

Hookworm infestation is often associated with severe anaemia and abdominal discomfort, particularly when there is widespread malnutrition. The blood shows a marked eosinophilia, and diagnosis is confirmed by finding the ova in the stools. Treatment must include correction of anaemia and malnutrition. Bephenium hydroxynaphthoate is effective and is less toxic than tetrachloroethylene. Prevention of infestation is effected by the proper disposal of sewage.

Toxocariasis (*Visceral larva migrans*)

Adult toxocara worms commonly inhabit the intestine of dogs (*Toxocara canis*) and cats (*T. cati*). They produce eggs which, if swallowed by children, hatch into larvae. These penetrate the intestinal wall and are carried in the bloodstream to various viscera, where they form granulomata. Clinical features of infestation include eosinophilia, hepatomegaly, choroidoretinitis, pneumonitis and epilepsy. Diagnostic skin and fluorescent antibody tests are available. Thiabendazole, 25 mg per kg daily for seven days, may be effective in treatment.

CESTODES

The cestodes, or tapeworms, are flat segmented worms, having a scolex (head) armed with suckers or hooks with which they attach themselves to the intestinal mucous membrane of their animal host. The peripheral segments, each of which contains a reproductive but no alimentary system, are shed off, passed in the faeces, and infect an intermediate host. The life cycle differs in different species, *Diphyllobothrium latum* passing first through a crustacean host and subsequently infecting fish and so man, while *Taenia solium* and *Taenia saginata* pass through a cysticercus stage in pigs and cattle respectively. Since cysticerci are destroyed by heat, infection of man is only likely to occur when meat or fish is eaten improperly cooked. Tapeworm infestation is uncommon in Britain, and is recognized when the flat, writhing segments of the worm are passed in the faeces. The purpose of treatment is to detach the scolex from the intestinal mucosa so that the worm is passed complete. A preliminary period of 24 to 48 hours fluid diet is indicated, and no fats should be given during this

time. Following a saline purge the previous evening, mepacrine (0·3 to 0·6 g depending on weight) is taken on an empty stomach. After a further saline purge, the stools should be carefully examined for the presence of the scolex. If this is not passed, the treatment will have to be repeated at a later date. An alternative drug is dichlorophen (70 mg per kg in divided doses over 24 hours). Tetrachloroethylene and extract of male fern are also used.

Hydatid disease

The presence of hydatids, the cystic stage of *Echinococcus granulosus* in man, is most likely to occur in sheep-rearing countries. Infection is from ova passed in the faeces of dogs. The larvae pass through the wall of the intestine, and become encysted in the liver or other tissues, where they gradually enlarge in size and form daughter cysts. The infection tends to be very chronic, but large cysts may rupture or become secondarily infected. In the liver they often project from the lower surface of the right lobe, but any part may be involved; hydatids may also occur in the lungs, kidneys, or nervous system. Surgical removal is the only treatment of value.

ARTHROPOD PARASITES

These may be divided for practical purposes into those which live externally to the body and cause symptoms by bites, stings, or local irritation; and those which burrow into the tissues. The former include lice, fleas, and bed-bugs, and the latter harvesters and the mite of scabies. In tropical areas the arthropods are of great importance both as vectors and as direct causes of disease, but in temperate regions their variety and significance is much more limited.

Pediculosis (*Lousiness*)

Louse infestation is closely related to low standards of personal hygiene and cleanliness. Of the three varieties of louse, *Pediculus capitis* (head-louse), *Ped. corporis* (body-louse), and *Phthirus pubis* (crab-louse), only the first is commonly found in childhood. The head-louse lays its eggs on the hair of the scalp; the eggs, or 'nits', are adherent to the individual hair, and appear as small whitish ovoid objects, projecting upward, and firmly attached by chitin at the base. The adult lice live in the hair and suck blood from the scalp. Their bites frequently become infected, and this will result in cervical and occipital lymph node enlargement. Pediculosis becomes of very great importance in areas where louse-borne typhus is endemic or epidemic. In general it is a measure of overcrowding and neglect, but head infestation is readily acquired by contact and children of all social strata may be affected.

TREATMENT. Pediculosis capitis must be treated by removal of nits with a fine comb and killing the adult lice with gamma benzene hexachloride or dicophane (DDT) application or with malathion lotion. This should be rubbed into the hair adjacent to the scalp and allowed to remain for 24 hours before washing. Subsequent applications will kill lice hatching from any nits which have not been removed.

Scabies (*The itch*)

The disease is due to infestation with a mite, *Sarcoptes scabiei*. The great majority of cases are due to close contact with an infested individual. The condition often affects several members of a family or institution, particularly when washing facilities are inadequate.

The six-legged larva hatches from an egg laid in the skin, migrates, and burrows into the skin to moult, reappearing as an eight-legged nymph. After further moults, the adult female mates and extends the skin-burrows in which the eggs are laid.

CLINICAL FEATURES. The presenting symptom is intense itching, worst at night, which results in scratching of lesions often followed by secondary pyogenic infection. Scratching spreads the disease to other areas.

The lesions occur most commonly between the fingers, around the wrists, on the anterior axillary wall, lower part of the buttocks, thighs, and ankles; the genitalia and umbilicus are often involved. Skin sepsis occurring in these areas should always suggest the likelihood of underlying scabies. The lesions consist of vesicles and linear burrows, the latter best seen in the webs of the fingers, but it is generally found that excoriations resulting from scratching are more obvious than the primary lesions by the time that the patient comes under observation. The diagnosis can be confirmed by examination of a mite removed from a skin-burrow.

TREATMENT. The patient should first be given a hot bath and the skin well scrubbed to open the vesicles and remove crusts. The whole body surface below the neck should then be treated with benzyl benzoate application B.P., using a soft brush, or with gamma benzene hexachloride cream. Repeated treatment may be necessary. Disinfestation of clothes and bedding is advisable.

BIBLIOGRAPHY AND REFERENCES

GENERAL

BUTLER, N. R. & BENSON, P. F. (1965). Immunization in general practice. *British Medical Journal*, i, 841.

CRUICKSHANK, R. (1970). Protection against specific infections. In *Child Life and Health*, 5th edn. Edited by R. G. Mitchell. London: Churchill.

DEPARTMENT OF HEALTH AND SOCIAL SECURITY (1968). *Immunization against Infectious Disease*. London: H.M.S.O.

DICK, G. (1971). Routine smallpox vaccination. *British Medical Journal*, iii, 163.

GALE, A. H. (1945). A century of changes in the mortality and incidence of the principal infections of childhood. *Archives of Disease in Childhood*, 20, 2.

KRUGMAN, S. (1971). Measles and rubella immunization. *Journal of Pediatrics*, 78, 1.

MEDICAL RESEARCH COUNCIL (1956). B.C.G. Report. *British Medical Journal*, i, 413.

MEDICAL RESEARCH COUNCIL (1962). Comparative trial of British and American oral poliomyelitis vaccines. *British Medical Journal*, ii, 142.

MEDICAL RESEARCH COUNCIL (1965). Report by the measles vaccination committee. *British Medical Journal*, i, 817.

MILLAR, E. L. M. (1971). The current immunization schedule. *Practitioner*, 206, 451.

POLLOCK, T. M. (1964). Control of measles by vaccination. *Proceedings of the Royal Society of Medicine*, 57, 849.

RAMSAY, A. M. & EDWARD, R. T. D. (1967). *Infectious Diseases*. London: Heinemann.

TUBERCULOSIS

BARCLAY, W. R. (1959). BCG vaccination. *Pediatrics, Springfield*, 24, 478.

BENTLY, F. J., GRZYBOWSKI, S. & BENJAMIN, B. (1954). *Tuberculosis in Childhood and Adolescence*. London: N.A.P.T.

CAMMOCK, R. M. & MILLER, F. J. W. (1953). Tuberculosis in young children. *Lancet*, i, 158.
CROFTON, J. (1959). Chemotherapy of pulmonary tuberculosis. *British Medical Journal*, i, 1610.
DANIELS, M. C. (1949). Tuberculosis in Europe during and after the Second World War. *British Medical Journal*, ii, 1065, 1135.
HORNE, N. W. (1971). Epidemiology and control of tuberculosis. *British Journal of Hospital Medicine*, 5, 732.
HUDSON, F. P. (1956). Clinical aspects of congenital tuberculosis. *Archives of Disease in Childhood*, 31, 136.
HUTCHISON, J. H. (1949). Bronchoscopic studies in primary tuberculosis in childhood. *Quarterly Journal of Medicine*, 69, 21.
LANCET (1972). Shorter chemotherapy in tuberculosis. *Lancet*, i, 1105.
LINCOLN, E. M. & VERA CRUZ, P. G. (1960). Progress in treatment of tuberculosis. *Pediatrics, Springfield*, 25, 1035.
LLEWELYN, D. M. & DORMAN, D. (1971). Mycobacterial lymphadenitis. *Australian Pediatric Journal*, 7, 97.
LORBER, J. (1954). The results of treatment of 549 cases of tuberculosis meningitis. *American Review of Tuberculosis*, 69, 13.
LOTTE, A., NOUFFLARD, H., DEBRÉ, R. & BRISSAUD, H. E. (1960). The treatment of primary tuberculosis in childhood. *Pediatrics, Springfield*, 26, 641.
MILLER, F. J. W., SEAL, R. M. E. & TAYLOR, M. D. (1963). *Tuberculosis in Children*. London: Churchill.
NAISH, P. F. (1969). Erythema nodosum. *Practitioner*, 202, 637.
RICH, A. R. (1944). *Pathogenesis of Tuberculosis*. Springfield, Ill.: Thomas. (With extensive bibliography.)
ROSENBERG, M. & GOTTLIEB, R. P. (1968). Current approach to tuberculosis in childhood. *Pediatric Clinics of North America*, 15, 513.
SORSBY, A. (1942). The aetiology of phlyctenular ophthalmia. *British Journal of Ophthalmology*, 26, 159.
WALLGREN, A. (1938). Erythema nodosum and pulmonary tuberculosis. *Lancet*, i, 359.
WORLD HEALTH ORGANIZATION (1964). Eighth report of expert committee on tuberculosis. Technical Report Series, W.H.O., no. 290.

OTHER BACTERIAL INFECTIONS

BIGGER, J. W. & HODGSON, G. A. (1943). Impetigo contagiosa. *Lancet*, i, 544.
BLACK, J. A. (1970). Treatment of bacterial meningitis in children. *Practitioner*, 204, 80.
BLATT, M. L. & SHAW, N. G. (1938). Bacillary dysentery in children. *Archives of Pathology*, 26, 216.
GALLOWAY, W. H., CLARK, N. S. & BLACKHALL, M. (1966). Paediatric aspects of the Aberdeen typhoid outbreak. *Archives of Disease in Childhood*, 41, 63.
GANADO, W. (1965). Human brucellosis. *Scottish Medical Journal*, 10, 451.
GREEN, J. H. (1967). Cloxacillin in treatment of acute osteomyelitis. *British Medical Journal*, ii, 414.
HAGGERTY, R. J. & ZIAI, M. (1964). Acute bacterial meningitis. *Advances in Pediatrics*, 13, 129.
HUTCHINSON, R. I. (1956). Some observations on the method of spread of Sonne dysentery. *Monthly Bulletin of the Ministry of Health and Public Health Laboratory Service*, 15, 110.
INSLEY, J. & HUSSAIN, Z. (1964). Listerial meningitis in infancy. *Archives of Disease in Childhood*, 39, 278.
WALDVOGEL, F. A., MEDOFF, G. & SWARTZ, M. N. (1970). Osteomyelitis. *New England Journal of Medicine*, 282, 198.

VIRUS INFECTIONS

BLATTNER, R. J. (1966). Infectious mononucleosis. *Journal of Pediatrics*, 69, 480.
BLATTNER, R. J. (1967). Paralytic poliomyelitis. *Journal of Pediatrics*, 71, 759.
BLATTNER, R. J. (1969). Bell's palsy in children. *Journal of Pediatrics*, 74, 835.
BLATTNER, R. J. & HEYS, F. M. (1962). Viral encephalitis. *Advances in Pediatrics*, 12, 11.
VAN BOGAERT, L. (1959). Acute encephalitis in childhood. *British Medical Journal*, i, 1199.
CLAXTON, R. C. (1963). A review of 31 cases of Stevens-Johnson syndrome. *Medical Journal of Australia*, 1, 963.
FENICHEL, G. M. & HATGER, W. (1965). Guillain-Barré syndrome. *Clinical Proceedings of the Children's Hospital, Washington*, 21, 158.
HORSTMANN, D. M. (1968). Viral exanthems and enanthems. *Pediatrics, Springfield*, 41, 867.
JAMES, W. & FREIER, A. (1949). Roseola infantum. *Archives of Disease in Childhood*, 24, 54.
KNYVETT, A. F. (1966). Pulmonary lesions of chickenpox. *Quarterly Journal of Medicine*, 34, 313.
MILLER, D. L. (1964). The public health importance of measles in Britain today. *Proceedings of the Royal Society of Medicine*, 57, 843.
NEFF, J. M. *et al.* (1967). Complications of smallpox vaccination. *Pediatrics, Springfield*, 39, 916.
SEVER, J. L. & ZEMAN, W. (1968). Conference on measles virus and subacute sclerosing panencephalitis. *Neurology*, 18, 1.
SMITH, C. H. (1947). Acute infectious lymphocytosis. In *Advances in Pediatrics*, vol. 2. London: Interscience Publishers.
STUART-HARRIS, C. H. (1966). Influenza and its complications. *British Medical Journal*, i, 149, 217.
WELLER, T. H. (1971). The cytomegaloviruses of man. *New England Journal of Medicine*, 285, 203.

MYCOTIC INFECTIONS

RYAN, T. J. (1969). Ringworm and thrush infection. *British Journal of Hospital Medicine*, **2**, 497.
STRELLING, M. K., RHANEY, K., SIMMONS, D. A. R. & THOMSON, J. (1966). Fatal acute pulmonary aspergillosis. *Archives of Disease in Childhood*, **41**, 34.
TILLEY, R. F. (1962). Present status of antifungal antibiotics. *Pediatric Clinics of North America*, **9**, 377.

PARASITIC INFESTATIONS

ALEXANDER, J. O. (1968). Scabies and pediculosis. *Practitioner*, **200**, 632.
BEATTIE, C. P. (1964). *Toxoplasmosis*. Edinburgh: Royal College of Physicians.
COLE, A. C. E. (1967). Parasitic infections in the United Kingdom. *British Journal of Hospital Medicine*, **1**, 692.
GILLES, H. M. (1966). Malaria in children. *British Medical Journal*, ii, 1375.
HUNTER, G. W., FRYE, W. W. & SWARTZWELDER, J. C. (1960). *A Manual of Tropical Medicine*, 3rd edn. Philadelphia: Saunders.
VEGHELYI, P. (1940). Giardiasis. *American Journal of Diseases in Children*, **50**, 793.
WOODRUFF, A. W. (1970). Toxocariasis. *British Medical Journal*, iii, 663.

16 Chronic Handicap in Childhood

Persisting disabilities causing handicap have become more important in childhood with the decline in frequency and severity of infections, nutritional deficiencies and other acute disorders. Handicap may be considered as a limitation imposed on the activities required of a child and the degree of handicap must therefore be assessed in relation to his circumstances and the demands made on him by society. Thus a disability which penalizes a child in the competitive atmosphere of a large urban college might cause little or no handicap in a village school. For administrative purposes, a disability can be said to constitute a handicap when special educational or social arrangements have to be made for the child.

The prevalence of handicap among children in different communities cannot be compared, because a disability causing a handicap in one community may not do so in another; it is probable, however, that in this country between 2 and 3 per cent of all children have a disability which constitutes a substantial handicap. Many more have minor disabilities which do not cause handicap in ordinary circumstances but require extra effort on the part of the child. In such cases the effect of the disability may only become apparent when additional demands are made on the child, who has no reserves left to meet them.

CAUSES

The pattern of disabilities causing chronic handicap is constantly changing. Rheumatic carditis and poliomyelitis, which until recently were responsible for many cases, now play a much smaller part, whereas congenital abnormalities are assuming increasing importance in many countries. One of the reasons for this is the increased survival rate among malformed infants as a result of better medical and surgical treatment. Almost any longstanding disability can constitute a handicap but the most important are those affecting the central nervous system. Malformation of the brain or damage sustained during its development is likely to cause a disturbance of function, due partly to loss of normal activity and partly to aberrant action of maldeveloped parts of the brain. Disorders of cerebral function may be grouped under five headings: (1) intellectual subnormality; (2) motor disability (cerebral palsy); (3) epilepsy; (4) sensory disturbances; (5) disorders of emotion and personality. Since the defect or lesion of the brain is seldom confined to one area, more than one function is usually disturbed and the possible combinations are endless. Thus one child may show intellectual subnormality and epilepsy, another cerebral palsy with sensory impairment and so on. The various clinical pictures have collectively been called 'the syndromes of cerebral dysfunction' and constitute a very important group of handicapping conditions.

Hydrocephalus and spina bifida (p. 117) are another major cause of chronic handicap, increasing in importance because of improving survival rates. Advances in surgery have also permitted the survival of children with cardiac and other malformations who would formerly have died but now live with some degree of disability. While improved obstetric care has diminished the number of infants with severe birth injury to the brain, more are surviving the newborn period, so that this cause of chronic disability may not be less frequent. Crippling diseases have greatly diminished in relative importance, but asthma and rheumatoid arthritis are two which are not yet fully amenable to therapy and may necessitate special educational and social provision over many years. Other less common diseases, especially neuromuscular disorders, contribute to the total of chronic handicap. Deafness and blindness are serious disabilities in childhood which have become less common. Longstanding psychiatric disturbance constitutes a special form of handicap.

GENERAL MANAGEMENT OF THE HANDICAPPED CHILD

Comprehensive management should start as early as possible. This implies early diagnosis which depends on neonatal screening techniques, anticipation of handicap in infants at risk, developmental examination of young children and other means of early ascertainment. The main objective of management is to help the child to make the most of his abilities and ultimately to achieve as great a degree of independence as possible. The disability may interfere with the ordinary activities of living, so that the child uses up much energy on such prosaic tasks as dressing and feeding himself. His education and later his employment are interfered with by both mental and physical disabilities and also by frequent absences because of illness or treatment. He may be estranged from other children because he is unable or too self-conscious to play with them or because they reject him on account of his appearance or behaviour. Management must take account of all these difficulties and help the child to overcome them, so that he achieves as much as he is capable of and does not develop secondary personality disturbances which add to the total handicap. It must also be constantly borne in mind that, in addition to his special requirements, the handicapped child has the same needs for care as any child and these must be met as well.

All children differ in their behavioural characteristics and reactions to stressful situations and handicapped children are no exception. Each child will therefore need careful handling attuned to his own personality and temperament. While behaviour disorders are more common among handicapped than among non-handicapped children, they are not dissimilar in kind. Disturbed behaviour may be due to abnormal brain function, the effect of the disability itself, e.g. bizarre mannerisms in blind children, the frustration of being handicapped and faulty adult attitudes. The prevention or amelioration of emotional disturbances will therefore depend on effective treatment, the provision of a wide range of experience and opportunity for self-expression and the maintenance of good parent–child relationships by sympathetic counselling and by strengthening the family's resources in every way possible.

Special methods of play will help the young handicapped child to develop his sensorimotor skills and creative instincts and combat social isolation. Special education should start early and continue long to help compensate for slow progress, and must be realistically related to the child's abilities and probable occupation in adult life. Therapy will depend on the nature of the disability. Full assessment and a co-ordinated programme of management planned by a team of experts from many fields will be required, especially when disabilities are multiple. Throughout childhood, but particularly in the early years, the parents will need constant support, encouragement and advice if they are to adapt successfully to life with a handicapped child.

CEREBRAL DYSFUNCTION
Mental subnormality

This is considered in Chapter 5. Mental subnormality is the commonest cause of chronic handicap in childhood, occurring either alone or with other disabilities such as cerebral palsy or epilepsy. The degree of associated mental handicap will determine not only the child's ability to benefit from treatment of these disabilities but also the extent to which he can be educated and can make use of such abilities as he has. It is therefore the most important single factor in assessing the child's future.

Cerebral palsy

This is defined as a persistent but not unchanging disorder of movement and posture, appearing in the early years of life and due to a non-progressive disorder of the brain, the result of interference during its development. While this definition emphasizes the motor disability, it must be remembered that most affected children also have other disorders of cerebral function, in varying combination and degree, so that the clinical picture is often extremely complex and requires careful and comprehensive assessment.

INCIDENCE. Recent estimates have suggested an incidence of between 2 and 2·5 per 1000 of the childhood community, and while some cases are so mild as to suffer little serious disability, the remainder represent a major social and educational problem.

ETIOLOGY. The group as a whole has no common etiology. In the majority of cases the abnormality of the brain originates at or before birth; perinatal anoxia probably represents the most important single factor, though others include malformation of genetic or early embryonic origin, prenatal infection, and birth trauma. In approximately 10 to 15 per cent of cases the condition is acquired after birth as the result of kernicterus, intracranial infection, thrombosis, embolism, or trauma. In many cases the etiology is obscure. Cerebral palsy is commoner in males and a high proportion of cases are firstborn.

CLASSIFICATION. Numerous different classifications are at present in use. The basis of classification may be the motor disorder, of which there are three main types, viz. spastic (80 per cent of all cases), athetoid and ataxic. Other less common types are flaccid, rigid and tremor. Cases may be further categorized by anatomical distribution, e.g. hemiplegia (limbs on one side of the body), paraplegia (both lower limbs) or tetraplegia (all four limbs), and by severity (slight, moderately severe or severe). Thus, complete diagnoses would be 'severe spastic hemiplegia' or 'moderately severe athetoid tetraplegia'.

Another classification, which recognizes neurological syndromes, has certain advantages, if it is realized that not all patients with cerebral palsy fit into these categories and that more than one may be present in the same patient. This classification is as follows.

Hemiplegia and double hemiplegia. In hemiplegia (paresis of one half of the body), the paresis is likely to affect the upper limb more severely than the lower, and to be associated with spasticity and retarded growth of the affected side. In double hemiplegia, all four limbs are affected, but the upper limbs to a greater extent than the lower; most children with double hemiplegia are mentally subnormal and many have epilepsy.

Diplegia. Here both lower limbs are principally and symmetrically affected, though in addition one arm (triplegia) or both arms (tetraplegia, quadriplegia) may be involved. The 'scissors gait' (Fig. 16.1) is characteristic and contractures of the adductor muscles of the thighs and of the calf muscles are liable to occur early. The distinction from double hemiplegia rests principally on the major involvement of the legs in diplegia. There is frequently a history of preterm birth or perinatal anoxia, and mental subnormality is common.

Ataxic diplegia. This condition occurs much less commonly than pure diplegia and may be present in more than one member of the family. Patients suffering from ataxic diplegia show spastic paralysis of the limbs in association with ataxia of cerebellar type. On account of their unsteadiness they tend to walk on a broader base and show less 'scissoring' than children with pure diplegia.

Ataxia. This may be either unilateral or symmetrical. The degree of functional disability varies from mild clumsiness to a degree of incoordination and impaired balance which interferes with all normal activities. Some ataxic patients are of normal or high intelligence.

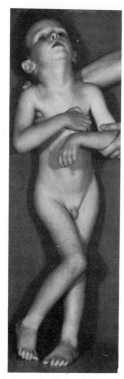

Fig. 16.1   Spastic tetraplegia, showing adductor spasm of thighs and characteristic position of left hand.

Athetoid cerebral palsy (*dyskinesia*). This is generally a sequel of severe intrapartum asphyxia or of kernicterus, and is consequently less common than formerly. In athetoid cerebral palsy voluntary and postural control of the limbs and trunk is disturbed by the presence of involuntary movements and alterations in muscle tone. While these movements are generally athetoid, consisting of involuntary writhing of the limbs, they may be choreoid, when they are shorter and sharper in character. Frequently they can only be described as choreoathetoid. Dystonic movements, involving the trunk, occur less frequently.

Involuntary movements and hypertonus disappear during sleep and may be abolished when the child has been trained to relax. In contrast, true spasticity, for example in hemiplegic patients, can be elicited during sleep and is not under voluntary control. Pure flaccid types of paralysis are uncommon.

DIAGNOSIS AND COURSE. Cerebral palsy may be looked for in infants with a history of abnormal pregnancy or delivery, suggestive signs in the newborn period or postnatal disease of the nervous system; often, however, it develops in the absence of such antecedents. The infant may appear normal until the age of a few months, when he is noted to be unusually 'floppy', so that he cannot support his head or sit up at the expected times. Spasms of extensor hypertonus (dystonia) may occur in some cases but as time passes the early hypotonia is gradually replaced by spasticity or athetoid movements. In hemiplegia, failure to use the affected hand may be noted early, while in severe tetraplegia spasticity is sometimes evident from the first.

PROGNOSIS. The prognosis as regards life depends so largely on the extent and nature of the cerebral damage, the age onset of symptoms, the degree of mental development, the quality of home management, and the occurrence of intercurrent infection, that generalization is impossible. The most severely affected patients are likely to die in infancy, while many others survive to adult life. Prognosis as regards functional improvement is largely governed by the intelligence of the patient and the age at which intensive rehabilitation and education are commenced. Little improvement can be expected in patients with severe mental subnormality, whereas in those with normal or superior intelligence prolonged training may render them useful members of the community, even when the initial physical disability is great.

TREATMENT. The best results are obtained when children considered suitable on selection by intelligence and age are treated by a team giving attention to education, physiotherapy, occupational therapy, speech training and social integration. This may best be carried out in a residential school devoted entirely to the purpose, but since the accommodation for this type of case falls very far short of the demand, the majority must still be treated at home under medical supervision. Moreover, for many children the advantages of a warm family environment outweigh those of residential care, while in home care the parents can be more effectively included in the team. Surgery may be of great value in correcting deformities, e.g. in lengthening the tendo achillis when contraction of the calf muscles has occurred, but if treatment aimed at the prevention of deformity is started in the first three years of life, surgery is rarely necessary.

Since the emphasis in treatment is predominantly on educating the patient to overcome the physical disability, treatment is likely to be prolonged and require patience and enthusiasm on the part of all concerned. A programme of exercises and occupation must be specially designed to develop such motor power as exists, and should be revised periodically in the light of progress.

In the case of spastic cerebral palsy, action patterns are normal and there is less trouble from paresis than from spasticity. Some movements can therefore be taught in an upside-down position so that gravity does not throw the usual muscles into spasm. Passive movements also have value in preventing muscle-shortening. Splinting may be necessary to stabilize the legs and also to prevent deformities occurring.

The treatment of athetoid patients includes the preliminary teaching of conscious relaxation. Movements are then consciously learnt from the relaxed state; this must be done almost muscle by muscle, since action patterns are undeveloped. Subsequently occupational therapy will develop the action patterns already learnt.

Speech therapy will be carried out in association with other treatment when necessary. Correction of visual or hearing disorders is especially important. Learning difficulties must be identified and analysed, so that special educational methods can be built into the therapeutic programme. In all cases, whether the children are treated at home or in institutions, special appliances are likely to be required. These include special chairs, toilet arrangements, feeding utensils (e.g. a spoon bent so that the child does not spill food when putting it into his mouth), tricycles, or walking-chairs, etc.

Other disorders of cerebral function

Sensory defects may affect peripheral sensation, e.g. the loss of touch in the hemiplegic hand, or central receptive mechanisms, e.g. perceptual disorders, in which the child is unable to interpret incoming stimuli correctly. The behaviour of a child with a defect or lesion of the brain may be characterized by lack of concentration, distractibility, hyperactivity and temper tantrums. Such pathological personality traits must not be confused with antisocial and other behaviour disturbances which result from handicap.

In some cases, central failure of recognition or execution (agnosia or apraxia) or difficulties with spatial relationships may add to the child's handicap. There may be specific difficulty in reading, in which the child has no visual defect but cannot easily recognize words (dyslexia), or

in writing (dysgraphia). These are often associated with impaired numbering and spelling, defective speech and language, and right–left confusion. When such disorders occur without gross motor or other disability, the organic origin of the disturbed behaviour may go unrecognized. Similarly, very slight degrees of cerebral palsy or clumsy movements due to delayed maturation of the neuromotor system may be mistaken for deliberate awkwardness and the child punished on this account. These various disabilities are a major cause of educational and social difficulty in apparently normal children: in order to focus attention on the need to identify and make allowance for them, they have been grouped together under the general title '*minimal disorders of cerebral function*'. While their recognition is important, however, they must not be used as convenient labels for behaviour which has complex physical, intellectual, emotional and social origins (see also p. 387).

CONVULSIONS AND EPILEPSY

Recurrent convulsions, or 'fits', due to abnormal electrical discharges in the brain constitute epilepsy, which is an important manifestation of cerebral dysfunction, occurring alone or in combination with intellectual subnormality, cerebral palsy, etc. Convulsions in general are considered here for convenience, though not all are recurrent or constitute a chronic disability. They may be generalized from the onset, when discharges occur simultaneously throughout the cerebral cortex, or focal, remaining localized or spreading to become generalized.

Convulsions

Convulsions are commoner during infancy than in any other age period, but there is much that remains obscure in their etiology. Experimental evidence suggests that the immature nervous system of the infant is less, rather than more, responsive to electrical stimulation than that of the adult. Nevertheless there appears to be a greater degree of instability, which is reflected in electroencephalographic studies.

The major causes of convulsions in infancy and childhood are acute infection, cerebral malformation and acquired lesions of the brain, while in a proportion of cases the cause is unidentified (idiopathic). The relative importance of different etiological factors is likely to vary in different localities and even in the same locality over a period of years. In using the following classification, it must be remembered that two or more factors may operate simultaneously and that the infant may have a 'lowered convulsive threshold' which is passed as the result of various stimuli.

INFECTION OUTWITH THE CENTRAL NERVOUS SYSTEM
    Tonsillitis; pneumonia; otitis media; urinary infection; dysentery; exanthemata.
INFECTION OF THE MENINGES AND/OR BRAIN
    Purulent meningitis; brain abscess
    Encephalitis; virus meningitis
    Cerebral malaria; cysticercosis
    Tuberculosis (meningitis and tuberculoma).
CEREBRAL INJURY AND HAEMORRHAGE
    Birth injury; postnatal trauma; rarely, pertussis
    Haemorrhagic diseases.
CEREBRAL THROMBOSIS AND EMBOLISM
METABOLIC DISORDERS
    Hypocalcaemia; hypoglycaemia; hypomagnesaemia; uraemia; anoxia; pyridoxine dependency.
CEREBRAL TUMOURS
CONGENITAL CEREBRAL AND CEREBROVASCULAR ABNORMALITIES
    E.g. hydrocephalus; microcephaly; microgyria; tuberous sclerosis; Sturge-Weber syndrome; congenital aneurysm.
PROGRESSIVE CEREBRAL DEGENERATION
    Tay-Sachs disease; Schilder's disease.
TOXINS
    Lead encephalopathy; the exotoxin of tetanus; strychnine, camphor, and other drugs and poisons.
MISCELLANEOUS
    Sunstroke: photic stimulation.
IDIOPATHIC EPILEPSY

CLINICAL FEATURES. Most of the above conditions have already been considered, and it will be realized that the primary cause will colour the clinical picture in the individual case. Fits vary from slight twitching (a common manifestation in the newborn) to generalized convulsions, in which the infant loses consciousness and becomes cyanotic, with stertorous breathing, deviation of the eyes, and urinary incontinence. The attack may last a few seconds, or convulsions may be semicontinuous over a long period (*status epilepticus*).

Convulsions are usually followed by sleep, though this is not invariable, consciousness sometimes being immediately regained. A generalized convulsion or series of convulsions is occasionally followed by a transient paralysis.

DIAGNOSIS. The occurrence of twitching or clonic movements is usually sufficient to indicate that a child is suffering from a convulsion, and the problem of diagnosis is rather one of determining the primary cause. Nevertheless, a breath-holding attack, masturbation or other disturbance of behaviour can easily be mistaken for a fit, as can a simple faint in an older child. Less common sources of error are the anoxic faints of congenital aortic stenosis and the painful cramps of tetany: hypocalcaemia may of course cause a true convulsion as well as the muscular twitching of tetany. The advisability of diagnostic lumbar puncture must depend on the presence or absence of other clinical findings, the danger of producing a pressure cone when there is increased intracranial pressure (e.g. from the presence of a tumour) being borne in mind. The procedure should never be carried out during a convulsion.

The age of the child is of considerable help in reaching a diagnosis, convulsions occurring first in early infancy being most commonly due to birth injury, congenital abnormality or metabolic disorder; febrile convulsions due to infection predominating in late infancy and early childhood, but seldom occurring after 5 years; and idiopathic epilepsy becoming increasingly important with increasing age. Cerebral tumours are seldom responsible for convulsions in early infancy, but the possibility must be considered at all ages.

TREATMENT. While treatment is essentially that of the primary cause, immediate treatment of the convulsions will be required when they are continuous or repeated. Diazepam 0·25 mg per kg by intramuscular injection, is the drug of choice, being both effective and safe. Another useful drug is paraldehyde given intramuscularly in a dose of 0·2 ml per kg, up to a maximum of 6 ml. Intramuscular sodium phenobarbitone 5 mg per kg or intravenous sodium phenytoin 5 mg per kg are also effective. If convulsions persist, a general anaesthetic may be necessary. Tepid sponging is indicated in the case of infants with high pyrexia.

Febrile convulsions

A child with a genetically determined low threshold to seizures may respond to sudden pyrexia by convulsing. Such a febrile convulsion commonly occurs at the onset of an extracranial infective illness, is generalized and lasts less than 10 minutes. In most cases the prognosis is good and the child is unlikely to develop epilepsy later, though he may have further febrile convulsions.

A prolonged, focal or severe seizure, very frequent episodes, especially if precipitated by only slight fever, a perinatal history suggesting the likelihood of brain damage, a family history of epilepsy and an abnormal electro-encephalogram in the interval between episodes are adverse features which make the prognosis more guarded.

Febrile convulsions affect about 4 per cent of children under 5 years of age and occur mainly between 1 and 5 years. There is frequently a family history of febrile convulsions, which has a good prognostic significance, unlike an epileptic family history.

Since the convulsion will usually have ceased by the time the child comes under medical care, the immediate need is to identify and treat the infection. A convulsion continuing more than 15 minutes must be stopped as soon as possible (see above), since hypoxic brain damage may occur. Phenobarbitone may be given for a day or two after the convulsion but continuous anti-convulsant prophylaxis is not required unless adverse prognostic features are present. A child known to be subject to febrile convulsions may be given an anticonvulsant or antipyretic drug at the onset of an infective illness, but this is often impracticable since the convulsion may be the first indication that the child is ill. If adverse factors are present, it will generally be advisable to prescribe phenobarbitone and to continue anti-convulsant therapy for two years after the last convulsion. Phenytoin may be preferrred if phenobarbitone causes excitement.

Idiopathic epilepsy

By definition, the cause of idiopathic epilepsy is unknown but it is not possible to distinguish it sharply from symptomatic epilepsy, since the distinction will often depend on the intensity with which the cause is sought. Moreover, the popula-tion cannot be clearly divided into epileptic and non-epileptic, because whether a person develops epilepsy or not depends not only on his personal predisposition but also on the strength of the provocation.

Epilepsy affects about 6 per 1000 of the school population. A family history is sometimes ob-tained, more commonly in petit mal than in grand mal, but direct inheritance from a parent is exceptional.

While electroencephalography has helped to define the condition, abnormal records are not consistently found in, or confined to, epileptic patients or their relatives, and their interpretation in early childhood is often difficult.

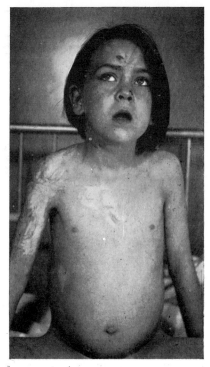

Fig. 16.2   Epilepsy and mental defect; dull facies, scarring of forehead from frequent falls, and keloid scarring of trunk from extensive burn.

CLINICAL FEATURES. The classical major attack (*grand mal*) may be preceded by an aura, or subjective warning, and consists of sudden loss of consciousness associated with tonic spasm which gives way to generalized clonic movements, followed by deep sleep; a period of disorientation (*post-epileptic state*) in which be-haviour may be grossly abnormal and memory affected, sometimes follows the attack. During the attack the child is liable to injure himself by falling to the ground or into the fire, bite his tongue, and pass urine or (much less commonly) faeces. The face is suffused or cyanotic during the attack, and frothing at the mouth often occurs.

The *petit mal* attack consists of transient loss of consciousness of very short duration in which the child neither falls nor shows tonic spasm, though slight rhythmic movement of the head or eyelids may occur. The child proceeds immedi-ately with whatever action was interrupted by the attack. Thus a spoon will be held momentarily poised on the way to the mouth, and the nature of the attack may only be recognized by observ-ing the staring or blinking of the eyes by which it is accompanied. Many such episodes may occur every day. The EEG shows a characteristic 3 per second spike-and-wave pattern. In case of doubt, a petit mal attack can sometimes be induced by asking the child to hyperventilate by breathing deeply and quickly for 2 minutes.

When attacks start in early life and are uncontrolled by sedatives, there may be progressive mental deterioration, while major seizures may supervene later. In some cases, however, petit mal attacks show spontaneous remission at puberty.

The same individual often suffers from both grand mal and petit mal epilepsy. Nocturnal epilepsy may pass unrecognized when there is little clonic spasm, or the child comes under observation with a diagnosis of enuresis. Epileptic seizures may be provoked in some children by flickering light, as from a television screen (photic epilepsy), or by other sensory or emotional stimuli. *Pyknolepsy* is the name sometimes given to very frequent petit mal attacks which may occur a hundred or more times a day. *Minor epileptic status* is caused by continuing epileptic discharges resulting in a state of variable stupor with unsteadiness and isolated muscle twitches. Intravenous diazepam may arrest the status.

Many other varieties of epilepsy occur. Seizures may be focal, characterized by localized movements limited to one limb or part of a limb, or by automatisms such as smacking of the lips, inappropriate speech or other semipurposeful activities (temporal lobe epilepsy). Paroxysmal attacks of abdominal pain may be epileptic in nature, in which case they will be accompanied by mental confusion and EEG abnormalities and will respond to anticonvulsant therapy. The Jacksonian type of seizure starts with focal twitching and the movements subsequently spread in a regular order and may pass into a general convulsion. Myoclonic seizures are muscular spasms of very short duration. Sudden loss of postural tone may cause the head to fall forward (salaam spasm) or the child to fall to the ground (drop seizure). Frequently recurring spasms beginning before the age of two years (infantile spasms) generally indicate diffuse cerebral damage of poor prognosis, with a chaotic EEG pattern (hypsarrhythmia): ACTH followed by prednisolone may lead to improvement in some cases.

DIAGNOSIS. When a child presents with a history of recurrent fits, every possible effort must be made to identify the cause (see list above) before the diagnosis of idiopathic epilepsy is made. It is particularly important that an intracranial tumour should not be overlooked when fits start suddenly in middle childhood. In atypical cases, difficulty may arise in distinguishing between syncope (faints) and epilepsy; indeed, there is evidence that in some cases repeated fainting attacks may in fact be a manifestation of epilepsy. In general, however, the following points will often help to distinguish between fainting attacks and fits in individual cases.

Age. Faints are rare in young children, though not unknown. They are common after the age of 10 years, especially in girls.

Onset. The onset of a fit is sudden, and the child is likely to fall, often striking his forehead on the ground (healed scars on the brow are sometimes a useful diagnostic point). The child who is about to faint feels dizzy beforehand, will usually be able to reach a chair or sink gradually to the ground without hurting himself, and often remembers afterwards what has happened.

Colour. In a fit the face is usually suffused, whereas during a fainting attack there is obvious pallor, due to fall in blood pressure.

Environment. A fit may occur in any place and at any time. A faint is more likely to occur in a hot and stuffy room, during prolonged standing or as a result of emotional stress.

MANAGEMENT. Children with epilepsy are a great danger to themselves and to others, since an attack may occur without warning in traffic or at any other time. They must never be left by an unguarded fire or open window or engage in any occupation in which sudden loss of consciousness would endanger life. When seizures are completely controlled or very infrequent, as few restrictions as possible should be imposed. Swimming can be permitted in the presence of an adult swimmer who knows the child is liable to seizures. Cycling may be allowed where there is no other traffic. Children with severe uncontrollable epilepsy are likely to require treatment in residential schools (about 2 per cent of all cases).

The immediate attack is treated as described for convulsions, and particular care must be taken to prevent the tongue being bitten by inserting a well-padded wooden gag between the side teeth. No attempt should be made to hold the limbs rigidly during the clonic movements, but

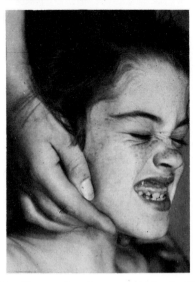

Fig. 16.3   Hypertrophy of gums and hirsuties following prolonged phenytoin administration to an epileptic girl aged 10 years.

the child should be prevented from hurting himself.

The success of drug therapy in controlling attacks over a long period is very variable, petit mal attacks often proving particularly resistant. Drugs should be introduced in small doses and gradually increased to full dosage, which should be maintained for several weeks before being pronounced ineffective. If fits are not completely controlled, another drug should be added (not substituted) and increased slowly in the same way. A combination of several drugs may ultimately be required to achieve control in some cases. An anticonvulsant drug should never be withdrawn abruptly, since status epilepticus may be precipitated.

Phenobarbitone is generally used in the first instance for major attacks. The optimum dosage must be found by trial, but initially 3 mg per kg body weight may be given daily in divided doses. Resistant cases will sometimes respond dramatically to phenytoin in doses up to 5 mg per kg daily or primidone in an initial dose of 125 mg b.d., which can be increased to 25 mg per kg daily. Overdosage of either drug may be indicated by ataxia or nausea, or rarely by megaloblastic anaemia due to folic acid deficiency. Prolonged high dosage with phenytoin may cause hypertrophy of the gums, hirsuties and possibly permanent cerebral damage. For petit mal attacks unassociated with major seizures the most effective drug is ethosuximide 125 to 250 mg b.d. Troxidone may also be given in a dose of 150 to 300 mg b.d. Troxidone often causes photophobia, while skin rash or leucopenia may occur with either drug; the latter may necessitate stopping the drug temporarily. Therapy in all cases of epilepsy should be as regular as possible and long-continued. Freedom from attacks for two years may justify a trial period without therapy, but in the majority of cases spontaneous remission cannot be expected.

OTHER NEUROLOGICAL DISORDERS

The disorders considered here may cause cerebral damage or disease leading to chronic neurological handicap. Some of the diseases are progressive but the rate of progress may be so slow that the child requires the same general management as any chronically handicapped child, though the long-term aims will necessarily be modified by the prognosis.

Cerebral thrombosis

Thrombosis of the longitudinal or other sinuses occasionally occurs in marasmic infants but in the majority of cases sinus thrombosis is the result of otitis media or mastoiditis, jugular thrombosis being followed by lateral sinus thrombosis which may extend to other intracranial sinuses.

Thrombosis of the longitudinal sinus will interfere with the normal absorption and circulation of cerebrospinal fluid and patients who survive are liable to develop hydrocephalus.

Cavernous sinus thrombosis is a rare complication of septic lesions of the nose and face and gives rise to severe toxaemia. The eyelids on the affected side become oedematous and there are unilateral exophthalmos and dilatation of superficial veins. Ocular paralysis and papilloedema may also occur. Treatment should be directed to the primary infection and should include intensive antibiotic therapy.

Thrombosis or *embolism of cerebral arteries* is very much rarer in childhood than in adult life. Occasionally sudden hemiplegia ushered in by convulsions is found to be due to embolism or thrombosis of a cerebral artery or vein without obvious cause. Recovery from the paralysis usually occurs in surviving children, though it may not be complete and there may be residual mental impairment.

Head injuries

Apart from birth injury, trauma to the skull in childhood is of very frequent occurrence, and the great majority of children suffer no serious effects. Compound fractures of the skull require immediate surgical treatment, but a more conservative attitude can be adopted to depressed fractures, while simple stellate or linear fractures require no intervention. The effects on the brain vary from transient loss of consciousness (concussion) due to alteration of intracranial pressure, to haemorrhage or laceration. Haemorrhage may be subdural resulting in the formation of a subdural haematoma (p. 44), subarachnoid, or rarely intracerebral or extradural. The last is commonly due to tearing of the middle meningeal arteries, and gives rise to symptoms of increasing intracranial pressure occurring some hours after the injury. Surgical intervention is required.

Subarachnoid haemorrhage results in free bleeding into the cerebrospinal fluid, which can be diagnosed by lumbar puncture, and localizing symptoms depending on the site of the injury. Relief is usually afforded by withdrawal of cerebrospinal fluid.

Although the prognosis of head injury will clearly depend on the site and severity of the lesion, late results are in general better in children than in adults. The complaint of post-traumatic headache following minor injury is less common, no doubt owing to the fact that compensation is seldom a matter of direct concern. It must be remembered that fractures through the frontal sinuses and tearing of the dura may provide a portal of entry for pneumococcal infections of the meninges.

Hypoglycaemia

Clinical manifestations of hypoglycaemia may occur in the newborn period or during insulin treatment but are otherwise relatively rare. Hypoglycaemia should be suspected if twitching, fainting or headache occurs after fasting or active exercise and the symptoms are promptly relieved by sugar. Confirmation is obtained by estimation of the blood glucose at the onset of an attack. Investigation should include tests of adrenaline response, glucose tolerance, insulin sensitivity, response to ACTH and leucine sensitivity (since some children are leucine-sensitive and protein feeding may cause hypoglycaemia). If glycogenosis, endocrine insufficiency, intracranial disease, hepatic cirrhosis, fructosaemia,

and severe renal glycosuria can be excluded, a laparotomy is advisable to exclude hyperplasia or adenoma of the islet cells of the pancreas.

Certain otherwise healthy children react to food deprivation by hypoglycaemia and ketonuria (ketotic hypoglycaemia). The syndrome affects mainly boys over 1 year of age who were disproportionately light for gestational age at birth. The sporadic attacks, which respond to glucose but not glucagon, become less frequent in later childhood. The cause is unknown.

There remain cases described as 'idiopathic hypoglycaemia' occurring most commonly in male infants and showing a familial incidence with a tendency to spontaneous recovery. In these, good results have been claimed for careful spacing of carbohydrate intake and diazoxide or steroid therapy.

Lead encephalopathy

In cases of chronic lead poisoning (p. 21), encephalopathy may occur insidiously or be precipitated by infection. Convulsions, mental deterioration, and the appearance of peripheral nerve palsies are likely to be associated with papilloedema or optic atrophy. Treatment is that of lead poisoning but when encephalopathy has occurred, the long-term prognosis is poor as there is likely to be permanent mental impairment.

Acute cerebral demyelinization and necrosis

In addition to post-infective encephalomyelitis (p. 361), in which demyelinization is liable to occur as part of an antigen—antibody reaction, acute cerebral degeneration may result from the direct action of a virus. Thus the herpes virus can probably cause necrotizing cerebral lesions in either of these two ways. There is also a group of acute necrotizing (van Bogaert) or acute polioclastic (Greenfield) encephalitides in which the etiology is obscure, though possibly viral. In these cases the onset may be marked by intestinal, respiratory, or general symptoms, followed by disturbances of consciousness, agitation, convulsions, and possibly death within two weeks of onset. Inflammatory necrosis of the superficial layers of the brain is found at necropsy.

Schilder's disease (*Encephalitis periaxialis diffusa*)

In this rare disease of infancy, progressive demyelinization of the cerebral hemispheres is likely to be associated with cerebral oedema and evidence of raised intracranial pressure. It is in some cases familial. Symptoms commonly start in infancy or early childhood in a patient who has previously developed normally. Convulsions and a wide variety of neurological manifestations, including blindness, hemiplegia or monoplegia, ataxia, and aphasia lead on to progressive mental defect and finally to a condition of decerebrate rigidity. Death often occurs after a period of 12 months, though the rate of progress may be slower than this and there may be short periods of arrest. No effective treatment is known.

Degenerative nervous disorders

A great variety of syndromes due to degenerative lesions of the nervous system have been described, but apart from those considered in previous sections, none are at all common in childhood. Of those which are primarily diseases of adult life, disseminated sclerosis, progressive muscular atrophy of adult type, and syringomyelia occasionally occur before puberty.

Heredofamilial conditions, of which Friedreich's ataxia, hereditary amyotrophic lateral sclerosis, hereditary spastic paraplegia, familial periodic paralysis and peroneal muscular atrophy are examples, are more likely to be detected in childhood when an affected family is being investigated. All of these are rare.

Friedreich's ataxia

The lateral and dorsal columns of the spinal cord are involved in a primary degeneration of neurones with secondary neuroglial proliferation. The disease starts insidiously in childhood, the presenting symptom being ataxia, which is followed by the appearance of weakness of the legs, intention tremor, nystagmus, disorders of speech, and progressive deformities, of which pes cavus is the most characteristic. The knee and ankle jerks are lost and the plantar reflex is extensor. The disease is gradually progressive and uninfluenced by treatment.

MUSCULAR DISORDERS

The muscular dystrophies

This group of heredofamilial disorders of the skeletal muscles is characterized by progressive weakness and wasting of various muscle groups, the presenting symptoms and mode of inheritance differing in different families. In all cases there is swelling of individual muscle fibres, which may reach great size, followed by hyaline degeneration and replacement of muscle fibres by connective tissue. Clinically the muscles may appear atrophied or firm and enlarged; in the latter case the hypertrophy is due to the presence of fat and connective tissue, and muscular elements are greatly reduced. Estimations of serum aldolase and serum creatine kinase may help in the early diagnosis of the muscular dystrophies, since the levels of these enzymes are frequently raised before clinical signs appear. Transmitting females of the Duchenne type of muscular dystrophy may in many cases be identified by estimation of serum creatine kinase also.

The conditions are usually familial, but sporadic cases are not very uncommon. Several clinical types have been described, of which the first two are the most characteristic.

In the *facio-scapulo-humeral type of Landouzy-Dejerine* the facial muscles are involved early, and the muscles of the shoulder girdle later, or vice versa. There is a mask-like facies, inability to close the eyes and extreme weakness of the shoulder muscles. The forearms, hips, and lower extremities are ultimately affected, though sometimes years may elapse before they are involved. This type is commonly inherited as an autosomal dominant with incomplete penetrance, and both sexes are affected.

Pseudohypertrophic type of Duchenne is the form most commonly seen in childhood. It appears typically as a sex-linked recessive with a high mutation rate affecting primarily males and transmitted by females. Here the lower extremities and buttocks are first affected, usually during the first years of life, and the calf muscles show well-marked pseudohypertrophy. The method adopted in rising from the supine position is characteristic, the child first rolling on to his side and raising his thorax on his arms ('dying gladiator' position). The legs are brought into the kneeling and then the standing position, after which the child 'climbs up his legs with his hands', i.e. raises his thorax by grasping the legs at successively higher levels, until finally the erect position is reached (Fig. 16.4).

The *limb–girdle type* of muscular dystrophy is a heterogeneous group of disorders affecting the proximal muscles of the limbs and generally inherited as an autosomal recessive. Boys and girls are equally affected, and the condition progresses very slowly, ending in severe disability after 20 or more years.

The onset of muscular dystrophy is very insidious, and symptoms commonly appear before the tenth year, though later in the limb–

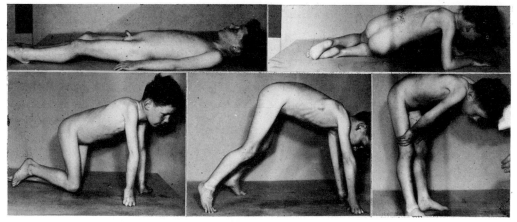

Fig. 16.4   Pseudohypertrophic muscular dystrophy. Serial photographs showing method of rising from supine to erect position. Calves pseudohypertrophic.

girdle type. The Duchenne type is first manifested by increasing inability to walk upstairs, or in cases which begin very early, by delay in standing erect and walking. The condition is slowly progressive; children in whom the lower extremities are first affected often become obese owing to inactivity and finally bedridden. There appears to be an association between the Duchenne type and mental subnormality, though most patients are of normal intelligence. Although muscular dystrophy is compatible with life for many years, a proportion of patients succumb to cardiac failure or respiratory infection. No form of treatment has been found effective, but regular exercise is desirable and occupational therapy and education are of great help in rendering the child's increasing disability more tolerable.

Myasthenia gravis

This is characterized by recoverable weakness of voluntary muscle following exercise. It occurs at all ages, including the newborn period, is occasionally familial and affects females predominantly. Weakness commonly involves the muscles of the eyes, neck, and face but the clinical picture is variable. Ptosis, diplopia, and bulbar signs are frequent and a typical 'snarling' facies may be observed. Involvement of shoulder and hip muscles may cause difficulty in raising the limbs, especially towards the end of the day when the muscles are fatigued. Such loss of power may be mistaken for hysterical paralysis, but the rapid recovery after intramuscular injection of 0·04 mg neostigmine methyl sulphate per

kg body weight enables the differentiation to be made. Transient myasthenia, characterized by general weakness, feeble cry and difficulty in sucking and breathing, may occur in some newborn infants of myasthenic mothers.

The disease is due to a block in neuromuscular transmission apparently due to defective synthesis or storage of acetyl choline. An autoimmune reaction involving the thymus gland has been held responsible and thymectomy sometimes effects improvement. Medical treatment consists of the oral administration of neostigmine bromide (one to ten 15 mg tablets daily as required) or pyridostigmine bromide (60 mg tablets).

SKELETAL DISORDERS

Many of the congenital malformations of bone described in Chapter 5 will cause chronic handicap if sufficiently severe. Degenerative bone diseases can also lead to disability, though this is not always permanent. Under the general title *osteochondritis deformans juvenilis* are included a number of clinical types of degenerative osteochondrosis. With the exception of osteochondritis of the spine, all are commoner in boys than girls. While trauma is thought to be a factor in the etiology of many cases, it does not provide a complete explanation for the local circulatory disturbances which follow, and a history of trauma is not always obtained. Endocrine disturbance, a neurotrophic factor, mild infection, and allergy have also been postulated to explain the etiology. In most instances there is associated swelling of soft tissues, pain, and limita-

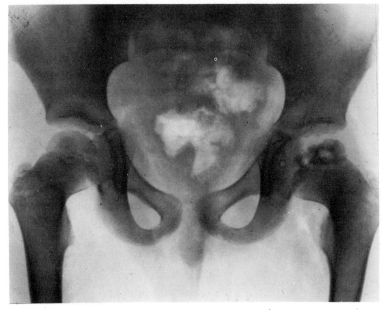

Fig. 16.5   Perthes' disease showing fragmentation and flattening of left femoral head. Boy aged 9 years.

tion of movement. The age-incidence of certain classical types of osteochondritis is usually limited as follows:

> *Perthes' Disease*—2 to 10 years.
> *Osteochondritis of tibial tubercle* (Osgood-Schlatter disease)—early adolescence.
> *Osteochondritis of tarsal navicular* (Kohler's disease)—4 to 6 years.
> *Osteochondritis of the spine* (Scheuermann's disease)—12 to 16 years.
> *Osteochondritis of the second metarsal head* (Freiberg's disease)—12 to 15 years.

Of the above, only Perthes' disease and osteochondritis of the spine can be considered at all common in childhood and the latter is less frequently seen before than after puberty.

Perthes' disease (*Coxa plana*)

The disease consists essentially of degenerative changes in the head of the femur resulting in flattening and irregular rarefaction of the epiphysis and decalcification at the junction of the neck and epiphysis. Healing is associated with recalcification of the head and neck of the femur, though there is often some persistent 'mushrooming' of the head and slight deformity of the acetabulum. The condition may be unilateral or bilateral. Boys are affected six times as commonly as girls; the average age of onset is approximately 6 years.

CLINICAL FEATURES. Limping is almost always the presenting symptom, the limp at first being slight and subsequently more persistent. Pain is a common complaint, but is seldom severe and is relieved by rest. It is usually referred to the knee, thigh or groin. In the early stages, examination reveals limitation of movement at the affected hip, pain on abduction and rotation, and possibly some soft-tissue swelling. As the disease progresses there is more marked limitation of movement, shortening of the femur, and atrophy of the muscles of the thigh and buttock. The erythrocyte sedimentation-rate may be slightly raised during the acute phase.

Radiological examination shows first a widening of the joint space, and subsequently flattening of the femoral head with increased density. As the disease progresses, irregular areas of decalcification appear in the head and neck of the femur (Fig. 16.5). Subsequent healing is shown by increasing density.

TREATMENT. It is uncertain how far prolonged immobilization affects the ultimate prognosis, but bed rest and traction are advisable so long as there are pain and spasm; some authorities recommend this treatment for a much longer period. Subsequently the child is usually allowed a walking caliper which prevents weight-bearing until the condition has fully healed.

COURSE AND PROGNOSIS. Spontaneous recovery occurs in two or more years, and even when there is persistent deformity of the femoral head the functional result is usually good.

Osteochondritis of the spine

Irregular ossification of the vertebral bodies and epiphyseal plates results in wedge-shaped deformities affecting several vertebrae, usually in the dorso-lumbar region. The child comes under observation on account of postural defects, of which round shoulders and a moderate degree of kyphosis are the most common (Fig. 16.6). There is often complaint of backache after prolonged standing. The general health and activity are apt to be affected.

Radiological examination shows that the epiphyseal plates and vertebral bodies are irregularly ossified, principally in their anterior positions; the epiphyses may at first show increased density and subsequently fragmentation.

TREATMENT. Patients in whom pain is a marked feature should be immobilized for three to six months and bed rest should be advised for all early cases. Subsequently the wearing of a supporting brace and postural exercises are indicated.

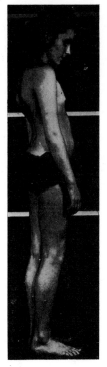

Fig. 16.6   Osteochondritis of spine causing juvenile kyphosis. Girl aged 12 years.

BIBLIOGRAPHY AND REFERENCES

BAKWIN, H. (1968). Developmental disorders of motility and language. *Pediatric Clinics of North America*, **15**, 565.
VAN BOGAERT, L. (1959). Acute encephalitis in childhood. *British Medical Journal*, i, 1199.
BOWER, B. D. (1969). Epilepsy in childhood. *British Journal of Hospital Medicine*, **2**, 454.
BRETT, E. M. (1966). Minor epileptic status. *Journal of Neurological Sciences*, **3**, 52.
BROWN, J. K., COCKBURN, F. & FORFAR, J. O. (1972). Clinical and chemical correlates in convulsions of the newborn. *Lancet*, i, 135.
BYERS, R. K. & LORD, E. E. (1943). Late effects of lead poisoning on mental development. *American Journal of Diseases of Children*, **66**, 471.
DENHOFF, E. & ROBINAULT, I. (1960). *Cerebral Palsy and Related Disorders*. New York: McGraw-Hill.
DOWBEN, R. M. (1961). Diagnosis and treatment of muscle diseases. *Archives of Internal Medicine*, **107**, 430.
FORD, F. R. (1966). *Diseases of the Nervous System in Infancy, Childhood and Adolescence*, 5th edn. Springfield, Ill.: Thomas.
FRIDERICHSEN, C. & MELCHIOR, J. (1954). Febrile convulsions in children. *Acta paediatrica, Stockholm*, **43**, S.100, 307.
HENDERSON, J. L. (1961). *Cerebral Palsy in Childhood and Adolescence*. Edinburgh: Livingstone.
ILLINGWORTH, R. S. (1966). Diagnosis of cerebral palsy in the first year of life. *Developmental Medicine and Child Neurology*, **8**, 178.
ILLINGWORTH, R. S. (1968). The clumsy child. *Clinical Pediatrics*, **7**, 539.
INGRAHAM, F. D. & MATSON, D. D. (1949). Subdural haematoma in infancy. In *Advances in Pediatrics*, vol. 4. London: Interscience Publishers.
INGRAM, T. T. S. (1964). *Paediatric Aspects of Cerebral Palsy*. Edinburgh: Livingstone.
INGRAM, T. T. S. (1966). The neurology of cerebral palsy. *Archives of Disease in Childhood*, **41**, 337.
JEAVONS, P. M. & BOWER, B. D. (1964). *Infantile Spasms*. London: Heinemann.
KERSHAW, J. D. (1966). *Handicapped Children*, 2nd edn. London: Heinemann.
KOGUT, M. D., BLASKOVICS, M. & DONNELL, G. N. (1969). Idiopathic hypoglycemia. *Journal of Pediatrics*, **74**, 853.
LENNOX, W. G. (1960). *Epilepsy and Related Disorders*. Boston: Little Brown.

MILLICHAP, J. G. (1960). Diagnosis and management of convulsive disorders. *Pediatric Clinics of North America*, **7**, 583.

MILLICHAP, J. G. (1968). *Febrile Convulsions*. NewYork: Macmillan.

MILLICHAP, J. G. & DODGE, P. R. (1960). Diagnosis and treatment of myasthenia gravis in infancy, childhood and adolescence. *Neurology*, **10**, 1007.

MITCHELL, R. G. (1966). Chronic handicap in childhood. *Post-Graduate Medical Journal*, **42**, 428.

MITCHELL, R. G. (1966). Minimal disorders of cerebral function. *British Journal of Disorders of Communication*, **1**, 109.

MITCHELL, R. G. (1971). The prevention of cerebral palsy. *Developmental Medicine and Child Neurology*, **13**, 137.

PAPPAS, A. M. (1967). The osteochondroses. *Pediatric Clinics of North America*, **14**, 549.

WALTON, J. N. (1969). Muscular dystrophies and their management. *British Medical Journal*, iii, 639.

WALTON, J. N. & NATTRASS, F. J. (1954). On the classification, natural history and treatment of the myopathies. *Brain*, **77**, 169.

WERTHEIM, E. (1967). The school-aged child with multiple minimal handicaps. *Australian Pediatric Journal*, **3**, 1.

17   Behaviour Disorders

Anxiety about the behaviour of a child is one of the commonest reasons for parents to seek medical advice. The parents are concerned because they believe the behaviour to be abnormal, because they do not know how to handle the situation or cannot agree about the management, or because the behaviour is creating difficulties with neighbours or bringing the family into conflict with authority, such as school or police. Sometimes the child is referred directly for medical opinion by the school, by a social work agency or by a juvenile court or children's hearing. The type of disorder tends to vary with the origin of referral. Although parents may seek advice for any disturbance of behaviour and sometimes require only reassurance, they are especially likely to be concerned over disorders which are most manifest in the home, such as enuresis, night terrors and disturbance of sleep, disobedience, lying, sexual interest, anorexia and displays of temper. In many cases, of course, more than one of these symptoms is present and parents also frequently show anxiety about educational or social failure. Among cases referred by the school, educational difficulties, social maladjustment and truancy predominate, while the juvenile court cases include behaviour problems which have brought the child into more serious conflict with society, e.g. stealing and house-breaking, wilful destruction of property, cruelty, vagrancy, living in moral danger and being beyond parental control.

HISTORY

A full history must be taken, including details of the family and school background, and the doctor must be prepared to listen patiently and sympathetically, no matter how trivial the symptom seems, for the process of unburdening themselves of the details helps to relieve the parents' anxieties. At the same time it must be remembered that the accuracy of recall by parents of disturbed children is notoriously unreliable, since unacceptable incidents are liable to be suppressed, the parents are on the defensive and they are trying to show their child in the best light despite the worry he has caused them. Moreover, false interpretations may already have been placed on the behavioural manifestations by the parents or others and these may prove misleading unless they are recognized as erroneous.

The first consideration is to decide whether the behaviour in fact requires attention or whether a normal phase of development has been misinterpreted by an overanxious mother, who may herself need help. The developing infant normally passes through a series of stages, each of which is characterized by behaviour which would be pathological if retained into later life. Thus bed-wetting, faecal soiling, interest in excreta, greed, aggression, temper tantrums, thumb-sucking, sexual curiosity and exhibitionism and destructiveness can only be considered as possibly pathological when they persist at an age when most children have outgrown or controlled them; similarly some children show a transient period of stammering while speech is being acquired, which disappears spontaneously when they have an adequate vocabulary to express their thought. As in the case of physical development, there are wide physiological variations in behaviour and emotional development, and it is not possible to draw a sharp distinction between acceptable and unacceptable behaviour.

ETIOLOGY

When behaviour is considered to be beyond the range of what is acceptable, it is necessary to explore how far it is the result of the child's own inborn temperament and how far it is related to continuing environmental stress. Some children have strong personality characteristics which are recognizable even in infancy and which make them more difficult to bring up than others. The child who shows intensity of emotional feeling, unwillingness to accept change and negative reactions to new experiences requires more careful, consistent and patient handling than the child who is adaptable and of equable temperament. The parents may be unable to give the required quality of care, sometimes because they themselves are anxious, demanding or insensitive, and the result is a tense, negative child who may show various disorders of behaviour.

Distorted parent/child relationships are thus of the first importance in the genesis of disturbed behaviour, but are often difficult to elicit in taking a history. Much may be learned from the doctor's assessment of the parents and observation of the interaction of parents and child during the interview, but more information must often be obtained from a social worker or other person in close contact with the family. One or both parents may be overprotective, punitive or intolerant in their attitude to child-rearing. The parents may be temperamentally unsuited to one another, and the child may then become the centre of quarrelling and aggression. Differing levels of intelligence between the parents, or between parents and child, must also be taken into consideration.

Behaviour is influenced by interaction between the child and many different factors in his environment. Early emotional stresses, such as deprivation or separation experiences, conflicts within the family and adverse conditions in neighbourhood or school all play their part. Once the child goes to school, new stresses arise as he adjusts to the social environment of the classroom and strives to establish his position in it. New relationships have to be made with teachers and other children and these may lead to new conflicts and difficulties in adaptation. Lesser degrees of mental retardation may become manifest at this stage and can cause feelings of inadequacy and low self-esteem. The child may behave irresponsibly because of his poor intelligence or may compensate for feeling intellectually inferior by restoring to delinquency. Intelligence testing is therefore essential to the elucidation of behaviour disorder, since backwardness in school is not a reliable index of low intelligence and may be due to emotional causes, while the specious 'brightness' sometimes seen in mentally backward children is often misleading. While intellectual subnormality is thus a cause of behaviour disorder, it is important to realize that the emotional problems of the retarded child are similar to those of children with normal intelligence and their behaviour disorders are therefore not of a different kind.

Disordered behaviour may be the direct result of organic disease. Almost any disease in childhood may result in an alteration of behaviour. A tendency to regress to a more infantile level and to make greater demands on the mother's affection is a normal response to acute disease: in chronic illness, e.g. coeliac disease, the child's behaviour and temperament will usually show marked variations depending on whether the disease is quiescent or active. Prolonged illness may itself introduce extrinsic factors such as immobilization, loss of schooling, confinement to hospital and separation from parents, which will inevitably have some effect on behaviour and emotional development; it is more surprising that so many children surmount these difficulties successfully than that others suffer some permanent disturbance from them.

Organic disease affecting the brain poses great difficulties in diagnosis. Rheumatic chorea and thyrotoxicosis may start with disturbed over-emotional behaviour before objective physical signs are clearly evident. Fretful irritability may be the first indication of a brain tumour or of tuberculous meningitis. The child whose brain is developmentally abnormal or has been damaged during pregnancy or delivery may show distractibility, short attention span, temper tantrums and restless hyperactivity. While easily recognized as abnormal in the severely 'brain-damaged' child, minor degrees of this hyperkinetic syndrome merge imperceptibly into the normal range of behaviour and the organic origin of the disturbance may easily be overlooked. Moreover, the difficulty is increased by the facts that such children require very patient and tolerant management and yet their characteristics are such as will arouse hostility and impatience in adults. Thus the 'brain-damaged' child is predisposed by his very nature to adverse environmental influences, which are likely to increase the abnormality of his behaviour still further. Learning difficulties in school often have a basis in organic brain damage and if this is overlooked the child may be unfairly punished for laziness or naughtiness. Some epileptic children show labile, over-emotional and unpredictable behaviour, which may be partly the direct result of brain damage and partly secondary to their having epilepsy. Moreover, it must not be forgotten that the drugs used to control epilepsy may themselves have adverse effects on behaviour.

When the child's personality is being considered, the possibility of psychosis must not be overlooked as a cause for disturbed behaviour. Infantile autism (see p. 400) may be manifest in the young child, and schizophrenic or other psychotic reactions in their early stages may be recognizable in the older child. These too have often an organic basis in brain damage. Immaturity of personality is extremely common and in such cases assessment must take account of the factors which have contributed to the child's failure to mature emotionally.

More serious personality disorders and psychoneuroses, manifest by such symptoms as anxiety, excessive fears and aggressiveness, usually require expert psychiatric diagnosis and treatment.

Children with psychopathic personalities form a small but socially important group, in whom there is apparently a constitutional lack of moral sense which may be coupled with normal or high intelligence. Their behaviour is characterized by an inability to resist immediate self-gratification often at the expense of the community. Although they will at times behave in a way calculated to please or disarm suspicion, such behaviour is designed to serve a purpose and is not based on affection or sense of responsibility. In later life their psychopathic personality renders them a serious menace to society.

PRESENTING SYMPTOMS

It is rare for a single symptom to be the sole manifestation of personality disturbance or behaviour disorder and while, for instance, enuresis or night terrors may provide the reason for the child's coming under observation, other symptoms will almost invariably come to light on further questioning. It will also commonly be found that the child is not the only member of the family whose behaviour is abnormal. Whatever the presenting symptom, therefore, full assessment is necessary. Preliminary enquiries will often disclose much deeper and far-reaching disturbance than was at first evident and in such cases, especially if there is anything to suggest a psychoneurotic or psychotic reaction, the child should be referred to a child psychiatrist. Nevertheless, family doctors and paediatricians see many lesser degrees of behaviour disturbance, usually of a transient nature, which are well within the scope of their diagnostic and therapeutic skills and do not require expert psychiatric help. When she seeks advice, the mother usually concentrates attention on one main complaint and it is wise to let her talk freely about this first before leading the discussion into a wider exploration of the problem. It is therefore appropriate to consider behaviour disorders in terms of presenting symptoms, provided it is realised that the symptom is only the tip of the iceberg.

Tic (*Habit spasm*)

In the differential diagnosis of chorea, with which condition tics are frequently confused, it was pointed out that a tic represents a co-ordinated series of muscular movements resulting in a performance such as blinking the eyes, twitching the face, jerking the head, coughing, grunting, or shrugging the shoulders, which could under certain circumstances serve a useful purpose, but is purposeless when carried out. The series of movements is always the same, is frequently repeated, and will sometimes be performed on request; after a time one form of tic may be replaced by another. The tic ceases during sleep and when the child's attention is distracted. The commonest age-incidence is between 5 and 11 years. A tic lasting for only a few weeks is a not uncommon indication of transient nervous tension usually requiring no action and best ignored. Persistent movements indicate more serious emotional disturbance and the history may provide evidence of sleep disorders, undue fears, tearfulness or other anxiety symptoms, often related to pressure of school-work or home conflict. It will usually be found that the child has been repeatedly reprimanded or punished without effect before he comes under observation; in such cases the parents and teacher should be advised to ignore the tic as far as possible and attempt to relieve any other cause of anxiety. Parents of these children are often tense and overanxious themselves and discussion may give them insight into the problem and lead to modification of their attitude. In some cases a holiday or change of environment will result in rapid improvement though relapse commonly follows return home. In such cases and in those where it is obvious from the beginning that the family is seriously disturbed, the advice of a child psychiatrist should be sought early. The prognosis is very variable, and if a tic has persisted for a year or more, the underlying disturbance is often less amenable to treatment; there is frequently an abnormal amount of repressed aggression in these cases.

Speech disorders

The average age at which most children start to use one or two words with meaning is about 1 year but the range is from 6 months to $2\frac{1}{2}$ years. Joining two or more words together is usually achieved at about 18 months, but again the range is wide, though the great majority of children are speaking in simple sentences by 3 years of age.

Delay in acquiring speech may be due to mental subnormality, deafness or specific developmental delay. Since the age at which speech is acquired varies so widely in normal children, it will sometimes be found that, if deafness (including high-tone deafness) and mental subnormality can be excluded, the parents of young children who are not yet speaking can be reassured. Delay beyond the range acceptable as normal is likely to be due to a specific developmental speech disorder. Occasionally failure to speak is not a disorder of speech but a manifestation of autism (see p. 400) or due to elective mutism, i.e. refusal to speak as a symptom of extreme negativism.

Imperfect speech, of which lisping and lalling are the commonest examples, is physiological in early childhood, when correct pronunciation of consonants is only being acquired piecemeal. Pronunciation will normally be greatly influenced by early training and environment. Persistent speech defects should suggest partial deafness, unless there is some gross abnormality of the mouth, nasopharynx or larynx to account for them. Persistence of infantile forms of speech may indicate regressive tensions or may be a symptom of anxiety, in which case they disappear without specific therapy when the source of anxiety is dealt with.

Stammering is dysrhythmic speech due to inco-ordination of breathing and speaking. It is generally a combination of hesitations, prolongations of sound and repetitions of the first consonant or syllable of words. Many children stammer for short periods during the normal acquisition of speech but persistent stammering affects rather less than 1 per cent of all children, is commoner in boys than in girls and generally appears between 2 and 8 years. Hereditary predisposition and emotional tension both play a part in the etiology of stammer, which may be accentuated by manifest parental anxiety about the disorder. Stammering may be associated with grimacing and posturing and the child becomes increasingly conscious of his disability, tending to avoid embarrassing situations and in some instances withdrawing from social contacts. In other children, the disorder is intermittent and only appears at times of emotional stress.

Speech training is necessary and sometimes gives good results but may be disappointing when there are such adverse features as a strong family history, psychological tension or parental overanxiety. When stammering is simply one symptom of a neurotic personality, successful treatment will often increase the child's self-confidence and so result in improvement in other respects.

Dysarthria. Abnormality of articulation due to malfunction of lips, tongue and palate may be caused by defective innervation or by local structural defects, such as cleft palate, abnormality of the nasopharyngeal airway or orthodontic malformation. Speech therapy usually produces improvement, although results are disappointing when the dysarthria is part of a general neurological disturbance such as athetoid cerebral palsy.

Specific delay in speech development. This varies in severity from immaturity of word sounds and slower than normal acquisition of spoken language to gross retardation of speech development, often with difficulty in comprehension of language. A proportion of affected children show poor lateralization of hand, leg and eye function and there may be associated manifestations of cerebral dysfunction such as reading and writing difficulties or clumsiness (see p. 374). Boys are more often affected than girls and there is frequently a family pattern of similar disorders. Intelligence is usually normal, though often in the lower range, and inability to communicate effectively leads to frustration, temper tantrums and avoidance of social relationships: Management must be aimed at preventing such secondary emotional disturbance, especially since many of these children will gradually acquire normal speech over the next few years, though some will have difficulty in using language even in adult life. Constructional toys and other means of self-expression must be provided and the parents should talk slowly, clearly and frequently to the child. Skilled speech therapy in a playroom environment is helpful in some cases.

Habit disorders

Under this heading may be included a variety of habitual manipulations of the body and other performances which are distinguished from tics in that they are carried out at a higher level of consciousness, may be performed continuously for long periods, can be interrupted, are under voluntary control, and are usually pleasurable. A large proportion of all children show one or more of these habits at some time, so their importance must not be exaggerated, but if frequent and persistent they may reasonably be regarded as indicating emotional disturbance. The commonest examples are

thumb-sucking, nail-biting, nose-picking, and chewing pencils or clothing; others are hair-plucking, ear-pulling, scratching and handling of the genitals (as distinct from masturbation). All are liable to provoke intense irritation in the adults who observe them, and this in turn is apt to lead to exaggeration of their physical effects, e.g. the attribution of malocclusion to thumb-sucking in early childhood requires much more critical appraisal than it has usually received.

Thumb-sucking or *finger-sucking* is a normal practice in infancy, and one which it is useless to try to prevent. It is usually relinquished gradually during the pre-school period, but children often continue to suck the thumb before going to sleep long after the habit has been abandoned at other times. Persistent thumb-sucking after school age has been reached is quite common and is particularly likely to be indulged in when the child is tired, lonely or unhappy.

Handling the genitals is also normal in the case of an infant who is still in the stage of exploring his own body. If he is sharply reprimanded for this he will soon realize that the act provokes a much greater reaction in his parents than when he touches his nose or ears, and his genitals will become more rather than less interesting in consequence.

Nail-biting and *nose-picking* may be regarded as signs of tension, but are so common in middle childhood that too much significance should not be attached to them at this age. The majority of children lose these habits before adolescence is reached.

Self-rocking and *head-banging* are indications of anxiety or other emotional disorder. They may be seen in young children of normal intelligence, especially when separated from their mothers, but are liable to be severe and persistent in the mentally subnormal.

Hair-plucking is a neurotic habit seen in young children, the hair being pulled out and often eaten (see p. 176). An extensive area of alopecia may result (Fig. 17.1), which must be distinguished from ringworm and from alopecia areata, a condition of unknown cause arising spontaneously in older children (Fig. 17.2).

Spasmus nutans, a rhythmical rolling of the head associated with a peculiar type of nystagmus, which may be horizontal, rotary or perpendicular, and may affect the two eyes differently, is occasionally seen in children under two years. When rickets and poorly-lit housing were

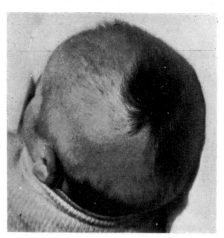

Fig. 17.1   Alopecia due to plucking out of hair with wetted thumb. Boy aged 3 years.

common, spasmus nutans was attributed to one or other of these causes but it is sometimes seen when neither of these is present and the cause must be considered unknown.

Disorders of sleep

Much anxiety can be avoided if it is realized that individual children vary considerably in their sleep requirements, and that, if allowed a certain latitude, they will normally establish the sleep rhythm that suits them best. If a child is happy and active during the day and appears healthy, it is most unlikely that he is suffering from lack of sleep even if he has not fulfilled theoretical requirements. The child who needs

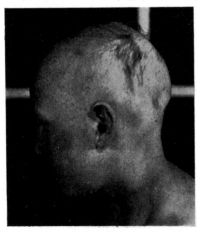

Fig. 17.2   Alopecia areata including the greater part of the scalp and eyebrows in a boy aged 11 years; hair growth normal one year previously.

little sleep may lie awake at night or waken early in the morning and read or otherwise amuse himself. He should be allowed to do so, provided that he is reasonably quiet and does not disturb the rest of the household.

Failure to go to sleep by the very young child is often a manifestation of negativism, which quickly becomes a habit if wrongly managed by overanxious parents. The child refuses to lie down or to go to sleep when he is put down, or he wakes after a few hours and cries or tries to get up. Different children require different handling but if the parents understand that negativistic behaviour is part of normal development, establish a good bedtime routine and try out various manoeuvres with patience and tolerance, the difficulty usually passes. They may leave the child to cry and fuss for a while in the hope that he will tire himself and fall asleep. If this is ineffective, picking him up and comforting him, possibly with a warm drink, may be more successful but should not become a regular practice. In persistent cases, or where parents are tense and anxious, the whole family situation should be looked at, for advice and support may be needed on many aspects of child-rearing.

Sedative drugs have little place in management but if the situation gets worse, sedation with chloral hydrate for a week or two may break the habit and establish a new sleep pattern. If drugs are used in this way, enough should be given to ensure a sound night's sleep for several nights in a row (e.g. up to 500 mg of chloral hydrate if necessary) and then the drug should be stopped. Inadequate sedation for longer periods does more harm than good. In some cases the habit may have to be accepted as a temporary phase and arrangements made for each parent in turn to get a night's sleep in another room or at a relative's house.

Failure to go to sleep by older children may be due to the child's being put to bed too early, to environmental causes (too hot or too cold a bed, disturbance by television, etc.), physical discomfort, hunger, or anxiety. Fear of the dark is an extremely common anxiety symptom, though it occurs in most normal children at some age. It may be sufficient to prevent or delay sleep unless the child can be provided with a shaded light. Many nervous children find a familiar ritual at bedtime essential for their peace of mind, and cannot readily fall asleep if it is broken. Worry over home-work, exciting play in the evening or late television viewing are other possible causes of insomnia in children who are emotionally unstable, while jealousy of a younger child sleeping in the parents' room will sometimes be found responsible.

Nightmares and night-terrors. Terrifying dreams are an occasional occurrence within the experience of most normal children, and it is only when they occur frequently that they require special consideration. In the case of nightmares, the child may talk or cry out or move violently during sleep, awaking frightened but fully conscious and able to recount his dream. The picture of night-terror, which is peculiar to childhood, is characterized by a period of terror after the child has woken, during which he fails to recognize his parents or peoples the room with imaginary figures. Full consciousness is only regained after a period of several minutes. Both are evidence of anxiety, and it may be possible to date their occurrence from some particularly frightening experience, such as being locked in a dark room, assault, or other episode. Sleep-walking is a closely related activity which, when frequent, also indicates serious emotional disturbance.

In some cases, abnormal repression of aggression is an important cause of these disorders. It is usually associated with high standards of social behaviour or achievement on the part of the parents, e.g. in the case of the consistently and excessively polite child or the boy who never dirties his hands or tears his clothes. While less emphasis is nowadays placed on purely visceral upsets as a cause of nightmares, there is no doubt that dietary indiscretion may precipitate them. It is also found that some cases will respond well to food last thing at night, supporting the view that hypoglycaemia is a possible factor. The child should be examined to exclude physical and mental defects, and the possibility of night-terrors being unusual manifestations of epilepsy borne in mind. An attempt should be made to assess whether the child is of constitutionally anxious type, i.e. whether anxiety symptoms preceded the attacks, or whether they are directly due to a single frightening experience, recent overpressure at school, or other single factor. With sympathetic handling, the prognosis in these cases is usually good.

Disorders of appetite

The commonest complaints are *lack of appetite* or *refusal to eat particular foods.* The child is usually brought for advice in the preschool or early school period, and it is significant that the complaint is much less common in the case of older children and those living in institutions. Frequently a previous history of feeding difficulty in infancy is obtained. Since normal appetite can readily be interfered with by wrong handling during early training it will often be found that the trouble is attributable to a parental attitude which has persisted over several years. Overanxiety or overseverity on the part of the parents, too scrupulous cleanliness, overloading the child's plate, insistence on finishing to the last mouthful may all be operative factors. Allowance must be made for the negativism which commonly occurs between the ages of 2 and 4 years, and the fact that refusal to eat is one way in which the young child can assert his independence.

The child's physical state should be carefully assessed, including the state of the teeth. If there is no evidence that he is in fact suffering from lack of adequate food, an explanation to the mother of the reasons for variation of appetite in childhood and encouragement of a more placid attitude to meals may be all that is required. The child's likes and dislikes should be respected and he should be neither hurried nor harried over his meal. In some cases, however, the difficulty is more deep-rooted, the result of years of struggle between parents and child, and the child may be suffering both physically and emotionally. In these cases more detailed investigation and therapy are required, though it should be remembered that the natural urge to eat associated with rapid growth is so strong that many children outgrow their difficulties spontaneously in later childhood.

Anorexia nervosa affects older children, generally adolescent girls, who resist eating for long periods and become extremely thin in consequence. They have immature, inhibited personalities and show excessive passivity or sometimes a bright overactivity. Difficulties in personal relationships and disturbed ideas about their bodies are common. The onset is insidious and so the condition may not be recognized for some time. Close nursing supervision is required to ensure that food is eaten and not concealed or regurgitated. Prolonged psychotherapy is usually necessary.

Pica is a perversion of appetite in children over the age of 1 year, who habitually eat substances unsuitable as food. Earth, coal, hair, paper, paint or the like may be consumed and there is a risk of poisoning, especially by lead. Pica is commonest under the age of 3 years but occasionally persists into later childhood, especially in emotionally disturbed children and the mentally subnormal, who cannot readily discriminate between food and non-food. Most children with pica are well nourished but some show iron deficiency anaemia, which should be corrected. The habit is often very resistant to treatment but tends to cease spontaneously in time. Enquiry should always be made about siblings, since there is frequently a familial incidence.

Excessive appetite may be due to organic lesions of the hypothalamus but is more commonly the result of overindulgence and associated with obesity (see p. 191). It is often imitative, when one or more members of the family habitually overeat, or due to a mistaken belief that a young child should be consistently stuffed. It may, however, be a symptom of deep-seated anxiety dating from mismanaged infant feeding and faulty mother–child relationship.

Disorders of bladder and bowel function

Enuresis is involuntary micturition in bed at night (nocturnal enuresis) or into the clothing during the day (diurnal enuresis) or both. Involuntary micturition is physiological in early infancy and becomes significant as enuresis only after the age at which bladder control is normally established. Since this control is acquired by a gradual stepwise process, which can be interrupted by a variety of disturbing events, the age at which a child may be expected to be dry can be defined only within wide limits. Thus an intelligent child receiving adequate but not excessive maternal attention will usually acquire diurnal control during the second year and cease to wet the bed, apart from occasional lapses, during the latter part of the third year. Some perfectly normal children continue to wet the bed intermittently during the fourth year and occasional lapses may be precipitated later than this by minor physical or emotional upsets or sudden changes in temperature. As a general rule, a policy of encouraging the child to make known his needs during the day and attending to them promptly, coupled with lifting him to pass urine once at night if necessary, will result in control being established over a period of about

18 months to 2 years (i.e. from the age of 1 to $2\frac{1}{2}$ or 3 years). Attempts to establish control by more vigorous disciplining are likely to defeat their own object, while parental overanxiety about continued wetting, or stressful episodes affecting the child, are also likely to delay the acquisition of this new skill. After the age of 4 years, training becomes more difficult, perhaps because the child has passed the sensitive period for learning. Persistent diurnal enuresis should be considered potentially abnormal after the age of 3 and persistent bed-wetting after the age of 4 years. During childhood, nocturnal enuresis is a much commoner symptom than diurnal enuresis alone. It is still present on entering school at 5 years of age in 10 per cent of all children and in an even higher proportion of children from residential homes or with disturbed family backgrounds. In the great majority of patients no organic abnormality will be found but, as organic disease is responsible for some 5 to 10 per cent of all cases, the history should be taken and the child and his urine examined with this in mind. If any of these procedures arouses the suspicion of organic disease, full urological investigation is necessary (see p. 284). In the majority of cases this is not indicated, however, because there is nothing to suggest the presence of physical disease. Should the condition fail to respond to medical or other treatment after a period of some months, however, it is always advisable to review the case fully to make certain that an organic cause has not been overlooked.

A full history of the child's development and behaviour should be taken, paying particular attention to the parents' attitude to habit training and the child's disability. The family history may reveal other examples of enuresis and a family pattern of late control of micturition may emerge. This might be taken to indicate a genetically determined delay in maturation or simply that the same factors of inadequate training and anxiety have operated in other members of the family.

Faulty habit training is undoubtedly an important factor in many cases dating from infancy, the mother either having been obsessed with trying to train the child rapidly or having paid too little attention to his requirements at a time when control could have been established comparatively easily. It must also be remembered that if the parental attitude has been at fault with regard to habit training in infancy, the lack of understanding is likely to persist in dealing with the enuretic child. Children who are late in becoming reliably dry might still do so with little trouble were it not that parental disapproval, teasing and rejection by other children, and the consequent anxiety combine to increase the difficulty of gaining control.

In some cases it will be found that a child who has previously been dry has become enuretic following an emotionally traumatic experience, such as the birth of another child in the family, a period in hospital or absence of the mother: here the condition is likely to be associated with other evidence of regression to infantile behaviour.

Evidence of lack of security, and particularly of split discipline and lack of parental affection, is commonly found in the histories of enuretic children and there may be a background of emotional instability in the family. Although the condition occurs in children of all social classes with parents who may be overindulgent or excessively severe, it is particularly common amongst children in institutions or those coming from broken homes.

MANAGEMENT. Since enuresis may be a symptom of a wide variety of emotional disturbances or represent failure to reach a normal phase of development at the expected time, every case must be considered individually. In a few instances removal from a hopelessly unsuitable home background may prove necessary but in the great majority the child should be treated in his own home and an attempt made to influence the parents' attitude appropriately. Punishment will almost inevitably make the condition more persistent and the aim should be to build up the child's confidence in himself and to establish the feeling of security which he lacks. The physician himself can do a great deal to make the child feel that his difficulties are sympathetically understood and that cure is expected. Some success is obtained with such a wide variety of treatments that the importance of suggestion is obvious. It will also be found that if the child succeeds in overcoming this distressing habit, his success will usually react favourably on his general emotional development.

In addition to investigating and where possible remedying the underlying cause, it is advisable to lay down a routine of treatment. The last drink should be taken at a fixed hour and the bladder emptied immediately before going to bed. Though the habit of drinking quantities of fluid

shortly before bedtime is not likely to cause enuresis in an otherwise normal child, it may be a contributory factor in one who already has enuresis and reduction in intake in the evening may help. In some children, however, the resulting concentration of urine increases the tendency to wet the bed and in these an adequate urinary output should be maintained.

Since enuresis often occurs within three hours of going to sleep, the mother should lift the child before she herself goes to bed, making quite sure that he is really awake and empties his bladder completely. She should ensure that the child is warm in bed, since cold will increase the tendency to enuresis. The bedding should be adequately dried if it has been wet the previous night, and the mattress covered with a rubber sheet. The child should be asked to keep a record of dry nights, not of those on which enuresis occurs, and reward for a high score will at least show that the emphasis is placed on encouragement rather than disapproval.

The use of drugs, e.g. imipramine or ephedrine, has a limited place in treatment if it is realized that the value is largely suggestive and that no specific drug is likely to prove uniformly successful. Amphetamine should no longer be used in the treatment of enuresis, because of the risk of addiction. Systematic attempts at bladder training, in which the child is required to pass urine during the day at specified short intervals which are gradually lengthened, may be successful in those children who have small bladder capacity and micturate very frequently.

An electric conditioning device, the 'buzzer alarm', which is designed to wake the child as soon as he begins to wet a pad on which he lies, is sometimes effective in older children who are co-operative and in younger children if they are not frightened by it. It cannot be expected to cure emotional disturbance when this is responsible for the symptom nor should it be used without proper investigation first. In favourable cases, the child quickly becomes dry at night and remains dry when treatment is stopped after a few weeks. If he does not, further use of the alarm is unlikely to prove successful.

PROGNOSIS depends on individual home circumstances, the degree of co-operation obtained from the parents, success in gaining the child's confidence and the age of the child when advice is first sought. Improvement or cure may be effected within a few months if the emotional disturbance is a superficial one, e.g. jealousy of a second child, which can be explained to the mother and appropriately handled. In other cases gradual improvement is interrupted by relapses relating to fresh emotional stresses. Selected cases may respond dramatically to the buzzer alarm or bladder training. In the most intractable cases enuresis may persist beyond puberty but in the majority control is established by late childhood.

Encopresis means emptying the bowel in inappropriate circumstances and should be distinguished from faecal incontinence, just as enuresis is distinct from urinary incontinence. Developmental delay may postpone the age at which a child gains control of his bowel, but habitual encopresis after the age of 3 or 4 years in a child of normal intelligence usually indicates serious psychiatric disturbance. Most children gain control of their bowel before the age of 2 years, by a combination of functional development and maternal training. At this age there is great interest in defaecation and a desire to handle and smear faeces, while at the same time negativism impels the child to resist his mother's persuasion to open his bowel into a pot. Training can therefore be a trying process but if the mother is firm but calm, showing what she expects of the child but betraying no anxiety when he is unresponsive or rebellious, the difficulties usually pass by the age of 3 years, though there may be occasional lapses thereafter. By this age a child usually opens his bowel once or twice a day and opportunity should be given for an unhurried visit to a clean, warm lavatory every morning after breakfast, especially once he has started school.

The stimulus to defaecation is filling of the rectum and if this is habitually ignored, because of negativism, faulty training or lack of opportunity, chronic constipation ensues. The origin in some cases is deliberate suppression of the desire to defaecate for fear of the pain caused by an anal fissure. Fermentation behind the retained faecal masses and mucus secreted in response to irritation of the intestinal wall cause liquefaction of bowel contents, which leak through the anus. This is *faecal incontinence* and treatment consists of emptying the bowel thoroughly and then training the child to empty it regularly, if necessary with the help of laxatives. When constipation is long present, the rectum becomes enlarged, atonic and insensitive, and ceases to

function properly (p. 83). In such an established condition, keeping the large bowel empty for a long period with laxatives, or in extreme cases by high colonic lavage, may allow it to regain tone but relapse is frequent and the prognosis for complete restoration of function is not good. Rarely, chronic constipation with paradoxical incontinence or faecal incontinence alone is due to a congenital anomaly of the intestine or anal sphincter and this possibility should always be excluded (p. 83). More commonly, disturbed behaviour and acquired functional abnormality are the main factors in etiology. Secondary emotional disturbance almost always accompanies faecal soiling, with its discomfort, unpleasant odour, social isolation and feelings of guilt and shame. It is therefore extremely difficult to determine the relative importance of physical and emotional factors, and successful management requires the close co-operation of family doctor, paediatrician and child psychiatrist.

In most cases of encopresis the child becomes clean at the usual age and starts soiling when 5 or 6 years old, the amount varying from faecal staining to complete evacuation of his bowel into his clothing. The child may seem oblivious to his state and continue playing, though other children will often refuse to associate with him because of the smell. For the same reason, difficulties arise in class and may result in the school refusing to accept him. Symptoms of emotional disturbance, such as enuresis, lying, stealing or aggressive behaviour are frequently associated. The parents of such children are often tense and authoritarian, demanding much of their families and reacting by extreme resentment and guilt to the child's habit. There may be a history of family disharmony or a broken home.

Psychotherapy is nearly always necessary in encopresis, but organic factors should first be excluded, or treated if present in consultation with the child psychiatrist. Admission to hospital is often necessary in the first place. It is a common experience that the child is not encopretic in hospital and remains clean for some time after returning home, though relapse usually occurs sooner or later.

Educational difficulties

Every schoolchild is subjected to conflicting pressures to conform to his peer group, to meet the demands of his teachers, to accede to his own desires and impulses. Children differ greatly in the ease with which they adapt to these stresses, some fitting readily into the life of the classroom and others remaining insecure and isolated by their own low self-esteem or rejected by other children. The social tensions of school life are an important source of anxiety and disturbed behaviour, which in turn will affect academic achievement and the mastery of new skills.

Poor progress at school is a complex phenomenon which can seldom be attributed to a single cause. Low intelligence and defective vision or hearing are obviously important in some cases but even then are usually associated with social and emotional disabilities which must also be taken into consideration. Similarly, emotional disturbance which seems adequate to account for poor achievement may have its origin in developmental reading disability (see p. 374). Home circumstances have a powerful influence on school progress. Children from poor socioeconomic backgrounds often start with the disadvantage of a culturally starved home and an atmosphere of indifference or even hostility towards education. Emotional disturbance due to parental disharmony, lack of affection or neglect shows itself as anxiety and low motivation for school work. Children who are naturally sensitive and of nervous temperament will suffer more from such adverse circumstances than will the bolder or more placid child. An overanxious child who finds it a struggle to keep up with the others in his class will tend to translate 'I can't compete' into 'I won't compete' and is often difficult to rescue from his position of hopelessness. Dread of an individual teacher or of bullying, dislike of school meals or other fears will affect his ability to learn. The same child may arrive at school having eaten little or no breakfast and hunger will then add to his difficulties. Large classes make it hard for the nervous child who lacks self-confidence to do himself justice and for the teacher to give him the personal attention and encouragement he needs. He tends to become withdrawn and in consequence to appear stupid and inattentive. Phantasy, which should play an important and constructive part in the child's emotional development, can in these circumstances become an escape mechanism and the child is then described as continually day-dreaming.

When a child is experiencing learning difficulties, a careful intellectual and physical assessment should be made and the possibility of

specific reading disability or other functional cerebral disorder ruled out. Where there are obvious emotional and social problems, psychiatric investigation and social casework may show how the situation can be improved. A great deal depends on the quality of teaching the child receives. The young child from a poor home will gain much from enrichment of his intellectual environment, especially if he is encouraged to follow his own inclinations and seek out what interests him under the guidance of the teacher, rather than being expected to perform correctly in a fixed programme. It is not easy to allow for the varying capacities and inclinations of older children but every effort should be made to do so, since lack of attention and boredom are likely if the child is placed in too high or too low a class for his abilities or if he is forced to study subjects which do not interest him. In some cases a special class or a different school may be desirable, though such a change should not be advised without a thorough analysis of the reasons for unsatisfactory progress and a clear idea of how the child's particular needs can be met.

Truancy and school phobia

The school truant is frequently a child of robust or adventurous personality who prefers other activities to school-work and is prepared to risk the consequences. Truancy may be associated with lack of adequate home care and with delinquent behaviour. A clear distinction should be made between the truant and the child with neurotic breakdown resulting in refusal to go to school (school phobia). In the case of the latter, fear and anxiety, sometimes amounting to panic when the time to enter school arrives, are the predominating features. Obsessional or hysterical symptoms sometimes occur also; the children are usually of good intelligence, timid, and dependent. The parents may be educationally ambitious and overdemanding and there is frequently a family history of neurotic illness. The prognosis is not good in severe cases of either truancy or school phobia, but is liable to be especially poor in truancy when there is associated wandering from home.

Sexual difficulties

It is now generally recognized that a phase of infantile sexuality, manifested by curiosity, sex play and exhibitionism, is a normal stage in the development of the young child. The concept has been extended to include the oral and anal regions as zones of erotic satisfaction in the infant, but we are here concerned with the more specific interest in the genitals which is commonly manifest between the ages of 3 and 5 years. Many sexual difficulties of childhood and later life arise from the failure of adults to recognize the essentially normal and healthy nature of sexual interest at this age. It is most important that the child should pass through his sexual phase (as also the anal phase which precedes it) without unnecessary feelings of guilt being inculcated. If the young child's interest is continually thwarted by replying to sexual questions with answers which are palpably untrue, and if every sexual manifestation is regarded as perverse or precocious and made the object of sharp reprimand, the foundations are laid for an unhealthy attitude to sex subsequently. The child at this age is also dependent on the affectionate response of love objects (normally the mother in the first instance and subsequently the father as well) for his normal emotional development; if he is deprived of this, he will turn inward for his gratification and come to depend to an increasing extent on auto-erotic habits. The child passes into a more latent period with regard to sex towards the end of the pre-school period lasting to the onset of puberty, but the latency period is certainly not universal.

Sexual curiosity and sex play. The child who is a member of a mixed family will normally have much of his curiosity satisfied by seeing his brothers and sisters naked in the home. In the case of only children and those who are not members of mixed families, there is a likelihood that they will try to see and compare the genitals of children of the opposite sex. Since this behaviour is liable to provoke feelings of intense hostility and guilt in adults, it frequently becomes secret and furtive and is then more likely to be carried over into school age. In such cases, i.e. when the child is of school age, it will usually be found that the parents find themselves too embarrassed or inadequate to undertake an objective discussion and explanation, since they have commonly baulked or mishandled the matter previously. It is then best for a physician or trained adult to give a sympathetic explanation that sexual interest is neither morbid nor disgraceful, and to describe sexual function as fully as is compatible with the child's understanding. The greater attention now paid to sex education

in schools helps to cultivate a healthy and informed attitude to sex. If the child is continually being stimulated by older or more precocious companions, a change of environment may be desirable.

Masturbation. This should be distinguished from simple handling of the genitals, since at whatever age masturbation occurs (and it may be observed in infancy), it is characterized by pleasurable excitation of the genitals associated with tension usually leading to climax and followed by relaxation. In infants, the effect is achieved by thigh-rubbing; the infant becomes flushed, with a look of intense concentration on his face, and angrily resents interference with the activity, which may be mistaken by parents for a form of fit. In older children, gratification is commonly obtained by manual or other means. The practice is common in later childhood, particularly amongst boys, and considerably less so before the age of 10 years. Thus Kinsey *et al.* (1948, 1953) found that 21 per cent of boys had experience of masturbation at the age of 12, and 82 per cent at 15 years, while corresponding figures for girls were 12 per cent and 20 per cent. Since the practice is frequently taught by companions, the incidence in different schools and communities is likely to differ widely. It is generally classified as a compulsive habit, but while it may represent a symptom of personality disturbance, e.g. when occurring to excess in the lonely, introspective type of child, or when associated with intense feelings of guilt, it must be recognized that it is common amongst otherwise normal and emotionally stable children. There is no evidence that masturbation causes permanent physical or mental damage, though it will induce temporary fatigue and apathy; the guilt feelings with which it is often associated, however, may be of considerably more consequence. Mutual masturbation and more systematized homosexual practices are considerably less common before than after puberty, though in some cases younger children will be initiated by older ones. When masturbation is practised by an older child publicly before adults and without apparent shame, it may prove to be a symptom of a psychotic personality. Such cases are rare.

Since advice is often asked by parents and others with regard to the attitude to be adopted to masturbation, consideration must be given to the age group concerned. When the habit has already been learnt by infants or younger children, the aim should be to provide alternative amusement and to help the introspective and withdrawn child to adapt to community life and interests. Attention should never be focused on the symptom, and mechanical restraints and punishments are useless.

In the case of older children, more good can be done by attempting to relieve guilt or fears which may be associated with the practice than by campaigning against it. Indeed, if the child is happy and stable, interference by a prying adult is only likely to do harm. It must always be remembered that the great majority of normal children of this age pass through a phase of sexual phantasy associated with masturbation which is outgrown when maturity is reached. If advice is asked by the child himself, it is probably best to point out that masturbation is not in itself harmful, and any existing feeling of guilt should not be added to directly or by implication.

Lying

Untruthfulness in children is often a matter of great concern to adults, sometimes when they themselves regard fabrications on their own part as entirely normal. The history will usually show whether 'lying' is in fact phantasy translated into story-telling, the reaction of an anxious or inadequate personality hoping to escape punishment or loss of parental affection; the 'wishing-away' of a crime; or a deliberate means of obtaining a particular end. In the case of very young children, it will be realized that phantasy is so near reality that a circumstantial account of having had tea with a tiger or having flown off the roof will be treated with proper interest. In middle childhood the reception of phantasy is often less sympathetic, largely because the adult is apt to be taken in by a more probable story; but for the child the distinction between fact and phantasy is still often much less clear.

In the case of the frightened child lying to avoid punishment, the best prospects of truthfulness lie in removing the penalty (whether punishment or loss of affection, more particularly the latter) which truthfulness is thought to involve, though even then the truth may not be elicited. The child who lies deliberately in order to gain his own ends is more closely related to the 'responsible delinquent', and the symptom may be associated with theft, truancy, or other antisocial behaviour.

Cruelty and aggression

Since aggression is a fundamental component of the child's emotional make-up, many behaviour problems stem from failure to canalize aggressive instincts in a manner acceptable to society. No infant is a 'born mixer', and the child under 2 years of age will commonly show more or less open hostility to another who invades his nursery or his parents' affection. Both parents are likely to experience aggressive behaviour from children during the pre-school period. Normally social adaptation is gradually learnt, the rough-and-tumble of school, outdoor games, and other activities providing an outlet for aggression which is socially harmless. It is the docile, overprotected child lacking in aggression who is most likely to suffer during school life.

Uncontrolled aggression will be shown by bullying, fighting, destruction of property, defiance of authority and the like. In schools where supervision is lax, bullying may assume formidable proportions, and while a few children are usually found to be the ring-leaders, it is surprising how many others will join in persecuting a 'lame duck'. Since aggression in the child is not associated with an adult appreciation of consequences, serious or fatal injuries may be inflicted on younger children.

The motivation of bullying, and of cruelty to younger children or animals, can also be based on a feeling of inadequacy and repression, children who have themselves suffered at the hands of older children or adults passing on the suffering to others. The oversimplified conception of the bully as a coward will apply to children of this type.

Crying and temper displays

Crying is a part of normal behaviour in infancy and childhood and has many causes, such as hunger, discomfort, pain, tiredness, loneliness, boredom, frustration, fear or anger. Crying is universal in early infancy but children vary greatly in the amount they cry, some doing so frequently and others only occasionally for good reason. The child who is constantly whining and girning is often insecure and in need of love and attention, though he is more likely to arouse anger and resentment in his parents. Discussion about the needs of young children and the reasons why children cry will help the parents to tolerate their child's behaviour and show him the affection he is asking for.

Most young children have occasional violent outbursts of temper, especially when they are thwarted or seeking attention. If *temper tantrums* are very frequent, and especially if they persist beyond the age of 5 years, it will usually be found that the parents are overindulgent or excessively dominating, though the temperament of the child must also be taken into account. In some cases the child has learnt that a display of temper is an effective method of getting his own way, while in other instances tantrums will be a symptom of negativism or of hostility to a particular person. The attacks may be imitative (when one parent is of violent temper) or related to physical ill-health or severe emotional disturbance.

Occasionally in the first three years they are associated with *breath-holding attacks*, which typically start with crying caused by anger or pain. At the end of a long expiratory cry, the child seems unable to 'get his breath back', becomes cyanosed and loses consciousness. After a short period, during which he may show opisthotonos and clonic twitching, normal breathing is resumed with prompt recovery thereafter. Breath-holding attacks are often familial and generally start during the first year. They are not in themselves dangerous and the mother can be assured that they generally cease before school age and always by 7 years of age. She should be cautioned not to indulge the child simply to avoid precipitating an attack. The mother's description generally serves to distinguish these attacks from epileptic seizures: rarely, however, the hypoxia of a breath-holding attack will precipitate a true epileptic fit.

Periodic disorders

It has long been recognized that certain children are prone to recurrent vomiting, headache, abdominal pain, pyrexia or limb pains, occurring at irregular intervals either alone or in combination. While the physical symptoms are striking and the etiology probably multifactorial, there are grounds for considering this group of disorders as primarily of psychogenic origin. Thus the affected children often show characteristic personality traits, being unusually sensitive and conscientious and no causative disease is demonstrable. These recurrent symptoms are generally considered to be different manifestations of a common disorder, which has been called the 'periodic syndrome' of childhood. The etiology is unknown but attacks may be precipitated by

emotional stress, fatigue or dietary indiscretion. There is an association between this syndrome and migraine, for both may occur in the same family and periodic disorders in childhood may be followed by migraine in later life. The best known of the periodic manifestations is vomiting, generally called *cyclical vomiting*, although the attacks are seldom strictly cyclical but occur at irregular intervals.

Recurrent vomiting in childhood is a common symptom, and one which calls for careful investigation. Organic obstruction and cerebral tumour must be excluded, and the possibility of any individual attack being due to appendicitis must be kept in mind. In a relatively small proportion of cases there will be a family history of migraine, and the occurrence of severe headache preceding the vomiting, associated with visual disturbances, should suggest the diagnosis of abdominal migraine.

In some children vomiting attacks are precipitated extremely readily, either by minor infections, by dietetic excesses (particularly over indulgence in fatty foods), or by excitement or anxiety, such as return to school, children's parties or the like. The 'nervous child' in whom vomiting attacks are clearly of psychogenic origin is sometimes a recognizable personality type, being intelligent, introspective, and a prey to a variety of minor neurotic symptoms such as food-fads and disturbances of sleep. A history of train- or car-sickness is often given. The general nutrition is poor, the build slender, and the posture characteristic, the child standing with rounded shoulders and with the abdomen sloping forward. The exact mechanism by which emotional disturbance precipitates vomiting is unknown.

The attack of cyclical vomiting is commonly ushered in by a short period of nausea, abdominal discomfort, and malaise. Vomiting then occurs, and is occasionally so severe and intractable that within a few hours the child is collapsed, dehydrated, and smelling strongly of acetone. The face is pale and dark circles appear beneath the eyes. Urinary output is reduced, and ketonuria is very marked. The bowels are usually constipated, but one or more pale stools may be passed. The upper abdomen is diffusely tender owing to the constant retching and vomiting.

Attacks usually last from one to three days and are followed by spontaneous recovery; but the degree of prostration which occurs may be such as to cause considerable anxiety. The condition rarely occurs before the age of 3 years and tends to disappear with the approach of puberty.

TREATMENT. At the first indication of an impending attack, the child should be put to rest in a darkened room and kept warm. When vomiting has started, it will usually be found that no solids can be retained, and nothing should then be given by mouth except orange juice or glucose-saline; it is advisable to start with minimal amounts (5 to 10 ml), doubling the amount each half-hour as long as it is not vomited. Sodium bicarbonate may be given in small dosage (120 mg two-hourly), but larger amounts carry a risk of producing an alkalosis. In the most severe and intractable cases it may be necessary to administer glucose-saline intravenously.

As soon as solids can be retained, dry toast and honey should be given and a gradual return to a normal diet made. It is advisable to limit fats throughout the period of recovery.

Migraine

The term migraine (derived from hemicrania) is applied to severe paroxysmal headache, which may be unilateral and is frequently associated with visual disturbances.

ETIOLOGY. There is probably no one cause of migraine, which should be thought of as a symptom complex rather than a disease entity. It is considered here for convenience, because of its close relationship to the periodic syndrome of childhood. As in the latter, a conscientious, introspective personality is common, while in some cases there may be an atopic background. With such a constitution, migraine may be precipitated by a variety of agents, especially emotional stress. Errors of refraction are sometimes said to be a precipitating cause but their importance has been overestimated. Migraine is believed to result from constriction followed by dilatation of cerebral and cranial blood vessels; some authorities consider that there is a relationship between migraine and epilepsy, but the evidence for this is unconvincing.

Migraine may occur in several generations. In childhood there appears to be little difference in incidence in the two sexes, though in older patients it is seen more frequently in females than in males. The symptoms often date from early childhood and the incidence at puberty is thought to be as high as 5 per cent.

CLINICAL FEATURES. The headache is prostrating and often accompanied by nausea. Abdominal pain and vomiting may dominate the picture and in younger children the condition is apt to be regarded as a 'bilious attack'. In typical cases in older children, however, the severity of the headache and the fact that this precedes the vomiting serve to establish the diagnosis. Visual disturbances may take the form of flashing lights, coloured figures or blurring of vision with transient diplopia or scotoma, though these are seldom accurately described by young children. The attack may last for several hours or for a day or longer, and is followed by a sense of depression and fatigue.

MANAGEMENT. The child should be investigated from both the physical and psychological aspects, and if a precipitating cause is found, e.g. sinus infection or overwork at school, this should be dealt with. Major errors of refraction should be corrected, but it is unlikely that a minor error discovered on routine examination will be responsible. If organic disease, particularly cerebral tumour, has been excluded, the child and parents should be reassured, and an attempt made to relieve anxiety.

The general treatment of the attack is similar to that of cyclical vomiting. Some patients obtain relief from aspirin or codeine, and if so this should always be given as soon as possible. The drug having the most specific effect, however, is ergotamine tartrate, a subcutaneous injection of 0.25 mg given early in the attack usually causing a dramatic relief of symptoms. Inhalation of ergotamine may be tried before resorting to injection; oral administration of ergotamine with caffeine is less effective.

Hysterical symptoms

Conversion hysteria is very much less common before puberty than in adolescence and adult life. An hysterical limp or weakness following a trivial injury is the most usual manifestation in childhood, but fits, aphonia, sensory disturbances, and choking attacks occur more rarely. The true hysteric is both highly suggestible and obstinate, and shows a characteristic complacency about his or her symptoms. Behaviour is comparable to that of a 4-year-old child, and is dramatic, posturing, and demanding attention. Hysteria must be distinguished both from *malingering*, which is a fully conscious complaint of non-existent symptoms, and from *anxiety symptoms* such as nausea, abdominal discomfort, or diarrhoea, which are produced by a frightening situation, and may appear regularly before the child sets off for school.

Infantile autism

This is a disturbance of interpersonal relationships, characterized by apparent lack of interest in other people and inability to establish emotional rapport with them. It becomes apparent in infancy or early childhood and is commoner in males. Autistic children give an impression of aloofness and isolation, with little expression of feeling. They may show ritualistic and stereotyped mannerisms, and their perception and comprehension are defective. These children fail to use speech normally and do not pay attention to the spoken word. They are therefore often thought to be deaf or mentally subnormal and indeed mental subnormality may frequently co-exist, although it is not an essential part of the syndrome. In many cases the parents are above average in intelligence and they are said to lack emotional warmth. Even with special education and skilled psychiatric treatment, the prognosis in infantile autism is poor and most children remain dependent throughout their lives.

CAUSATIVE FACTORS AND TREATMENT

It will be clear that many of the symptoms described may arise in children of widely different types, and that treatment must be appropriate to the problems of the individual child rather than directed to particular symptoms. In many cases it will be found that treatment of a parent is at least as important as treatment of the child, and the situation may be greatly improved if the overanxious or obsessive parent is helped to see things in proper perspective. In other cases, the parent will only require reassurance or advice, e.g. when the child is passing through what may be regarded as a normal phase of development.

In assessing personality-type, the history and direct observation will usually show which characters predominate. The *inadequate personality* will tend to avoid difficulties, show excessive dependence on the mother, be easily led into trouble, and may later overcompensate by bullying or antisocial behaviour. Such children when suffering from an *anxiety state* frequently show excessive fear of the dark, disturbance of sleep,

enuresis, recurrent vomiting or headache, or fear of going to school and of separation from the mother. *Aggressive types* will show greater independence and love of adventure which may, if repressed, turn to defiance of authority and negativism, or may find expression in physical symptoms such as tics, stammering, or asthma. The *withdrawn, solitary* child given to daydreaming may be of inadequate or psychotic personality or suffering from anxiety. It will be realized that these generalizations cannot be too strictly applied, since the child's behaviour will depend not only on constitution but also on the nature of the subsequent stress to which his personality is subject and the *age* at which conflict occurs.

Environmental and other factors affecting the child's emotional development are so numerous that only a few of the commoner patterns can be mentioned. Quarrelling parents and split discipline, e.g. one parent overindulgent and the other too severe, parents who are divorced or separated, return of a parent after a long absence, drunken, psychotic, or immoral parents, too high parental demands on a child unable to fulfil them, jealousy of a younger child, early separation experiences, institutional life with lack of personal affection, interference by neighbours or relatives, frequent changes of foster home, illegitimacy and rejection by the mother or relatives, are factors which appear repeatedly in case histories. It is exceptional in the case of a disturbed child to find that both parents are emotionally stable and happily married, or that there is no family history of behaviour disorders. (When there is no evidence of family disturbance, the child will probably be found to be constitutionally unstable, e.g. because he shows the hyperactive restlessness of organic cerebral damage or is a potential psychotic.) Extrinsic factors, such as pressure of school work, are only likely to cause severe disturbance in a child whose home background fails to give him the sense of security and affection which is required for normal development.

TREATMENT. The broad lines which treatment may follow in appropriate cases are: (1) advice and reassurance; (2) adjustment or change of environment, either at home or school; (3) group play therapy, which not only serves to release conflict and repressed desires but which may be of great value to the therapist in clarifying the nature of the disturbance, and will make possible a more direct approach to the child; (4) treatment of one or both parents, which may run parallel with that of the child; (5) treatment of the child by individual play therapy in which reassurance, suggestion, or interpretation according to analytical theory and technique may be used.

Speech therapy and education suitable for visual or auditory disability involve special techniques, and in the case of stammerers general psychotherapy may be required in addition.

In the case of a seriously disturbed child whose home environment is beyond remedy, it may be found advisable to admit him to a residential school or specially selected foster home where he can receive appropriate attention. The aim is essentially to provide the sense of security lacking in the child's own home, while individual attention can be given to educational problems which frequently co-exist with emotional difficulties even in children of high intelligence. In the case of children who are beyond parental control or living in moral danger, there are legal facilities for bringing the child before a juvenile court which has the power to order admission to an approved school, to direct guardianship, or to arrange other disposal. The court has power to make full use of the Child Guidance Service and suitable voluntary organizations. In Scotland, some of the functions of the juvenile court have been taken over by children's panels of lay people qualified by knowledge and experience to consider the problems of children requiring care or control.

BIBLIOGRAPHY AND REFERENCES

APLEY, J. & MACKEITH, R. (1967). *The Child and his Symptoms. A Psychosomatic Approach*, 2nd edn. Oxford: Blackwell.
BAKWIN, H. (1965). Learning problems and school phobia. *Pediatric Clinics of North America*, 12, 995.
BAKWIN, H. & BAKWIN, R. M. (1972). *Behaviour Disorders in Children*, 4th edn. Philadelphia: Saunders.
BAKWIN, H. (1965). Learning problems and school phobia. *Pediatric Clinics of North America*, 12, 995.
BELLMAN, M. (1966). Studies on encopresis. *Acta paediatrica* suppl. 170.
BENTLEY, J. F. R. (1971). Constipation in infants and children. *Gut*, 12, 85.
BERG, I. & JONES, K. V. (1964). Functional faecal incontinence in children. *Archives of Disease in Childhood*, 39, 465.
BOWLBY, J. (1951). *Maternal Care and Mental Health*. Geneva: W.H.O.
CAMERON, H. C. (1945). *The Nervous Child*, 5th edn. Oxford University Press.
FENICHEL, G. M. (1968). Migraine in childhood. *Clinical Pediatrics*, 7, 192.
HERSOV, L. A. (1960). Refusal to go to school. *Journal of Child Psychology and Psychiatry and Allied Disciplines*, 1, 137.
INGRAM, T. T. S. (1959). Specific developmental disorders of speech in childhood. *Brain*, 82, 450.
KANNER, L. (1972). *Child Psychiatry*, 4th edn. Springfield: Thomas.
KANNER, L. (1960). Do behavioural symptoms always indicate psychopathology? *Journal of Child Psychology and Psychiatry and Allied Disciplines*, 1, 17.
KINSEY, A. C., POMEROY, W. B. & MARTIN, C. E. (1948). *Sexual Behaviour in the Human Male*. Philadelphia: Saunders.
KINSEY, A. C., POMEROY, W. B., MARTIN, C. E. & GEBHARD, P. H. (1953). *Sexual Behaviour in the Human Female*. Philadelphia: Saunders.
LAXDAL, T., GOMEZ, M. R. & REIHER, J. (1969). Cyanotic and pallid syncopal attacks in children (breath-holding spells). *Developmental Medicine and Child Neurology*, 11, 755.
LEWIS, H. (1954). *Deprived Children*. London: Nuffield Foundation.
LIVINGSTON, S. (1970). Breath-holding spells in children. *Journal of the American Medical Association*, 212, 2231.
MACKEITH, R. (1960). Faecal incontinence in children. *British Medical Journal*, ii, 1451.
MACKEITH, R. & SANDLER, J. (1961). *Psychosomatic Aspects of Paediatrics*. Oxford: Pergamon Press.
MORLEY, M. E. (1972). *The Development and Disorders of Speech in Childhood*, 3rd edn. Edinburgh: Churchill Livingstone.
RUTTER, M. (1968). Concepts of autism. *Journal of Child Psychology and Psychiatry and Allied Disciplines*, 9, 1.
SCOTT, P. D. (1965). Delinquency. In *Modern Perspectives in Child Psychiatry*. Edited by J. G. Howells. Edinburgh: Oliver & Boyd.
SPENCE, J. C. (1946). *The Purpose of the Family*. London: National Children's Home.
STONE, F. H. (1970). Emotional development. In *Child Life and Health*, 5th edn. Edited by R. G. Mitchell. London: Churchill.
WHITE, M. (1968). A thousand consecutive cases of enuresis. *Medical Officer*, 120, 151.
WILKINS, L. T. (1960). *Delinquent Generations*. London: H.M.S.O.
WING, L. (1970). The syndrome of early childhood autism. *British Journal of Hospital Medicine*, 4, 381.
YOUNGHUSBAND, E. L. (1970). Children in trouble. In *Child Life and Health*, 5th edn. Edited by R. G. Mitchell. London: Churchill.

18 Procedures and Therapy

OBTAINING BLOOD AND MARROW

Venepuncture is a procedure dreaded by children and the number performed should be kept to a minimum by skilful technique and by carrying out as many as possible of the necessary tests on the same sample of blood. Fortunately, venepuncture should be less frequent in future owing to the increasing application of microchemical techniques using capillary blood. Obtaining venous blood from infants and young children may present difficulty owing to the small size of the veins, particularly in cases with dehydration and collapse. The umbilical vessels can only be utilized for a short time following birth. The antecubital vein is often invisible and impalpable in early infancy, though it is a site of choice if it can be entered. Careful examination may show other superficial veins, e.g. on the scalp, wrist, or ankle, from which 1 or more ml of blood can be withdrawn. The risk of venepuncture is small in experienced hands but, in general, superficial veins are to be preferred to deep ones because the potential complications of using the latter are more serious.

Capillary blood

Small quantities of blood (0·5 to 1·0 ml) may be obtained from infants by heel stab. The ankle is grasped in the left hand so that the forefinger lies across the sole of the foot, the thumb across the tendo achillis, and the third, fourth, and fifth fingers around the anterior surface of the tibia. After warming and cleansing the skin of the heel, the latter is stabbed with a disposable stilette, and the blood collected in a tube by capillary attraction. Squeezing the heel should be avoided. In older children, capillary blood may be obtained from the finger or the lobe of the ear.

Venepuncture

Failing the antecubital veins, larger quantities of blood may be aspirated from one of the following sites, the skin being first carefully prepared with chlorhexidine.

EXTERNAL JUGULAR. In the case of the right external jugular, the infant should be wrapped in a blanket securing the arms, and held lying on the left side. The neck is flexed to the left, and the infant's chin held by the assistant's right hand. In this position the external jugular is brought into prominence as it crosses the sternomastoid, and its engorgement will be increased by crying. The needle is most readily inserted from below upward (Fig. 18.1).

INTERNAL JUGULAR. Internal jugular puncture requires accurate attention to the positioning of the infant, and care to avoid damage to other structures in the neck. In the position described, the vein lies superficially and is usually entered at a depth of 0·5 cm. With proper precautions there

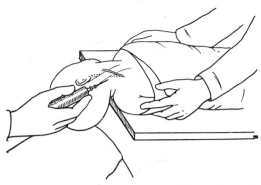

Fig. 18.2   Internal jugular puncture. Infant supine with both shoulders on table; neck extended, chin turned to left.

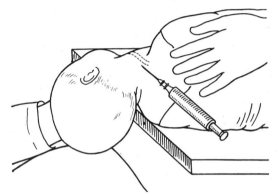

Fig. 18.1   External jugular puncture. Infant on left side and neck flexed to left.

is little risk of damage to the carotid artery or vagus nerve, both of which tend to slip away from the needle; only deep and indiscriminate needling is liable to puncture the trachea.

The infant is held in the supine position by an assistant; it is important that both shoulders should lie flat on the table. The infant's head should project beyond the end of the table; the neck is fully extended, and the chin turned fully to the left (when the right internal jugular is being approached), being kept in position by the assistant or by the operator's left wrist. The needle is entered obliquely, pointing toward the sterno-clavicular junction of the same side, at the junction of the middle and lower thirds of the posterior border of the sternomastoid (Fig. 18.2). The point of the needle should pass just underneath the belly of the sternomastoid; failure to enter the vein is usually due to the needle being directed too deeply.

FEMORAL VEIN. This has the disadvantage that venepuncture must be made in an area subject to faecal contamination, and also that the femoral artery may be punctured since it is immobilized at the level of the inguinal ligament.

The infant's thigh is abducted, externally rotated, and slightly extended. The pulsation of the femoral artery is palpated, and the needle entered immediately internal and parallel to the artery, 1 cm distal to and pointing towards the inguinal ligament.

SUPERIOR SAGITTAL SINUS. This is not recommended as a site of choice for taking blood, and should never be used for giving intravenous injections. The dangers of cerebral haemorrhage or sinus thrombosis are so serious that, although both these eventualities are rare, other sites should be used whenever possible.

The scalp over and surrounding the anterior fontanelle is shaved, the infant placed in the supine position, and the head held firmly by an assistant. A short sinus-needle, e.g. 1 cm in length, is inserted exactly in the midline at the posterior angle of the fontanelle, and may be directed anteriorly or posteriorly. Care must be taken to avoid puncturing the inferior walls of the sinus or deflecting the needle to right or left of the midline. The posterior fontanelle is sometimes used as an alternative site of entry.

Marrow puncture

Examination of bone marrow is required in the investigation of many types of blood disorder. The best site for obtaining marrow is the iliac crest, but a vertebral spinous process may also be used and the upper end of the tibia is a suitable site in infants. The sternum should not be used in children because of the risk of penetration. The child may require to be anaesthetized for the procedure, a useful method being rectal thiopentone in a dose of 40 mg per kg, with a local anaesthetic in addition if required. A dry-sterilized Sala-type needle is used, with an adjustable guard to control the depth of entry. After the needle is inserted, the stilette is removed and aspiration of marrow effected by use of a well-fitting 1 ml syringe.

BLOOD TRANSFUSION AND ADMINISTRATION OF FLUID

Blood transfusion

It is usually desirable to give blood or other intravenous fluids by slow drip through plastic tubing attached to a needle or cannula. The simplest method is to insert a needle into a superficial vein in the scalp or wrist: an intravenous catheter placement unit is convenient for introducing a plastic catheter into a vein but must be used with care for there is a risk that the end of the catheter may be accidentally cut and swept into the circulation. Occasionally it may be necessary to expose a vein and tie a cannula into position.

TRANSFUSION WITHOUT EXPOSURE OF A VEIN. The scalp veins are those of choice in young infants, since they are well supported by surrounding tissue and any leakage is clearly visible. They may be distended by application of a drop of xylol or by warmth or pressure. After shaving the hair and preparing the skin, the needle of a disposable scalp-vein transfusion set is introduced into the vein. When the appearance of blood in the tubing indicates entry into the lumen, the needle is fixed flat against the head with adhesive tape. Alternatively, a needle may be attached to a syringe for introduction into the vein. The rate of flow should not exceed 30 drops per minute and myocardial damage is an indication for greater caution.

The internal jugular and femoral veins should not be used, since the risk of over-distending the right side of the heart by internal jugular transfusion is considerable, while transfusion into the femoral vein may result in thrombosis or infection.

TRANSFUSION WITH EXPOSURE OF A VEIN. The internal saphenous or antecubital veins are usually found the most satisfactory. The limb must be immobilized by splinting before the procedure is started, care being taken to avoid impeding the circulation.

After injection of a local anaesthetic, the vein is exposed by an incision at right angles to the course of the vein. In the case of the internal saphenous, the incision is made slightly above and anterior to the internal malleolus. The incision is opened with artery forceps and the vein stripped for a distance of 1 to 1·5 cm, in order to avoid insertion of the cannula into the perivascular sheath. Ligatures should be loosely applied above and below the site chosen for opening the vein, but it is not always necessary subsequently to tie them off. The centre of the presenting surface of the vein is seized with mosquito forceps (or the vein drawn forward by gentle traction on one of the ligatures), and a V-shaped incision made with sharp-pointed scissors. In order to avoid tearing the vein, the incision should not include more than one-third of its circumference.

A Luer-fitting plastic catheter or length of polythene tubing connected to a glass drip and blood-reservoir is then inserted into the proximal portion of the vein for a distance of 3 cm or more (Fig. 18.3). Alternatively a small metal cannula, e.g. the outer portion of a Bateman needle, can be inserted, in which case the proximal ligature is tightened round the cannula to keep it in place. Plastic tubing has the advantage of being flexible, and greater mobility of the limb is possible during transfusion. For slow-drip transfusions, a closed flask should be used as a blood reservoir, with a graduated 100 ml cylinder below it to allow accurate measurement of the quantity of blood given. The rate of flow must be regulated by frequent adjustment of the screw clip or by means of an automated infusion unit, since a partial block may suddenly become cleared and the rate of flow increase dangerously. For infants, transfusion at the rate of 35 to 45 ml per hour (12 to 15 drops per minute) will usually be appropriate, although slower rates may be necessary for infants of low birth weight.

REPLACEMENT TRANSFUSION OF NEWBORN INFANTS. Although replacement transfusion is occasionally required in older children, the principal indication is haemolytic disease of the newborn. A suitable apparatus is shown in Figure 18.4; disposable sets of similar design are now available. Before use, the apparatus should be filled with saline and all air bubbles excluded. Joints in the apparatus must fit closely to avoid the risk of injecting air. The umbilical cord is cut off approximately 1·5 cm from the umbilicus, the

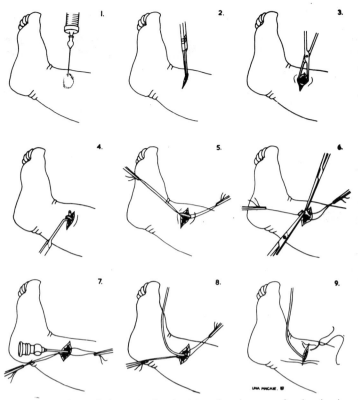

Fig. 18.3   Technique of transfusion, exposing the internal saphenous vein, showing insertion of cannula (7) or plastic catheter (8).

thin-walled umbilical vein identified, and held with mosquito forceps. A catheter with lateral apertures (A) is inserted into the umbilical vein. Some difficulty may be experienced in passing the catheter beyond the abdominal wall, in which case the stump of the cord should be drawn downward and the lower abdominal wall compressed. Further obstruction at the wall of the portal arch may be overcome by manipulation. The catheter should, if possible, be inserted for a distance of 5 to 8 cm. If the umbilical route is found impossible, the femoral vein may be approached through the long saphenous vein in the groin (1·5 cm below the inguinal ligament). Before starting the procedure, 20 ml of blood should be withdrawn, or up to 50 ml if venous pressure is high. Exchange transfusion is then carried out by withdrawing 10 ml blood into the syringe, turning the stop-cock and ejecting the blood through B; filling the syringe with fresh donor blood from the bottle through C, and injecting this through A. The process is repeated until a transfusion of 180 ml blood per kg body weight has been completed. This will effect an exchange of approximately 85 per cent, which is usually adequate. (Repeated exchange transfusions may be necessary if the bilirubin rises, and some authorities consider that two smaller exchange transfusions are preferable to one large one.) A second flask (H.S.) is kept filled with heparinized saline (1000 units per 500 ml) which may be aspirated into the syringe through D and used to wash out the apparatus at intervals to prevent clotting. The infant's stomach should be emptied before the transfusion, and the infant must be kept warm throughout. The procedure should be carried out slowly and a careful watch kept on the pulse, as cardiac failure is a very real danger in infants with a low haemoglobin and myocardial weakness. The infusion of large quantities of citrated blood may also depress calcium ionization (Farquhar and Smith, 1958), and 1 ml of 10 per cent calcium gluconate may be injected slowly after every 100 to 150 ml of blood.

In small or ill infants, a smoother replacement may be effected by umbilical arteriovenous ex-

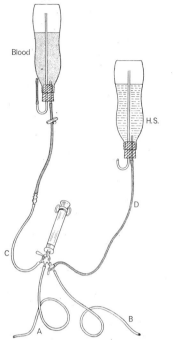

Fig. 18.4   Apparatus for replacement transfusion. (After J. W. Farquhar and I. C. Lewis, 1949.)

change, blood being withdrawn through a catheter in an umbilical artery and fresh blood being transfused through the umbilical vein. Other methods of replacement transfusion have been described but are generally more complicated and offer no great advantage over standard methods.

ADMINISTRATION OF SOLUTIONS. Fluids other than blood are best given by slow-drip infusion into a vein as described for blood. For very small infants, the use of a micro-drop cylinder delivering 80 drops per ml will help to avoid accidental overloading of the circulation. Subcutaneous injection of physiological saline is occasionally used in the treatment of mild degrees of salt and water depletion, but does not provide a substitute for intravenous therapy in moderate or severe dehydration. A reservoir is suspended above the bed, and connected by a Y-junction with two venepuncture needles, which are inserted subcutaneously into the axillae, thighs, or over the abdominal wall. As the injected area becomes distended with fluid, the direction or site of the needles should be changed from time to time. The rate of absorption can be increased by the use of hyaluronidase.

Fluids, including blood, may be given by intraperitoneal drip, inserting the needle through the skin of the flank. The administration of fluid by rectal drip has a limited value in the treatment of older children who are unable to take fluid by mouth, but even 5 per cent glucose solution is generally found irritating after a short while. The fluid is run into the rectum by slow drip, using a gravity apparatus and soft rubber catheter. A gastric drip infusion may occasionally be useful when feeding by mouth causes vomiting and the fluid cannot be given by the intravenous route.

STOMACH-WASHING AND GAVAGE

Washing out the stomach is sometimes indicated in the case of infants suffering from severe vomiting associated with mucous gastritis; to determine the amount of gastric residue in cases with partial obstruction; and in order to obtain swallowed sputum for bacteriological examination. Oral thrush is a contraindication, as the infection may be transmitted to the oesophagus or stomach.

A soft rubber or plastic catheter (14 French gauge) is passed over the back of the tongue. As insertion is gently continued, a sensation of release is felt when the end enters the stomach. It is very rare for the tube to pass through the glottis, but when this occurs a to-and-fro movement of air through the catheter will be obvious on respiration. Gastric residue can be siphoned off, or the stomach washed out by running in sterile water or saline through a funnel attached to the catheter, siphoning back the fluid after 50 to 100 ml have been injected. Bicarbonate solutions should never be used in cases where there has been vomiting, owing to the risk of precipitating alkalosis. Tube feeding is effected in a similar manner, passing the tube either by the mouth (10 French gauge) or through the nose (5 French gauge), though the latter is more liable to cause respiratory obstruction. Care must be taken in pouring the feed through the funnel to avoid large amounts of air entering the stomach at the same time.

LUMBAR, CISTERNAL, AND VENTRICULAR PUNCTURE

Lumbar puncture

The child should be laid on his right side on a flat surface. The assistant stands facing the child, and passes her right arm round and under the child's flexed thighs, holding the child's hands with her right hand. The assistant's left arm serves to flex the child's neck. It is important that the back should not be rotated. The spines of the vertebrae should be parallel with the surface of the table and the left shoulder and left hip should be vertically above the right. An alternative method is for the child to be held in the sitting posture with the back flexed; this has anatomical advantages, but it is less easy to prevent movement.

A 4 to 6 cm lumbar puncture needle is inserted in the midline between the spines of the third and fourth or fourth and fifth lumbar vertebrae, since the spinal cord in the young infant reaches a lower level (L3 in the newborn) than in the adult. Failure to obtain fluid uncontaminated by blood is most commonly due to the posterior dura being carried forward across the canal by the point of the needle until pinned against the anterior wall of the canal. The needle then penetrates the posterior dura, but it is not uncommon for the anterior dura to be punctured at the same time, and for the needle to penetrate the venous plexus, body of the vertebra, or disc, resulting in a bloody or dry tap. The use of sharp fine needles will reduce the likelihood of faulty taps, but when the fluid is purulent, a needle of adequate gauge will be necessary to obtain fluid whatever the age of the patient.

Fluid should always be withdrawn slowly and never during a convulsion. Manometer readings are only of value if the patient is quiet, as screaming or struggling will raise the pressure very greatly. It is occasionally necessary to perform lumbar puncture under general anaesthesia. In older infants and children, local anaesthesia should be used as a routine, but in young infants the injection of a local anaesthetic is likely to cause as much disturbance as lumbar puncture itself.

Cisternal puncture

The cisterna magna lies between the cerebellum and medulla, and owing to the immediate vicinity of vital centres and the ease with which adjacent structures may be displaced as a result of raised intracranial pressure, cisternal puncture should never be lightly undertaken. Previous practice on the cadaver is advisable.

The needle is introduced midway between the external occipital protuberance and the spine of the atlas, and directed forward along the under surface of the basi-occipital. It is usually possible to feel when the dura is punctured, but in any case of doubt the stilette should be repeatedly withdrawn until fluid is obtained.

Ventricular puncture

This is only practicable (without surgical procedure) in infants in whom the anterior fontanelle is still patent. It may be indicated when a block is suspected in the ventricular system.

The scalp is shaved, and the external angle of the fontanelle identified. A lumbar puncture needle is inserted at the external angle of the fontanelle, and directed either towards the inner canthus of the eye (to reach the anterior horn) or at right angles to the scalp (to enter the central cavity of the ventricle). It is most important that the direction of the needle should not be altered while it lies within cerebral tissue. Unless the ventricle is grossly dilated, the point of the needle may have to be inserted 4 to 5 cm from the surface before fluid is obtained. Air should not be injected directly into the ventricle unless preparations for immediate neurosurgery have been made.

Subdural tap

When the presence of a subdural collection of fluid is suspected, the scalp should be shaved and a short-bevelled needle inserted through the coronal suture about 1 cm lateral to the angle of the anterior fontanelle. The needle is advanced at right angles to the surface for not more than 1 cm, when any fluid present will drip or spurt out. The procedure should be repeated on the opposite side, not more than 20 ml of fluid being removed at each tap.

Air encephalography

This useful diagnostic procedure may be indicated when there is no evidence of raised intracranial pressure, and it is desirable to demonstrate radiologically the appearance of the ventricles or cortex. The child is sedated and lumbar puncture performed in the usual way. The child is then held in the sitting posture, with the head exactly in the midline and the neck slightly extended. 20 ml of cerebrospinal fluid are removed, and 10 ml of air then injected by syringe through the lumbar puncture needle. A further 10 ml fluid are removed, followed by the injection of 10 ml of air, the process being repeated until 60 to 100 ml fluid or less have been removed and a volume of air 10 ml less than that of the fluid removed has been injected. The skull is then X-rayed in the required positions, and careful positioning will reduce the necessity for injecting large volumes of air. Good visualization of the ventricles can often be obtained by this method, though frequently some air (which may demonstrate porencephaly or other abnormality) will come to lie over the cortex (Fig. 18.5).

DOSAGE OF DRUGS

Unfortunately no single rule of thumb can be applied indiscriminately for calculating the proportion of the adult dose appropriate for children of different ages, since some drugs produce toxic symptoms more readily in infants than in adults, while others are better tolerated by the young. Even when the weight rather than the age is used for calculating dosage, many examples will be found where a single formula is not applicable. Body surface area is a better yardstick but is complex for ordinary use. In practice, the dose of a drug may be calculated on the basis of a known number of mg or g per kg body weight, making allowance for the fact that the younger the patient the more drug is generally required per kg

body weight, though the total dose will of course be less. A valuable source of ready reference to the dosage of drugs used in paediatric practice is the vade-mecum maintained for many years by the staff of Birmingham Children's Hospital (Wood, 1970). This also contains much useful information on normal biological standards in infancy and childhood.

SULPHONAMIDES AND ANTIBIOTICS

In deciding on the treatment of choice in combating infection, the causative organism and its antibiotic sensitivities should be determined as soon as possible, though in the case of a severely ill child it is often necessary to start treatment before the results are available. Sensitivity testing has assumed major importance in view of the increasing incidence of resistance to the antibiotics in general and to penicillin in particular, as the result either of the selective survival of naturally resistant variants or of the emergence of insensitive mutants. In some instances the best results are obtained by a combination of sulphonamide and antibiotic therapy, but as a general principle it is preferable not to combine a bacteriostatic agent, such as tetracycline, with a

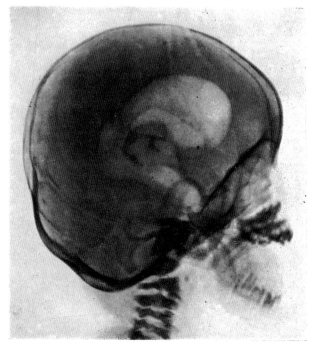

Fig. 18.5   Air-filled ventricles, showing dilatation of ventricular system, in an infant with hydrocephalus.

bactericidal one, e.g. penicillin. The drugs or antibiotics of choice will be ones with high therapeutic activity combined with low toxicity, while the method of administration (oral or parenteral, and single or multiple daily injections) will require particular consideration in the case of infants and young children.

Table 18.1 shows the order of preference of antibiotics in a number of infections, and the response to sulphonamides.

Where the response to sulphonamides is good and where there is difficulty in an antibiotic reaching the infecting organisms (e.g. meningococcal meningitis), sulphonamide treatment is the method of choice, with supportive antibiotic therapy.

THE SULPHONAMIDES

Toxic manifestations

All patients under sulphonamide therapy should be carefully watched for toxic manifestations. Infants are, on the whole, more tolerant of sulphonamides than are older children, but since dehydration and acidosis are commoner in infancy, the risk of renal blockage in this group must be borne in mind and the urine regularly examined. Care must be taken to maintain an adequate fluid intake. Drug fever is not very uncommon, and if the temperature fails to settle within five days of commencing treatment, the possibility of its being a sensitization phenomenon should be tested by withholding the drug for 24 hours. Drug rashes, erythema nodosum and agranulocytosis are now less common than with the earlier preparations. Sulphonamide preparations should not be applied to the skin owing to the risk of sensitization. Sulphonamides should be avoided in the newborn, since they may cause kernicterus in the presence of hyperbilirubinaemia, possibly by dissociating indirect bilirubin and albumin. They may also give rise to haemolytic anaemia in infants with G-6-PD deficiency.

Long-acting sulphonamides, e.g. sulphamethoxypyridazine, are now seldom used because they may precipitate Stevens-Johnson syndrome (p. 354).

ADMINISTRATION

Oral administration (of a flavoured suspension for infants and younger children) is generally adopted. If vomiting or the necessity for attaining a high blood-level quickly makes an alternative route preferable, sulphadimidine sodium may be given intravenously or intramuscularly.

Table 18.1 Choice of antibiotics and response to sulphonamides
A=ampicillin, C=chloramphenicol, Ca=carbenicillin, Cl=cloxacillin, Co=colistin, E=erythromycin, Ne=neomycin, P=penicillin G or V, Px=polymyxin, S=streptomycin, SULPH=sulphonamides, T=tetracyclines. This table is intended as a guide pending results of sensitivity testing: penicillin should be used when organism proved penicillin-sensitive.

Infecting organism		Choice of antibiotic			Response to sulphonamide
		1	2	3	
Brucella		T	C	S or Px	+
Corynebacterium diphtheriae		P	T	C	0
Haemophilus influenzae		C or A	T or Px	S	+
Bordetella pertussis		T	C	...	0
Escherichia coli	parenteral	A	T	S	+
	intestinal	N	Co	A	+
Gonococci		P	A	T	+
Meningococci		SULPH	P	A	+ +
Peumococci		P	Cl or E	T	+
Proteus	parenteral	S	A	C	0
	intestinal	Px	A	Ne	0
Pseudomonas pyocyanea		Px	Co	Ca	0
Salmonella typhi		C	A	...	0
Shigella sonnei		T	Ne or Co	S	+
Shigella dysenteriae		T	Px	Ne or Co	+
Streptococcus haemolyticus or viridans		P	A	E or S	±
Enterococci		T	C	Px	0
Staphylococcus pyogenes		Cl	T	E	±
Treponema pallidum		P	...	T or C	0

Intrathecal administration should never be attempted.

DOSAGE

The dosage of sulphonamide can be calculated on the basis of 0·2 g per kg body weight per day, although rather higher doses may be required at the onset of severe infections. The initial loading dose should be double that of subsequent doses, and the total daily dosage is divided into four doses, given at six-hourly intervals. After a period of two to three days, the maintenance dose can usually be reduced. A child weighing 15 kg would thus receive 3 g in each 24 hours, i.e. 0·75 g six-hourly. To this would be added a loading dose on the first day.

CHOICE OF DRUG

Sulphadimidine is the sulphonamide most suitable for general use, since the risk of toxicity or crystalluria is low and an adequate blood level can readily be maintained. The causative organism and site of infection may sometimes indicate the choice of another preparation, such as a poorly absorbed sulphonamide in intestinal infections. Trimethoprim enhances the response of infections to sulphonamides, and the combination of sulphamethoxazole and trimethoprim is very effective in urinary and respiratory infections in childhood.

Meningococcal meningitis (see p. 344).

Urinary tract infection

Sulphadimidine is the preparation of choice owing to the low risk of renal complications. The fluid intake should be high.

Acute rheumatism

Sulphadimidine may be used for prophylaxis (p. 270).

Ulcerative colitis

Sulphasalazine may sometimes be of value.

Gastrointestinal infections

The insoluble sulphonamide phthalylsulphathiazole may be used in the treatment of bacillary dysentery, e.g. when the more effective antibiotics are not available.

THE ANTIBIOTICS

Toxic effects

Harmful side effects may complicate the use of any of the antibacterial substances. Penicillin remains the least toxic but may produce stomatitis, allergic dermatitis and rare fatal anaphylactic reactions. Streptomycin may produce febrile disturbances and proteinuria, and is toxic to the eighth cranial nerve. Chloramphenicol (see below) is liable to depress or completely suppress one or more of the blood-forming components of the bone marrow, and in newborn and pre-term infants may produce collapse (the 'grey syndrome') if the recommended dosage is exceeded. Thrombocytopenic purpura, liver damage and meningeal irritation have followed the use of tetracyclines which may also cause yellow staining of the first dentition. A number of intestinal disorders, ranging from an irritating proctitis to intractable diarrhoea or a fatal staphylococcal enterocolitis, may be produced by interference with normal intestinal flora. Most antibiotics may predispose the alimentary and respiratory tracts to invasion by *Candida albicans*.

The severe side effects of antibiotics are admittedly uncommon, but the unpredictability of their occurrence should exert a restraining influence on the indiscriminate use of antibiotic therapy. Even greater importance should be attached to the fact that the more an antibiotic is used in a community the more rapidly do resistant strains emerge. In general, therefore, antibiotics should only be used when clearly indicated and it should be borne in mind that many respiratory infections in childhood are caused by viruses which will not respond to antibiotic therapy. Only in infants is immediate treatment commonly required before the infecting organism and its resistance can be determined.

THE PENICILLINS

Benzylpenicillin (penicillin G) is active against the Gram-positive cocci, the meningococci, gonococci, the organisms of anthrax, diphtheria, tetanus, gas gangrene, actinomycosis, Vincent's angina, and the spirochaetes of syphilis, yaws, relapsing fever, and Weil's disease. There has been steady increase in the incidence of penicillin resistance of pathogenic staphylococci, however, with the practical result that in staphylococcal infections of early infancy benzylpenicillin is no longer the antibiotic of choice.

The use of benzylpenicillin is limited by four factors, viz. its destruction by gastric acidity makes oral administration unreliable except possibly in the newborn infant; its rapid elimination by the kidney makes frequent injections the only alternative to continuous infusion; it is inactivated by penicillinase-producing organisms including some strains of *Staphylococcus aureus*; and it is relatively inefficient against many Gram-negative organisms.

The development of slowly-released penicillin salts has made possible long-acting injections of depot penicillin which will maintain effective levels for one day to two or more weeks. Isolation of the penicillin nucleus has led to biosynthetic preparations falling into three main groups: those which resist acid destruction, those which resist penicillinase, and those which are effective not only against Gram-positive but also against a wider range of Gram-negative organisms. Of penicillins which are acid-resistant and suitable for oral administration, phenoxymethylpenicillin (penicillin V) approximates most closely to the activity of benzylpenicillin, but is less suitable for the treatment of very acute infections or those in which resistance may be encountered.

Cloxacillin, which is active against most penicillinase-producing organisms and is a very valuable antistaphylococcal agent, is indicated in staphylococcal infections resistant to benzylpenicillin. Methicillin is also effective but must be given by injection.

Ampillicin has been described as a broad-spectrum penicillin because it is effective not only against those organisms which are sensitive to benzylpenicillin but also against *Haemophilus influenzae* and some species of salmonella, while it is moderately active against *E. coli* and some strains of *Proteus* and *Shigella*.

Carbenicillin is active against *Ps. pyocyanea* and some strains of *Proteus* and *E. coli*. It is given by intravenous or intramuscular injection in a dosage of 200 mg per kg daily.

PREPARATIONS of penicillin available for systemic therapy include benzylpenicillin for intermittent intramuscular injection, various depot penicillins, and a number of preparations for oral administration. Penicillin is also prepared as an ointment for local application to the skin. Solutions of benzylpenicillin may be employed in the pleura, in the conjunctiva, in abscess cavities, for inhalation and for intrathecal injection.

Benzylpenicillin. In severe infections, benzylpenicillin in aqueous solution should be injected intramuscularly at six-hourly intervals. Although the dosage will be influenced by the sensitivity of the organism, a total daily dosage of 500,000 units in children under 5 years of age and 1 mega unit in older children will generally be adequate.

Depot penicillin. Procaine penicillin, benethamine penicillin, and benzathine penicillin, in that order, provide intramuscular depots from which effective plasma levels may be maintained for one to two days, three to six days, and two weeks or more respectively. Of these the procaine salt remains the most generally useful and may be administered in a single daily dose of 150,000 to 300,000 units, depending on the age of the child.

The longer-acting preparations may cause more or less painful local reactions. Benzathine penicillin has been employed successfully in the prophylaxis of streptococcal infections in rheumatic children.

ORAL PENICILLIN. Phenoxymethylpenicillin (penicillin V), cloxacillin or ampicillin may be given six-hourly, 62·5 to 250 mg up to the age of 10 years, after which the adult dosage is applicable. Larger doses may be required in severe infections. Penicillin lozenges should not be used, owing to the risk of producing stomatitis.

INTRAVENOUS INJECTION. Administration of penicillin by intravenous drip is most likely to be required at the onset of treatment in fulminating infections, e.g. meningococcal meningitis. Benzylpenicillin in solution is incorporated in the fluid selected for intravenous infusion.

TOPICAL THERAPY. Injection of penicillin into infected cavities may usefully be combined with intensive systemic therapy. In the case of an empyema, aspiration of pus should be followed by injection through the same needle of penicillin solution containing 50,000 to 250,000 units, depending on the size of the patient. This is continued daily until the fluid is sterile or no further pus can be withdrawn.

STREPTOMYCIN

The major value of this antibiotic lies in the treatment of selected tuberculous conditions, the indications for its use in tuberculosis being considered in Chapter 15. In non-tuberculous conditions it is now mainly used in the treatment of Proteus infections of the urinary tract and in combined therapy with other antibiotics.

ADMINISTRATION AND DOSAGE. *Systemic therapy* is effected by intramuscular injection of 40 mg per kg body weight daily in two divided doses, up to a total daily dose of 1 g. The risks of overdosage are considerably less in the case of non-tuberculous infections where systemic therapy is used only for short periods.

Oral therapy. Since absorption from the bowel is slight, oral therapy is only indicated in infections of the gastrointestinal tract. In bacillary dysenteric infections, particularly those due to *Sh. sonnei*, rapid clearing of the stools has been obtained, using 1 g per day in divided doses for five days in the case of infants.

Combined therapy. The use of para-aminosalicylic acid (PAS) and isoniazid in combination with streptomycin in tuberculous conditions has been found to reduce the tendency to development of streptomycin resistance. Schemes of combined therapy are outlined on p. 325.

CHLORAMPHENICOL

Now prepared synthetically, this is effective against a wide range of Gram-negative and Gram-positive organisms, spirochaetes, and Rickettsiae. Unfortunately its potential toxicity (see above) makes it unsuitable for prolonged or repeated use, particularly in infants of low birth weight. Chloramphenicol remains the antibiotic of choice in typhoid fever and in the initial treatment of pyogenic meningitis. It may prove superior to others in the treatment of laryngo-tracheobronchitis, and in proteus and other resistant Gram-negative infections.

Oral administration results in adequate blood and cerebrospinal fluid levels in children when a total daily dosage of 25 to 50 mg per kg body weight is given in four doses, six-hourly. In pre-term infants and during the first week of life, the dosage should not exceed 25 mg per kg body weight daily, in divided doses. An intramuscular preparation, 1 per cent skin and eye ointments and 10 per cent ear drops (for treatment of otitis externa) are available.

THE TETRACYCLINES

Tetracycline, oxytetracycline, and chlortetracycline are all 'broad-spectrum' antibiotics with a wide range of antibacterial activity. All are effective by mouth in a dosage of 25 to 50 mg per kg body weight daily, given in four doses six-hourly, the larger dosage being indicated in the initial treatment of severe infections. When given parenterally the dose is approximately half that required by mouth. Demethylchlortetracycline is given in an oral dosage of 7 to 14 mg per kg body weight daily, in four divided doses. Tetracyclines should not be given to infants and children under 7 years of age because of their undesirable side effects (see above).

ERYTHROMYCIN

This is effective against most Gram-positive and a limited number of Gram-negative organisms. It is particularly valuable in treating staphylococcal infections which have proved resistant to other antibiotics, and should be kept in reserve for such infections. The oral dosage is 30 to 40 mg per kg body weight daily, given six-hourly.

POLYMYXIN

Polymyxin is most effective against *Ps. pyocyanea*, *H. influenzae*, and the Salmonella-Shigella organisms. Its main clinical value is in the treatment of infections with *Ps. pyocyanea*, e.g. in infected burns and in urinary and meningeal infections. It may also be effective orally in clearing the bowel of serological types of *E. coli* associated with infantile gastroenteritis when these have resisted other antibiotics.

The intramuscular dose is 2·5 mg per kg body weight daily in four divided doses. The oral dose is 15 mg per kg daily in five or six divided doses.

OTHER ANTIBIOTICS

Colistin (colomycin) is closely related to polymyxin and is valuable in gastrointestinal infections, including dysentery and those due to pathogenic strains of *E. coli*. The oral dose is 150,000 units per kg body weight daily, divided into three doses. Its low toxicity makes it suitable for parenteral use and it is effective against *Ps. pyocyanea* infections, the dose being 50,000 units per kg daily, in two intramuscular injections. Neomycin is unfortunately too toxic to be used systemically, but as it is not absorbed from the bowel, it has a place in treating gastrointestinal infections. The oral dose is 50 to 100 mg per kg daily, in four doses. Kanamycin is also nephrotoxic and ototoxic, but may be life-saving in septicaemia due to Gram-negative organisms. Toxic effects are very rare in early infancy and kanamycin is therefore often used in neonatal infections. The systemic dosage is 15 mg per kg daily, in two intramuscular injections.

Novobiocin is effective against staphylococci and some strains of *Proteus*, but resistance develops rapidly. It is usually combined with erythromycin, the oral dosage being 25 mg per kg daily, in four doses. Cephaloridine, 25 to 50 mg per kg daily, is a valuable broad-spectrum antibiotic for parenteral injection, which is mainly useful in penicillin-resistant staphylococcal infection, since it is not susceptible to the action of penicillinase. Fusidic acid salts and lincomycin may also be useful against resistant staphylococci.

Proprietary preparations which contain two of the less widely used antibiotics are available for use on the skin or conjunctiva or in the nose. Either polymyxin B or neomycin (effective against a wide range of Gram-negative organisms) is combined with tyrothricin, bacitracin or gramicidin (effective against Gram-positive organisms). The use of two antibiotics hinders the development of bacterial resistance, but even so there is a risk in their routine use, particularly in hospital practice. A combination of neomycin and bacitracin in an ointment has proved effective in the treatment of neonatal conjunctivitis.

Although antibiotic therapy is principally of value in combating bacterial infection, its use extends to *Candida albicans*, which is sensitive to nystatin, 100,000 units orally four times a day, and to chronic fungus infections of the skin, nails or scalp, which respond to griseofulvin in a dose of 10 mg per kg daily.

STEROID THERAPY

Adrenocorticotrophic hormone (corticotrophin, ACTH), which is derived from the anterior pituitary gland, is the stimulator of adrenocortical steroid hormone production, and its therapeutic effect is therefore dependent on the existence of sufficient adrenal cortex to secrete these hormones. Of the effective adrenal steroids, hydrocortisone or compound F is the most potent released naturally in response to stress. Cortisone or compound E resembles hydrocortisone in its action, and is probably a precursor or degradation product of the latter. The principal indications for administration of steroids in paediatric practice are related to their anti-inflammatory effects, the electrolytic effects only being required in cases with adrenal insufficiency. Prednisone and prednisolone are synthetic analogues of cortisone and hydrocortisone. They also cause less electrolyte disturbance than cortisone or hydrocortisone, and prednisone is the one generally preferred when an anti-inflammatory action is the therapeutic effect required. Of the various preparations available,

the relative potency and salt-retaining action is shown in Table 18.2.

Unwanted effects

The systemic administration of any of these compounds is accompanied by side effects, the milder of which are scarcely avoidable. Patients on prolonged treatment with cortisone will become oedematous and potassium-deficient unless the sodium intake is restricted and the potassium intake increased: these effects of water and salt retention and excessive potassium excretion are only slight with the newer corticosteroids. The clinical picture of Cushing's syndrome (moonfacies, hypertension, obesity, hirsuties, striae, pigmentation, and reduced carbohydrate tolerance) may be reproduced in a varying degree. Although small doses produce a positive nitrogen balance, the therapeutic doses usually employed are liable to result in a negative nitrogen balance calling for a high protein intake. The risk of osteoporosis, due to increased calcium excretion, necessitates an increased calcium intake. The suppressive effect of the hormones on the body's resistance to infection is a real danger, and may result in silent abscess formation at injection sites, death from unsuspected septicaemia or viraemia, or activation of a tuberculous focus. Haemorrhage from a peptic ulcer is an uncommon but serious complication while severe abdominal pain may indicate acute pancreatitis. Interference with growth may occur and dwarfism is the major adverse effect of prolonged therapy. The risk of adrenal atrophy persisting after therapy may necessitate subsequent corticosteroid administration, e.g. during operations.

INDICATIONS. Owing to the potency and dangers of corticosteroids, their use in paediatric practice should never be embarked on lightly. Apart from Addison's disease (which is ex-

Table 18.2

	Relative potency by weight	Salt retaining action
Cortisone	1	Marked
Hydrocortisone	1·2	Marked
Prednisone	5	Slight
Prednisolone	5	Slight
Methyl prednisolone	6	None
Triamcinolone	6	None
Dexamethasone	35	Very slight
Betamethasone	35	Very slight

(From J. D. N. Nabarro, 1961)

tremely rare in childhood), replacement therapy is indicated in the Waterhouse-Friderichsen syndrome. In adrenal hyperplasia, steroids are used both for replacement and to suppress the production of abnormal androgenic hormones. Although dramatic results may sometimes be obtained in asthma, therapy should be restricted to severe attacks endangering life and to intractable cases where serious interference with education or social life is likely. Hydrocortisone by intravenous or intramuscular injection may also be life-saving in the emergency treatment of very severe infections. The long-term results in rheumatism and other collagen disorders are equivocal, though in rheumatic carditis steroids are indicated and in dermatomyositis and most cases of Still's disease there is little alternative to steroid therapy. Good results have been obtained from maintenance therapy in the nephrotic syndrome, where it is thought that the action may be hormonal interference with an antibody–antigen reaction. Remissions may be produced by steroid therapy in most patients suffering from acquired haemolytic anaemia or idiopathic thrombocytopenic purpura, and may be maintained by prolonged therapy. The hormones are ineffective in spherocytosis and do not influence the course of anaphylactoid purpura although they are useful in alleviating symptoms. In the leukaemias of childhood they produce temporary remission, and may be very effective in causing shrinkage of lymphatic tissue in both leukaemia and lymphosarcoma.

Of the numerous other conditions in which steroid therapy has been used systemically, exfoliative dermatitis and certain exudative eczematous conditions have been found to respond while topical therapy in interstitial keratitis and iritis has been effective. Corticosteroid retention enemata are valuable in ulcerative colitis. In conditions which are usually self-limited and in which therapy produces remission, the risks make the use of corticosteroids doubtfully justifiable.

ADMINISTRATION. ACTH is theoretically preferable to corticosteroids for long-term treatment, since it does not have the same growth-retarding effect, but the need for parenteral administration and the risk of sensitization limit its usefulness. It is usually administered as an intramuscular preparation, either six-hourly (when large amounts must be used owing to local extravascular inactivation), or as a slowly released gel

which is given once daily. The synthetic compound tetracosactrin is available in depot form which may be given twice weekly. The greatest response from the lowest dosage of ACTH is obtained when it is given by slow intravenous infusion greatly diluted in normal saline.

Cortisone, prednisone, and prednisolone are as rapidly effective when given orally as intramuscularly, but the latter route is preferable when there is vomiting or delay in gastric emptying: in these circumstances, soluble prednisolone phosphate is useful. Hydrocortisone may be given intravenously and in emergencies may be the steroid of choice. All these preparations may be employed topically, e.g. in ointment or eye-drops.

The dosage of any of the hormones will depend on whether a physiological (replacement) or pharmacological effect is required. In adrenal hyperplasia, cortisone is effective in a daily dose of 25 mg by mouth in infants and double this in older patients. The dose must be adjusted according to clinical progress and urinary excretion of 17-ketosteroids. In patients with salt loss, a mineralocorticoid effect may be produced by the oral administration of fludrocortisone, 0·1 to 0·2 mg daily. In very severe cases it may be necessary to give DOCA in addition. This can be implanted after treatment is established, or may be given as an injection of deoxycortone trimethylacetate at three- to six-weekly intervals. Prednisone is used in one-fifth to one-quarter the dosage of cortisone, and betamethasone in about one-tenth that of prednisone. The course of treatment advocated in acute rheumatism is given on p. 269, and that in the nephrotic syndrome on p. 289.

While on corticosteroid therapy, children should be weighed frequently and excessive weight gain controlled by dietary measures. With the newer preparations it is not necessary to add extra potassium to the diet. In long-term treatment, the spine should be X-rayed periodically to detect early osteoporosis. If acute bacterial infections occur they must receive intensive antibiotic therapy and the dose of steroid should be maintained. Severe viral infections for which no specific therapy is available are a greater danger.

When corticosteroids are administered over long periods, the dosage must be tailed off gradually. When withdrawal is more rapid, it is advisable to stimulate the natural production of adrenal corticosteroids by the injection of ACTH before cessation of treatment.

BIBLIOGRAPHY AND REFERENCES

ALLEN, F. H. & DIAMOND, L. K. (1957). *Erythroblastosis Fetalis including Exchange Transfusion Technic.* London: Churchill.

ATA, M. & HOLMAN, C. A. (1966). Simultaneous umbilical arteriovenous exchange transfusion. *British Medical Journal*, ii, 743.

CLYMO, A. B. (1971). Antecubital venepuncture in neonates. *Lancet*, ii, 1235.

DUNLOP, D. M. & MURDOCH, J. M. (1960). Dangers of antibiotic treatment. *British Medical Bulletin*, **16**, 67.

EMERY, J. L. (1957). The technique of bone marrow aspiration in children. *Journal of Clinical Pathology*, **10**, 339.

FARQUHAR, J. W. & SMITH, H. (1958). Clinical and biochemical changes during exchange transfusion. *Archives of Disease in Childhood*, **33**, 142.

FARQUHAR, J. W., SHANNON, D. W. & BATCHELOR, A. D. R. (1961). Equipment for intravenous fluid therapy of children. *Lancet*, ii, 537.

FONKALSRUD, E. W. (1966). Clinical uses of the small plastic catheter in pediatric patients. *Clinical Pediatrics*, **5**, 68.

FRIEDMAN, M. & STRANG, L. B. (1966). Effect of long-term corticosteroids and corticotrophin on the growth of children. *Lancet*, ii, 568.

GARROD, L. P. & SCOWEN, E. F. (1960). Antibiotics in medicine: principles of therapeutic use. *British Medical Bulletin*, **16**, 23.

GLASER, J. (1928). The cerebrospinal fluid of premature infants. *American Journal of Diseases of Children*, **36**, 195.

LANGE, K., SLOBODY, L. & STRANG, R. (1955). Prolonged intermittent ACTH and cortisone therapy in the nephrotic syndrome. *Pediatrics, Springfield*, **15**, 156.

LEACH, R. H. & WOOD, B. S. B. (1967). Drug dosage for children. *Lancet*, ii, 1350.

McCRACKEN, G. H., EICHENWALD, H. F. & NELSON, J. D. (1969). Antimicrobial therapy in theory and practice. *Journal of Pediatrics*, **75**, 742, 923.

McKAY, R. J. (1964). Current status of use of exchange transfusion in newborn infants. *Pediatrics, Springfield*, **33**, 763.

McKAY, R. J. (1966). Risks of obtaining samples of venous blood in infants. *Pediatrics, Springfield*, **38**, 906.

MARTIN, W. J. (1967). Antimicrobial research and therapeutics. In *Modern Trends in Pharmacology and Therapeutics.* Edited by W. F. M. Fulton. London: Butterworths.

MITCHELL, R. G. (1970). The sulphonamides in childhood. *Practitioner*, **204**, 20.

MOLLISON, P. L. (1967). Blood Transfusion in Clinical Medicine, 4th edn. Oxford: Blackwell.

NABARRO, J. D. N. (1961). Systemic cortico-steroid therapy. *Prescriber's Journal*, **1**, 1.

PHIBBS, R. H. (1966). Advances in the theory and practice of exchange transfusions. *California Medicine*, **105**, 442.

PLAUT, T. F. (1968). Lumbar puncture in children. *Clinical Pediatrics*, **7**, 130.

RILEY, H. D. (1970). The new penicillins and cephalosporins. *Advances in Pediatrics*, **17**, 227.

SIEGEL, S. C. (1965). ACTH and the corticosteroids in the management of allergic disorders in children. *Journal of Pediatrics*, **66**, 927.

WOOD, B. S. B. (1970), *A Paediatric Vade-mecum.* 7th edn. London: Lloyd-Luke.

Index